TUBERCULOSIS

GUY P. <u>YOUMANS</u>, M.D., Ph.D.

Professor Emeritus, Northwestern University Medical School,
Chicago, Illinois; Visiting Professor,
Department of Microbiology,
University of Arizona, Tucson, Arizona

1979

W. B. SAUNDERS COMPANY *Philadelphia • London • Toronto*

W. B. Saunders Company: West Washington Square
Philadelphia, PA   19105

1 St. Anne's Road
Eastbourne, East Sussex BN21 3UN, England

1 Goldthorne Avenue
Toronto, Ontario M8Z 5T9, Canada

Front cover illustration is an electron photomicrograph of cells of
the H37a strain of *M. tuberculosis,* courtesy of Dr. Ray Crispen.

TUBERCULOSIS   ISBN   0-7216-9641-4

Last digit is the print number: 9   8   7   6   5   4   3   2   1

TO ANNE
Without whose help and encouragement
this book could never have been written

CONTRIBUTORS

PATRICK J. BRENNAN, Ph.D. Senior Research Associate, National Jewish Hospital and Research Center; Assistant Professor, Department of Microbiology, University of Colorado School of Medicine, Denver, Colorado.

LEONARD DOUB, B.S. Formerly, Section Director, Infectious Diseases, Chemistry Department, Research Division, Parke, Davis & Company, Ann Arbor, Michigan.

MAYER B. GOREN, Ph.D. Margaret Regan Investigator in Chemical Pathology, National Jewish Hospital and Research Center; Associate Professor of Microbiology, University of Colorado School of Medicine, Denver, Colorado.

H. CORWIN HINSHAW, M.D., Ph.D., D.Sc. Clinical Professor of Medicine, University of California Medical School, San Francisco, California.

HERBERT M. SOMMERS, M.D. Professor of Pathology, Northwestern University Medical School; Director of Clinical Microbiology, Northwestern Memorial Hospital; Consultant Pathologist, Veterans Administration Research Hospital, Chicago, Illinois.

ANNE S. YOUMANS, Ph.D. Formerly, Professor of Microbiology, Northwestern University Medical School, Chicago, Illinois; Visiting Professor, Department of Microbiology, The University of Arizona, Tucson, Arizona.

GUY P. YOUMANS, M.D., Ph.D. Professor Emeritus, Northwestern University Medical School, Chicago, Illinois; Visiting Professor, Department of Microbiology, The University of Arizona, Tucson, Arizona.

PREFACE

The following statement appears in the preface to the first edition of the monumental book by Arnold Rich, *The Pathogenesis of Tuberculosis*, published in 1944:

> In every field of science, as in all other forms of human endeavor, it is desirable and advantageous periodically to take stock of the state of the endeavor. During the past sixty years, clinicians, pathologists, bacteriologists, immunologists, roentgenologists, epidemiologists and geneticists have devoted an immense amount of work to the attempt to understand the disease tuberculosis and the factors which influence its progression or arrest. Out of this vast effort have come the views and conclusions which are used as guiding principles by those who today have the responsibility of dealing with tuberculosis in the individual patient, in the community or in the laboratory. Everyone knows that many of these views and conclusions, though often dogmatically expressed, are countered by equally dogmatic, contrary opinions. What is the actual evidence upon which these opposing views are based, and how sound is that evidence? Even in the case of views that are more generally agreed upon, it is of value to re-examine the evidence, for it is an old story that opinions supported by little more than the weight of early authority have often remained embedded for years in the corpus of science through the failure to enquire carefully into the validity of the observations upon which the opinions rest.
>
> The purposes of this work are to present, in a clear and orderly manner, the basic factors and principles which influence the occurrence of tuberculous infection or determine its progression or arrest; to examine carefully the evidence relating to those matters and, from that analysis, to attempt to define clearly the present limits of our knowledge regarding the influence of each of those factors upon the pathogenesis of the disease; and, finally, to attempt to accomplish this survey in a manner that will correlate into a unified whole the basic, interdependent, but at present often isolated, facts that have been given to us by bacteriology, immunology, pathology, clinical observation, experimental investigation, epidemiology and genetics.

It is probably even more desirable today to take stock of the situation in tuberculosis. The increase in knowledge and understanding of the pathogenesis of tuberculosis in the years since the publication of Rich's book has probably been greater than in all of the years preceding that event. For example, at that time, the impact of chemotherapy upon tuberculosis had not been felt. Now, this governs our thinking in a number of areas of tuberculosis. In addition, these intervening years have seen the development of almost our entire knowledge of the role of atypical mycobacteria in the production of pulmonary and other disease in human beings. This, in turn, has greatly altered our understanding of the epidemiology of tuberculosis and the factors concerned in its prevention. At the present time, we have a much greater knowledge of the physiology of the tubercle bacillus and of the biologic activities produced by mycobacterial components. The influence of these on the pathogenesis of the disease in some cases can be reasonably well-defined. Finally, enormous advances have been made in our understanding of the immunologic responses of mammalian hosts. It is clear that immunologic responses are of at least two kinds — humoral and cellular — and that these responses are mediated by different lymphocyte populations. We also know that resistance to infection with facultative intracellular parasites such as *Mycobacterium tuberculosis* is determined primarily, if not exclusively, by cellular factors. At the time of publication of Rich's book, there was still reason to believe that circulating antibody might be involved in immunity to tuberculosis; and the role of lymphocytes in immune responses was hardly even suspected.

For these reasons, and for others too numerous to mention here, we feel that a systematic presentation of some of our knowledge concerning the tubercle bacillus and the host-parasite interaction in tuberculosis, and a critical examination of the significance of these findings, would not only promote a greater understanding of the host-parasite relationship in the disease itself but also would help point the direction for profitable lines of research in the future.

The major focus of this book will be on the host-parasite interaction and, in particular, on host responses. Some of the data to be presented will be that of our own laboratory. The major portion, however, will be provided by the published results of other investigators. Because of the voluminous literature, some selection had to be made. Realizing that many important contributions had to be omitted, we have attempted to include those references which we feel are the most significant. In addition, we have made no attempt to cover, in detail, the literature that appeared before publication of the second edition of *The Pathogenesis of Tuberculosis* by Rich in 1951. Rich more than adequately covers the literature up to that time, and we recommend his book as a source for the earlier literature.

A number of the views expressed in this book are primarily those of the authors and are not necessarily shared by all workers in the field. For any book to achieve the purposes stated by Rich, we feel that it should involve a critical analysis of the available evidence upon which views are based and a re-evaluation of the validity of interpretations. It is our strong feeling that this is the only way in which real progress in science can be made. Uncritical acceptance of the "conventional wisdom" of the day leads too frequently to stagnation rather than to progress.

Our aims in writing this book, then, remain much the same as those expressed by Rich in the preface to the first edition of *The Pathogenesis of Tuberculosis* (1944) and quoted here.

ACKNOWLEDGMENTS

As the senior author of this volume (Guy P. Youmans), I wish to acknowledge my indebtedness to a number of people who significantly contributed to the publication of this volume. The individual whom I would like to acknowledge first is Dr. John Weinzirl (deceased) who, as Chairman of the Department of Bacteriology at the University of Washington while I was a graduate student in that department, markedly stimulated my interest in the mycobacteria and the host-parasite relationship in tuberculosis. Dr. Weinzirl's own research in the field of tuberculosis set an example of thoughtfulness and meticulousness which I have tried always to emulate. Second, I am greatly indebted to the many graduate students who trained with me in the Department of Microbiology at Northwestern University Medical School. The efforts of these students are in part responsible for generating much of the data that has improved our understanding of the nature of the host-parasite relationships in mycobacterial disease. Third, I wish to thank my former fellow faculty members in the Department of Microbiology, Northwestern University Medical School, for their interest in my work, their many helpful suggestions, and their encouragement in the preparation of this volume. It would have been difficult, indeed, to have made such substantial progress over the years without their help.

I also wish to express my appreciation to Miss Sharon Stafford, Secretary, Department of Microbiology, Northwestern University Medical School, for her invaluable help in the preparation and typing of the manuscript. Particular thanks should go to Miss Katie Matthysse, Secretary, Department of Microbiology, The University of Arizona, not only for her preparation of the typed manuscript but also for her dedication and devotion to the many details involved in researching the bibliography, correcting the manuscript, and reading the proof, as well as for her very real interest in all of the aspects of the preparation of a book of this nature.

My thanks also go to the many people of the W. B. Saunders Company for their help—to Mr. John Hanley, for his initial interest in the subject and his desire to publish the volume; to Ms. Susan Hunter for her editorial services and general helpfulness; to Ms. Joanne Shore, for her work as copy editor; to Mr. Herb Powell, for his management of the production process; and to the others in the W. B. Saunders organization who contributed so much to the preparation of this volume.

In addition, I wish to acknowledge the following organizations and their generous financial support over a period of many years for my research program on tuberculosis:

Canal Zone Tuberculosis Association

Illinois Tuberculosis Association (Now the Illinois Lung Association)

National Institutes of Health, United States Public Health Service

National Tuberculosis Association (Now the American Lung Association)

Northwestern University Medical School

Parke, Davis & Company, Detroit, Michigan

Tuberculosis Institute of Chicago and Cook County (Now the Chicago Lung Association)

GUY P. YOUMANS, M.D., PH.D.

CONTENTS

1

Introduction

TUBERCULOSIS IN THE WORLD TODAY

Of all the infectious diseases that have plagued man, tuberculosis has probably been responsible for the greatest morbidity and mortality. It has apparently plagued man ever since human beings emerged as a species on this planet. Its depredations, especially over the last several hundred years, have earned it the epithet, "The captain of all the men of death."[7] Readers interested in the history of tuberculosis, and how it has ravaged successive generations of human beings beginning with the early years of the Industrial Revolution, should consult the beautifully written and descriptive book entitled *The White Plague*, by René and Jean Dubos.[7] (See also Chapter 16.)

Even today, when the incidence of tuberculosis in the Western nations has markedly decreased and the mortality is less than ten per hundred thousand population, tuberculosis still remains one of the world's most prevalent infec-

tious diseases. It is found, at the present time, primarily in the developing areas of the world.[19] The World Health Organization estimates that there are probably as many as 20 million active cases, which annually infect from 50 to 100 million people in the areas of highest prevalence.[17] It has been estimated that on a world-wide basis approximately 3 million people die every year of tuberculosis and, of this total, 80 percent or more are in the developing nations.[17] As a cause of death among human beings, tuberculosis is still at the forefront of infectious diseases. Thus, on a world-wide basis, tuberculosis remains one of the important infectious diseases with which human beings have to cope.

In spite of the enormous amount of research that has been done since Koch first reported the isolation of the etiologic agent in 1882,[13] we still have a very incomplete understanding of the nature of the virulence of the tubercle bacillus and the nature of the host response to the tuberculous infection. Nor do we have a very clear un-

1

derstanding of the reason for the rise and fall in the number of cases of tuberculosis, nor is there a general appreciation of the inadequacies of the public health control methods that have been used to combat the disease. However, in recent years there has been great improvement in our understanding of the host-parasite interaction in tuberculosis. It is hoped that in the not-too-distant future, continued research will point the way toward better methods for the control and treatment of tuberculosis. Our present knowledge and the implications for future control of the disease will be brought out in detail in subsequent chapters in this book.

There are those who feel that tuberculosis may eventually be eradicated as an infectious disease of human beings.[10, 12] This ideal conclusion to the war between the parasite *Mycobacterium tuberculosis* and its human host is indeed a very unlikely prospect, as we will demonstrate later on in the text (see especially Chapters 16 and 17). Nevertheless, we must always harbor the hope that our increasing knowledge and understanding of both parasite and host reaction will eventually put us in a position to completely control this infectious disease.

THE MYCOBACTERIAL WORLD

As far as disease in human beings is concerned, *Mycobacterium tuberculosis* is by far the most important of the mycobacterial pathogens, and the one that has been responsible over the centuries for most of the mycobacteria-caused morbidity and mortality among human beings. However, readers should be aware that *M. tuberculosis* is only one member of a microbial family that includes many microorganisms with certain common properties. For example, all mycobacteria are acid-fast; to the best of our

knowledge, they are all obligate aerobes; they all grow and metabolize rather slowly; and all share the property of being appreciably more resistant to a variety of deleterious influences than most other bacteria. However, the mycobacteria vary markedly in their metabolic activities and are found in widely different habitats. For example, *M. tuberculosis* is an obligate parasite of human beings and certain other warm-blooded animals and grows best at 37° C. On the other hand, *M. avium,* which is a parasite of fowl, has an optimum growth temperature of 42° C; thus, it is able to grow and produce disease in fowl, which have a higher body temperature than human beings. Disease is seldom produced in man by *M. avium,* although a related microorganism, *M. intracellulare,* frequently does so. (More will be said about *M. intracellulare* in Chapter 18.) There are other mycobacteria, such as *M. leprae, M. marinum,* and *M. ulcerans,* which have lower optimal growth temperatures. In fact, *M. marinum* and *M. ulcerans* will not grow in temperatures over 35° C. This does not prevent them from producing disease in man, but it does limit the tissues that will be affected. In addition, there is a large group of mycobacteria usually referred to as saprophytes. These are found widely distributed in nature — in soil, in water, and so forth — and do not produce disease in man or other animals except under the most abnormal conditions.

The pathogenic properties of mycobacteria range from those of the saprophytes, which ordinarily do not produce disease, to those of the obligate intracellular parasites (such as *M. leprae* and *M. lepraemurium*), which will not grow at all except in a suitable host or, under certain conditions, in cells in tissue cultures. In between these two extremes are microorganisms, such as *M. tuberculosis,* which are facultative intracellular parasites; that is, they can grow within cells or outside of cells, depending upon the conditions that prevail in the host. There also are species of mycobacteria that produce disease in a variety of lower animals. *M. bovis,* for example, produces disease primarily in cattle and other domestic animals but can and will infect human beings if the opportunity arises.

The mycobacterial world, therefore, is a large one containing diverse species of mycobacteria with greatly differing potentials for producing disease.

THE CLASSIFICATION OF THE MYCOBACTERIA

In this section, a brief classification of the mycobacteria will be presented. This is done primarily to indicate some of the characteristics of the major mycobacterial species. The names and the disease-producing potential of a much wider number of species, which do on occasion produce disease in man, can be found in Chapters 18 and 19.

Included in this section for purposes of orientation are some of the species of mycobacteria listed in *Bergey's Manual of Determinative Bacteriology,*[6] together with their important characteristics and disease-producing potential. This list emphasizes the variety of species of mycobacteria and the considerable differences in their characteristics.

1. *Mycobacterium tuberculosis.* Type species. We will say relatively little about this microorganism here, since the major portion of the subsequent chapters of this book will be devoted to the characteristics and disease-producing potential of *M. tuberculosis* and the host reaction to infection with this parasite.

2. *Mycobacterium microti.* Common name: Vole bacillus. Slow-growing facultative intracellular parasite, with an optimal growth temperature of 37° C. Produces disease in rodents, such as the vole and guinea pig, in rabbits, and sometimes in calves.

3. *Mycobacterium bovis.* Optimal growth temperature of 37° C. Facultative intracellular parasite. Produces tuberculous disease in cattle and in other domestic and wild ruminants. Pathogenic in man and other primates, in carnivores (including dogs and cats), in swine, in parrots (and possibly other birds), and in hamsters and mice.

4. *Mycobacterium africanum.* Occasionally causes pulmonary tuberculosis in human beings in tropical Africa. Optimal growth temperature apparently 37° C.

5. *Mycobacterium kansasii.* Optimal growth temperature 37° C. Produces pulmonary disease in human beings (see Chapter 18).

6. *Mycobacterium marinum.* Found in swimming pools, aquaria, and other water sources. May produce disease in fish. Grows only in temperature range of 25° to 35° C. In human beings, causes cutaneous granulomas ("swimming pool granulomas"). Lesions found on the elbows, knees, feet, fingers, and toes; heals spontaneously.

7. *Mycobacterium gastri.* Grows in the temperature range of 25° to 40° C. Found originally in gastric contents of human beings. Not considered to be pathogenic.

8. *Mycobacterium nonchromogenicum.* Saprophyte.

9. *Mycobacterium terrae.* Also found in gastric contents. Not considered to be pathogenic.

10. *Mycobacterium triviale.* Found in sputum. Thought to be a saprophyte.

11. *Mycobacterium gordonae.* Common name: Tap water scotochromogen (see Chapter 18). Found in human sputum and gastric lavage specimens. Also found in water and soil. Rarely, if ever, implicated in disease processes.

12. *Mycobacterium scrofulaceum.* Causes cervical lymphadenitis in children. Not particularly pathogenic for experimental animals. (See Chapter 18.)

13. *Mycobacterium intracellulare.* An

important pathogen, which may produce pulmonary disease in man (see Chapter 18).

14. *Mycobacterium avium.* Causes tuberculosis in fowl.

15. *Mycobacterium xenopi.* Mostly a saprophyte. Has occasionally been isolated from human excretions and from disease of the genitourinary tract.

16. *Mycobacterium ulcerans.* Temperature growth range between 30° and 33° C. In man, causes skin ulcers that may be severe. Found in Australia, Mexico, New Guinea, Malaysia, and Africa.

17. *Mycobacterium phlei.* Saprophyte found in soil and water.

18. *Mycobacterium vaccae.* Occasionally seen in skin lesions in cattle. Widely distributed in nature; found in water and soil. Mostly a saprophyte.

19. *Mycobacterium diernhoferi.* Isolated from water and found in environments where there are domestic cattle. Apparently not pathogenic.

20. *Mycobacterium smegmatis.* Found in soil, in water, and in the smegma of man. Not pathogenic.

21. *Mycobacterium thamnopheos.* Has a temperature growth range of 10° to 35° C. Produces generalized disease in snakes, frogs, lizards, and fish, but not pathogenic for guinea pigs, rabbits, or fowl.

22. *Mycobacterium flavescens.* A rapidly growing saprophyte.

23. *Mycobacterium fortuitum.* Produces disease in man, in cattle, and even in the frog. Found in soil and in some cold-blooded animals.

24. *Mycobacterium peregrinum.* Isolated from the sputum of man, though its possible role as a pathogen is obscure.

25. *Mycobacterium chelonei.* Rarely produces infection in man. Growth temperature range of 22° to 40° C.

26. *Mycobacterium paratuberculosis.* Common name: Johne's bacillus. Facultative intracellular parasite that produces disease primarily in cattle and sheep. Lesion produced is a regional ileitis. Disease is serious in cat-

tle and sheep, and mortality can be high. Does not produce disease in man.

27. *Mycobacterium leprae.* Produces leprosy (Hansen's disease) in man. An important obligate intracellular parasite. Has an optimal growth temperature that is apparently lower than 37° C. Lesions produced in skin and in other organs, such as the testes, where temperature is lower; internal organs not affected.

28. *Mycobacterium lepraemurium.* Obligate intracellular parasite that produces leprosy in rodents, such as rats and mice. Serves as an important experimental model for the study of leprosy.

For a detailed consideration of the very complicated problems involved in the classification of mycobacterial species, the following references should be consulted: Barksdale and Kim;[2] Bradley and Bond;[5] Juhlin;[11] Kubica;[14] Ratledge;[20] Runyon et al.;[22] Tsukamura and Mizuno;[32] and Tsukamura et al.[33]

MYCOBACTERIAL DISEASES OF MAN

From the descriptions given in the preceding list of species, it should be clear that there are many nonpathogenic as well as disease-producing mycobacteria. Some mycobacteria are capable of producing disease in certain lower animals; other species, besides *M. tuberculosis,* can and do produce disease in human beings.

Tuberculosis in human beings is, by definition, disease caused by *M. tuberculosis.* However, it is now clear that a number of mycobacteria can produce pulmonary or other disease in man that is indistinguishable from that produced by *M. tuberculosis.* In particular, these include *M. kansasii* and *M. intracellulare.* More will be said about these pathogens and the disease they cause in Chapter 18. We wish to emphasize here that tuberculosis can no longer be regarded simply as a disease caused by *M. tuberculosis*. In fact, in certain areas of the country (see Chapters 16 and 18), as many as 10 to 15 percent of the pulmonary disease cases diagnosed as tuberculosis may be caused by *M. kansasii*. Thus, even though in this book we are concerned primarily with disease produced by *M. tuberculosis* and with the particular host-parasite relationship involved when *M. tuberculosis* is the etiologic agent, we must always keep in mind that certain other mycobacteria produce disease that is similar in every respect to that produced by *M. tuberculosis*. Fortunately, insofar as we can determine, the major features of the host-parasite relationship are the same for all of these species.

No mention of human mycobacterial disease would be complete without some reference to *M. leprae* and leprosy (Hansen's disease).[3, 21] A disease that is probably as old as tuberculosis, leprosy over the centuries has afflicted tens of millions of human beings. It was more prevalent at one time, since the disease has now almost disappeared from Western Countries; nevertheless, a few cases of leprosy are detected each year in the United States. In many of the developing countries, leprosy is still a major infectious disease affecting a high proportion of the population.

We have no intention here of discussing leprosy to any great extent, but we would like to point out that the host-parasite relationship in leprosy is apparently very similar to that found in tuberculosis. The lesions of leprosy occur primarily in the skin, peripheral nerves, and mucous membranes of the upper respiratory tract. It is assumed that this localization occurs because the causative organism requires lower temperatures for growth. *M. leprae* has never been isolated and cultured in vitro. Experimental infections with *M. leprae* can be induced in the footpad of the mouse[23-26] and more recently, in a cold-blooded animal — the nine-banded armadillo.[27-31]

For many years it has been assumed that *M. leprae* is strictly a parasite of human beings and that the disease is transmitted only from human to human by close contact. However, very recently, a natural disease caused by a microorganism that cannot be distinguished in any way from *M. leprae* has been detected in the nine-banded armadillo.[4, 18, 34, 35] This raises the important question of whether there is, by chance, a reservoir of infection with *M. leprae* in cold-blooded animals such as the armadillo, thereby explaining some of the peculiar epidemiologic features of leprosy. With tuberculous disease, it has also been assumed that it is only transmitted from human to human and that there is no reservoir of infection with *M. tuberculosis* except in man. We now may have cause to wonder, or at least to keep in mind, the possibility that eventually an animal reservoir of tuberculous infection might be found. It is well known that domestic animals, particularly pets, may become infected with *M. tuberculosis* and serve as sources of infection for human beings; however, to date, no natural infection with *M. tuberculosis* in wild animals has been detected.

Other mycobacterial infections of man that should be mentioned are those caused by *M. marinum* and *M. ulcerans*. *M. marinum* infections can occur epidemically from either natural waters, such as ocean beaches, or from swimming pools.[1, 15] *M. ulcerans* infections are limited geographically, as previously indicated.[8, 9, 16] Other bacteria that occasionally produce disease in man, such as *M. scrofulaceum* and *M. fortuitum* and some of the others, will be covered to a greater extent in Chapter 18.

Thus, while *M. tuberculosis* is still the major culprit for the production of human disease, increasingly, we are finding that other mycobacteria found in nature can also cause troublesome clinical problems in man. In this book our emphasis will be on *M. tuberculosis,* because most of our knowledge about the mycobacteria and the host-parasite relationship in mycobacterial disease has been derived from studying this microorganism. However, most of what we will have to say, particularly about host-parasite interaction, can be applied to infection produced in man by the other mycobacteria as well.

THE HOST-PARASITE RELATIONSHIP IN MYCOBACTERIAL DISEASE

A good part of the book will be devoted to the host-parasite relationship in tuberculosis. In this chapter, we only wish to emphasize two points that readers should always keep in mind. First, the pathogenicity of *M. tuberculosis* and the other mycobacteria depends primarily upon the capacity of these microorganisms to resist the natural defensive mechanisms of the infected host. Second, in view of the insusceptibility of these mycobacteria to normal defense mechanisms, the host has developed a special and rather unique way of responding to the presence of these parasites, so that it has the power to inhibit the multiplication of the infecting mycobacteria. This unique defense mechanism is known as cellular immunity to infection and is invoked by the body primarily against facultative or obligate intracellular parasites. As we will see, it is a potent antimicrobial immunologic response. Yet the mechanism is a very inadequate one because it does not readily bring about destruction of all of the infecting mycobacterial cells.

Cellular immunity to infection not only is the major immunologic defense reaction to infection of man and lower animals with *M. tuberculosis* or other mycobacteria but also is a major immunologic defense reaction against

a variety of other bacterial parasites and viruses. We need only mention such diseases as histoplasmosis, coccidioidomycosis, pasteurellosis, brucellosis, and Listeria infection. Most of our knowledge of cellular immunity to infection has come from study, under experimental conditions, of host-parasite relationships in tuberculosis. Apparently, the same general mechanisms that operate in defense against tuberculosis also operate in defense against these other parasites. Thus, knowledge of the nature of the host-parasite relationship in tuberculosis is important for students interested in cellular immune responses to many other infectious diseases. It is very likely that when the exact nature of acquired cellular immunity to infection is determined, the knowledge will have been derived from a study of the host-parasite relationship in tuberculosis.

REFERENCES

1. Aronson, J. D.: Spontaneous tuberculosis in salt water fish. J. Infect. Dis. *39*:315, 1926.
2. Barksdale, L., and Kim, K.: *Mycobacterium.* Bacteriol. Rev. *41*:217, 1977.
3. Beeson, P. B., and McDermott, W.: Textbook of Medicine. 14th ed. Philadelphia, W. B. Saunders Co., 1975.
4. Binford, C. H., Meyers, W. M., Walsh, G. P., Storrs, E. E., and Brown, H. L.: Naturally acquired leprosy-like disease in the nine-banded armadillo (*Dasypus novemcinctus*): histopathologic and microbiologic studies of tissues. J. Reticuloendothel. Soc. *22*:377, 1977.
5. Bradley, S. G., and Bond, J. S.: Taxonomic criteria for mycobacteria and nocardiae. Adv. Appl. Microbiol. *18*:131, 1974.
6. Buchanan, R. E., and Gibbons, N. E. (eds.): Bergey's Manual of Determinative Bacteriology. 8th ed. Baltimore, The Williams & Wilkins Company, 1974.
7. Dubos, R., and Dubos, J.: The White Plague. Tuberculosis, Man and Society. Boston, Little, Brown and Co., 1952.
8. Fenner, F.: Homologous and heterologous immunity in infections of mice with *Mycobacterium ulcerans* and *Mycobacterium balnei.* Am. Rev. Tuberc. *76*:76, 1957.
9. Fenner, F.: The pathogenic behavior of *Mycobacterium ulcerans* and *Mycobacterium*

balnei in the mouse and the developing chick embryo. Am. Rev. Tuberc. *73*:650, 1956.

10. Horne, N. W.: Epidemiology and control of tuberculosis. Br. J. Hosp. Med. *5*:732, 1971.

11. Juhlin, I.: Contribution to the classification of mycobacteria and nocardias. Acta Pathol. Microbiol. Scandinav. *70*(Suppl. 189):1, 1967.

12. Kaplan, A. I.: Tuberculosis treatment in Massachusetts in 1977. N. Engl. J. Med. *297*:616, 1977.

13. Koch, R.: Die Aetiologie der Tuberkulose. Berl. Klin. Wochenschr. *19*:221, 1882.

14. Kubica, G. P.: Differential identification of mycobacteria. VII. Key features of identification of clinically significant mycobacteria. Am. Rev. Respir. Dis. *107*:9, 1973.

15. Linell, F., and Norden, A.: *Mycobacterium balnei;* new acid-fast bacillus occurring in swimming pools and capable of producing skin lesions in humans. Acta Tuberc. Scandinav. (Suppl. 33):1, 1954.

16. MacCallum, P., Tolhurst, J. C., Buckle, G., and Sissons, H. A.: A new mycobacterial infection in man. J. Pathol. Bacteriol. *60*:93, 1948.

17. Mahler, H. T.: Tuberculosis in the world today. Bull. Int. Union Tuberc. *43*:19, 1970.

18. Myers, W. M., Walsh, G. P., Brown, H. L., Reese, R. J. W., and Convit, J.: Naturally acquired leprosy-like disease in the nine-banded armadillo (*Dasypus novemcinctus*): reactions in leprosy patients to lepromins prepared from naturally infected armadillos. J. Reticuloendothel. Soc. *22*:369, 1977.

19. Okada, H., Aoki, K., Ohno, Y., and Kodama, K.: Global Epidemiology of Tuberculosis. Japan, Department of Preventive Medicine, Nagoya University School of Medicine, 1967.

20. Ratledge, C.: The Mycobacteria. Durham, England, Meadowfield Press Ltd., 1977.

21. Robbins, S. L.: Pathological Basis of Disease. Philadelphia, W. B. Saunders Company, 1974.

22. Runyon, E. H., Karlson, A. G., Kubica, G. P., and Wayne, L. G.: *Mycobacterium. In* Lennette, E. H., Spaulding, E. H., and Truant, J. P. (eds.): Manual of Clinical Microbiology. 2nd ed. Washington, D.C., American Society for Microbiology, 1974.

23. Shepard, C. C.: The experimental disease that follows the injection of human leprosy bacilli into foot-pads of mice. J. Exp. Med. *112*:445, 1960.

24. Shepard, C. C.: Leprosy bacilli in mouse foot-pads. *In* Wolstenholme, G. E. W., and O'Connor, M. (eds.): Pathogenesis of Leprosy. Ciba Found. Study Group *15*:80, 1963.

25. Shepard, C. C.: Multiplication of *Mycobacterium leprae* in the foot-pad of the mouse. Int. J. Lepr. *30*:291, 1962.

26. Shepard, C. C.: The nasal excretion of *Mycobacterium leprae* in leprosy. Int. J. Lepr. *30*:10, 1962.

27. Storrs, E. E.: Growing points in leprosy research. 1. The armadillo as an experimental model for the study of human leprosy. Lepr. Rev. *45*:8, 1974.

28. Storrs, E. E.: Leprosy in the nine-banded armadillo. Z. Tropenmed. Parasitol. *24* (Suppl. 1):53, 1973.

29. Storrs, E. E.: The nine-banded armadillo. A model for biomedical research. *In* Spiegel, A. (ed.): The Laboratory Animal in Drug Testing. 5th Symposium of the International Committee on Laboratory Animals, Hannover, 19–21, September, 1972. Stuttgart, Gustav Fisher Verlag, 1973.

30. Storrs, E. E.: The nine-banded armadillo: a model for leprosy and other biomedical research. Int. J. Lepr. *39*:703, 1971.

31. Storrs, E. E., Walsh, G. P., Burchfield, H. P., and Binford, C. H.: Leprosy in the armadillo: a new model for biomedical research. Science *183*:851, 1974.

32. Tsukamura, M., and Mizuno, S.: "Hypothetical mean organisms" of mycobacteria. A study of classification of mycobacteria. Jpn. J. Microbiol. *12*:371, 1968.

33. Tsukamura, M., Mizuno, S., and Tsukamura, S.: Classification of rapidly growing mycobacteria. Jpn. J. Microbiol. *12*:151, 1968.

34. Walsh, G. P., Storrs, E. E., Burchfield, H. P., Cottrell, E. H., Vidrine, M. F., and Binford, C. H.: Leprosy-like disease occurring naturally in armadillos. J. Reticuloendothel. Soc. *18*:347, 1975.

35. Walsh, G. P., Storrs, E. E., Meyers, W., and Binford, C. H.: Naturally acquired leprosy-like disease in the nine-banded armadillo (*Dasypus novemcinctus*): Recent epizootiologic findings. J. Reticuloendothel. Soc. *22*:363, 1977.

2

The Morphology and Metabolism of Mycobacteria

INTRODUCTION

The metabolism of *Mycobacterium tuberculosis* has been of great interest to physicians and scientists ever since the report of its isolation by Koch in 1882.[52] In fact, probably no other pathogenic bacterium has been studied so intensely. As a result, books have appeared over the years devoted almost exclusively to the metabolism of the tubercle bacillus. Volumes include *The Chemistry and Chemotherapy of Tuber-*

culosis by Long (1958);[58] *The Bacteriology of Tuberculosis* by Darzins (1958);[15] and *The Metabolism of the Tubercle Bacillus* by Drea and Andrejew (1953).[21] A more recent view of the metabolism of mycobacteria will be found in *Topley and Wilson's Principles of Bacteriology, Virology, and Immunity* by Wilson and Miles (1975);[92] and a review of the intermediary metabolism of mycobacteria will be found in Ramakrishnan and associates (1972).[68]

Extensive treatment of certain aspects of the morphology, physiology, and genetics of mycobacteria also will be found in Barksdale and Kim (1977),[3] Iwainsky and Kappler (1974),[46] Ratledge (1976, 1977),[69, 70] and in Chapter 4 of this volume.

Interest in the metabolism of *M. tuberculosis* stemmed not only from its importance as a pathogen but from the hope that such studies would reveal the factor or factors responsible for its ability to produce disease. This hope was fostered by the success that had been achieved by studying *Corynebacterium diphtheriae*. Here, it was quickly learned that the virulence of *C. diphtheriae* resides primarily in its capacity to produce a potent exotoxin. This discovery rapidly led to successful specific therapy of diphtheria and to effective prevention by vaccination. Unfortunately, in spite of the intensive efforts and the enormous amount of information acquired, such success has not been achieved in the case of tuberculosis. We still do not understand fully the nature of the factor or factors that are responsible for the virulence of tubercle bacilli (see Chapters 4 and 5), nor do we fully understand the nature of the immune response of the infected host (see Chapters 8, 10, 11, 12, and 13).

In view of the situation just outlined, the present chapter will be devoted not only to those morphologic and metabolic features of the mycobacteria that separate this family of microorganisms from other bacteria but, in addition, to those metabolic characteristics that may bear some relationship to the power to produce disease. The references cited at the beginning of this chapter should be consulted for the more detailed aspects of the metabolism and genetics of the tubercle bacillus.

MORPHOLOGY

In *Bergey's Manual of Determinative Bacteriology*,[10] *M. tuberculosis*, type species of the genus *Mycobacterium*, is described as follows:

Rods ranging in size from 0.3 to 0.6 by 1–4 μm, straight or slightly curved, occurring singly and in occasional strands. Stain uniformly or irregularly, often showing banded or beaded forms. Strongly acid-fast and acid-alcohol-fast as demonstrated by Ziehl-Neelsen or fluorochrome procedures.

Similar descriptions will be found in most textbooks of microbiology and medicine that deal with the mycobacteria. Although correct, they tell us relatively little about the tubercle bacillus or about the morphology of mycobacteria. In the first place, such descriptions are made from observations of Ziehl-Neelsen stained smears[63, 112] of *M. tuberculosis*, or other mycobacteria, grown in vitro on a variety of artificial media. They tell us little or nothing about the morphology of the microorganism in its natural habitat. Ziehl-Neelsen stains of infected tissues or sputum frequently show cells that are much longer, more curved, and sometimes more beaded than cells found in culture. For some reason cells found in culture tend to be shorter. Also, the chemical treatment of infected tissues or sputum samples (see Chapter 19) may change the morphology of a mycobacterial species.

It would be much better if live mycobacteria could be observed directly while growing in vivo; unfortunately, this is impossible. Direct observation of mycobacteria within cells in tissue culture, however, can be made. Figures 2–1, 2–2, 2–3, and 2–4 show *M. tuberculosis* within peritoneal macrophages. Here, when stained by the Ziehl-Neelsen procedure, the cells are longer than the 3 to 4 microns mentioned earlier and can be seen to be more curved and, of greater importance, cord formation is quite pronounced. "Cord factor" is a lipid material (trehalose 6,6'-dimycolate) found on the surface of the cells of many mycobacterial species.[34] This sub-

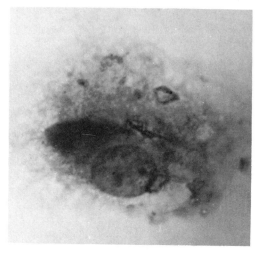

FIGURE 2–1. Peritoneal macrophage in tissue culture containing small clump of tubercle bacilli. (From Youmans, G. P., Paterson, P. Y., and Sommers, H. M.: The Biologic and Clinical Basis of Infectious Diseases. Philadelphia, W. B. Saunders Co., 1975.)

stance appears to be responsible for the cells of *M. tuberculosis* sticking together and growing in "cords" (Fig. 2–3). See Chapters 3 and 4 for further information about "cord factor" and its biologic properties.

Attenuated mycobacterial cells are difficult to observe within macrophages either because they may not grow or because their morphology may be altered by the antimycobacterial action of this phagocyte. Mycobacteria, however, will infect cells such as HeLa cells or human amnion cells.[78-81] Within these cells a wide variety of pathogenic or attenuated mycobacteria will grow readily.

Shepard has examined the growth and morphology of a variety of mycobacteria within HeLa cells, kidney cells, and human amnion cells.[78-81] Figures 2–5, 2–6, and 2–7 provide a picture of *M. tuberculosis* in all three types of cells. Figure 2–8 shows the R1Rv strain (an attenuated strain of *M. tuberculosis*) in HeLa cells. Figures

(*Text continued on p. 17*)

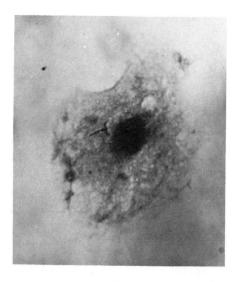

FIGURE 2–2. Periotoneal macrophage in tissue culture containing two tubercle bacilli. (From Youmans, G. P., Paterson, P. Y., and Sommers, H. M.: The Biologic and Clinical Basis of Infectious Diseases. Philadelphia, W. B. Saunders Co., 1975.)

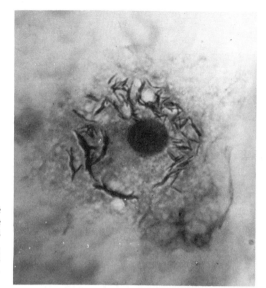

FIGURE 2–3. Peritoneal macrophage in tissue culture containing numerous tubercle bacilli. Note the alignment of the tubercle bacilli in the clumps as "cords." (From Youmans, G. P., Paterson, P. Y., and Sommers, H. M.: The Biologic and Clinical Basis of Infectious Diseases. Philadelphia, W. B. Saunders Co., 1975.)

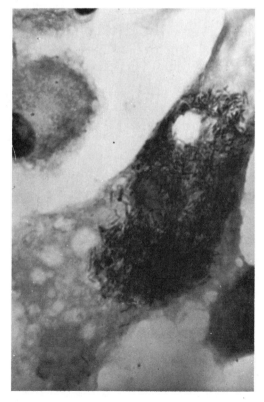

FIGURE 2–4. Peritoneal macrophage in tissue culture containing enormous numbers of tubercle bacilli. (From Youmans, G. P., Paterson, P. Y., and Sommers, H. M.: The Biologic and Clinical Basis of Infectious Diseases. Philadelphia, W. B. Saunders Co., 1975.)

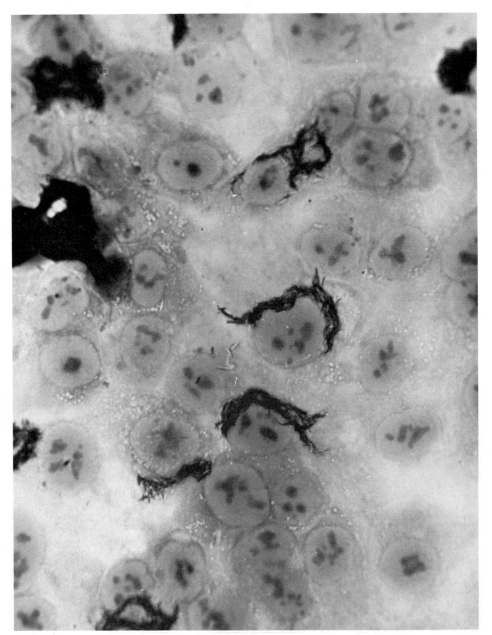

FIGURE 2–5

FIGURES 2–5 to 2–7. Human tubercle bacilli, strain H37Rv, five days after inoculation with HeLa (Fig. 2–5), monkey kidney (Fig. 2–6), and human amnion cells (Fig. 2–7). × 825. (From Shepard, C. C.: A comparison of the growth of selected mycobacteria in HeLa, monkey kidney, and human amnion cells in tissue culture. J. Exp. Med. *107*:237, 1958.)

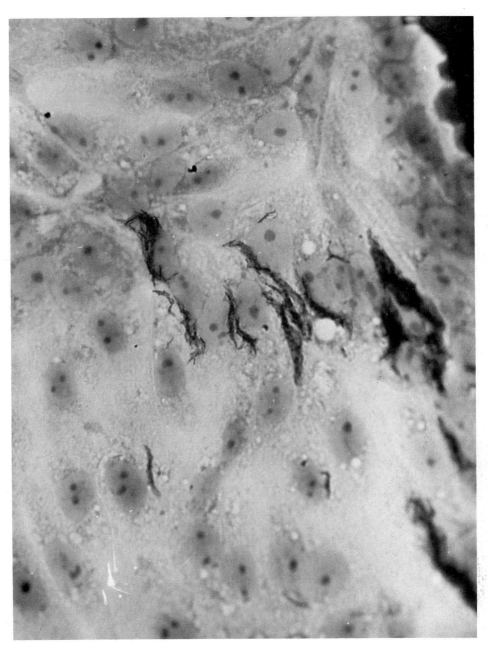

FIGURE 2–6. *Legend on opposite page.*

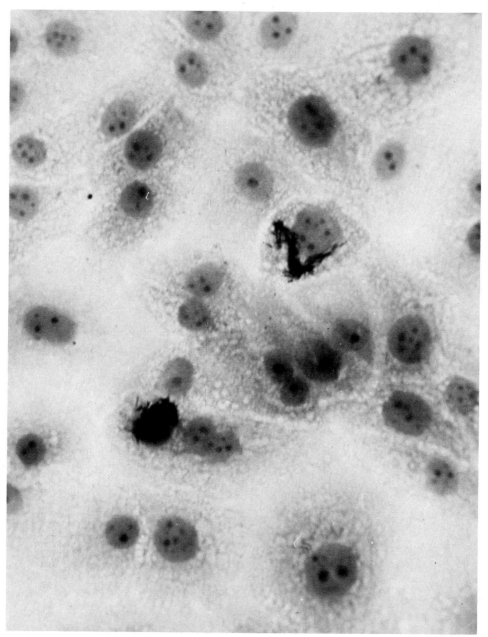

FIGURE 2–7. *Legend on page 12.*

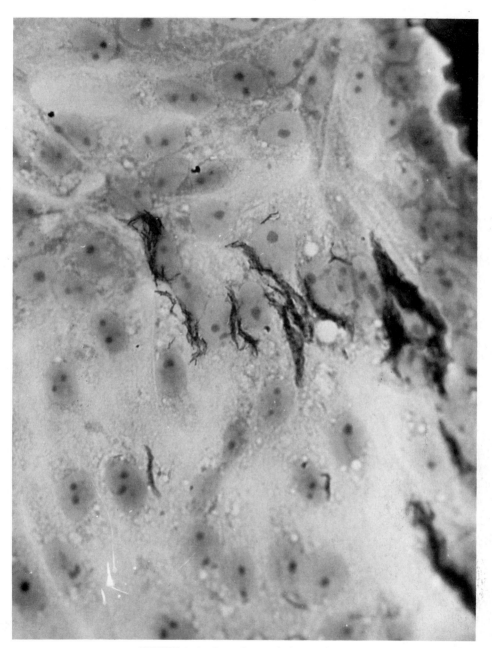

FIGURE 2–6. *Legend on opposite page.*

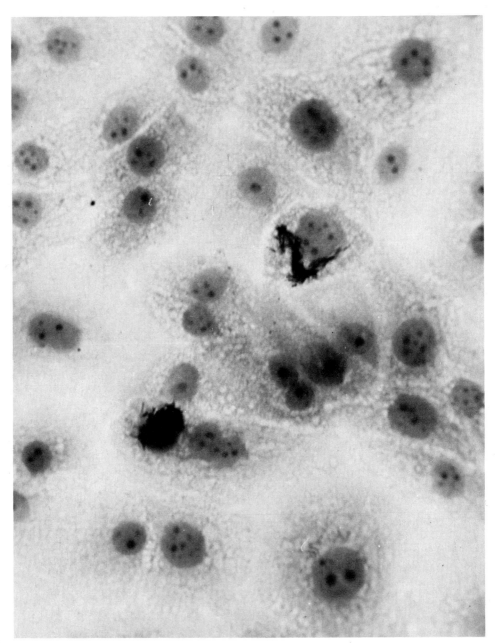

FIGURE 2–7.   *Legend on page 12.*

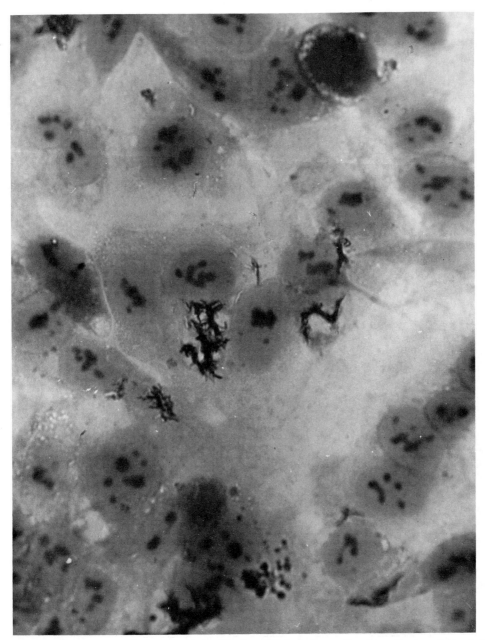

FIGURE 2–8. R1Rv, a strain of tubercle bacilli of modified virulence, five days after inoculation into HeLa cells. × 825. (From Shepard, C. C.: A comparison of the growth of selected mycobacteria in HeLa, monkey kidney, and human amnion cells in tissue culture. J. Exp. Med. *107*:237, 1958.)

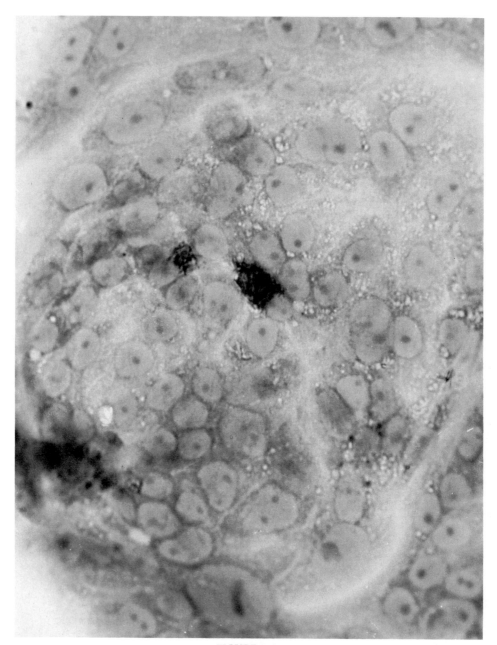

FIGURE 2–9

FIGURES 2–9 and 2–10. RlRv, five days after inoculation into monkey kidney (Fig. 2–9) and human amnion cells (Fig. 2–10). × 825. (From Shepard, C. C.: A comparison of the growth of selected mycobacteria in HeLa, monkey kidney, and human amnion cells in tissue culture. J. Exp. Med. *107*:237, 1958.)

2–9 and 2–10 picture the same R1Rv strain in monkey kidney and in human amnion cells, respectively. The morphologic appearance of *M. kansasii* within HeLa cells can be seen in Figure 2–11. Note the marked beading or banding that is characteristic of this species and that is far more pronounced in HeLa cells than in an artificial culture medium.

Figure 2–12 shows *M. intracellulare* in HeLa cells, and one of the charac-

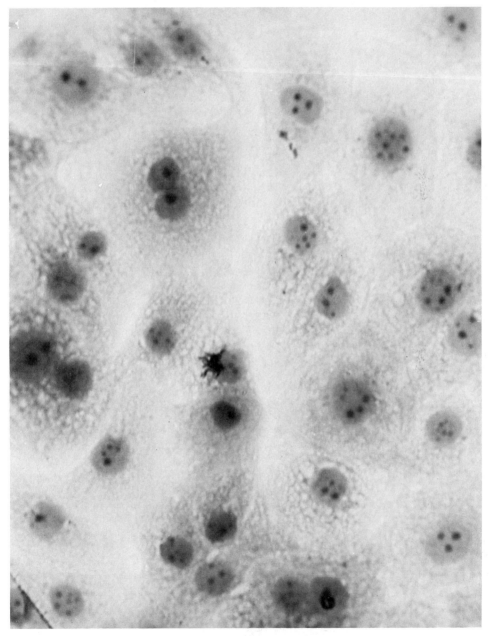

FIGURE 2–10. *Legend on opposite page.*

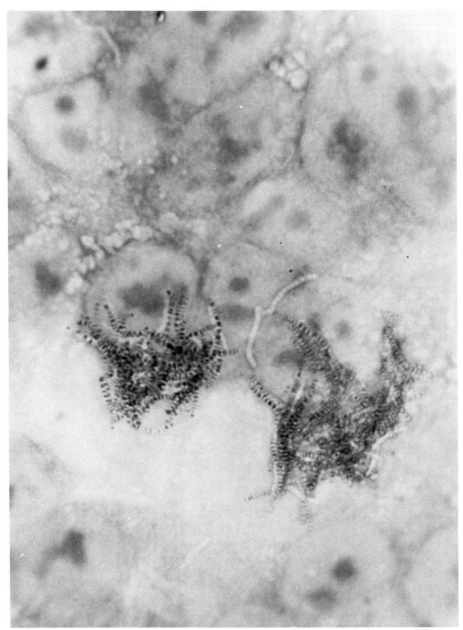

FIGURE 2–11. "Yellow" bacilli in HeLa cells. Growth in five days. There is characteristically spaced beading along the entire length of nearly every organism. (From Shepard, C. C.: Behavior of the "atypical" mycobacteria in HeLa cells. Am. Rev. Tuberc. 77:968, 1958.)

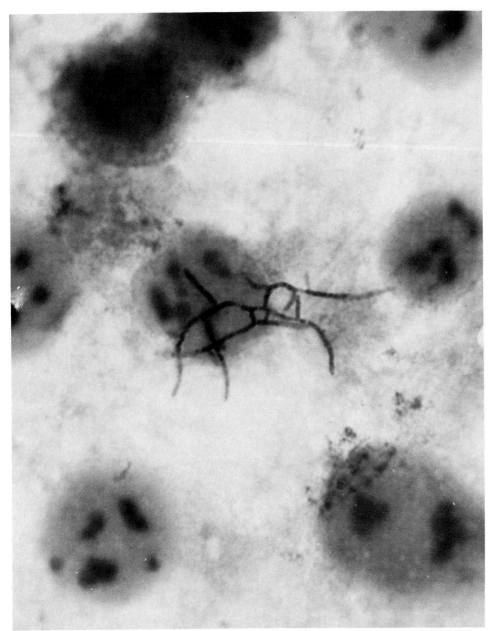

FIGURE 2–12. "Battey" type, strain No. 3, three days after inoculation into HeLa cells. Branching is distinct and gives rise to a characteristic arrangement of the bacilli. × 880. (From Shepard, C. C.: Behavior of the "atypical" mycobacteria in HeLa cells. Am. Rev. Tuberc. 77:968, 1958.)

teristics of this strain is the branching that occurs. This is also seen more characteristically within HeLa cells than in smears from culture. In preparation of smears of this microorganism from cultures, the mechanical processes involved may fragment the cells and minimize the appearance of branching. Figure 2–13 is another example of the appearance of this microorganism growing within HeLa cells. Note that neither *M. kansasii* nor *M. intracellulare* shows the cord formation that is characteristic of *M. tuberculosis*. The morphologic appearance of *M. marinum* and *M. ulcerans* within monkey kidney cells can be seen in Figures 2–14 and 2–15. There is nothing particularly characteristic about the morphology of these cells, but one should note again that there is no cording.

Shepard[80] found that the rapidly growing saprophytic species *M. phlei* and *M. smegmatis* did not grow within HeLa cells but that *M. fortuitum*, an occasional pathogen of humans, did. He also pointed out[80] that the distinctive appearance of many mycobacteria when grown within tissue culture cells could be used as an aid in the identification of several of these species. Unfortunately, in the intervening years since the Shepard observations, little or no use has been made of this elegant technique for studying the growth of mycobacteria or the identification of species.

The morphology of many mycobacterial species varies considerably, depending upon the conditions under which the cells are grown. As far as *M. tuberculosis* is concerned, there is nothing distinctive about the morphologic appearance no matter how the cells are cultured except for the occurrence of cording. This property, though, is shared by other species, such as *M. bovis*, and on occasion even by attenuated species such as bacillus Calmette-Guérin (BCG).

Staining of Mycobacteria

Mycobacterial cells do not stain easily by the Gram method or by simple staining procedures. Probably because of the very high lipid content of these cells, they resist penetration of the stain. This resistance can be overcome by heating the staining solution during the staining process. Under ordinary conditions of applying the Gram stain, mycobacterial cells stain a faint blue color and resist decolorization with alcohol or acetone. For this reason, they have been described as gram-positive. However, in other respects such as lipid content, cell wall composition (see Chapters 3 and 4), and antibiotic resistance, they resemble gram-negative bacteria more closely. The violet color of the Gram stain apparently is retained for the same reasons as the red color is in the acid-fast stain rather than because of some intrinsic property of gram-positiveness.

Acid-Fastness

By far the most distinctive feature of all species of mycobacteria is the capacity to retain certain stains even when vigorously decolorized with acid or acid-alcohol. This characteristic is referred to as acid-fastness, and the mycobacteria are frequently referred to as acid-fast bacteria. Most of the staining procedures that are used to demonstrate this property are modifications of the methods devised by Ziehl[112] and Neelsen.[63] All, however, are acid-fast staining procedures, and we shall refer to them as such in this text. (See Chapter 19 for technical details.)

The property of acid-fastness is shared by the mycobacteria with a few other microorganisms. Some nocardia strains, as well as some strains of corynebacteria, can at times be acid-fast.[56] It is of interest that these two

(Text continued on p. 24)

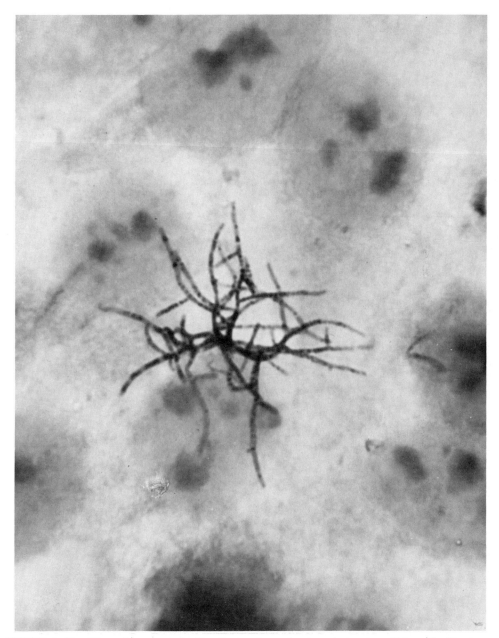

FIGURE 2–13. "Battey" type, strain No. 7, two days after inoculation into HeLa cells. The long, branched filaments also may be seen in this figure. × 880. (From Shepard, C. C.: Behavior of the "atypical" mycobacteria in HeLa cells. Am. Rev. Tuberc. 77:968, 1958.

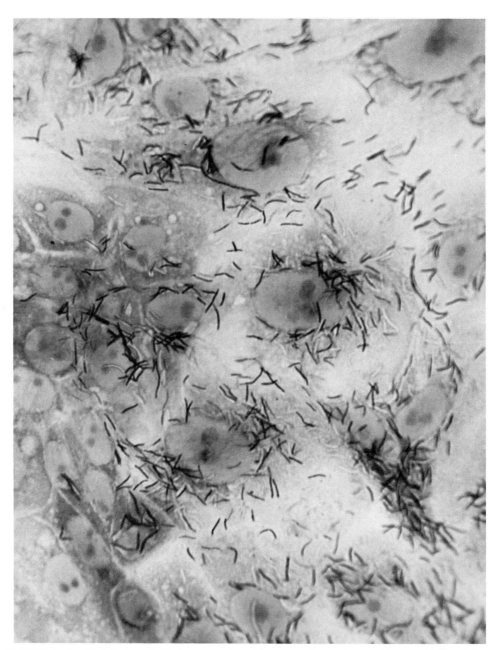

FIGURE 2–14.   *M. balnei*, strain X, the cause of "swimming pool granuloma," three days after inoculation into monkey kidney. × 825. (From Shepard, C. C.: A comparison of the growth of selected mycobacteria in HeLa, monkey kidney, and human amnion cells in tissue culture. J. Exp. Med. *107*:237, 1958.)

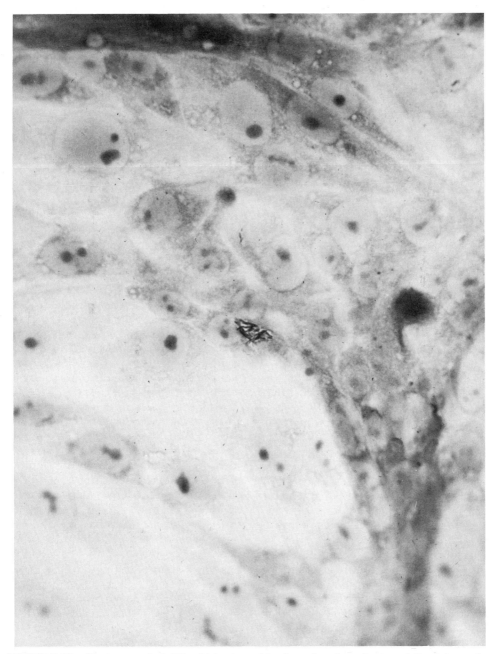

FIGURE 2–15. *M. ulcerans,* strain RS, which causes skin ulcers, four days after inoculation into monkey kidney cultures. No apparent growth at this time. × 825. (From Shepard, C. C.: A comparison of the growth of selected mycobacteria in HeLa, monkey kidney, and human amnion cells in tissue culture. J. Exp. Med. *107*:237, 1958.)

microorganisms have been thought to be closely related phylogenetically to the mycobacteria.

The property of acid-fastness is not limited to those bacteria just mentioned in the preceding paragraph. The heads of the spermatozoa of man and of some lower animals have been found to be acid-fast.[56] Ascospores of certain yeasts may be acid-fast, and bacterial endospores frequently are.[56] The exoskeletons of insects, as well as the inclusions sometimes found in the lungs of lipid pneumonia patients, may be acid-fast;[56] also, the oxidation of unsaturated fatty acids may yield acid-fast materials. The mechanism whereby these miscellaneous materials stain acid-fast is thought to be different from that responsible for the acid-fastness of mycobacteria.[56]

The property of acid-fastness in mycobacterial cells is not fully understood. Basic dyes are required; basic fuchsin, a mixture of the triphenylmethane dyes, rosanilin and pararosanilin, is by far the best. It is of interest that either phenol or aniline is required, although the exact role that these substances play is not clear.

It has been reported that mycolic acids,[84] when isolated from mycobacterial cells, show acid-fastness. Some workers have felt that the mycolic acids comprise the acid-fast material in the mycobacterial cell (see Chapter 4 for further details). The property of acid-fastness is completely lost if the mycobacterial cell is broken. This fact is not in keeping with a role for mycolic acids since these compounds are found in the cell walls. Cell walls isolated by centrifugation and purified from all intact mycobacterial cells are clearly not acid-fast.[50] It seems more reasonable that the basic fuchsin forms a complex with some substance within the mycobacterial cell. This complex is retained, even in the face of vigorous decolorization. The cell membrane may form a barrier that is impenetrable to the escape of the dye complex. This dye complex, though, may be soluble in organic solvents within the cell.[50]

Mycobacteria do not always stain uniformly by the Ziehl-Neelsen procedure, since the mycobacterial cells may appear beaded — i.e., the retention of the red dye seems to be limited to certain locations within the cells. The cause of this beading is not known.

Recently, results from our own laboratory suggest a possible role for mycobacterial RNA in the acid-fast staining process. Mycobacterial RNA in young cultures can comprise approximately 25 percent of the bacterial cell mass.[101] When a mycobacterial RNA protein complex[98, 100] is isolated from mycobacterial cells and stained by the Ziehl-Neelsen method, it becomes bright red; then, when exposed to acid-alcohol, it does not decolorize. In other words, a basic fuchsin-RNA protein complex is formed in which the basic fuchsin is so firmly bound that it cannot be dissolved readily in acid-alcohol. It is not known why mycobacterial RNA should bind so firmly to basic fuchsin, when the RNA in most other bacterial species does not. However, mycobacterial RNA has been found to be unique in a number of characteristics,[97] and this firm retention of basic dyes may be another unique property (see Chapter 9).

Barksdale and Kim[3] feel that acid-fastness is due to the trapping of fuchsin-mycolate complexes within the mycobacterial cell. The trapping, they feel, is the result of the barrier furnished by the peptidoglycolipid of the outer cell wall. Barksdale and Kim[3] also reported that delipidated mycobacterial cells, although non-acid-fast, are gram-positive; thus, mycobacteria are truly gram-positive.

Regardless of the mechanisms involved, acid-fastness is a very useful characteristic by which the mycobacteria as a family can be separated from the majority of other bacteria. When used with care and judgment in the diagnostic laboratory, it can be very helpful in the isolation and identification of pathogenic mycobacteria (see Chapter 19 for further discussion).

Electron Microscopy

No matter what staining procedure is used, examination of mycobacterial cells by light microscopy reveals little or none of the interior or surface structures. Electron microscopy, on the other hand, has been used extensively for the examination of bacterial cells because it does reveal many internal structures. Such examination of mycobacterial cells is appreciably more difficult because the high lipid content of the cell walls makes these bacteria difficult to imbed and section.[14] There have been, however, a number of reports on the electron microscopy of intact mycobacterial cells and of thin sections.*

Figures 2–16 and 2–17 show electron photomicrographs of intact cells of the H37Ra strain of *M. tuberculosis*. The obviously rugose surface illustrated in Figure 2–16 is similar to that seen on many gram-negative bacteria, again indicating that tubercle bacilli are more closely related to gram-negative bacteria than to gram-positive. Figures 2–18, 2–19, and 2–20 show thin sections of cells of the H37Ra strain of *M. tuberculosis*. Most of the structures and inclusions seen in other bacterial species also appear in mycobacterial cells. Mesosomes appear in Figure 2–18, and ribosomes of typical size and shape are visible in Figure 2–19. The trilaminar cell wall shows up particularly well in Figure 2–20. A detailed description of the structure and chemical composition of the mycobacterial trilaminar cell wall will be found in Chapter 4. Figures 2–21 and 2–22

---

*For further discussion concerning electron microscopy, see the following references (at end of chapter): 3, 4, 9, 11, 13, 14, 22, 31, 32, 33, 39, 40, 44, 45, 55, 60, 61, 64, 72, 82, 83, 85, 86, 87, 94, 111

represent a picture taken of ribosomal material isolated from broken H37Ra cells (see Chapter 9). Other electron photomicrographs of mycobacterial cells can be found in Chapter 4.

CULTIVATION OF MYCOBACTERIA

M. tuberculosis, and probably all other mycobacteria, is a strict aerobe. It can be grown on a variety of media, some of which are very simple in composition. For example, *M. tuberculosis* will grow quite readily on a medium containing only asparagine (as a nitrogen source), glycerol (as a carbon source), magnesium citrate, and phosphates. A number of these so-called chemically defined media have been devised and utilized for the growth of *M. tuberculosis.*

The formula for the one that we have used most extensively, a modified Proskauer and Beck medium, is as follows:

Asparagine	0.5 percent
Monopotassium phosphate	0.5 percent
Potassium sulfate	0.5 percent
Glycerol	2.0 percent

The above ingredients are dissolved in the order given in distilled water, care being taken that each ingredient is completely dissolved before the next is added. The hydrogen ion concentration is then adjusted to pH 6.8 to 7.0 with 40 percent sodium hydroxide;

Magnesium citrate	0.15 percent

is then added. This constitutes the basic medium, which is sterilized in the autoclave at 15 pounds for 20 minutes.

The utilization of a modified Proskauer and Beck medium for the growth of mycobacteria requires that certain precautions be taken. First, ad-

(Text continued on p. 33)

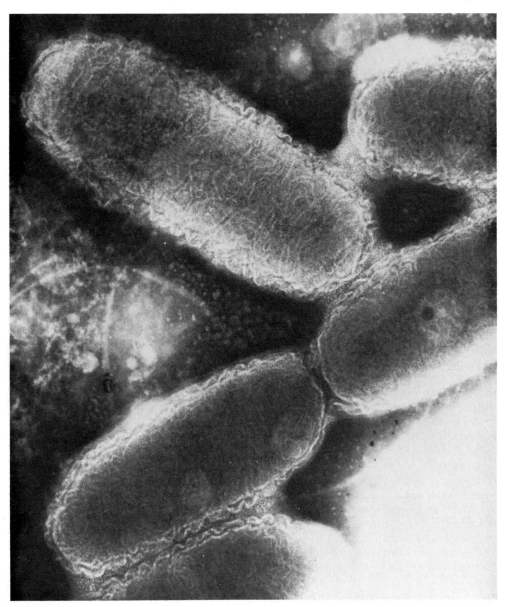

FIGURE 2–16.   *Mycobacterium tuberculosis* cells, strain H37Ra. × 100,000. (From Crispen, R. G.: Biological and ultrastructural characteristics of *Mycobacterium tuberculosis* cells and cell components. Northwestern University Medical School, Ph.D. thesis, June, 1967.)

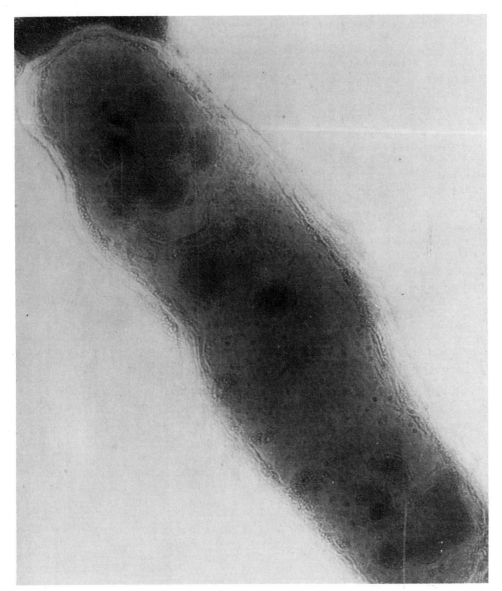

FIGURE 2–17. A cell of *Mycobacterium tuberculosis*, strain H37Ra. × 100,000. (From Crispen, R. G.: Biological and ultrastructural characteristics of *Mycobacterium tuberculosis* cells and cell components. Northwestern University Medical School, Ph.D. thesis, June, 1967.)

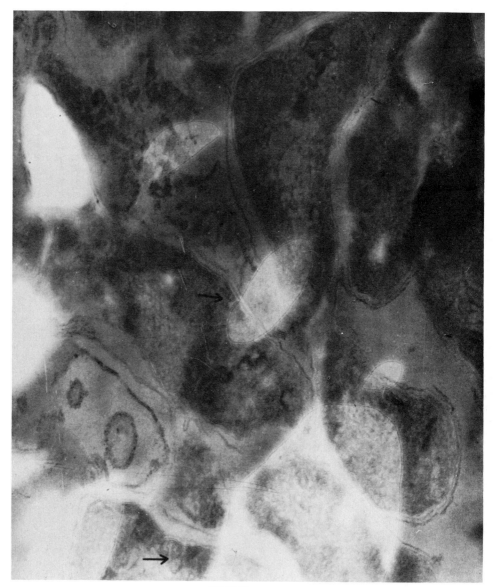

FIGURE 2–18

FIGURES 2–18 to 2–20.   Thin section of cells of *Mycobacterium tuberculosis,* H37Ra strain. × 100,000.
(From Crispen, R. G.: Biological and ultrastructural characteristics of *Mycobacterium tuberculosis* cells
and cell components. Northwestern University Medical School, Ph.D. thesis, June, 1967.)

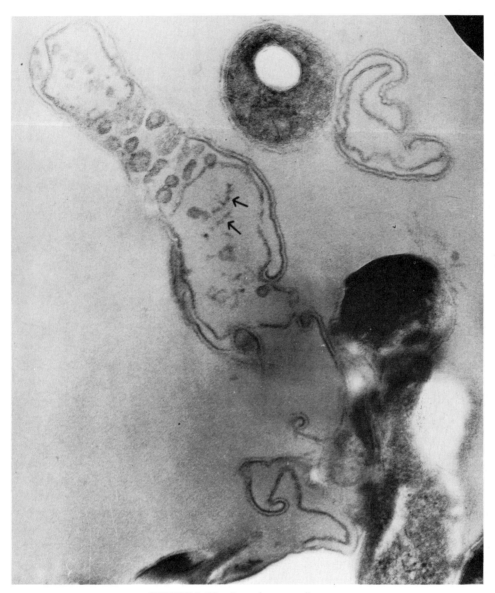

FIGURE 2–19. *Legend on opposite page.*

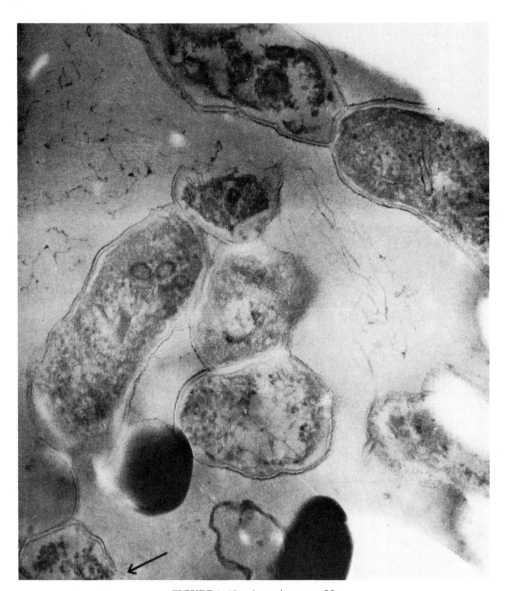

FIGURE 2–20.   *Legend on page 28.*

FIGURE 2–21. Ribosomes of *Mycobacterium tuberculosis,* strain H37Ra. × 30,000. (From Crispen, R. G.: Biological and ultrastructural characteristics of *Mycobacterium tuberculosis* cells and cell components. Northwestern University Medical School, Ph.D. thesis, June, 1967.)

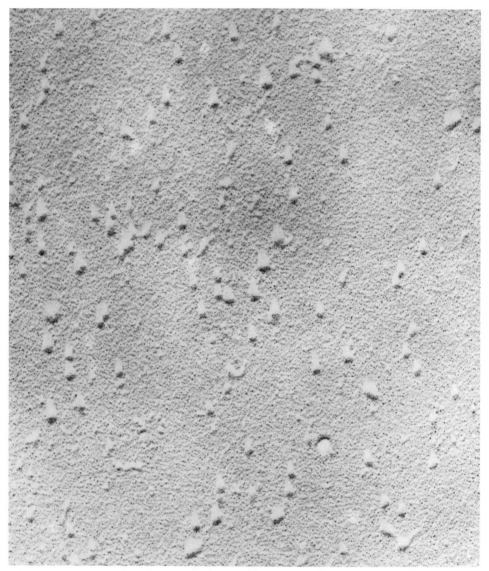

FIGURE 2–22.   Ribosomes of *Mycobacterium tuberculosis,* strain H37Ra. × 100,000. (From Crispen, R. G.: Biological and ultrastructural characteristics of *Mycobacterium tuberculosis* cells and cell components. Northwestern University Medical School, Ph.D. thesis, June, 1967.)

equate zinc must be present. When glycerol that comes from zinc-lined containers is utilized, there is usually enough zinc dissolved to allow vigorous growth of *M. tuberculosis.*[20, 90, 101] On the other hand, if glycerol is put up in glass containers, it may not contain enough zinc and the medium may not support good growth of *M. tuberculosis.* Second, the distilled water used in the preparations of the medium must be pure; otherwise, contaminating materials, such as heavy metals or organic acids, may seriously impede the growth of tubercle bacilli.[18] Third, glassware in which the medium is dispensed must be especially clean. It has been shown[19] that glassware sterilized by hot air, and especially glassware in which cotton plugs have been inserted, will not be suitable containers for the growth of tubercle bacilli on synthetic media. Dry heat sterilization produces distillates of organic acids that may condense as films on the interior surfaces of the tubes or flasks in sufficient quantity to inhibit or prevent the growth of tubercle bacilli. These matters are critical; unless the person attempting to grow tubercle bacilli on such a simple medium is aware of these factors and allows for them, it may be impossible to initiate growth from small numbers of tubercle bacilli.

In the semisynthetic medium, the simplest way of obviating the difficulties just discussed is to incorporate sterile serum or albumin in sufficient quantity to bind the deleterious ions, thus preventing the inhibition of growth of tubercle bacilli.[26, 96] However, in many experimental situations, it is undesirable to have proteins of any kind in the medium in which the tubercle bacillus is to be grown. In such cases, the only alternative is to be scrupulously careful about the state of the glassware and the nature of the distilled water and, if one has some question about the glycerol, to add very small amounts of zinc chloride.[90, 101]

Traditionally, mycobacteria have been grown as pellicles on the surface of liquid media. It was not until 1942, when Drea[18, 19] in an elegant series of experiments showed that tubercle bacilli would grow within the depths of liquid media, that any extensive use of this technique was made. Earlier investigators had occasionally observed subsurface growth, but the general opinion remained that tubercle bacilli would only grow on the surface. Drea clearly showed that this was a misconception, and his papers can be referred to for the earlier literature on the subject.

Youmans[106, 107] in 1944 studied the subsurface growth of *M. tuberculosis* and utilized this form of cultivation for the determination of the antimycobacterial action of drugs. He found that modified Proskauer and Beck medium could be put into tubes in 4 or 5 mm amounts, sterilized by autoclaving, and inoculated with suspensions of tubercle bacilli. The suspensions were prepared mechanically by grinding pellicle growth in a mortar with a pestle and then diluting these to the desired number of cells. Serial dilutions of bacteriostatic drugs were made in tubes of this medium; then each tube, together with the appropriate control tubes, was inoculated with small numbers of tubercle bacilli. The tubercle bacilli grew at the bottom of the liquid in the tube in a characteristic fashion. This subsurface growth was granular, and when the tubes were shaken, particles of mycobacterial growth would swirl through the medium in a characteristic manner. Bacteriostatic end points were recorded as the least amount of drug in the serial dilution that would completely prevent the appearance of this kind of growth. The procedure greatly accelerated the search for potential chemotherapeutic agents for the treatment of tuberculosis in humans. Over the next several years Sattler and Youmans[73] and Youmans and Youmans and coworkers extended the use of this procedure to a number of other areas, including extensive studies on the nutrition and physiology of mycobacteria.[37, 38, 62, 99, 102–105, 108–110] (These will be reported in greater detail at more appropriate places in the book.) It is worth pointing out here that with careful attention to the elimination of the deleterious factors just mentioned and to the careful handling of cultures, it was possible to secure growth from an inoculum consisting of only one viable tubercle bacillus in the Proskauer and Beck medium without serum or albumin.

In a tube containing 4 or 5 mm of Proskauer and Beck medium, after inoculation with cells of *M. tuberculosis,* the appearance of the developing growth is typical. The growth first appears as a slight sediment, which adheres to the tube at the bottom of the column of medium. Over a period of days, this film-like growth, which actually appears to be between the liquid and the surface of the glass tube, extends up the sides of the tube until it reaches the surface of the medium. When the surface of the medium is reached, this growth extends across the surface from all sides, and a heavy pellicle of growth eventually forms on the surface. Apparently, the surface growth is greater not only because of the greater oxygen supply but because the mycobacterial cells are not physically restricted in any way. When small numbers of tubercle bacilli are used as an inoculum, three or four (or sometimes more) weeks of incubation at 37° C may be required to form a fairly heavy pellicle.[107]

Aeration of liquid cultures can increase appreciably the yield of mycobacterial cells.[57]

A distinct advance in the handling of mycobacterial cultures and of growing mycobacteria came in 1947 when Dubos[25] and Dubos and Davis[26] reported that when the nonionic detergent Tween 80 was added to a liquid medium, the tubercle bacilli would grow in a dispersed fashion. Initially, it was also reported that Tween 80 greatly accelerated the rate of growth of tubercle bacilli. However, it became apparent that the increased rate of growth was more an illusion than a reality. Because the tubercle bacilli grew in a dispersed fashion with Tween 80, it was possible for investigators to detect the turbidity earlier than they were able to recognize the more film-like granular growth that occurred on the bottom of the tube without Tween 80. Sattler and Youmans[73] accurately measured the quantity of growth at different times after inoculation of a medium containing Tween 80 and the same medium without Tween 80. They showed that the growth was actually slower in the medium containing Tween 80 than in the one lacking it. This inhibition of growth by Tween 80 was subsequently shown to be caused by the hydrolysis of the Tween 80 with the production of small amounts of oleic acid.[16, 23, 24, 26, 27]

Organic acids, particularly oleic acid, can be very inhibitory for growth of tubercle bacilli. This led to the incorporation of bovine serum albumin into the Dubos' Tween 80 medium.[16, 23, 24, 26, 27] The bovine serum albumin combined with the oleic acid and eliminated its toxicity. When this was done, tubercle bacilli were found to grow at approximately comparable rates in medium without Tween 80 and medium with Tween 80.[73]

Growth of tubercle bacilli in a diffuse manner can be a distinct advantage. It permits direct turbidity measurements of the amount of growth, and the greater separation between the mycobacterial cells makes the application of plating procedures more feasible. As a matter of fact, the dispersed growth of tubercle bacilli in medium containing Tween 80 is not due to the separation of the mycobacteria into separate single cells. Microscopic examination shows that in a well-dispersed growth in Tween 80 medium, the mycobacteria are in small clumps of two to ten cells. This should be kept in mind whenever Tween 80 medium is used for inoculation of animals or for any other purpose in which enumeration of mycobacterial cells is desired.

It is important to realize that even in the presence of bovine serum or albumin, both of which neutralize the oleic acid, the results of tests may be altered because of the presence of the surface-active agent, Tween 80. For example, bacteriostatic activity of a compound may appear to be much greater in the Tween-albumin medium than in a medium that does not contain the detergent.[28] Presumably, the detergent permits more ready penetration of the bacteriostatic agent into the mycobacterial cell.[91] This phenomenon was first recognized by Fisher,[28] who noted that Tween 80 would markedly increase the bacteriostatic action of streptomycin for *M. tuberculosis*.

ARITHMETIC LINEAR GROWTH

Fisher and colleagues in 1951[30] first described the arithmetic linear growth

of *M. tuberculosis*. Under ordinary circumstances, since the mycobacteria divide by binary fission, one would expect growth to be exponential, and it is. However, if mycobacteria are cultivated in tubes containing liquid media, to which has been added a dispersing agent such as Tween 80, an initial period of exponential growth is followed by an arithmetic linear growth period, in which the number of tubercle bacilli increase at a constant rate. This is illustrated in Figure 2–23. Fisher and coworkers[30] and Fisher and Kirchheimer[29] felt that this peculiar type of growth pattern was a unique characteristic of mycobacteria, and since the increase in number of bacilli is very slow when compared to that obtained by exponential growth, they also felt that this might account for the very slow rate of growth exhibited by most mycobacterial species.

However, Volk and Myrvik[88] pointed out in 1953 that the arithmetic linear growth pattern of mycobacteria did not result from some peculiar manner of multiplication of tubercle bacilli but was a consequence of oxygen

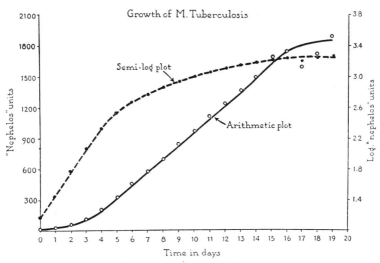

FIGURE 2–23. Arithmetic and semilogarithmic plots of nephelometric measurements of the growth of *Mycobacterium tuberculosis*, strain H37Rv, illustrating the "arithmetic linear" growth phase. (From Fisher, M. W., Kirchheimer, W. F., and Hess, A. R.: The arithmetic linear growth of *Mycobacterium tuberculosis* var. *hominis*. J. Bacteriol. 62:319, 1951.)

deprivation. These authors claimed that if the same cultures that showed arithmetic linear growth were well aerated by constant shaking, the growth pattern changed from arithmetic linear to exponential. They also were able to show that the lower two-thirds or more of a tube of medium containing tubercle bacilli that was maintained in an incubator without shaking did not have enough oxygen to provide for the growth of all of the tubercle bacilli present. Therefore, only those bacilli in the upper 10 percent of the tube were able to multiply. These tubercle bacilli multiplied exponentially, but since the growth measurements were turbidimetric, the total mass of cells in the tube would reflect the number of both multiplying and nonmultiplying bacteria. The increase in the turbidity would be accounted for by only those cells with enough oxygen to multiply exponentially, i.e., those at the top of the tube. In the case of tubercle bacilli, atmospheric oxygen is essential for growth. When the oxygen available is less than the minimal amount necessary, tubercle bacilli will stop growing. If the cultures of mycobacteria are

aerated adequately, exponential growth will occur (Figs. 2–24 and 2–25)[36] until further growth is limited by factors other than the availability of molecular oxygen. Arithmetic linear growth can be seen with other bacteria when there is a limited amount of some absolutely essential nutrient.[88]

SYNCHRONOUS GROWTH

Wayne[89] has recently shown that when *M. tuberculosis* is grown in Tween-albumin broth without any agitation, the bacilli replicate in the upper oxygen-rich portion of the medium at a rate that is just balanced by the rate at which the bacilli settle toward the bottom of the tube. When the organisms that accumulate in the sediment are resuspended and diluted with fresh medium, they exhibit synchronous replication (Fig. 2–26).

Wayne suggests that the resting state of the tubercle bacilli in the bottom of the tube may be analogous to that of tubercle bacilli in vivo where, under certain circumstances, they may remain viable but nonmultiplying for

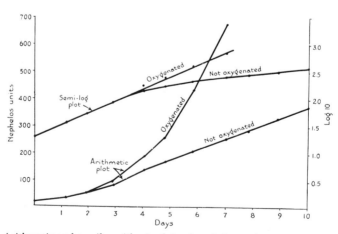

FIGURE 2–24. Arithmetic and semilogarithmic plots of nephelometric measurements of the *Mycobacterium tuberculosis*, strain H37Ra, in oxygenated and in nonoxygenated medium. (From Halpern, B., and Kirchheimer, W. F.: Studies on the growth of mycobacteria. II. The effect of oxygenation and aeration on the growth pattern of mycobacteria. Am. Rev. Tuberc. 70:665, 1954.)

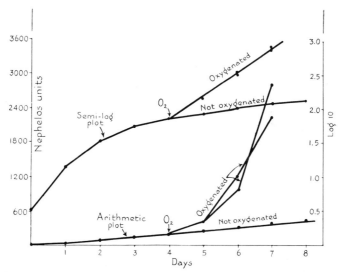

FIGURE 2–25. The effect of oxygenation during arithmetic linear growth on the growth pattern of *Mycobacterium sp.*, strain 607. (From Halpern, B., and Kirchheimer, W. F.: Studies on the growth of mycobacteria. II. The effect of oxygenation and aeration on the growth pattern of mycobacteria. Am. Rev. Tuberc. 70:665, 1954.)

long periods. If so, use of these resting cells would provide a means of testing in vitro the effect of environmental factors, including drugs, on dormant tubercle bacilli equivalent to those found in vivo. Using synchronous growth, it should also be possible to measure the effect of drugs or other factors on mycobacteria at different stages of their replicative cycle.

GROWTH ON SOLID MEDIA

Solid media also can be used for the cultivation of *M. tuberculosis* and other mycobacteria. Media containing egg yolk or whole egg have long been favorites for the isolation of mycobacteria from clinical specimens because egg yolk apparently stimulates the

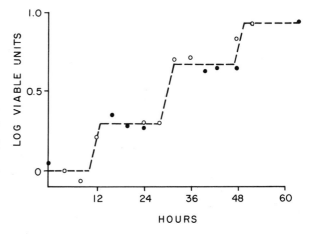

FIGURE 2–26. Synchronous replication of *M. tuberculosis* on resuspension and dilution of microaerophilic sediments. The curve is a composite of normalized points from two experiments, indicated by open and closed circles. (From Wayne, L. G.: Synchronized replication of *Mycobacterium tuberculosis*. Infect. Immun. 17:528, 1977.)

growth of *M. tuberculosis*. However, efforts to isolate the growth-stimulating factor from egg yolk have not been particularly rewarding.[58] These egg yolk media can be complex (see Chapter 19) and usually have not employed agar as a solidifying agent because of its toxicity. Agar can be toxic to a variety of microorganisms but is particularly so for mycobacteria. Therefore, most egg yolk media used for isolation of tubercle bacilli have been solidified and sterilized by inspissation. Such media are excellent for the growth of mycobacteria but are difficult to prepare and sterilize.

As a matter of fact, perfectly satisfactory solid media for the growth of tubercle bacilli can be made by solidifying Proskauer and Beck medium with agar and adding bovine albumin or bovine serum. The albumin and serum tend to neutralize the toxicity of the agar. Serum should not be used in a concentration greater than 5 or 10 percent because high concentrations of serum can inhibit mycobacterial growth.[96, 108]

One of the most commonly used solid media for both research and diagnostic purposes is Middlebrook's 7H10 or 7H11.[12, 71] These are excellent media, which are easy to prepare since they can be obtained commercially in dehydrated form. Agar media detoxified by the addition of serum or albumin are particularly useful because, being semitransparent, they permit the detection of colony morphology. Their usefulness as media for the isolation of *M. tuberculosis* from clinical specimens is covered in Chapter 19.

Thus, it is apparent that mycobacteria, including *M. tuberculosis*, can be cultivated in both liquid and solid media. Although their hydrophobic nature makes cultivation and handling difficult, mycobacteria, by appropriate procedures, can be grown in much the same manner as other, less hydrophobic bacteria. The use of pellicle cultures of mycobacteria has now largely been abandoned. Pellicle growth, however, can be useful for the preparation of large masses of mycobacterial cells, and as we will see in Chapter 5, is essential for the in-vitro maintenance of the virulence of certain strains of mycobacteria.

METABOLISM OF MYCOBACTERIA

An enormous amount of work has been done on the metabolism of *M. tuberculosis* and the other mycobacteria. No attempt will be made to cover this literature in detail, since it will be found completely reviewed in a number of excellent books and monographs.[3, 15, 21, 46, 58, 68–70, 92] We will focus upon the characteristics that distinguish the mycobacteria from many other microorganisms and those features that may be of particular importance in their capacity to produce infection and disease.

Compared to most bacteria, mycobacteria grow very slowly. The free-living saprophytic species have generation times of four to six hours. *M. tuberculosis* in vitro requires a generation time of at least 10 to 15 hours on the most favorable medium,[1, 108] and 20 to 24 hours on the modified Proskauer and Beck synthetic medium.[107, 109] *M. leprae*, which will only grow in vivo, needs approximately 12 days for a single generation. No reasonable explanation has yet been offered to account for these relatively slow rates of growth.

Role of Oxygen

M. tuberculosis is a strict aerobe. Although entirely dependent upon the presence of molecular oxygen for growth, *M. tuberculosis* will multiply at reduced oxygen tensions. There is some evidence that the capacity of tubercle bacilli to produce disease may depend in part upon the amount of oxygen available. For example, in reinfection, tuberculosis occurs more frequently in the poorly aerated parts of the lung (the apices) where the blood flow is least rapid. This reduced blood flow results in less oxygen exchange and, therefore, in a higher alveolar oxygen tension. Also, if animals are infected with *M. tuberculosis* and housed in atmospheres containing different concentrations of oxygen, the rate at which the disease will develop is directly proportional to the concentration of oxygen in the inspired air.[76] (See Chapter 5 for more information on this subject.) The predilection for *M. tuberculosis* to produce disease in the lung can be explained in this way.

Not all mycobacterial species, or strains, have the same molecular oxygen requirements. For example, it has been shown that the attenuated H37Ra mutant of the H37Rv strain of *M. tuberculosis* will not grow in an oxygen tension quite as low as its virulent parent strain. Perhaps the virulence of the H37Rv strain might be accounted for by its capacity to multiply at lower oxygen tensions; this has been suggested by Guy and associates.[35] Conversely, the lack of virulence of the H37Ra mutant might arise from its inability to grow at the low oxygen tension found in cells and tissues.[35] (See also Chapter 5.)

Glycerol and *M. tuberculosis*

One of the unique features of *M. tuberculosis* is its preference for glycerol as a source of carbon; no other alcohols can be substituted.[110] In this connection, it appears that glucose may be oxidized by the anaerobic glycolytic system,[5, 41, 42, 43, 65, 67, 68] or it may be oxidized aerobically to glucuronic acid and then, by a series of decarboxylations via the alphaketo acids, to pyruvic acid.[68, 103] No other monosaccharides or disaccharides can be effectively utilized as carbon and energy sources by *M. tuberculosis*. Other mycobacteria, insofar as they have been tested, appear to follow the same pattern. The exception is *M. bovis*, which does not readily utilize glycerol or glucose and prefers pyruvate as a carbon source.[3, 17] There is some evidence that *M. tuberculosis* may also prefer pyruvate when available.[3, 17]

The preference of *M. tuberculosis* for glycerol is of some importance as far as virulence is concerned. Glycerol, of course, is a common tissue constituent. The concentration of glycerol available to the tubercle bacillus may, in part, regulate its capacity to metabolize and multiply in vivo. Long and Vorwald,[59] in fact, found an unmistakable increase in the number of bacilli and extent of disease in experimentally infected rats fed large quantities of glycerol over a long period of time, as compared with the controls.

Extensive work from our own laboratory has shown that *M. tuberculosis* possesses a citric acid terminal respiratory cycle.[110] Carbon compounds are oxidized by *M. tuberculosis* to carbon dioxide and water.[68, 102]

Sources of Nitrogen

On the one hand, *M. tuberculosis* is very particular in the sources of nitrogen it can utilize, on the other, very elemental in its requirements. Asparagine is by far the best nitrogen source for the growth of tubercle bacilli. Glutamic acid can substitute for asparagine but only over a more limited range of concentrations.[105] Histidine, aspartic acid, and L-proline can be utilized to a limited extent, but the growth rate will be slower. Some growth will occur, at a greatly reduced rate, on the Proskauer and Beck medium to which no nitrogen-containing compound has been added;[95] apparently, traces of ammonia in the air may be utilized or atmospheric nitrogen may be fixed. When the sole source of nitrogen in a synthetic medium is either ammonium malate[93] or ammonium phosphate, growth is somewhat better, though it is still not comparable with the amount or rate of growth that occurs in the presence of asparagine.

Importance of Enzymes and Lipids

Mycobacteria, including M. tuberculosis, produce a variety of enzymes, many of which are very useful in the characterization and identification of the various species (see Chapters 18 and 19).

The lipid metabolism of M. tuberculosis and the other mycobacteria is of particular importance. The major portion of many mycobacterial cells is composed of lipids of one kind or another. Many of these lipids have important biologic effects (see Chapter 4).

Effects of Iron on Mycobacteria

A variety of elements — in particular, metals in trace amounts — are also required for the growth of mycobacteria. (The nature of these elements can be found in the general references listed at the beginning of this chapter.) One of them — zinc — we have already discussed; another element of critical importance is iron. Traces of iron are essential. If iron is removed from a medium, growth of tubercle bacilli will cease. This is of particular importance when serum is included in a medium for growth of mycobacteria, as frequently occurs. Serum from dif-

ferent species of animals or different batches of serum from a single species may contain variable amounts of transferrin. Transferrin will bind iron, and if there is sufficient binding of iron by transferrin, growth of tubercle bacilli may be inhibited. Kochan and his colleagues[53, 54] have analyzed exhaustively the role of iron in serum on the growth of tubercle bacilli as well as the competing activity of transferrin for iron. Kochan believes the availability of iron in animal tissue plays a significant role in the virulence of tubercle bacilli and perhaps in the induction of acquired immunity. This is discussed in more detail in Chapter 5.

IN VIVO-GROWN MYCOBACTERIAL CELLS

The possibility that tubercle bacilli might metabolize differently or have a different chemical composition when growing in vivo rather than in vitro was a subject of some speculation in the early literature.[2, 77] In 1956, Segal and Bloch[74] attempted to answer this question by studying tubercle bacilli isolated from the lungs of infected mice. When mice are infected intravenously with tubercle bacilli, the resulting disease is primarily pulmonary. Therefore, the lungs of moribund mice will contain enormous numbers of tubercle bacilli. Segal and Bloch harvested the tubercle bacilli by homogenizing the lungs and then separating the tubercle bacilli by differential centrifugation.

The initial observations of these two researchers indicated that in morphology, in staining properties, in colonial characteristics or rate of growth on oleic acid-albumin agar plates, and in pathogenicity for mice, there was no significant difference between the bacilli grown in vitro and those grown in vivo. However, there was a marked difference in hydrogen transfer activity between the two types of cells as measured on a number of substrates, such as glycerol, glucose, pyruvate, and acetate. The tubercle bacilli grown in vivo showed almost no hydrogen transfer capacity, as compared with the very active cells grown in vitro. It is noteworthy that the endogenous respiration for both types was the same.

Continuing their investigations, Segal and Bloch[75] in 1957 reported that tubercle bacilli grown in vivo actually were somewhat more virulent for mice than those grown in vitro. When tubercle bacilli grown in vitro were killed with phenol, they produced a greater degree of immunity to infection than did bacilli grown in vivo under similar circumstances. The H37Rv strain of *M. tuberculosis* was used in all of Segal and Bloch's studies.

In 1959 Bekierkunst and Artman[6] examined the hydrogen transfer capacity of cell-free extracts of tubercle bacilli obtained from the lungs of mice. They noted that such extracts had low dehydrogenase activity in the presence of lactate, malate, or pyruvate, even though similar extracts prepared from the same mycobacteria grown in vitro were active. In follow-up studies in 1960 and 1962,[7, 8] these two workers found that the lack of oxidative activity resulted from the presence of an inhibitor. This inhibitor was identified as a NADase that came from mouse pulmonary tissue. The inhibition of the respiration of the tubercle bacilli apparently occurs because of the action of the NADase, which is adsorbed to the surface of the mycobacterial cells. It is of interest here to note that the NADase activity of mouse tuberculous lung tissue is two to three times as high as that found in lung tissue of noninfected mice.

Pokorny and Sulova,[66] quoted in Kanai,[49] examined the lipid composition of tubercle bacilli obtained from the lungs of mice by using density gradient centrifugation. They found that, in general, the bacilli grown in

vivo synthesized fewer lipids than those grown in artificial media; there were also some changes in the composition of the higher fatty acids. However, Kanai and colleagues[51] found that tubercle bacilli grown in vivo produce mycolic acids and phthiocerol dimycocerosate, as did cells grown in artificial culture medium.

Thus, it appears that tubercle bacilli grown in vivo may differ somewhat in composition and possibly in certain metabolic activities from those grown in vitro. Some of these alterations of metabolic activity are brought about by adsorbed host enzymes. This, in turn, indicates that host constituents adsorbed to the surface of mycobacterial cells may play an important role in infection. It is quite possible that the adsorption of such materials to mycobacterial surfaces might make the mycobacteria more like the host and thus interfere with the host response to the infection. For a more detailed discussion of growth and metabolism of in vitro- and in vivo-grown tubercle bacilli, see Chapter 4. The papers of Kanai[47, 48] and the reviews of Kanai[49] and Barksdale and Kim[3] should be consulted as well.

REFERENCES

1. Abramson, S.: The failure of chick embryo extract to accelerate the growth of tubercle bacilli. Am. Rev. Tuberc. 65:783, 1952.
2. Anderson, R. J., Reeves, R. E., Creighton, M. M., and Lothrop, W. C.: The chemistry of the lipids of tubercle bacilli. LXV. An investigation of tuberculous lung tissue. Am. Rev. Tuberc. 48:65, 1943.
3. Barksdale, L., and Kim, K.: *Mycobacterium.* Bacteriol. Rev. 41:217, 1977.
4. Bassermann, F. J.: Neueste Forschungsergebnisse über das *Mycobacterium tuberculosis.* Beitr. Klin. Erforsch. Tuberk. 132:60, 1965.
5. Bastarrachea, F., Anderson, D. G., and Goldman, D. S.: Enzyme systems in the mycobacteria. XI. Evidence for a functional glycolytic system. J. Bacteriol. 82:94, 1961.
6. Bekierkunst, A., and Artman, M.: Effect of

cell-free extracts from *Mycobacterium tuberculosis* H$_{37}$Rv on lung succinooxidase. Nature *184*:458, 1959.

7. Bekierkunst, A., and Artman, M.: Studies on *Mycobacterium tuberculosis* H37Rv grown *in vivo*: Inhibitor of lactic acid dehydrogenase in normal and infected mice. Proc. Soc. Exp. Biol. Med. *105*:605, 1960.

8. Bekierkunst, A., and Artman, M.: Tissue metabolism in infection. DPNase activity, DPN levels, and DPN-linked dehydrogenase in tissues from normal and tuberculous mice. Am. Rev. Respir. Dis. *86*:832, 1962.

9. Brieger, E. M.: Structure and Ultrastructure of Microorganisms. New York, Academic Press, 1963.

10. Buchanan, R. E., and Gibbons, N. E. (eds.): Bergey's Manual of Determinative Bacteriology. 8th ed. Baltimore, The Williams & Wilkins Company, 1974.

11. Chapman, G. B., Hanks, J. H., and Wallace, J. H.: An electron microscope study of the disposition and fine structure of *Mycobacterium lepraemurium* in mouse spleen. J. Bacteriol. *77*:205, 1959.

12. Cohn, M. L., Waggoner, R. F., and McClatchy, J. K.: The 7H11 medium for the cultivation of mycobacteria. Am. Rev. Respir. Dis. *98*:295, 1968.

13. Cole, R. M.: Bacterial structure and replication. Science *146*:554, 1964.

14. Crispen, R. G.: Biological and ultrastructural characteristics of *Mycobacterium tuberculosis* cells and cell components. Ph. D. Thesis, Northwestern University Medical School, June, 1967.

15. Darzins, E.: The Bacteriology of Tuberculosis. Minneapolis, University of Minnesota Press, 1958.

16. Davis, B. D., and Dubos, R. J.: Interaction of serum albumin, free and esterified oleic acid and lipase in relation to cultivation of the tubercle bacillus. Arch. Biochem. *11*:201, 1946.

17. Dixon, J. M. S., and Cuthbert, E. H.: Isolation of tubercle bacilli from uncentrifuged sputum on pyruvic acid medium. Am. Rev. Respir. Dis. *96*:119, 1967.

18. Drea, W. F.: The growth of human tubercle bacilli, H37, in synthetic medium with and without agar. J. Bacteriol. *39*:197, 1940.

19. Drea, W. F.: Growth of small numbers of tubercle bacilli, H37, in Long's liquid synthetic medium and some interfering factors. J. Bacteriol. *44*:149, 1942.

20. Drea, W. F.: Traces of zinc in glycerol. Am. Rev. Tuberc. *74*:145, 1956.

21. Drea, W. F., and Andrejew, A.: The Metabolism of the Tubercle Bacillus. Springfield, Ill., Charles C Thomas, 1953.

22. Drews, G.: Elektronenmikroskopische untersuchungen an *Mycobacterium phlei*. Archiv Mikrobiol. *35*:53, 1960.

23. Dubos, R. J.: The effect of lipids and serum albumin on bacterial growth. J. Exp. Med. *85*:9, 1947.

24. Dubos, R. J.: Effect of long chain fatty acids on bacterial growth. Proc. Soc. Exp. Biol. Med. *63*:56, 1946.

25. Dubos, R. J.: Rapid and submerged growth of mycobacteria in liquid media. Proc. Soc. Exp. Biol. Med. *58*:361, 1945.

26. Dubos, R. J., and Davis, B. D.: Factors affecting the growth of tubercle bacilli in liquid media. J. Exp. Med. *83*:409, 1946.

27. Dubos, R. J., Davis, B. D., Middlebrook, G., and Pierce, C.: The effect of water soluble lipids on the growth and biological properties of tubercle bacilli. Am. Rev. Tuberc. *54*:204, 1946.

28. Fisher, M. W.: Sensitivity of tubercle bacilli to streptomycin. An *in vitro* study of some factors affecting results in various test media. Am. Rev. Tuberc. *57*:58, 1948.

29. Fisher, M. W., and Kirchheimer, W. F.: Studies on the growth of mycobacteria. I. The occurrence of arithmetic linear growth. Am. Rev. Tuberc. *66*:758, 1952.

30. Fisher, M. W., Kirchheimer, W. F., and Hess, A. R.: The arithmetic linear growth of *Mycobacterium tuberculosis* var. *hominis*. J. Bacteriol. *62*:319, 1951.

.31. Fukushi, K., Suzuki, T., Sato, T., Hasebe, E., and Ebina, T.: Intracytoplasmic membranous organelles in cell division of mycobacteria. *In* Breese, S. S., Jr., (ed.): Electron Microscopy. New York, Academic Press, 1962, RR-6.

32. Giesbrecht, P.: Über "organisierte" Mitochondrien und andere Feinstrukturen von Bacillus megaterium. Zbl. Bakt. [Orig.] *179*:538, 1960.

33. Glauert, A. M., and Glauert, R. H.: Araldite as an embedding medium for electron microscopy. J. Biophys. Biochem. Cytol. *4*:191, 1958.

34. Goren, M. B.: Mycobacterial lipids: Selected topics. Bacteriol. Rev. *36*:33, 1972.

35. Guy, L. R., Raffel, S., and Clifton, C. E.: Virulence of the tubercle bacillus. II. Effect of oxygen tension upon growth of virulent and avirulent bacilli. J. Infect. Dis. *94*:99, 1954.

36. Halpern, B., and Kirchheimer, W. F.: Studies on the growth of mycobacteria. II. The effect of oxygenation and aeration on the growth pattern of mycobacteria. Am. Rev. Tuberc. *70*:665, 1954.

37. Holmgren, N., Millman, I., and Youmans, G. P.: Studies on the metabolism of *Mycobacterium tuberculosis*. VI. The effect of Krebs' tricarboxylic acid cycle intermediates and precursors on the growth and respiration of *Mycobacterium tuberculosis*. J. Bacteriol. *68*:405, 1954.

38. Holmgren, N. B., and Youmans, G. P.: Studies on the metabolism of virulent and

avirulent mycobacteria. Am. Rev. Tuberc. 66:416, 1952.

39. Imaeda, T., and Convit, J.: Electron microscope study of *Mycobacterium leprae* and its environment in a vesicular leprous lesion. J. Bacteriol. 83:43, 1962.

40. Imaeda, T., and Ogura, M.: Formation of intracytoplasmic membrane system of mycobacteria related to cell division. J. Bacteriol. 85:150, 1963.

41. Indira, M.: Studies on the glucose metabolism of the virulent and avirulent strains of *Mycobacterium tuberculosis* H37Rv and H37Ra. Doctoral Thesis, Indian Institute of Science, Bangalore, India, 1964. (As cited in Ramakrishnan et al.[67])

42. Indira, M., and Ramakrishnan, T.: Glucose dissimilation by *Mycobacterium tuberculosis* H37Ra. J. Sci. Industr. Res. 21C:1, 1962.

43. Indira, M., and Ramakrishnan, T.: Metabolism of micro-organisms. *In* Biology and Biochemistry of Micro-organisms, Golden Jubliee Symposium, Indian Institute of Science, Bangalore, 1959, p. 26.

44. van Iterson, W.: Membranous structures in micro-organisms. *In* Gibbons, N. E. (ed.): Recent Progress in Microbiology. Eighth International Congress for Microbiology. Canada, University of Toronto Press, 1963.

45. van Iterson, W.: Symposium on the fine structure and replication of bacteria and their parts: II. Bacterial cytoplasm. Bacteriol. Rev. 29:299, 1965.

46. Iwainsky, H., and Kappler, W.: Mykobakterien: Biochemie und Biochemische Differenzierung. Leipzig, J. A. Barth, 1974.

47. Kanai, K.: Detection of host-originated acid phosphatase on the surface of "*in vivo* grown tubercle bacilli." Jpn. J. Med. Sci. Biol. 20:73, 1967.

48. Kanai, K.: Resistance to sodium hydroxide treatment of "*in vivo* grown tubercle bacilli." Jpn. J. Med. Sci. Biol. 20:91, 1967.

49. Kanai, K.: Acquired resistance to tuberculous infection in experimental model. Jpn. J. Med. Sci. Biol. 20:21, 1967.

50. Kanai, K.: The staining properties of isolated mycobacterial cellular components as revealed by the Ziehl-Neelsen procedure. Am. Rev. Respir. Dis. 85:442, 1962.

51. Kanai, K., Wiegeshaus, E., and Smith, D. W.: Detection of lipids of *in vitro* grown mycobacteria in bacilli separated from infected tissues. Die Variabilitat der Mycobakterien unter experimentellen und klinischen Bedingungen, Kolloquium im Forschungsinstitut Borstel, 13, 14 und 15 Oktober, 1965.

52. Koch, R.: Die Aetiologie der Tuberkulose. Berl. Klin. Wochenschr. 19:221, 1882.

53. Kochan, I., Cahall, D. L., and Golden, C. A.: Employment of tuberculostasis in serum-agar medium for the study of production and activity of mycobactin. Infect. Immun. 4:130, 1971.

54. Kochan, I., Pellis, N. R., and Golden, C. A.: Mechanism of tuberculostasis in mammalian serum III. Neutralization of serum tuberculostasis by mycobactin. Infect. Immun. 3:553, 1971.

55. Koike, M., and Takeya, K.: Fine structures of intracytoplasmic organelles of mycobacteria. J. Biophys. Biochem. Cytol. 9:597, 1961.

56. Lamanna, C., and Mallette, M. F.: Basic Bacteriology, Its Biological and Chemical Background. 2nd ed. Baltimore, The Williams & Wilkins Company, 1959.

57. Lenert, T. F., Stasko, I., and Hobby, G. L.: The cultivation of the Bacille-Calmette-Guerin strain of *M. tuberculosis* (BCG). Am. Rev. Tuberc. 78:934, 1958.

58. Long, E. R.: The Chemistry and Chemotherapy of Tuberculosis. 3rd ed. Baltimore, The Williams & Wilkins Company, 1958.

59. Long, E. R., and Vorwald, A. J.: An attempt to influence the growth of the tubercle bacillus in the animal body by modifying the concentration of growth-promoting substance (glycerol) in the tissues. Am. Rev. Tuberc. 22:636, 1930.

60. Merckx, J. J., Brown, A. L., Jr., and Karlson, A. G.: An electron-microscopic study of experimental infections with acid-fast bacilli. Am. Rev. Respir. Dis. 89:485, 1964.

61 Merckx, J. J., Brown, A. L., Jr., and Karlson, A. G.: Morphology of two strains of mycobacteria grown in artificial media as studied with the electron microscope. Acta Tuberc. Scandinav. 45:204, 1964.

62. Millman, I., and Youmans, G. P.: Studies on the metabolism of *Mycobacterium tuberculosis*. VII. Terminal respiratory activity of an avirulent strain of *Mycobacterium tuberculosis*. J. Bacteriol. 68:411, 1954.

63. Neelsen, F.: Ein casuistischer Beitrag zur Lehre von der Tuberkulose. Centralbl. f. d. Med. Wissensch. Berl. 21:497, 1883.

64. Niklowitz, W.: Mitochondrienaquivalente bei Escherichia coli. Zbl. Bakt. I. Abt. Orig. 173:12, 1958.

65. O'Barr, T. P., and Rothlauf, M. V.: Metabolism of D-glucose by *Mycobacterium tuberculosis*. Am. Rev. Respir. Dis. 101:964, 1970.

66. Pokorny, J., and Sulova, J.: Cultivation of mycobacteria *in vivo*. Rozhl. Tuberk. 22:241, 1962.

67. Ramakrishnan, T., Indira, M., and Maller, R. K.: Evaluation of the routes of glucose utilization in virulent and avirulent strains of *Mycobacterium tuberculosis*. Biochim. Biophys. Acta 59:529, 1962.

68. Ramakrishnan, T., Suryanarayana Murthy, P., and Gopinathan, K. P.: Intermediary metabolism of mycobacteria. Bacteriol. Rev. 36:65, 1972.

69. Ratledge, C.: The Mycobacteria. Durham, England, Meadowfield Press Ltd., 1977.
70. Ratledge, C.: The physiology of the mycobacteria. Adv. Microb. Physiol. *13*:115, 1976.
71. Russell, W. F., and Middlebrook, G.: Chemotherapy of Tuberculosis. Springfield, Ill., Charles C Thomas, 1961.
72. Sato, T.: Electron microscopic studies on the intracytoplasmic membranous organelles of mycobacteria. Sci. Rep. Res. Inst. Tohoku Univ. [Med.] *11*:143, 1963.
73. Sattler, T. H., and Youmans, G. P.: The effect of "tween 80," bovine albumin, glycerol, and glucose on the growth of *Mycobacterium tuberculosis* var. *hominis* (H37Rv). J. Bacteriol. *56*:235, 1948.
74. Segal, W., and Bloch, H.: Biochemical differentiation of *Mycobacterium tuberculosis* grown *in vivo* and *in vitro*. J. Bacteriol. *72*:132, 1956.
75. Segal, W., and Bloch, H.: Pathogenic and immunogenic differentiation of *Mycobacterium tuberculosis* grown *in vitro* and *in vivo*. Am. Rev. Tuberc. *75*:495, 1957.
76. Sever, J. L., and Youmans, G. P.: The relation of oxygen tension to virulence of tubercle bacilli and to acquired resistance in tuberculosis. J. Infect. Dis. *101*:193, 1957.
77. Sheehan, H. L., and Whitwell, F.: The staining of tubercle bacilli with sudan black B. J. Pathol. Bacteriol. *61*:269, 1949.
78. Shepard, C. C.: Behavior of the "atypical" mycobacteria in HeLa cells. Am. Rev. Tuberc. *77*:968, 1958.
79. Shepard, C. C.: A comparison of the growth of selected mycobacteria in HeLa, monkey kidney, and human amnion cells in tissue culture. J. Exp. Med. *107*:237, 1958.
80. Shepard, C. C.: Growth characteristics of tubercle bacilli and certain other mycobacteria in HeLa cells. J. Exp. Med. *105*:39, 1957.
81. Shepard, C. C.: Phagocytosis by HeLa cells and their susceptibility to infection by human tubercle bacilli. Proc. Soc. Exp. Biol. Med. *90*:392, 1955.
82. Shinohara, C., Fukushi, K., and Suzuki, J.: Mitochondrialike structures in ultrathin sections of *Mycobacterium avium*. J. Bacteriol. *74*:413, 1957.
83. Shinohara, C., Fukushi, K., Suzuki, J., Sato, K., Suzuki, T., and Motomiya, M.: Fine structure of Mycobacterium. A morphological and enzymatical study of mycobacterial mitochondria. Ann. Report Jap. Soc. Tuberculosis *4*:10, 1959.
84. Stodola, F. H., Lesuk, A., and Anderson, R. J.: The chemistry of the lipids of tubercle bacilli. LIV. The isolation and properties of mycolic acid. J. Biol. Chem. *126*:505, 1938.
85. Takeya, K., and Hisatsune K.: Mycobac-

86. terial cell walls: I. Methods of preparation and treatment with various chemicals. J. Bacteriol. *85*:16, 1963.
86. Takeya, K., Hisatsune, K., and Inoue, Y.: Mycobacterial cell walls: II. Chemical composition of the "basal layer." J. Bacteriol. *85*:24, 1963.
87. Takeya, K., Koike, M., Hisatsune, K., Hagiwara, Y., and Inoue, Y.: Fine structure of mycobacterial cell. *In* Breese, S. S., Jr. (ed.): Electron Microscopy. New York, Academic Press, 1962. RR5.
88. Volk, W. A., and Myrvik, Q. N.: An explanation for the arithmetic linear growth of mycobacteria. J. Bacteriol. *66*:386, 1953.
89. Wayne, L. G.: Synchronized replication of *Mycobacterium tuberculosis*. Infect. Immun. *17*:528, 1977.
90. Williston, E. H., Bingenheimer, J., and Rosenthal, S. R.: Trace elements and BCG cultures. Ann. Inst. Pasteur (Paris) *94*:49, 1958.
91. Williston, E. H., and Youmans, G. P.: Factors affecting the sensitivity *in vitro* of tubercle bacilli to streptomycin. Am. Rev. Tuberc. *59*:336, 1949.
92. Wilson, G. S., and Miles, A.: Topley & Wilson's Principles of Bacteriology, Virology and Immunity. Vol. 1. 6th ed. Baltimore, The Williams & Wilkins Company, 1975.
93. Wong, S., and Weinzirl, J.: An inexpensive synthetic medium for growing *Mycobacterium tuberculosis*. Am. Rev. Tuberc. *33*:577, 1936.
94. Yamaguchi, J., Ariji, F., Fukushi, K., Hasebe, E., and Oka, S.: Electron microscopic observations on the sites of ATPase, acid phosphatase, and succinic dehydrogenase activity in *Mycobacterium tuberculosis*. J. Electron Microsc. (Tokyo) *14*:339, 1965.
95. Youmans, A. S., and Youmans, G. P.: The development *in vitro* of an avirulent, immunogenic variant of *Mycobacterium tuberculosis* var. *hominis*. Proc. Soc. Exp. Biol. Med. *92*:566, 1956.
96. Youmans, A. S., and Youmans, G. P.: The effect of bovine plasma fractions on the growth of *Mycobacterium tuberculosis* var. *hominis*. J. Bacteriol. *60*:561, 1950.
97. Youmans, A. S., and Youmans, G. P.: The effect of metabolic inhibitors and hydroxylamine on the immune response in mice to mycobacterial ribonucleic acid vaccines. J. Immunol. *112*:271, 1974.
98. Youmans A. S., and Youmans, G. P.: Effect of trypsin and ribonuclease on the immunogenic activity of ribosomes and ribonucleic acid isolated from *Mycobacterium tuberculosis*. J. Bacteriol. *91*:2146, 1966.
99. Youmans, A. S., and Youmans, G. P.: The effect of "Tween 80" *in vitro* on the bac-

teriostatic activity of twenty compounds for *Mycobacterium tuberculosis*. J. Bacteriol. *56*:245, 1948.

100. Youmans, A. S., and Youmans, G. P.: Preparation of highly immunogenic ribosomal fractions of *Mycobacterium tuberculosis* by use of sodium dodecyl sulfate. J. Bacteriol. *91*:2139, 1966.

101. Youmans, A. S., and Youmans, G. P.: Ribonucleic acid, deoxyribonucleic acid, and protein content of cells of different ages of *Mycobacterium tuberculosis* and the relationship to immunogenicity. J. Bacteriol. *95*:272, 1968.

102. Youmans, A. S., and Youmans, G. P.: Studies on the metabolism of *Mycobacterium tuberculosis*. II. The effect of compounds related to the Krebs' tricarboxylic acid cycle on the growth of *Mycobacterium tuberculosis* var. *hominis*. J. Bacteriol. *65*:96, 1953.

103. Youmans, A. S., and Youmans, G. P.: Studies on the metabolism of *Mycobacterium tuberculosis*. III. The growth of *Mycobacterium tuberculosis* var. *hominis* in the presence of various intermediates of the dissimilation of glucose to pyruvic acid. J. Bacteriol. *65*:100, 1953.

104. Youmans, A. S., and Youmans, G. P.: Studies on the metabolism of *Mycobacterium tuberculosis*. IV. The effect of fatty acids on the growth of *M. tuberculosis* var. *hominis*. J. Bacteriol. *67*:731, 1954.

105. Youmans, A. S., and Youmans, G. P.: Stud-
ies on the metabolism of *Mycobacterium tuberculosis*. V. The effect of amino acids on the growth of *M. tuberculosis* var. *hominis*. J. Bacteriol. *67*:734, 1954.

106. Youmans, G. P.: An improved method for testing of bacteriostatic agents using virulent human type tubercle bacilli. Proc. Soc. Exp. Biol. Med. *57*:119, 1944.

107. Youmans, G. P.: Subsurface growth of virulent human tubercle bacilli in a synthetic medium. Proc. Soc. Exp. Biol. Med. *57*:122, 1944.

108. Youmans, G. P., and Youmans, A. S.: The growth of recently isolated strains of *Mycobacterium tuberculosis* var. *hominis* in liquid media. J. Bacteriol. *60*:569, 1950.

109. Youmans, G. P., and Youmans, A. S.: A method for the determination of the rate of growth of tubercle bacilli by the use of small inocula. J. Bacteriol. *58*:247, 1949.

110. Youmans, G. P., and Youmans, A. S.: Studies on the metabolism of *Mycobacterium tuberculosis*. I. The effect of carbohydrates and alcohols on the growth of *Mycobacterium tuberculosis* var. *hominis*. J. Bacteriol. *65*:92, 1953.

111. Zapf, K.: Vergleichende Untersuchungen zur Morphologie und Zytologie des Mycobakterium tuberculosis (BCG). II. Licht- und elecktronenmikroskopische Befunde zum Kernproblem. Zbl. Bakt. I. Abt. Orig. *174*:253, 1959.

112. Ziehl, F.: Die Farbung des Tuberkelbacillus. Deutsche Med. Wochenschr. *8*:451, 1882.

3

Biologic Activities of Mycobacterial Cells and Cell Components

INTRODUCTION

Mycobacteria are of particular interest because of the wide range of biologic effects produced by the cell and some of its components. The mycobacterial cell is extremely rich in lipids, and many of its biologic activities can be related to one or more of the lipid substances. For a complete discussion of the nature of mycobacterial lipids and their biologic effects, Chapter 4 should be consulted.

Early workers in the field of tuberculosis were primarily concerned with the effect of the tubercle bacillus and its constituents on the cellular response. The tubercle is the typical initial lesion in tuberculosis. The occur-

rence in the tubercle of abnormal cell types, including epithelioid and giant cells, is not pathognomonic for tuberculosis because such cells are also found in lesions produced by other microorganisms or by foreign bodies. These cellular changes, which were reported in the earlier literature, have been reviewed by Rich,[64] so there is no need to consider them in detail here except to say that there is some evidence that phosphatides found in mycobacterial cells may be responsible for the formation of epithelioid cells.[64, 65]

Of much greater importance today are the several biologic effects produced by certain mycobacterial constituents. Recent research has shown that some of these mycobacterial constituents have a

46

profound effect on the reticuloendo-thelial system, on the lymphocytic system, and on neoplastic cells. Some of these constituents will be described in this chapter.

THE TUBERCLE

The primary lesion in tuberculosis is the tubercle, or nodule. Even though it is not characteristic of this disease alone, all people interested in tuberculosis or working in the field should have a knowledge of the morphology and genesis of the tubercle because whenever the morphologic features typical of a tubercle are encountered in tissues, mycobacteria must be suspected as the possible cause. We can do no better for this purpose than to quote the description of the genesis of the tubercle bacilli given by Arnold Rich[64] in 1951 and entitled *The Manner of Formation of the Tubercle.*

All types of tubercle bacilli, whether virulent or avirulent, and, indeed, even certain nonpathogenic acid-fast bacilli such as the grass bacillus, will cause the formation of a fundamentally identical type of nodular tubercle. Tubercles may be formed intravascularly or extravascularly. Within the liver lobule, for example, they always arise within the sinusoids. Indeed, the hepatic sinusoids offer one of the most favorable sites for the study of the manner of development of the tubercle. For this purpose one may inject a thin suspension of tubercle bacilli intravenously in a group of animals, kill animals of the group at frequent intervals between five minutes and several weeks, and stain sections of the livers with acid-fast stains to reveal the tubercle bacilli. The study of the development of the lesions shows plainly that the mononuclear phagocytes of the hepatic sinusoids begin to ingest the bacilli within a few minutes. A phagocyte that has ingested a bacillus soon undergoes the transformation into an epithelioid cell. It may then become a multinuclear giant cell, so that single Langhans giant cells, unaccompan-ied by any other cells may be found in the sinusoids after a day or two. Within several days other mononuclear cells will have clustered about the original one that had ingested a bacillus, and these, too, become epithelioid cells. That the epithelioid cells which make up the tubercle are altered mononuclear phagocytes was clearly recognized by Metchnikoff half a century ago, and has been amply confirmed by subsequent investigators. . . . The small epithelioid cell nodule enlarges progressively. Some of the new cells are blood monocytes which stop at the site and adhere to the little group of cells, but it seems evident that multiplication of the phagocytes *in situ* also occurs, for the tubercle continues to enlarge in a globular shape even after the sinusoid in which it arises has been completely filled up by the nodular mass so that no further access of blood-borne cells is possible. Other giant cells may or may not form from epithelioid cells in the mass. The adjacent liver cells are pushed aside by the growing nodule; their nutrition is interfered with, and they become thin and atrophic, and eventually die and disappear as the tubercle expands. When a strand of liver cells at the periphery of an expanding tubercle disappears in this manner, new cells can be added to the tubercle from the blood stream in the sinusoid that was on the opposite side of the liver cell strand, and which becomes adjacent to the tubercle when the intervening liver cells disappear.

When a tubercle has become well formed a network of argyrophile reticulum fibrils [Fig. 3–1], demonstrable by silver stains, appears between the epithelioid cells, and a gradual transition of the reticulum into collagen fibers can be observed. . . . Lymphocytes can often be found among the epithelioid cells in well formed tubercles, but they are scanty unless the tubercle has remained in a stationary state for some time. In these older, arrested tubercles lymphocytes are more numerous, particularly at the periphery, though not infrequently they wander into the central portions. If the multiplication of the bacilli is held in check no appreciable necrosis will occur in the tubercle. If multiplication proceeds, the central portion, where the bacilli are present in greatest numbers, will become necrotic. When

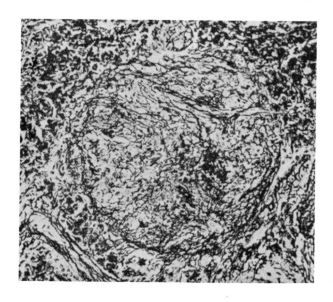

FIGURE 3–1. Reticulum framework of epithelioid cell tubercle in spleen (cells unstained). (From Rich, A. R.: The Pathogenesis of Tuberculosis. 2nd ed. Springfield, Ill., Charles C Thomas, 1951.)

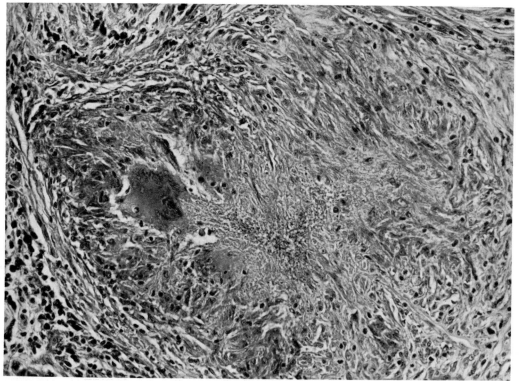

FIGURE 3–2. A typical tubercle with giant cell and central caseous necrosis. (From Robbins, S. L.: Pathologic Basis of Disease. 2nd ed. Philadelphia, W. B. Saunders Co., 1974.)

bacilli are numerous and necrosis occurs, polymorphonuclear leucocytes, sometimes in large numbers, may wander into the tubercle.

When tubercles are formed extravascularly, the constituent cells are ordinarily derived partly from the mononuclear phagocytes that are normally present in practically all tissues, and partly from those that migrate from the circulating blood (monocytes). The series of events in the development of the extravascular tubercle itself is, however, essentially the same as that described above in the case of the intravascular tubercle.

Figure 3–2 shows some of the morphologic features of a typical tubercle. It should be pointed out that while epithelioid and giant cell formations are seen in human beings and guinea pigs, they are not found in the tubercles of animals like the mouse or the rat. The pathology of tuberculosis in the mouse has been described in detail by Raleigh and Youmans,[63] by Mayer and coworkers,[49] and by Nyka.[58] In this animal, there is an accumulation of macrophages derived from circulating monocytes, which form the tubercles. The formation of epithelioid cells and giant cells is rare, if it occurs at all.

The tubercle is, of course, a granuloma because of the predominance of macrophages. It is now more common to refer to the cellular response, particularly in experimental tuberculosis, as granulomatous. This is especially appropriate when describing the response to mycobacterial cells or components in the mouse and the rat.

THE GRANULOMATOUS RESPONSE

As we have already noted, one of the outstanding features of the host-parasite relationship in tuberculosis is the granulomatous response — that is, the accumulation of macrophages at the site of infection.

Although virulent tubercle bacilli can multiply within the cytoplasm of macrophages, the granulomatous response has generally been regarded as a defensive reaction on the part of the host. Undoubtedly, limitation of spread and, in some cases, eventual resolution of the infection can be brought about simply as a consequence of the accumulation of large numbers of macrophages at the point of infection.

Recently developed techniques have permitted the induction of the granulomatous response in rabbits and mice under conditions that allow the degree of the response to be measured with some accuracy. This, in turn, has permitted the correlation of the relationship of the magnitude of the granulomatous response with the amount of resistance to infection. Myrvik and associates[32, 41-45, 54, 55] have shown that an intense granulomatous response can be induced in the lungs of rabbits by the intravenous injection of small numbers of killed BCG cells into rabbits that had been given a subcutaneous priming injection of BCG cells several weeks previously. The pulmonary granulomatous reaction is so great that the lungs can increase in weight severalfold within three or four days. Large numbers of alveolar macrophages for study can be washed easily from these granulomatous lungs by way of the trachea. If the killed mycobacterial cells are incorporated in Freund's incomplete adjuvant prior to intravenous administration, the preliminary priming subcutaneous injection of BCG cells is not needed.

Youmans and Youmans[78] obtained similar results using mice. When the animals were injected intravenously with large numbers of either living or heat-killed H37Ra mycobacterial cells, an intense pulmonary granulomatous response occurred in which the size and weight of the lungs would increase two- to threefold. As in the rabbit, the granulomatous response was slightly accelerated when the mice had

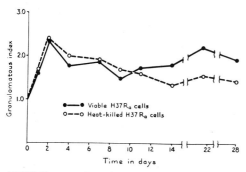

FIGURE 3–3. Granulomatous response in lungs of normal mice following intravenous injection of 5 mg H37Ra cells. (From Youmans, G. P., and Youmans, A. S.: An acute pulmonary granulomatous response in mice produced by mycobacterial cells and its relation to increased resistance and increased susceptibility to experimental tuberculous infection. J. Infect. Dis. *114*:135, 1964.)

been injected intraperitoneally or subcutaneously with H37Ra cells two or three weeks prior to the intravenous injection of mycobacterial cells. The pulmonary granulomatous response reached its height within two days and declined somewhat thereafter; however, it persisted for at least 28 days (Fig. 3–3).

The magnitude of the pulmonary response is directly proportional to the number of mycobacterial cells injected intravenously; heat-killed or living cells are equally effective for the induction. No grossly measurable, similar pulmonary response follows the intraperitoneal injection of large numbers of mycobacterial cells or the intravenous injection of *E. coli* endotoxin or of an emulsion of mineral oil (see, however, Chapter 4).

Youmans and Youmans in 1964[78] carried out extensive experiments in which the pulmonary granulomatous response was induced in mice by the procedure described previously. The mice then were infected with virulent tubercle bacilli, either intravenously or intranasally. These results can be briefly summarized as follows. Three and five days after receiving the injec-

tion to induce the intravenous granulomatous response, mice infected intravenously with virulent tubercle bacilli showed appreciably increased resistance. This was more marked in animals that had been given the initial intravenous injection of viable H37Ra cells than in those in which the pulmonary granulomatous response had been induced with heat-killed cells. When challenged by intranasal instillation of virulent mycobacteria, the granulomatous lungs withstood infection with several thousand times the infecting dose that would produce lesions in nongranulomatous mouse lungs. On the other hand, mice vaccinated intraperitoneally with the same numbers of H37Ra cells were just as susceptible as nonvaccinated animals to challenge by the intranasal route but were highly immune when challenged by the intravenous route.[83] Similar findings had been previously made by others.[40, 71]

The degree of increased resistance to infection with virulent tubercle bacilli was directly proportional to the magnitude of the pulmonary granulomatous response. This observation, coupled with the fact that the increased resistance appears concomitantly with the appearance of the granulomatous response, indicates that no immunologic mechanism is involved in the greater resistance to infection. Apparently, the sole factor that determines the degree of increased resistance to infection is the number of macrophages that accumulate. It must be emphasized that we are referring here only to the situation that exists in the first few days following induction of the granulomatous response. Later, immunologic forces will come into play and contribute to the immune response.

It would also be expected that the increased resistance due to the accumulation of macrophages would be nonspecific, that is, would be effective in combating infection due to other species of microorganisms, and this is apparently the case (see Chapter 13).

It should be kept in mind that we have been speaking primarily of the pulmonary granulomatous response because the lung is the organ in which the response can be most easily detected and measured. When mycobacteria are injected intravenously, a granulomatous response will also occur in other organs and tissues.

The kinetics of the pulmonary granulomatous response are of considerable interest. Figure 3–3 shows the development of a pulmonary granulomatous response in the lungs of mice after the intravenous injection with 5.0 mg moist weight of either living or heat-killed tubercle bacilli. At daily intervals thereafter, five mice were killed. Their lungs were removed and blotted free of blood; then each lung was weighed separately. The average weight of the lungs at each time was then calculated, providing the data used in Figure 3–3. Sections prepared and stained by hematoxylin-eosin from the same specimens confirmed that the increased weight of the lungs was due to the accumulation of enormous numbers of macrophages.

Figure 3–3 shows that the granulomatous response developed very rapidly and reached a height on the second day. The magnitude of the response at this time was similar whether living or heat-killed cells had been injected. Following this time, there was a decline in the lung weights, showing that the abnormal accumulation of macrophages was being resolved. This decline continued until about ten days after injection when the weight of the lungs obtained from the animals injected with the viable cells again increased. However, in those animals given the killed cells, the decline in lung weights continued over the length of the experiment.

We can assume that the secondary granulomatous response noted in those animals given the live mycobacterial cells was immunologic in nature (allergic?), since the beginning of the response corresponded roughly with the time an immune response might be expected to occur. Also, no marked immune response would be expected in animals given the heat-killed mycobacterial cells, because such cells are notoriously poor inducers of either delayed hypersensitivity or immunity to infection.

That the secondary granulomatous response was mediated by immunologic mechanisms was clearly demonstrated in other experiments in which mice injected intravenously with viable mycobacterial cells were treated with rifampin. Rifampin is a potent immunosuppressive drug; with the dosage used, the secondary granulomatous response, if it were truly immunologic, should be suppressed in the animals being treated. Reference to Figure 3–4 will show that animals in which the pulmonary granulomatous response had been induced by live cells, then treated with rifampin, showed no signs of a secondary granulomatous response. These animals, however, did show the initial granulomatous response, which reached a height on the second day.

Therefore, it would appear that the initial, or early, granulomatous response is merely the equivalent of a response to a foreign body. However, sensitization to an antigen, which results in the induction of delayed hypersensitivity, and subsequent exposure to this antigen will accelerate the accumulation of macrophages. This is known to occur readily in animals after injection with viable mycobacterial cells.

Accelerated pulmonary granulomatous response has also been noted in rabbits. Kawata and colleagues[37] initially felt that this phenomenon in rabbits was not due to delayed hypersensitivity, because no dermal tuberculin hypersensitivity could be detected in some of the animals in which it occurred. Subsequently, though, Galindo and Myrvik[29] found that lym-

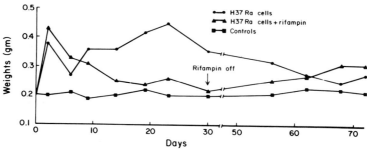

FIGURE 3–4. Effect of rifampin on the pulmonary granulomatous response. (From Youmans, A. S., Youmans, G. P., and Cahall, D.: Effect of rifampin on immunity to tuberculosis and on delayed hypersensitivity to purified protein derivative. Infect. Immun. *13*:127, 1976.)

phocytes taken from granulomatous lungs of animals showing no dermal tuberculin hypersensitivity would nevertheless inhibit macrophage migration when exposed to purified protein derivative (PPD). It is now known that lack of dermal hypersensitivity does not necessarily mean complete absence of lymphocytes that mediate delayed hypersensitivity. This will be further discussed in Chapter 7.

MACROPHAGE ACTIVATION

In the preceding discussion on the granulomatous response, we have been concerned in part with the influence of the number of macrophages on the resistance of the host to tuberculous infection. It is evident from the work of numerous investigators that macrophages exposed in vivo to killed or living, whole tubercle bacilli or to certain fractions of this microorganism also become altered qualitatively. Dannenberg[19] and Dannenberg and coworkers[20] have reviewed this extensive literature in detail. Macrophage activation includes increased irritability, motility, oxygen consumption, glycolysis, lipid turnover, and phagocytosis. Dannenberg refers to this early phase as "excitation."

Soon, longer lasting changes occur,

such as a marked increase in the number of mitochondria, lysosomes, and enzymes contained within lysosomes. Thus, the macrophage becomes rapidly poised to cope more efficiently with phagocytosed particles, such as bacterial cells. Although the activated state is reversed fairly rapidly, macrophages, if activated by contact with tubercle bacilli in vivo, will respond in a similar fashion upon second exposure, but more rapidly. This phenomenon may play a role in the accelerated granulomatous response (accelerated tubercle formation) mentioned previously.

Considering the review by Dannenberg[19] it is not necessary here to describe in detail the changes that have been noted in activated macrophages. The most important feature, from the standpoint of our discussion, is that such activated macrophages apparently have a greater capacity to destroy mycobacteria and other microorganisms (see Chapter 13).

Apparently, a number of substances from mycobacteria will activate macrophages but seem to have little capacity to induce macrophage accumulation and proliferation. These include lipopolysaccharides, wax D, cell wall hulls, and possibly other components. The evidence for this includes the fact that such substances induce a low-grade, nonspecific increase in resistance that is most likely caused by macrophage activation. On the other hand, if mycobacterial cells are injected by a route that permits some localization (i.e., subcutaneous or intraperitoneal), the increase in resistance due to the accumulation of macrophages would be more pronounced at the focus of infection. This accounts for the local nature of the increased resistance to tuberculous infection stressed by Dannenberg and fellow researchers.[21] Also, this probably accounts for the observations[40] just referred to that mice vaccinated intraperitoneally with mycobacterial cells exhibit no immunity when challenged by the pulmonary route. Apparently, insufficient vaccine reaches the lung to stimulate a significant granulomatous reaction. Furthermore, the very small numbers of virulent tubercle bacilli administered intranasally or by aerosol are probably not enough to stimulate the accelerated granulomatous response (accelerated tubercle formation) noted in animals having had previous experience with mycobacteria.

It should be emphasized that lipopolysaccharides from other microorganisms also have the capacity to activate macrophages and, in this manner, may induce increased resistance to both homologous and heterologous infection. In fact, the amount of resistance against tuberculous infection induced by the nondescript substances from tubercle bacilli is about the same as that produced by *E. coli* endotoxin.[81] Thus, macrophage activation cannot account for the high level of immune response noted following vaccination of animals with viable mycobacterial cells, with mycobacterial ribosomal fraction, or with RNA (see Chapters 8, 9, and 10).

CORD FACTOR: TREHALOSE 6,6'-DIMYCOLATE

Cord factor is a surface constituent of many mycobacterial strains and has been alleged or inferred to be responsible for the sticking together, in parallel fashion, of virulent cells during growth to produce the typical serpentine cords (see Chapter 4). It is toxic when repeatedly administered to mice; at one time, it was thought to play a role in virulence of mycobacteria.[9, 10, 57] However, it is also found in attenuated strains (such as BCG) and even in saprophytes (such as *M. phlei.*).

A number of investigators have attempted without success to induce increased resistance to tuberculous infection by injection of cord factor subcutaneously or intraperitoneally into mice and guinea pigs.[18, 60, 70] However, Bekierkunst recently has shown that purified cord factor dissolved in mineral oil and injected intravenously into mice in the form of 10 percent oil-in-water emulsion brought about a rapid and pronounced pulmonary granulomatous response.[6-8] The pulmonary granulomatous response was proportional to the amount of cord factor injected. The importance of the oil in the reaction was shown by the fact that when equal amounts of cord factor were administered in the form of a 1.0 percent oil-in-water emulsion, no granulomatous response could be detected.

These findings indicate that cord factor is one of the agents in mycobacterial cells responsible for the pulmonary granulomatous response. The necessity for mineral oil for the production of the granulomatous response by cord factor parallels the requirement for oil noted when mycobacterial cell walls are used to produce the granulomatous response.[5] It might also explain why the investigators previously mentioned[40, 71] were unable to produce any increased resistance to tuberculous infection by the injection of cord factor alone into experimental animals. The major role of the oil could well be to provide a mechanism whereby significant amounts of cell wall material or cord factor would be deposited in the lungs and retained for a long enough period to stimulate both macrophage accumulation and activation. In addition to the production of a pulmonary granulomatous response, the intravenous injection of mycobacterial cells or mycobacterial cell walls in mineral oil would, of course, provide a general stimulation of reticuloendothelial system and, therefore, induce a general increase in resistance. Cord factor is further discussed in Chapter 4.

ADJUVANT ACTIVITY

Dienes and Schoenheit[22] first demonstrated in 1927 that mycobacterial cells are potent immunologic adjuvants. The later work of Freund and his collaborators led to the development of water and oil emulsions containing mycobacterial cells and having a profound enhancing action on immunologic responses.[27] Today these adjuvants are known as *Freund's complete adjuvant* (FCA), when the water-in-oil emulsions contain mycobacterial cells, and *Freund's incomplete adjuvant* (FIA), when the myocbacterial cells are omitted. Freund's complete adjuvant not only will enhance antibody formation but also will so direct the immune response to protein antigens that delayed hypersensitivity will develop. Mycobacteria in the form of Freund's complete adjuvant also are necessary for the induction of experimental allergic encephalomyelitis and can be used to induce other forms of autoimmunity.[28]

Raffel in 1952[61, 62] was the first to demonstrate that the adjuvant activity of mycobacterial cells could be duplicated by using wax D (see Chapters 4 and 13) extracted from tubercle bacilli instead of using intact cells. This finding was confirmed by White and his associates.[75, 76] Since that time a major amount of effort has been expended in attempts to characterize the component of wax D that is responsible for adjuvant activity. In addition to wax D, Bekierkunst has reported that cord fac-

tor extracted from mycobacterial cells has adjuvant activity.[6-8] More recently, water-soluble extracts of mycobacterial cells have been found to have adjuvant activity.*

The smallest water-soluble molecules isolated from mycobacterial cells that have adjuvant activity are N-glycolyl-muramyl-dipeptides.[25] Synthetic N-glycolyl-muramyl-dipeptide also has adjuvant activity.[25]

Detailed consideration of the major mycobacterial lipids, their adjuvant activities, the water-soluble adjuvants, and the relationship of adjuvant activity to chemical structure will be found in Chapter 4. Recent reviews on adjuvants and adjuvant activity should be consulted for additional details.[16, 35, 46, 77] We will concentrate here on the adjuvanticity of another nonlipid mycobacterial component.

Youmans and Youmans[80] reported that mycobacterial RNA preparations have adjuvant activity, since they were found to enhance markedly antibody formation to bovine gamma globulin. Also, Gumbiner and his coworkers[30] found that mycobacterial RNA preparations could substitute for whole mycobacterial cells in Freund's complete adjuvant for the induction of experimental allergic encephalomyelitis in guinea pigs. Finally, Casavant and Youmans[14] found that mycobacterial RNA preparations could substitute for the whole mycobacterial cells in Freund's complete adjuvant for the induction of delayed hypersensitivity to tuberculoprotein or ovalbumin. In these studies, as little as 2 μg of RNA per animal induced either experimental allergic encephalomyelitis or delayed hypersensitivity to tuberculin or to ovalbumin.

The mode of action of immunologic adjuvants is not clearly understood. Possible mechanisms include the recruitment of reactive cells, the stimulation of proliferation and differentiation

*See in reference section at end of chapter:[1-4, 12, 15, 25, 33, 35, 39, 46, 50, 51, 53, 56, 59, 77]

of immunocompetent cells, the slowing of the release of antigen from the site of injection, and the entrapment of lymphocytes.[16, 35, 77] Certain adjuvants, such as *Bordetella pertussis,* affect both T- and B-lymphocytes; whereas lipopolysaccharide from *Salmonella typhosa* affects only B-lymphocytes. Therefore, different adjuvants need not act by exactly the same mechanism. The possible role of polyadenylic and polyuridylic acid complexes has been explored by Johnson and his colleagues.[34, 67] These investigators have shown that poly A:U exerts a direct effect on macrophages. It also expands a population of thymic cells capable of reacting with sheep erythrocytes in irradiated mice treated with antithymocyte serum and subsequently reconstituted with T- and B-lymphocytes. Campbell and Kind[13] reported enhanced plaque-forming cell responses to sheep erythrocytes in mice given poly A:U; this suggests that the adjuvant exerted its effect on antibody-producing cells derived from bone marrow. Mycobacterial RNA might act in a similar fashion.

Maillard and Bloom,[48] in an examination of pertussis vaccine and tubercle bacilli as immunologic adjuvants, found that spleen cells from mice primed with adjuvant produced enhanced secondary responses to sheep erythrocytes when specific adjuvant to which the donors had been primed, was added. An enhanced primary response was observed when supernatant fluids from specific adjuvant-primed spleen cells were added to normal spleen cells cultured in vitro with sheep erythrocytes. Mouse anti-isoantiserum completely prevented production of supernatant fluids that enhanced the primary response of normal spleen cells.

It is conceivable that mycobacterial RNA preparations might act by causing the release of a soluble mediator with "blastogenic" properties, which might act to expand the population of lymphoid cells; this would allow antigen to react with more cells, thus potentiating the response. Bloom and Bennett[11] also reported that normal lymphocytes cultured in supernatants rich in macrophage migration inhibitory factor (MIF) underwent blast transformation. Dumonde and coworkers[24] reported similar findings. We have found that the culturing of nonimmunized lymphocytes, in the presence of mycobacterial RNA, as well as intact viable H37Ra cells, produced supernatant fluids that inhibited migration of normal peritoneal exudate cells.[14]

The adjuvanticity of the mycobacterial RNA preparations also raises the question of the role these materials might play in the adjuvant activity of intact mycobacterial cells. As has already been mentioned (and reviewed more completely in Chapter 4), the lipid fractions have always been considered the principal adjuvant materials. In view, however, of the discovery of the water-soluble adjuvants and the results we have obtained showing adjuvanticity of mycobacterial RNA preparations, the possibility must be entertained that mycobacterial RNA as well as other nonlipid mycobacterial components may play a significant role in the adjuvanticity of intact mycobacterial cells.

INDUCTION OF NONSPECIFIC RESISTANCE TO INFECTION

It has been known for some years that the injection of mycobacterial cells and certain mycobacterial extracts into experimental animals will increase resistance to a wide variety of other microorganisms. The earlier literature on this has been beautifully reviewed by Crowle[17] and, later, by Kanai.[36] This interesting and important phenomenon will not be discussed at length in this chapter but will be examined in detail in the chapters dealing with the nature and development of immunity to tuberculosis. The subject is being approached in this manner because of a prevailing school of thought that considers immunity in tuberculosis to be nonspecific.[38, 47, 52] There is another school that feels that there are a number of mechanisms of increased resistance to tuberculous infection, including one that is highly specific.[26, 81, 82] Thus, the phenomenon of the induction of nonspecific immunity to infection by tubercle bacilli becomes an integral part of any discussion of the nature of the immune response to mycobacterial disease. We can state here, however, that the mechanisms involved in nonspecific immunity to infection, in our opinion, are primarily those we have just discussed, that is, macrophage activation, accumulation, and proliferation—the granulomatous response (see also Chapter 4).

EFFECT ON TUMOR GROWTH

A large volume of literature has accumulated on the effects of mycobacteria and, in particular, of viable BCG cells on the growth of tumors in experimental animals and in human beings. It is clear that under appropriate conditions, BCG cells will exert a profound suppressive and, in some cases, regressive effect on tumor growth. This is covered in detail in Chapters 4 and 9. It is sufficient to point out here that mycobacterial cells act in this manner probably because of their capacity to activate macrophages and bring about a granulomatous response and because of their adjuvanticity—in other words, because of their stimulation of the reticuloendothelial system.

ENHANCEMENT OF INFECTION

One of the most intriguing properties of mycobacterial cells and of certain mycobacterial products is that under the appropriate conditions, they can enhance infection not only by mycobacteria but also by microorganisms such as staphylococci. This phenomenon was first described by Schaedler and Dubos.[23, 66] These investigators mixed mycobacterial BCG cells with staphylococci and injected this combination intravenously into mice. They found that the staphylococcal infection was greater in the BCG-injected mice than in the animals that received no BCG cells. Furthermore, this enhancement of staphylococcal infection was manifested whether the subcutaneous or intravenous route of injection was used. Killed BCG cells also were effective in enhancing the staphylococcal disease. Similar enhancement of *M. fortuitum* infection was found when *M. fortuitum* cells were injected, one, three, and six hours after a preliminary injection of fairly large numbers of BCG cells. Of particular interest is the fact that in mice, in which a chronic infection has been established with small numbers of *Staphylococcus aureus*, *Mycobacterium tuberculosis*, or *M. fortuitum*, these infections could be reactivated three months later by the intravenous administration of killed mycobacterial cells. Similar results were obtained when *Haemophilus pertussis* vaccine was used instead of the mycobacterial cells to reactivate the infection.

This phenomenon was further investigated by Youmans and Youmans[79] in 1964. As described in the earlier section of this chapter on the granulomatous response, these investigators had noted that if large numbers of living or killed mycobacterial cells of the H37Ra strain were injected intravenously into mice, a pronounced pulmonary granulomatous response was obtained in which the degree of the granulomatous response was directly proportional to the number of microorganisms injected intravenously. In an attempt to determine the relation of this granulomatous response to susceptibility to infection, virulent mycobacteria of the H37Rv strain were administered to mice at daily intervals, beginning one day after the granuloma-tous response had been induced. They noted that injections given on the first day caused an acute rapid onset of convulsions, which rapidly led to death. These fatal reactions occurred in mice injected one or two days after the H37Ra cells. Following this time, the mice not only survived the injection of virulent tubercle bacilli (although many showed some signs of illness) but also lived much longer than animals that had not been given the injection of H37Ra cells. In other words, these mice had become more resistant to subsequent challenge with virulent tubercle bacilli. Even if the granulomatous response-inducing injections of both mycobacterial cells and the challenge with virulent tubercle bacilli were separated by only 30 seconds, the acute, shock-like fatal reactions still occurred.

In an attempt to circumvent these shocklike reactions, Youmans and Youmans[79] mixed the challenge dose of the virulent H37Rv cells with the granulomatous response-inducing dose of the H37Ra cells and injected this mixture intravenously into mice that had received no other treatment. These mice handled the injection well, since they showed no immediate or delayed reaction. However, when the survival time in these animals was compared with animals that had only received the virulent H37Rv cells, it was clear that they died much sooner. The disease had progressed much more rapidly in the animals that had also received the attenuated H37Ra cells. Heat-killed H37Ra cells acted in a similar fashion. Table 3–1 shows the results of a typical experiment. In these studies, the duration of the tuberculous infection was rather short. In order to determine whether the infection-enhancing effect would persist over a longer period of time, similar experiments were conducted in which a very small infecting dose of tubercle bacilli of the H37Rv strain was mixed with the attenuated mycobacterial cells and injected (see Table 3–1). Even though approximately

50 percent of the animals that received only the virulent cells survived longer than 50 days, the animals that received the attenuated mycobacterial cells died much sooner. Therefore, the infection-enhancing effect persisted over a period of at least seven weeks.

Attempts were made to determine what component of the mycobacterial cell might be responsible for this infection-enhancing action. Mycobacterial cells were broken mechanically,[82] and certain components separated by ultracentrifugation. The fractions obtained consisted of mycobacterial cell walls, a mycobacterial ribosomal preparation, and several cytoplasmic membrane fractions. Each of these fractions was then mixed with a standard infecting dose of the virulent H37Rv strain and injected intravenously into mice. The only component that duplicated the infection-enhancing effect of the intact mycobacterial cells was the cytoplasmic membrane preparation. To date, attempts to further localize the infection-enhancing action to some subcomponent of the membrane fraction have not been successful.[79]

These puzzling and contradictory results are difficult to explain. When attenuated mycobacterial cells are injected intravenously into mice and a pulmonary granulomatous response is induced, these mice are more resistant to infection if they are challenged with virulent tubercle bacilli three or more days after the injection of attenuated cells. On the other hand, if the virulent cells are given shortly after the administration of the attenuated cells, severe and usually fatal reactions are obtained. Furthermore, if virulent mycobacterial cells are mixed with the attenuated cells and given intravenously, no immediate reaction occurs, but the virulent cells apparently multiply much more rapidly and will produce death earlier than the same cells injected alone. The granulomatous response is the same in both cases, and theoretically, one would expect these activated macrophages to be able to cope

TABLE 3–1. **Response to Infection with Tubercle Bacilli of CF-1 Mice Injected Intravenously with Mixtures of Virulent and Attenuated Mycobacteria**

Mycobacterial Cells in Mixtures	Amount Injected, mg*	Number of Mice	S-30 Mice**		Median Survival Time (95% confidence limits)
			NUMBER	PERCENT	
H37Ra, living and H37Rv, living	4.0 1.0	25	0	0	9.2 (8.9 to 9.5)
H37Ra, living and H37Rv, living	2.0 1.0	24	0	0	12.5 (11.6 to 13.5)
H37Ra, living and H37Rv, living	1.0 1.0	21	0	0	15.5 (14.7 to 16.4)
H37Ra, heat-killed and H37Rv, living	4.0 1.0	25	0	0	10.2 (9.5 to 10.9)
BCG, heat-killed and H37Rv, living	4.0 1.0	23	0	0	11.8 (11.3 to 12.1)
H37Ra, living and H37Rv, living	4.0 0.1	28	3	10.7†	
H37Rv, living	1.0		0	0	15.2 (14.7 to 15.7)
H37Rv, living	0.1	30	15	50.0†	

From Youmans, G. P., and Youmans, A. S.: An acute pulmonary granulomatous response in mice produced by mycobacterial cells and its relation to increased resistance and increased susceptibility to experimental tuberculous infection. J. Infect. Dis. *114*:135, 1964.
   *Wet weight.
  **Mice that survived longer than 30 days.
   †Percent of mice that survived longer than 50 days.

more effectively with the virulent organisms. However, this is not the case, since the protective effect is reversed when the organisms are present from the time of induction of the granulomatous response. Why should this be?

The possibility that the virulent bacilli, in some manner, so affected the attenuated H37Ra cells that they, in turn, began to multiply and produce an overwhelmingly mixed infection would seem to be ruled out by the fact that heat-killed attenuated cells also enhanced the infection.

The more rapid mycobacterial multiplication of virulent bacilli following the simultaneous injection of virulent and attenuated mycobacteria suggests that the macrophage milieu may be more suitable for multiplication of virulent tubercle bacilli when they are injected along with the attenuated cells. Therefore, for some unknown reason, the macrophages produced under these conditions may be and may remain more susceptible. On the other hand, the increased susceptibility of the mice is dependent upon the number of attenuated mycobacterial cells present in the mixture. This suggests that attenuated mycobacterial cells that are being broken down by the macrophages within which they reside may be releasing metabolites that may provide a stimulus for the growth of the virulent cells. Attenuated H37Ra cells are readily destroyed in the mouse, while virulent cells are not.[68, 69] Why a comparable situation does not exist in mice challenged with virulent cells three days following the injection of attenuated cells is not readily apparent.

The possibility should not be ignored that an endotoxin of some kind plays a significant role in the production of one or more, or all, of the phenomena described.[74] Lipopolysaccharides (endotoxins) found in many gram-negative bacteria are known to produce shock in susceptible animals and to first decrease, then increase nonspecific resistance to infection.[74]

Neither virulent nor attenuated mycobacteria have been regarded as producers of endotoxin. However, it is known that endotoxins will increase somewhat the resistance of mice to infection with virulent tubercle bacilli[23] and that infection with attenuated mycobacteria (BCG) will markedly increase the susceptibility of mice to the lethal effect of endotoxin.[31, 73] Also, Stetson and colleagues[72] have reported that old tuberculin shows some endotoxic activity.

The following observations, based on the experiments of Youmans and Youmans, seem to contradict the theory that a classic type of endotoxin is the sole cause of the phenomena described previously. The shock-like reactions of the mice, as noted in their investigation, could be elicited only in those animals that had recently received a preliminary injection of mycobacterial cells. A single intravenous injection containing large amounts (3 to 5 mg) of living, attenuated mycobacterial cells had no effect. The convulsive reactions occurred within seconds after the second injection. The classical picture of delayed endotoxic shock was absent. An appreciable delay between the first and second injection was not necessary, since a second injection, given within 30 seconds of the first, elicited fatal reactions. The capacity of attenuated mycobacterial cells to sensitize and to elicit shock was reduced when the microorganisms were killed by heat. The heat lability of the responsible agent, or agents, in attenuated cells also argues against a classic type of endotoxin being the only factor in the increase in susceptibility to virulent tubercle bacilli noted under the conditions of these experiments.

The possibility that a Shwarzman-type reactivity might be involved in the production of the acute convulsive reactions would appear unlikely since no latent period is required for induction of the increased sensitivity to mycobacterial cells. Secondly, the onset of these reactions is not delayed; instead, it occurs immediately and death follows within a few seconds.

REFERENCES

1. Adam, A., Amar, C., Ciorbaru, R., Lederer, E., Petit, J. F., and Vilkas, E.: Activité adjuvant des peptidoglycanes de mycobactéries. C. R. Acad. Sci. [D] (Paris) 278:799, 1974.
2. Adam, A., Ciorbaru, R., Ellouz, F., Petit, J. F., and Lederer, E.: Adjuvant activity of monomeric bacterial cell wall peptidoglycans. Biochem. Biophys. Res. Commun. 56:561, 1974.
3. Adam, A., Ciorbaru, R., Petit, J. F., and Lederer, E.: Isolation and properties of a macromolecular, water-soluble, immunoadjuvant fraction from the cell wall of *Mycobacterium smegmatis*. Proc. Natl. Acad. Sci. U.S.A. 69:851, 1972.
4. Adam, A., Ciorbaru, R., Petit, J. F., Lederer, E., Chedid, L., Lamensans, A., Parant, F., Parant, M., Rosselet, J. P., and Berger, F. M.: Preparation and biological properties of water-soluble adjuvant fractions from delipidated cells of *Mycobacterium smegmatis* and *Nocardia opaca*. Infect. Immun. 7:855, 1973.
5. Barclay, W. R., Anacker, R., Brehmer, W., and Ribi, E.: Effects of oil-treated mycobacterial cell walls on the organs of mice. J. Bacteriol. 94:1736, 1967.
6. Bekierkunst, A.: Acute granulomatous response produced in mice by trehalose-6, 6'-dimycolate. J. Bacteriol. 96:958, 1968.
7. Bekierkunst, A., Levij, I. S., Yarkoni, E., Vilkas, E., Adam, A., and Lederer, E.: Granuloma formation induced in mice by chemically defined mycobacterial fractions. J. Bacteriol. 100:95, 1969.
8. Bekierkunst, A., Levij, I. S., Yarkoni, E., Vilkas, E., and Lederer, E.: Cellular reaction in the footpad and draining lymph nodes of mice induced by mycobacterial fractions and BCG bacilli. Infect. Immun. 4:245, 1971.
9. Bloch, H.: Studies on the virulence of tubercle bacilli. Isolation and biological properties of

a constituent of virulent organisms. J. Exp. Med. *91*:197, 1950.

10. Bloch, H., Sorkin, E., and Erlenmeyer, H.: A toxic lipid component of the tubercle bacillus ("cord factor"). I. Isolation from petroleum ether extracts of young bacterial cultures. Am. Rev. Tuberc. *67*:629, 1953.

11. Bloom, B. R., and Bennett, B.: Migration inhibitory factor associated with delayed-type hypersensitivity. Fed. Proc. *27*:13, 1968.

12. Borek, F.: Adjuvants. *In* Sela, M. (ed.): The Antigens. New York, Academic Press, 1977.

13. Campbell, P. A., and Kind, P.: Bone marrow-derived cells as target cells for polynucleotide adjuvants. J. Immunol. *107*:1419, 1971.

14. Casavant, C. H., and Youmans, G. P.: The adjuvant activity of mycobacterial RNA preparations and synthetic polynucleotides for induction of delayed hypersensitivity to purified protein derivative in guinea pigs. J. Immunol. *114*:1014, 1975.

15. Chedid, L., Parant, M., Parant, F., Gustafson, R. H., and Berger, F. M.: Biological study of a nontoxic, water-soluble immunoadjuvant from mycobacterial cell walls. Proc. Natl. Acad. Sci. U.S.A. *69*:855, 1972.

16. Ciba Foundation: Symposium 18 (new series): Immunopotentiation. Amsterdam, Associated Scientific Publishers, 1973.

17. Crowle, A. J.: Immunizing constituents of the tubercle bacillus. Bacteriol. Rev. *22*:183, 1958.

18. Crowle, A. J.: Tubercle bacillary extracts immunogenic for mice. 4. Lipids. Proc. Soc. Exp. Biol. Med. *109*:969, 1962.

19. Dannenberg, A. M., Jr.: Cellular hypersensitivity and cellular immunity in the pathogenesis of tuberculosis: Specificity, systemic and local nature, and associated macrophage enzymes. Bacteriol. Rev. *32*:85, 1968.

20. Dannenberg, A. M., Jr., Ando, M., and Shima, K.: Macrophage accumulation, division, maturation, and digestive and microbicidal capacities in tuberculous lesions. III. The turnover of macrophages and its relation to their activation and antimicrobial immunity in primary BCG lesions and those of reinfection. J. Immunol. *109*:1109, 1972.

21. Dannenberg, A. M., Jr., Meyer, O. T., Esterly, J. R., and Kambara, T.: The local nature of immunity in tuberculosis, illustrated histochemically in dermal BCG lesions. J. Immunol. *100*:931, 1968.

22. Dienes, L., and Schoenheit, E. W.: Local hypersensitiveness. I. Sensitization of tuberculous guinea pigs with egg-white and timothy pollen. J. Immunol. *14*:9, 1927.

23. Dubos, R. J., and Schaedler, R. W.: Reversible changes in the susceptibility of mice to bac-

terial infections. I. Changes brought about by injection of pertussis vaccine or of bacterial endotoxins. J. Exp. Med. *104*:53, 1956.

24. Dumonde, D. C., Howson, W. T., and Wolstencroft, R. A.: The role of macrophages and lymphocytes in reactions of delayed hypersensitivity. *In* Miescher, P. A., and Grabar, P. (eds.): Immunopathology, Fiftieth International Symposium, Mechanisms of Inflammation Induced by Immune Reactions. New York, Grune & Stratton, Inc., 1968.

25. Ellouz, F., Adam, A., Ciorbaru, R., and Lederer, E.: Minimal structural requirements for adjuvant activity of bacterial peptidoglycan derivatives. Biochem. Biophys. Res. Commun. *59*:1317, 1974.

26. Frenkel, J. K., and Caldwell, S. A.: Specific immunity and nonspecific resistance to infection: *Listeria*, protozoa, and viruses in mice and hamsters. J. Infect. Dis. *131*:201, 1975.

27. Freund, J., Casals, J., and Hosmer, E. P.: Sensitization and antibody formation after injection of tubercle bacilli and paraffin oil. Proc. Soc. Exp. Biol. Med. *37*:509, 1937.

28. Freund, J., and Walter, A. W.: Saprophytic acidfast bacilli and paraffin oil as adjuvants in immunization. Proc. Soc. Exp. Biol. Med. *56*:47, 1944.

29. Galindo, B., and Myrvik, Q. N.: Migratory response of granulomatous alveolar cells from BCG-sensitized rabbits. J. Immunol. *105*:227, 1970.

30. Gumbiner, C., Paterson, P. Y., Youmans, G. P., and Youmans, A. S.: Adjuvanticity of mycobacterial RNA and poly A:U for induction of experimental allergic encephalomyelitis in guinea pigs. J. Immunol. *110*:309, 1973.

31. Halpern, B. N., Biozzi, G., Howard, J., Stiffel, C., and Mouton, D.: Exaltation du pouvoir toxique d'*Eberthella typhosa* tuée chez la souris inoculée avec le B.C.G. vivant. Relation entre cette augmentation de la susceptibilité et l'état fonctionnel du système reticulo-éndothélial. C. R. Soc. Biol. (Paris) *152*:899, 1958.

32. Heise, E. R., Myrvik, Q. N., and Leake, E. S.: Effect of Bacillus Calmette-Guérin on the levels of acid phosphatase, lysozyme and cathepsin in rabbit alveolar macrophages. J. Immunol. *95*:125, 1965.

33. Hiu, I. J.: Water-soluble and lipid-free fraction from BCG with adjuvant and antitumor activity. Nature [New Biol.] *238*:241, 1972.

34. Johnson, H. G., and Johnson, A. G.: Regulation of the immune system by synthetic polynucleotides. II. Action on peritoneal exudate cells. J. Exp. Med. *133*:649, 1971.

35. Jolles, P., and Paraf, A.: Chemical and Biological Basis of Adjuvants. New York, Springer-Verlag, 1973.

36. Kanai, K.: Review. Acquired resistance to tu-

berculous infection in experimental model. Jpn. J. Med. Sci. Biol. *20*:21, 1967.

37. Kawata, H., Myrvik, Q. N., and Leake, E. S.: Dissociation of tuberculin hypersensitivity as mediator for an accelerated pulmonary granulomatous response in rabbits. J. Immunol. *93*:433, 1964.

38. Khoo, K. K., and Mackaness, G. B.: Macrophage proliferation in relation to acquired cellular resistance. Aust. J. Exp. Biol. Med. Sci. *42*:707, 1964.

39. Kotani, S., Watanabe, Y., Shimono, T., Kato, K., Kinoshita, F., Stewart-Tull, D. E. S., Shiba, T., Kusumoto, S., Tarumi, Y., Yokogawa, K., and Kawata, S.: Abstract, Symposium International, Les Immunostimulants Bactériens (Structures Chimiques, Mécanismes d'Action, Applications) Paris, Institut Pasteur, 14, 15 Octobre, 1974.

40. Larson, C. L., and Wicht, W. C.: Studies of resistance to experimental tuberculosis in mice vaccinated with living attenuated tubercle bacilli and challenged with virulent organisms. Am. Rev. Respir. Dis. *85*:833, 1962.

41. Leake, E. S., Gonzalez-Ojeda, D., and Myrvik, Q. N.: Enzymatic differences between normal alveolar macrophages and oil-induced peritoneal macrophages obtained from rabbits. Exp. Cell Res. *33*:553, 1964.

42. Leake, E. S., and Heise, E. R.: Comparative cytology of alveolar and peritoneal macrophages from germfree rats. In DiLuzio, N. R., and Paoletti, R. (eds.): The Reticuloendothelial System and Atherosclerosis. New York, Plenum Press, 1967.

43. Leake, E. S., and Myrvik, Q. N.: Changes in morphology and in lysozyme content of free alveolar cells after the intravenous injection of killed BCG in oil. J. Reticuloendothel. Soc. *5*:33, 1968.

44. Leake, E. S., and Myrvik, Q. N.: Differential release of lysozyme and acid phosphatase from sub-cellular granules of normal rabbit alveolar macrophages. Br. J. Exp. Pathol. *45*:384, 1964.

45. Leake, E. S., and Myrvik, Q. N.: Digestive vacuole formation in alveolar macrophages after phagocytosis of *Mycobacterium smegmatis in vivo*. J. Reticuloendothel. Soc. *3*:83, 1966.

46. Lederer, E., Adam, A., Ciorbaru, R., Petit, J., and Wietzerbin, J.: Cell walls of mycobacteria and related organisms; chemistry and immunostimulant properties. Mol. Cell. Biochem. *7*:87, 1975.

47. Mackaness, G. B.: The immunological basis of acquired cellular resistance. J. Exp. Med. *120*:105, 1964.

48. Maillard, J., and Bloom, B. R.: Immunological adjuvants and the mechanism of cell cooperation. J. Exp. Med. *136*:185, 1972.

49. Mayer, E., Jackson, E. R., Whiteside, E. S., and Alverson, C.: Experimental embolic pulmonary tuberculosis in mice. Am. Rev. Tuberc. *69*:419, 1954.

50. Merser, C., Sinay, P., and Adam, A.: J. Med. Chem. (In press, 1975). (As cited in Lederer et al.[46])

51. Migliore-Samour, D., and Jollès, P.: A hydrosoluble adjuvant-active mycobacterial "polysaccharide-peptidoglycan." Preparation by a simple extraction technique of the bacterial cells (strain *Peurois*). FEBS Lett. *25*:301, 1972.

52. Miki, K., and Mackaness, G. B.: The passive transfer of acquired resistance to *Listeria monocytogenes*. J. Exp. Med. *120*:93, 1964.

53. Modolell, M., Luckenbach, G. A., Parant, M., and Munder, P. G.: The adjuvant activity of a mycobacterial water soluble adjuvant (WSA) *in vitro*. I. The requirement of macrophages. J. Immunol. *113*:395, 1974.

54. Myrvik, Q. N., and Evans, D. G.: Effect of Bacillus Calmette Guerin on the metabolism of alveolar macrophages. In DiLuzio, N. R., and Paoletti, R. (eds.): The Reticuloendothelial System and Atherosclerosis. New York, Plenum Press, 1967.

55. Myrvik, Q. N., Leake, E. S., and Oshima, S.: A study of macrophages and epithelioid-like cells from granulomatous (BCG-induced) lungs of rabbits. J. Immunol. *89*:745, 1962.

56. Nauciel, C., Fleck, J., Martin, J. P., and Mock, M.: Activité adjuvante de piptidoglycanes de bactéries à Gram négatif dans l'hypersensibilité de type retardé. C. R. Acad. Sci. [D] (Paris) *276*:3499, 1973.

57. Noll, H.: The chemistry of cord factor, a toxic glycolipid of *M. tuberculosis*. Adv. Tuberc. Res. *7*:149, 1956.

58. Nyka, W.: Enhancement of resistance to tuberculosis in mice experimentally infected with *Brucella abortus*. Am. Rev. Tuberc. *73*:251, 1956.

59. Parant, M., and Chedid, L.: Biological properties of non-toxic water soluble immunoadjuvants from mycobacterial cells. Recent Results Cancer Res. *47*:190, 1974.

60. Philpot, F. J., and Wells, A. Q.: Lipids of living and killed tubercle bacilli. Am. Rev. Tuberc. *66*:28, 1952.

61. Raffel, S.: Chemical factors involved in the induction of infectious allergy. Experientia *6*:410, 1950.

62. Raffel, S.: The components of the tubercle bacillus responsible for the delayed type of "infectious" allergy. J. Infect. Dis. *82*:267, 1948.

63. Raleigh, G. W., and Youmans, G. P.: The use of mice in experimental chemotherapy of tuberculosis. I. Rationale and review of the literature. J. Infect. Dis. *82*:197, 1948.

64. Rich, A. R.: The Pathogenesis of Tuberculosis. 2nd ed. Springfield, Ill., Charles C Thomas, 1951.

65. Sabin, F. R., Doan, C. A., and Forkner, C. E.: Studies on tuberculosis. J. Exp. Med. *52* (No. 6 Suppl. 3):1, 1930.

66. Schaedler, R. W., and Dubos, R. J.: Effects of cellular constituents of mycobacteria on the resistance of mice to heterologous infections. II. Enhancement of infection. J. Exp. Med. *106*:719, 1957.

67. Schmidtke, J. R., and Johnson, A. G.: Regulation of the immune system by synthetic polynucleotides. I. Characteristics of adjuvant action on antibody synthesis. J. Immunol. *106*:1191, 1971.

68. Sever, J. L., and Youmans, G. P.: The enumeration of nonpathogenic viable tubercle bacilli from the organs of mice. Am. Rev. Tuberc. *75*:280, 1957.

69. Sever, J. L., and Youmans, G. P.: Enumeration of viable tubercle bacilli from the organs of nonimmunized and immunized mice. Am. Rev. Tuberc. *76*:616, 1957.

70. Smith, D. W., and Robertsen, J. A.: Immunogenicity in guinea pigs of lipid fractions of *Mycobacterium tuberculosis*. Am. Rev. Respir. Dis. *85*:398, 1962.

71. Smith, D. W., Wiegeshaus, E., Navalkar, R., and Grover, A. A.: Host-parasite relationships in experimental airborne tuberculosis. I. Preliminary studies in BCG-vaccinated and nonvaccinated animals. J. Bacteriol. *91*:718, 1966.

72. Stetson, C., Jr., Schlossman, S., and Benacerraf, B.: Endotoxin-like effects of old tuberculin. Fed. Proc. *17*:536, 1958.

73. Suter, E., Ullman, G. E., and Hoffman, R. G.: Sensitivity of mice to endotoxin after vaccination with BCG (Bacillus Calmette-Guérin). Proc. Soc. Exp. Biol. Med. *99*:167, 1958.

74. Westphal, O.: Recentes recherches sur la chimie et la biologie des endotoxines des bacteries à gram negatif. Ann. Inst. Pasteur (Paris) *98*:789, 1960.

75. White, R. G., Bernstock, L., Johns, R. G. S., and Lederer, E.: The influence of components of *M. tuberculosis* and other mycobacteria upon antibody production to ovalbumin. Immunology *1*:54, 1958.

76. White, R. G., Coons, A. H., and Connolly, J. M.: Studies on antibody production. IV. The role of a wax fraction of *Mycobacterium tuberculosis* in adjuvant emulsions on the production of antibody to egg albumin. J. Exp. Med. *102*:83, 1955.

77. Whitehouse, M. W.: The chemical nature of adjuvants. *In* Glynn, L. E., and Steward, M. W. (eds.): Immunochemistry. United Kingdom, John Wiley & Sons, Inc., 1978.

78. Youmans, G. P., and Youmans, A. S.: An acute pulmonary granulomatous response in mice produced by mycobacterial cells and its relation to increased resistance and increased susceptibility to experimental tuberculous infection. J. Infect. Dis. *114*:135, 1964.

79. Youmans, G. P., and Youmans, A.S.: Effect of mycobacterial cell components upon susceptibility of mice to infection with *M. tuberculosis*. Proc. Soc. Exp. Biol. Med. *120*:656, 1965.

80. Youmans, G. P., and Youmans, A. S.: The effect of mycobacterial RNA on the primary antibody response of mice to bovine gamma globulin. J. Immunol. *109*:217, 1972.

81. Youmans, G. P., and Youmans, A. S.: Nonspecific factors in resistance of mice to experimental tuberculosis. J. Bacteriol. *90*:1675, 1965.

82. Youmans, G. P., and Youmans, A. S.: Recent studies on acquired immunity in tuberculosis. Curr. Top. Microbiol. Immunol. *48*:129, 1969.

83. Youmans, G. P., and Youmans, A. S.: Unpublished data.

4

Mycobacterial Lipids: Chemistry and Biologic Activities

MAYER B. GOREN, Ph.D.
and PATRICK J. BRENNAN, Ph.D.

INTRODUCTION*

Tubercle bacilli in stationary liquid culture, in time, will seed the surface of the liquid and assume a myceliumlike aspect that eventually covers the entire surface (Fig. 4–1). This moldlike growth pattern is characteristic of the genus (hence, the name "Mycobacterium") and evidently derives from the extraordinarily high lipids content of the bacilli, constituting up to 40 percent of the dry weight.[11, 22] The mycobacterial cell wall contains up to 60 percent lipids, as compared with some 20 percent for the lipid-rich cell walls of gram-negative organisms. The lipids render the surface of Mycobacterium tuberculosis hydrophobic. This property facilitates seeding for optimum surface cultiva-

tion of these obligate aerobes. Vigorous but careful shaking to aerate and foam an inoculum collects the bacilli at the foamy air-water interface and deposits them on the surface in the same way that fine particles of many ores, when wet with oil (molybdenum sulfide is a good example), will collect at the surface in a minerals' flotation process.[132] The high lipid content has been associated with various other singular properties of mycobacteria. Although the response to the injection of dead tubercle bacilli is similar to that elicited in an infection, e.g., formation of tubercles, it was early demonstrated that this property is notably attenuated by delipidation of the cells. This raised the possibility that the activity might reside in individual components of the extracted substances. The property of mycobacterial acid-fastness is also clearly conferred by the lipid-rich cell and cell wall and will be discussed in

---

*See Appendix A at end of chapter for list of abbreviations referred to in text.

some detail in this chapter (see also Chapter 2).

In 1927, as part of a cooperative investigation on tuberculosis, the Medical Research Committee of the National Tuberculosis Association (United States) initiated an intensive program under the direction of R. J. Anderson at Yale University to study the lipids of acid-fast bacteria — "To secure compounds of reasonable purity for biological studies and to determine the chemical composition of the various substances as nearly quantitatively as possible."[11] The efforts of the Anderson group in mycobacterial lipids research inaugurated the first of several "golden ages," which in toto have yielded a rich harvest of insight and understanding of the tubercle bacillus and of mycobacteria in general. The participation of the mycobacterial lipids is indelibly imprinted in all of the following: structures and relationships of structure to biologic functions; biosynthetic pathways; host-parasite relationships and the singularity of the in vivo-grown organism; some assessments of factors involved in pathogenicity; the nature of biochemical lesions induced by toxic factors; mechanisms in antigenicity, immunogenicity, cellular hypersensitivity, and tuberculoimmunity; and it is hoped, in the areas of mycobacterial genetics.

The Anderson group delineated or encountered, in one way or another, most of the chemically and biologically significant mycobacterial substances that have been studied in the last half-century. The mycolic acids, the phosphatides, the arabinogalactans of cell wall and waxes, and the single branched and multibranched fatty acids and polyols all bear the imprimatur of that group of investigators. We have seen this legacy augmented by new substances or by variants of older ones. In some cases, significant functional or biologic activities are either evident or convincingly presumed. Examples of these are: trehalose 6, 6'-dimycolate — the "cord factor" of Bloch and Noll and of Asselineau and Lederer; Middlebrook's neutral-red-reactive sulfolipid; the 6-O-methylglucose-lipopolysaccharides of Ballou; and the variety of

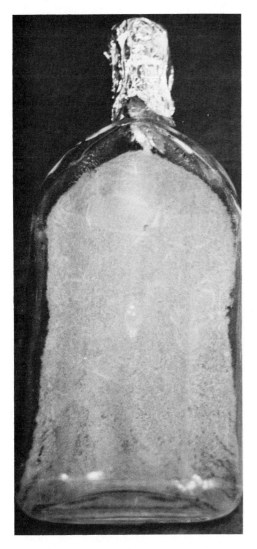

FIGURE 4–1. Veil growth of *M. tuberculosis* H37Rv on the surface of medium ten days after surface seeding by aeration-flotation. (From Goren, M. B.: Improved surface culturing of *Mycobacterium tuberculosis*. J. Bacteriol. 94:1258, 1967.)

"mycosides" first recognized by Randall and Smith.

The accelerating pace at which the structural problems associated with the mycobacterial lipids are being resolved stems largely from the sophistication of instruments and from techniques whose development we have all been privileged to witness: procedures for preparation and purification of subcellular fractions; specific enzymatic degradations used for macromolecules or for stereochemical analysis; broad categorization of chromatographic separations; automatic amino acid analysis and peptide sequencing; and determination of intimate structural details through ultraviolet and infrared spectrophotometry, nuclear magnetic resonance (NMR) spectrometry and mass spectrometry. Some of the examples are impressively dramatic, but most often this is so because of the fastidiousness and thoughtful judgment of the scientists who analyzed the data. We believe that the investigator has not been rendered obsolete by the instruments he has fashioned. A mass spectrum can indeed tell a complete structural tale; nevertheless, the words that tell the tale were originally created painstakingly in the longhand of traditional chemical research.

An abundant, indeed, a massive literature has accumulated on the mycobacterial lipids and related topics. Following the recapitulations of the early studies,[11] the most comprehensive reviews have come from the individual and collaborative efforts of J. Asselineau and E. Lederer, whose own research interests have embraced almost every important class of mycobacterial lipids. Their earlier review[25] and Asselineau's treatise[23] were devoted to bacterial lipids in general.[22] They have been concerned lately with cell wall constituents and with trehalose-containing glycolipids.[221-223] In Goren's review,[136] the "selected topics" particu-larly emphasized biologically relevant mycolic acids, glycolipids of trehalose and 6-O-methylglucose, mycosides, phospholipids and wax D. The reader is urged to refer to two superb reviews, which have recently appeared, by C. Ratledge[290] and by L. Barksdale and K.-S. Kim.[40]

Lipids Extraction and Separation

It was possible for the Anderson group to process, for the first time, very large quantities (50-pound batches, for example) of virulent cells of *M. tuberculosis* and other mycobacteria. These were grown on defined synthetic media, such as those of Sauton and Long, so that the bacilli were cultured under standard and uniform conditions. In Anderson's procedure, the bacteria were collected on Büchner funnels, then washed and, under inert atmosphere, immediately introduced into ethanol-ether and exhaustively extracted with this solvent for several weeks. The cells were then extracted several times with chloroform, leaving only traces of extractable free lipids. "Firmly bound lipids" were subsequently obtained by treatment of the residue with alcohol-ether-1% HCl, followed by additional extraction with chloroform and ether. Through various solvent treatments, the extracted lipids were separated into "phosphatide," "acetone-soluble fat," and various "wax" fractions. The Anderson procedure was ultimately modified by Aebi, Asselineau, and Lederer,[5] as depicted in Figure 4–2, to provide somewhat different gross primary fractions, which have been found more useful in the separation and ultimate purification of individual specific substances. Thus, for the preparation of fractions leading to the biologically important waxes D,

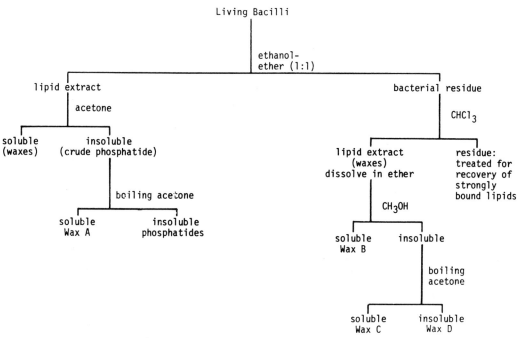

FIGURE 4–2.   Extraction of mycobacterial lipids.

phthiocerol mycocerosates, and "cord factor," this remains the procedure of choice.

The primary ethanol-ether extraction of the Anderson procedure also has been favored for extraction and recovery of several "mycosides" — glycolipids or peptidoglycolipids that have been utilized in characterizing some *Mycobacterium* species.[324] Some of these mycosides are only now assuming significant biologic prominence, after a "latent" period of some twenty years. Still other extraction processes were developed to accommodate the securing of select individual substances. The sulfatides (sulfolipids) of *M. tuberculosis* are recovered and separated from Anderson extracts only with great difficulty; instead, recovery and purification from contaminating phosphatides are dramatically facilitated if the moist bacilli are merely extracted with

hexane containing 0.1 percent decylamine.[133, 254]

Vilkas and coworkers[282] extracted cells with acetone to remove neutral lipids, followed by refluxing with methanol to solubilize phospholipids for recovery. Pangborn and McKinney[279] favored pyridine for the same purpose and cleverly employed solubility differences in methanol and acetone to separate cardiolipin and phosphatidylinositol as well as phosphatidylinositol mannosides. Brennan and Ballou[54] chose chloroform-methanol-water, according to the procedure of Folch, for the purpose of solubilizing all lipids. The apolar neutral lipids then were removed largely with cold acetone. Brennan and colleagues[59] quantitatively compared this Folch-based procedure with the traditional Anderson-Aebi method. The most striking difference was seen in the amount of recoverable phospholipids: extraction with chloroform-methanol yielded about 4 g of phospholipid per gram of cell nitrogen, and about 1.1 g of neutral lipid, whereas ethanol-ether solubilized only 0.25 to 0.45 g of phospholipid and comparable amounts of neutral lipids. In addition, the fractions obtained in the Anderson procedure were heterogeneous, with triglycerides distributed among many of them. Brennan and colleagues[59] concluded that chloroform-methanol extraction processes followed by chromatographic fractionations were much more suitable, at least for analytic purposes.

Mycolic acids, which are high molecular weight (80 to 90 carbons), α-branched, β-hydroxy acids of mycobacteria with a role in acid-fastness, are largely covalently linked (esterified) to polysaccharides in the mycobacterial cell wall. They are quite readily obtained by alkaline hydrolysis of either whole cells or neutral, solvent-extracted cell residues. The saponification is conducted with benzene-methanol-KOH; the mycolic acids are obtained partly as methyl esters, partly as K-salts. Because of high molecular weight, both of these are soluble in ether and insoluble in boiling methanol — a solvent process that yields a concentrate suitably enriched in mycolate components for subsequent chromatographic separations.

Chromatographic Processes

The separation techniques and their associated assemblages of columns, adsorbents, solvents, and fraction collectors have become the hallmark of lipid laboratories and are augmented by preparative adaptations of the more often analytic thin-layer chromatography (TLC), dry-column chromatography, gas-liquid chromatography (GLC), and high-performance-liquid chromatography (HPLC). These have notably facilitated the required separations and purification of mycobacterial lipids that were denied to the Anderson group and their contemporaries; of course, they have also allowed for manipulation on much smaller and convenient scales. However, column chromatography is by no means limited to laboratory scale operations. Extracts from 30 kg harvests of *M. tuberculosis* are currently being processed in pilot plants in the Institut de Chimie des Substances Naturelles (Gif-sur-Yvette, France), under E. Lederer's direction, to provide multigram quantities of cord factor for tumor immunotherapy studies. At the other end of the spectrum, E. Ribi and colleagues at the Rocky Mountain Laboratory in Hamilton, Montana, are processing milligram quantities of cord factor concentrates by high-pressure-liquid chromatography on microparticulate silica gel to prepare samples of cord factor (P_3) — by current criteria, some of the purest presently available — for tumor studies. Silicic acid, silica gel, magnesium silicate, and alumina are adsorbents of choice for many separations. In organic solvents, cellulose powder and diethylaminoethyl cellulose are useful in particular separation processes. Diethylaminoethyl cellulose is especially suitable for acidic lipids such as the mycobacterial sulfatides[133] and brain lipids.[297] Sephadex products, modified to render them sufficiently lipophilic, have also been exploited for specific lipid separations.[337]

Mycobacterial Surface Ultrastructure and Chemistry

The thick (about 20 nm), abundantly lipidic — and therefore hydrophobic — mycobacterial wall, extending from the murein to the cell surface, is almost unquestionably a result of the unusual composition of the mycobacterial *cell wall skeleton*. A more detailed discussion of the cell wall is included in another section; for the present, it is sufficient to say that in *Mycobacterium*, the hydrophilic peptidoglycan ground substance (which is not remarkably different from that of many other bacteria) is covalently linked to a polysaccharide (an arabinogalactan — also hydrophilic), which in turn is embellished by a multitude of covalently linked (esterified) mycolic acid residues that have high molecular weight (1200 to 1300 daltons) and are extremely hydrophobic. From thermodynamic considerations, it is unlikely that these lipophilic appendages would be buried in the mass of hydrophilic hydroxyl-substituted ring structures that comprise the arabinogalactan-peptidoglycan. Instead, they would be oriented away from this basal layer and thus would be able to attract and to associate with and hold lipophilic substances external to the murein layer. In accord with this perhaps simplified interpretation, prepared cell walls (as distinguished from *cell wall skeleton*) of certain species (for example, *M. bovis* BCG or *M. phlei*) contain some 60 per-cent of their dry weight as lipid,[204, 348] of which two-thirds is extractable by organic solvents, leaving cell wall skeleton. The remaining lipid (largely mycolic acid) is covalently bound and is released only after acid or alkaline hydrolysis.

From electron microscopy studies,[40, 159] the mycobacterial cell wall is considered to be constructed of several layers. A conception of this is given in Figure 4–3, which has been kindly provided to the authors by Barksdale and Kim. A somewhat similar representation by Imaeda and coworkers[159] is reproduced and analyzed in Ratledge's review. Numerous electron microscopic examples of fibrous or filamentous ropelike structures at or near the surface of mycobacteria have been documented, as shown in Figure 4–4.[348, 381] Somewhat similar structures are seen as well in nocardia and corynebacteria, and several examples are included in the review of Barksdale and Kim.[40]

In Barksdale and Kim's construction and interpretation (Fig. 4–3), which differ in several details from those of

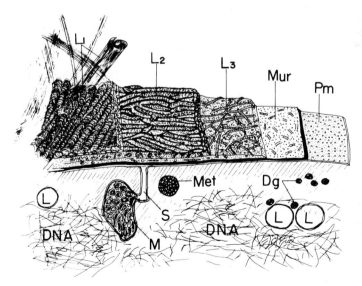

FIGURE 4–3. Section of mycobacterial cell wall. (From Barksdale, L., and Kim, K.-S.: *Mycobacterium.* Bacteriol. Rev. *41*:217, 1977.)

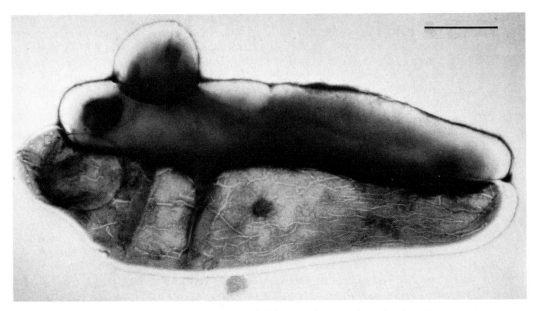

FIGURE 4-4. Ramified fibrous structures revealed by negative staining: *M. tuberculosis* H37Rv. Bar = 0.5 μm. (From Barksdale, L., and Kim, K.-S.: *Mycobacterium.* Bacteriol. Rev. *41*:217, 1977.)

Imaeda and colleagues, the peptidoglycan layer (Mur) shows remnants of fibrous, ropelike structures; these are very prominent in the adjacent layer L_3. In L_2, which is continuous with L_3, the ropes appear fatter and more wrinkled, according to Barksdale and Kim. These may represent folds of glycolipid or peptidoglycolipid that are wrinkled in postlog-phase cells and are more stretched out in actively growing cells. Evidence gathered individually by White, Takeya, and Imaeda unequivocally implicates the mycolic acids in delineating these fibrillar and ropelike aspects. It is important to recognize that in the mycobacterial cell wall, mycolic acids are present in at least four forms: esterified to the rigid insoluble murein-arabinogalactan complex, esterified to (presumably) autolytically derived "soluble" murein-arabinogalactan (adjuvant-active wax D), esterified to "soluble" arabinogalactan (adjuvant-inactive wax D), and as free mycolic acid. Ratledge estimates the amount of free mycolic acid in the cell to be quite meager. We consider that the facile visualization of the ropy structures in electron microscopy is rendered so because of the "soluble" mycolates' associating with each other and with the species linked to the cell wall and because their form is further augmented by adsorption of various other free mycobacterial lipids. The disappearance of the ropelike patterns ("paired fibrous structures" in Takeya's terminology) after simple solvent extraction with either pyridine or $CHCl_3$ is in accord with this interpretation. These solvents would *not* remove mycoloyl residues covalently linked to the cell wall ground substance but, instead, would extract the free lipid, which is merely physically associated with these mycoloyl esters. In the absence of associated soluble lipids, therefore, the mycoloyl esters alone do not appear as fibrous structures. The fibrillar configuration is also destroyed by alkaline hydrolysis, which cleaves the mycolate esters; alkaline degradation of whole cells renders them nonacid-fast as well.

From chemical and ultrastructural studies, Imaeda, Kanetsuna, and Galin-

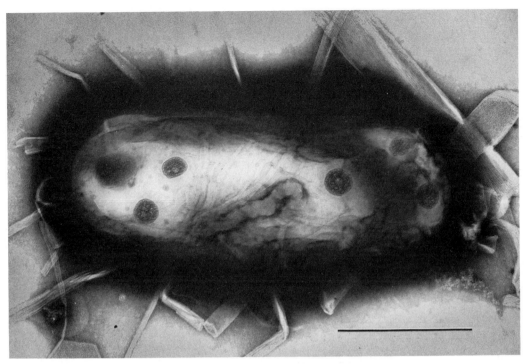

FIGURE 4–5. Tapelike integuments of mycosidic material, extending from the surface of still-grown *Mycobacterium sp.* NQ and corresponding to layer L_1 of Figure 4–2. Bar equals 0.5 μm. (From Barksdale, L., and Kim, K.-S.: *Mycobacterium.* Bacteriol. Rev. *41*:217, 1977.)

do[159] concluded that in the innermost layer of cell wall (a lipopolysaccharide-arabinogalactan-mucopeptide complex), the fibrillar structures are conferred by the mycolate residues. They characterized the adjacent layer as a membranous matrix of fibrillar mycoloyl arabinogalactan and lipoprotein; whereas the outermost layer (corresponding to L_2 of Barksdale and Kim) evidently consists of two lipopolysaccharides: mycoloyl-glucose-rich fibrils and a component rich in arabinogalactan.

In Figure 4–5, the most superficial layer, L_1, is most readily recognized as filaments, tapes, or ribbons, as revealed by negative-staining techniques in specimens from still-grown cultures. The L_1 filaments may cover up the succeeding layer, L_2, so that the adornment of ropy structures in L_2 is hidden and becomes visible only after the cells are repeatedly washed or subjected to sonic vibration to eliminate the outer layer. In *M. lepraemurium* (Fig. 4–6),[91] in *M. avium*,[90] and, by inference, in *Mycobacterium NQ*,[197] the most superficial layer is composed of 5 nm diameter filaments of C-mycosides — ordinarily, not very complex peptidoglycolipids. We infer from studies currently in progress in our laboratories[57] that *M. intracellulare* species would present a similar picture. L_1 cannot, of course, be constituted of C-type mycosides in all mycobacterium species since not all mycobacteria synthesize that particular mycoside. Also, there is no evidence as yet that L_1 is ubiquitous in mycobacteria.

Figure 4–7, taken from Kim, Salton, and Barksdale,[197] is a micrograph of freeze-etched *Mycobacterium NQ*. The ribbonlike mycoside (refer to Fig. 4–5) has just been shaken away to expose various features of the wall. The arrow indicates a fracture through L_1, reveal-

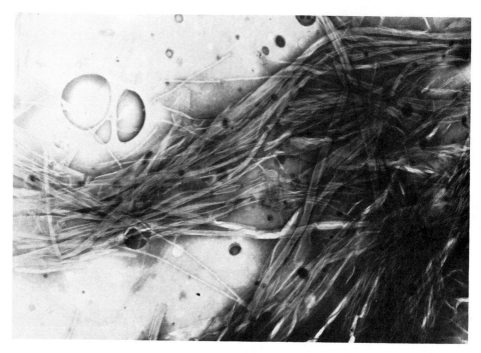

FIGURE 4–6. Electron micrographs of the C-mycosidic fibrillar material isolated from mouse liver infected with *M. lepraemurium*. Fibrillar material from a urea gradient, negatively stained with sodium silicotungstate. × 62,200. (From Draper, P., and Rees, R. J. W.: The nature of the electron transparent zone that surrounds *Mycobacterium lepraemurium* inside host cells. J. Gen. Microbiol. 77:79, 1973.)

ing in profile the ropelike structures of L_2 and L_3 adhering to the rigid murein layer. We would perhaps be more content with the interpretation if the "rigid murein layer" might instead be seen as the *cytoplasmic membrane* from which the thick cell wall has separated, with the ropelike structures and their complement of mycoloyl arabinogalactan-peptidoglycan intact. We find it difficult to conceive of such a clean fracture of the murein away from extensively covalently linked mycoloyl arabinogalactan. Indeed, in Takeya's studies, following disruption of frozen cells with glass beads, numerous examples of saclike membrane, apparently cytoplasmic, were seen.[347] However, Drs. Barksdale and Salton kindly informed us that in their interpretation, as based on studies of *Pseudomonas*,[129] the

"powerful physically induced cleavage . . . (by) freeze fracture (would) separate this surface decoration (covalently linked mycoloyl arabinogalactan) like an earthquake breaks off superstructures . . ." to expose the murein.

Acid-Fastness

The ability to form (albeit with difficulty) deeply colored acid-stable complexes with the cationic triphenylmethane dyes, fuchsin (*i*) and crystal violet (*ii*) is "regarded by many as the hallmark of mycobacteria."[40] The cationic (basic) nature of these dyes is conferred by the amino substituents that they bear and favors their complexing with acidic substances—especially polyanionics, such as DNA and acidic proteins.

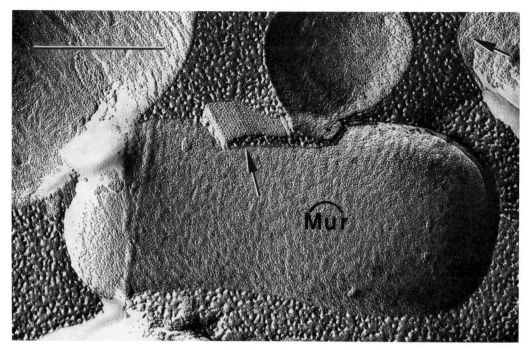

FIGURE 4–7. Micrograph of freeze-etched *Mycobacterium* sp. *NQ*. Mycosidic filaments of Figure 4–5 have first been removed by either vigorous shaking or brief sonication. The vertical arrow indicates a fracture through L_1, revealing in profile the ropelike structures, L_2 and L_3, adhering to the rigid murein layer (MUR). Direction of shadowing is indicated by arrow (top right). Bar = 0.25 μm. (From Barksdale, L., and Kim, K. S.: *Mycobacterium*. Bacteriol. Rev. *41*:217, 1977.)

i   Pararosanilin (Fuchsin)

ii   Crystal Violet

The important taxonomic and diagnostic tool of acid-fastness has been surrounded by such an aura of mystery that for many informed scientists, the phenomenon has completely evaded comprehension. In contrast to most other bacteria, mycobacteria in their native state are difficult to stain with polar water-soluble dyes. The reason for this seems to be found in the hydrophobic lipid-rich layers, which are substantially impervious to penetration by aqueous solutions. Koch prolonged the contact with dyes for 12 hours in order to achieve staining; Ehrlich incorporated into the dyeing solution organic substances having both polar and nonpolar qualities (for example, aniline and phenol) so as to aid penetration of the dye; this is further facilitated by heating. Once this is achieved, the dye, with few exceptions, is very likely complexed by the same kinds of cellular components in mycobacteria as complex the dyes in other cells where penetration is not hindered. According to Yegian and Vanderlinde,[395] much of the intracellular dye is present in a free, uncomplexed form. The resistance of stained mycobacteria to bleaching by the acid alcohol is also reasonably explained by the same barrier principle. Cold ethanol is a notably poor solvent for mycobacterial lipids. It is probably no more successful than an aqueous acid solution in penetrating the lipid layers. Our anticipation, on this basis, that facilitated penetration of the acid should achieve bleaching is readily demonstrated (see below). Barksdale and Kim suggest that the barrier to penetration of the bleaching acid is augmented still further by the acid-fast complex that is known to form between the dye and mycolic acid. They state, "Once the mycolic acid of the cell is complexed with an arylmethane dye, the cell surface becomes extremely hydrophobic."[40] The Anderson group showed mycolic acid to be "acid-fast," but its contribution to the depth of color is demonstrably meager. As reviewed by Asselineau[22] and by Barksdale and Kim,[40] *only free* mycolic acid is capable of complexing the dye. The bulk of mycolates, which are found esterified to arabinose in the cell wall, and in the varieties of wax D, are incapable of this complexing. In our interpretation, it seems sufficient that the *totality* of mycobacterial lipids — mycolic acid, its dye complex, and especially its esterified forms, such as the mycoloyl arabinogalactan-mucopeptide — all contribute to impeding penetration of the bleaching acid, and loss of acid-fastness can be correlated with a breach of this barrier.

Our interpretation is in accordance with many diverse observations. Only the intact bacillus is acid-fast. Simple grinding of dried bacilli in a mortar does not affect the mycolic acid; nevertheless, it destroys acid-fastness. This probably occurs because the cytoplasmic components that complex the dye are no longer protected from the bleaching acid by an intact lipids barrier. According to Murohashi, Kondo, and Yoshida,[265] disruption of the cells also allows association of acid-fast, free mycolic acid with released cell proteins; this diminishes the contribution of the mycolate in dye complexing.

The relative importance of free lipids, including mycolic acids, as compared with the mycolate esterified to cell wall may be discerned from the observations that acid-fastness is only *diminished* when the free lipids are extracted by neutral solvents.[102, 265, 395] However, when intact cells are delipidated by *ethanolic alkali* or by prolonged contact with acidic solvents (which will hydrolyze even the mycoloyl arabinogalactan linkages), acid-fastness is completely lost. The chemical treatments release the so-called "bound lipids" of mycobacterial cell wall; these contain about 50 percent mycolic acid.[11] The undeniable contribution of mycolates, *as distinguished* from mycolic acid, is further attested to in the loss of acid-fastness accompanying exposure of *M. tuberculosis* to isonicotinic acid hydrazide. As discussed later on in this chapter, the mode of action of INH very likely involves inhibition of mycolic acid synthesis.

We have been able to demonstrate that the so-called "acid-fastness" of the mycolic acid-dye complex is an artifact of the physical state of this lipid component and depends upon the same barrier principle. Films of mycolic acid deposited on glass slides, then stained, appear to be acid-fast. In contrast, when a mycolate salt is dissolved in an organic solvent, such as xylene, and shaken with an aqueous solution of, for example, crystal violet, it complexes the water-soluble aryl-methane dye and solubilizes it into the organic phase, which becomes vividly colored. But the complex in solution is demonstrably *not* acid-fast; the organic phase is immediately bleached on contact with fairly dilute, aqueous HCl. This bleaching occurs even with aqueous citric or acetic acid! In such cases, there is no "barrier" to the acid contact.[144a]

Accordingly, if the failure of acid alcohol to bleach the stained cells is due to the penetration barrier imposed by free lipids and especially by the mycoloylated cell wall, it can be predicted that an appropriate solvent, which allows the mineral acid to breach the barrier, should effect destaining; this is readily demonstrated. If the stained preparation is briefly contacted with a more effective acidified solvent [$CHCl_3$:CH_3OH:HCl (75:25:2)], the cells are almost completely bleached. Under these conditions, it is unlikely that the mycoloyl-arabinogalactan-peptidoglycan is disturbed; therefore, we consider the bleaching as resulting from a mere penetration of the lipid barrier by the acid and lipid solvent. On the other hand, free lipids may well be extracted by even brief solvent contact. The residue, however, is still acid-fast according to convention; in a second Ziehl-Neelsen staining, the dye is once again complexed and still resists bleaching with acid alcohol; but the stained bacilli can again be bleached with the acidic solvent.[144a]

We suggest that the demonstration just described uniquely delineates the lipid species that is particularly relevant to acid-fastness—the mycolic acid residues, which are covalently linked to the arabinogalactan-peptidoglycan basal layer and are thus integral to the cell wall skeleton. The soluble lipids, which we suggest are a part of the cell wall because of the lipophilic characteristics conferred by the mycoloyl esters, contribute to and enhance acid-fastness, but in their absence, the residue of mycoloyl arabinogalactan appears to be sufficient.

FATTY ACID BIOSYNTHESIS

Synthetases of *Mycobacterium smegmatis*

The most characteristic feature of mycobacterial fatty acid biosynthesis is the functionality of a single homogeneous multienzyme synthetase, as occurs in *M. smegmatis* (formerly *M. phlei* ATCC) and probably in other mycobacteria. The prototype of this enzyme complex for fatty acid synthesis is found in yeast and in liver and was generally regarded as being specifically eukaryotic, since in most bacteria, fatty acid synthesis is catalyzed by individual nonaggregating enzymes.[374] Whether independent multienzymes or a multienzyme complex is involved, acyl carrier protein (ACP) serves as an anchor to which the acyl intermediates are esterified during the synthetic processes that build up the aliphatic chain. With acetyl-S-ACP as the primer, the fatty acid is successively elongated by condensation with malonyl-S-ACP, followed by the transformations outlined in Figure 4–8. Sequential additions of malonate — produced from acetyl coenzyme A (CoA) via the carboxy-biotin enzyme, acetyl CoA carboxylase — are followed by the same repeated series of reductions, dehydrations, and reductions. These series serve to build up the fatty acid chain by 2-carbon units to the lengths characteristic of the individual organism.

The multienzyme complex as depicted by Lehninger is reproduced with permission in Figure 4–9.

Brindley, Matsumura, and Bloch[60] and Vance and colleagues[363] isolated from *M. smegmatis* a 340-fold purified complex which was similar to that from eukaryotic systems, both in its size (MW 1.38×10^6) and in its association with complexed ACP. However, it was rela-

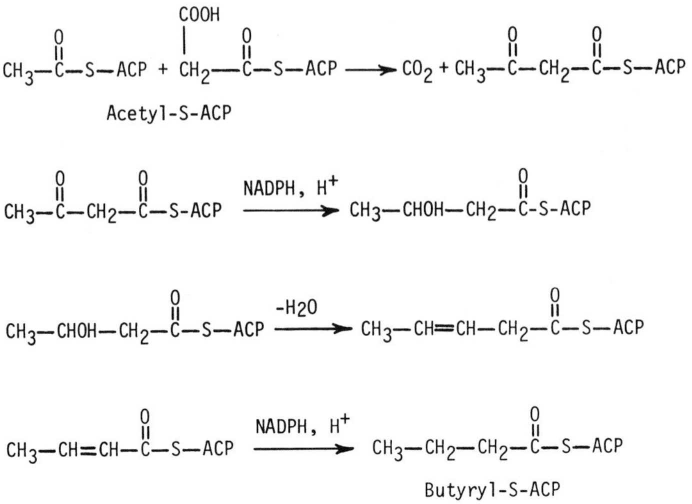

$$\underset{\text{Acetyl-S-ACP}}{CH_3-\overset{O}{\overset{\|}{C}}-S-ACP} + \underset{}{\overset{\text{COOH}}{\overset{|}{CH_2}}-\overset{O}{\overset{\|}{C}}-S-ACP} \longrightarrow CO_2 + CH_3-\overset{O}{\overset{\|}{C}}-CH_2-\overset{O}{\overset{\|}{C}}-S-ACP$$

$$CH_3-\overset{O}{\overset{\|}{C}}-CH_2-\overset{O}{\overset{\|}{C}}-S-ACP \xrightarrow{\text{NADPH, H}^+} CH_3-CHOH-CH_2-\overset{O}{\overset{\|}{C}}-S-ACP$$

$$CH_3-CHOH-CH_2-\overset{O}{\overset{\|}{C}}-S-ACP \xrightarrow{-H_2O} CH_3-CH=CH-CH_2-\overset{O}{\overset{\|}{C}}-S-ACP$$

$$CH_3-CH=CH-\overset{O}{\overset{\|}{C}}-S-ACP \xrightarrow{\text{NADPH, H}^+} \underset{\text{Butyryl-S-ACP}}{CH_3-CH_2-CH_2-\overset{O}{\overset{\|}{C}}-S-ACP}$$

FIGURE 4–8.   *De novo* synthesis of even-chain fatty acids.

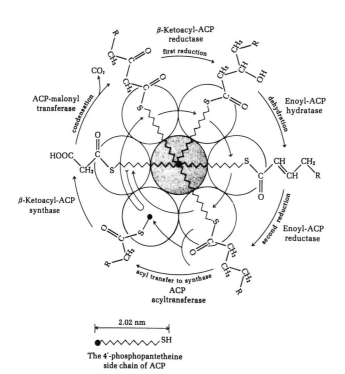

FIGURE 4–9.   A schematic representation of the fatty acid synthetase complex. The central protein molecule is ACP. Its long phosphopantetheine side chain apparently serves as a swinging arm to carry acyl groups from one enzyme molecule to the next to accomplish the six steps needed for addition of each 2-carbon unit. (From Lehninger, A. L.: Biochemistry. 2nd ed. New York, Worth Publishers, 1975, p. 664.)

tively unstable since it could be dissociated by low concentrations of buffer into inactive fragments. The *M. phlei* synthetase has several unique features: it requires NADH and NADPH; it has relative nonspecificity for acyl CoA primers; and it requires a heat-stable stimulatory factor. Moreover, it exhibits a bimodal pattern of fatty acid production; i.e., fatty acids with shorter (mostly C_{16}) and longer (mostly C_{24}) chains are simultaneously synthesized. Ilton and coworkers[158] demonstrated that the heat-stable cofactor material consisted of two fractions: flavine mononucleotide (FMN), which probably dissociates from the complex during its purification, and three polysaccharides (S_1, S_2, S_3). S_1 contains considerable amounts of 3-O-methylmannose; it is now recognized as being identical with the 3-O-*M*ethyl*M*annose-containing *P*olysaccharide (MMP) described in detail by Gray and Ballou[150] and by Maitra and Ballou.[241] S_2 and S_3 appear to be identical with some of the 6-O-*M*ethyl*G*lucose-containing *L*ipo*P*olysaccharides (MGLP), also described by Ballou and colleagues (see p. 82).

Both MMP and MGLP stimulate the fatty acid synthetase complex. MMP is the more effective of the two, especially in lowering the K_m for acetyl and malonyl CoA. Since the polysaccharides did not alter any of the individual activities of the synthetase complex, it was proposed that they function by associating with the long-chain acyl CoA end-products of the reaction, thereby rendering them ineffective as end-product inhibitors of fatty acid synthesis. In support of this interpretation, Knoche and colleagues[198] and Machida

and Bloch[238] described the formation of stable complexes consisting of palmitoyl CoA and MMP or MGLP. A model has been proposed in which hydrophobic interactions between the paraffin chains of the fatty acid CoA and the 6-O-methyl groups of MGLP ensure the stability of the complex, as illustrated in Figure 4–10 (taken from Machida and Bloch).[238]

Bloch and collaborators have suggested schemes to explain the control of overall fatty acid synthesis, the bimodal nature of the fatty acids produced, and the effects of the mycobacterial polysaccharides. According to their most recent interpretation,[51] the rate-limiting step is termination of long-chain fatty acid synthesis — specifically, release of C_{24}-CoA from the synthetase complex. Termination in the presence or absence of MMP occurs as shown at the bottom of the page.

Reaction 2 is the ordinarily slow, rate-limiting release of C_{24}-CoA from the fatty acyl elongation step. Reaction 3 represents diffusion facilitated by complex formation between enzyme-bound acyl CoA and polysaccharide. The presence of MMP (and presumably MGLP) considerably enhances the sum of reactions 2 and 3, thereby promoting overall synthesis by as much as 100-fold.

The product pattern of *M. smegmatis* fatty acid synthesis is consistently bimodal, if highly variable.[103] Shifts in favor of the shorter acids occur at high concentrations of acetyl CoA or in the presence of MGLP or MMP. The latter (MMP) alters the equilibrium of the transacylase reaction palmitoyl synthetase $\rightleftharpoons$ palmitoyl CoA in the direction of CoA. This favors early C_{16}-

Reaction 1. C_{24} — synthetase + CoA $\rightleftharpoons$ C_{24} — CoA—synthetase
Reaction 2. C_{24} — CoA—synthetase $\rightleftharpoons$ C_{24} — CoA + synthetase

or

Reaction 3. C_{24} — CoA—synthetase $\rightleftharpoons$ $[C_{24}$—CoA·MMP] + synthetase

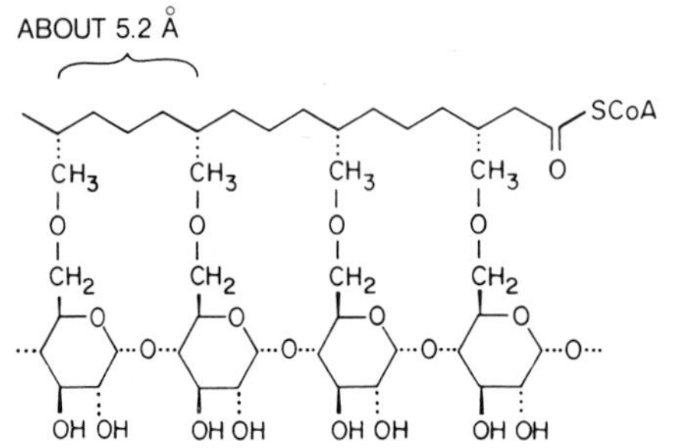

ABOUT 5.2 Å

FIGURE 4–10. Proposed hydrophobic interaction between the paraffin chain of fatty acyl CoA and the 6-O-methyl groups of MGLP. (From Machida, Y., and Bloch, K.: Complex formation between mycobacterial polysaccharides and fatty acyl CoA derivatives. Proc. Natl. Acad. Sci. U.S.A. 70:1146, 1973.)

chain termination and, therefore, suppression of its elongation. Accordingly, in *M. smegmatis* a combination of metabolites and regulatory molecules exists that is capable of exerting both negative and positive controls over fatty acid synthesis.

In addition to these controls, Flick and Bloch[104] postulate that palmitoyl CoA is capable of dissociating the fatty acid synthetase complex (MW 1.4×10^6) into inactive subunits (MW about 2.5×10^5) to which it binds; however, this binding can be prevented or reversed and activity restored by MMP and MGLP.

When Brindley and coworkers[60] first described the fatty acid synthetase complex of *M. smegmatis*, they also presented evidence for a second *soluble* synthetase — a carrier protein similar, in most respects, to that found in other bacteria. The second system, which apparently can operate alongside the multienzyme complex but remain completely independent of it, is primarily an additional means for chain elongation since it is primed by palmitoyl CoA and stearoyl CoA but cannot use acetyl CoA. The free ACP and other features of this fatty acid elongation mechanism have been examined and compared with those of its prototype, the ACP-requiring system from *E. coli*.[245, 246] The amino acid composition

of the *M. smegmatis* ACP differs slightly from its counterpart in *E. coli* and in other bacteria. The *M. smegmatis* product, except for its amino acid composition and its exceptional chain length specificity, is rather like the *E. coli* synthetase.

Etemadi and coworkers have also examined de novo fatty acid synthesis in another strain of *M. smegmatis* and have reported only single separable enzymes, such as malonyl CoA:ACP transacylase, acetyl CoA:ACP transacylase, caprylyl CoA:ACP transacylase, and palmitoyl CoA:ACP transacylase.[194] To explain the apparent discrepancy between the results from the laboratories of Bloch and those of Etemadi, Ratledge[290] has suggested that the instability of the synthetase complex in *M. smegmatis* may become even more exaggerated in another mycobacterium, to such a point that the quaternary structure is no longer retained. However, the report of a fatty acid synthetase complex in *Corynebacterium diphtheriae*[199] seems to indicate its widespread occurrence among the actinomycetales.

Previously, Goren[136] reviewed the evidence from D. S. Goldman and colleagues for the existence of several fatty acid-synthesizing mechanisms in *M. tuberculosis* H37Ra. Perhaps some of these observations can now be accommodated by the various de novo and elongation pathways described above. However, an additional system described by Kanemasa and Goldman[176] is apparently unique. It involves the head-to-tail condensation of two or three moles of a fatty acid such as octanoate to yield palmitate and tetracosanoate, respectively. An intermolecular condensation of this sort would almost certainly entail ω-oxidation of participant molecules. No mechanistic details of this intriguing biochemical pathway (Fig. 4–11) have appeared, but the postulated ω-oxidations–condensations have recently been embraced as possibly contributing to mycolic acid synthesis. Mechanisms as unique as the one just postulated deserve further clarifica-

1) $CH_3—(CH_2—CH_2)_3—COOH \xrightarrow{?} HOOC—(CH_2—CH_2)_3—COOH$

2) $CH_3—(CH_2—CH_2)_3—COOH + HOOC—(CH_2—CH_2)_3COOH + HOOC—(CH_2—CH_2)_3—COOH$

$$\downarrow ?$$

$CH_3—(CH_2—CH_2)_3—CH_2—CH_2—(CH_2—CH_2)_3—CH_2—CH_2—CH_2—(CH_2—CH_2)_3—COOH$

FIGURE 4–11. Proposal for synthesis of fatty acids by head-to-tail condensation.

tion, and an unambiguous confirmation of this pathway in mycobacteria seems warranted.

Varieties of Fatty Acids in *Mycobacterium*

Saturated and Unsaturated Acids

Cason and Miller[69] and Asselineau[23] have thoroughly explored and reviewed the complexity of mycobacterial fatty acids. Straight-chain carboxylates, ranging from C_8 to C_{26} (the most abundant being palmitic acid), have been identified. The formidable technique of combined gas-liquid chromatography–mass spectroscopy has revealed the inordinate complexity of still more products. Campbell and Naworal[66, 67] reported over 30 fatty acid esters from methanolysis of only the neutral lipids of *M. phlei*. All of the odd carbon fatty acids from C_{11} to C_{23} have now been recognized in mycobacteria. It is unlikely that any of these acids occur in substantial quantities in the free form; instead, they are found in the form of esters and amides as part of the lipids that are described further on in this chapter. Campbell and Naworal[66, 67] and Hung and Walker[156] have established the structures of the large variety of monounsaturated fatty acids from *M. smegmatis*, *M. phlei*, and *M. bovis* BCG. Asselineau and coworkers[17] also have

isolated from *M. phlei* monounsaturated fatty acids containing from 20 to 27 carbon atoms. These include normal Δ^5—monoeneic acids of 22, 24, or 26 carbon atoms; branched-chain Δ^5 derivatives of 25 and 27 carbon atoms; and a series that includes 4-eicosenoic, 6-docosenoic, and 8-hexacosenoic acids.

Fulco[107] has reviewed the topic of unsaturated fatty acid biosynthesis, and many of his observations are relevant to mycobacteria. There are two distinct biochemical mechanisms for the introduction of *cis* double bonds into fatty acids. In the more common bacterial system (the so-called "anaerobic" pathway shown in Fig. 4–12) a *cis*-3 double bond is introduced into the β-hydroxydecanoyl thioester. Chain elongation of the *cis*-3-derivative gives rise to longer-chain, unsaturated fatty acids. However, *M. phlei*, and possibly other mycobacteria, does not use this pathway but instead employs direct, oxygen-dependent desaturation of long-chain fatty acids. This pathway is traditionally associated with higher phyla. The overall reaction in *M. phlei* has been established by Fulco and Bloch,[108, 109] as shown below.

Desaturation is catalyzed by a particulate enzyme and shows absolute requirements for O_2, NADPH, Fe^{2+}, and flavine adenine dinucleotide (FAD) or FMN. The end-product may perhaps be an oleyl-phospholipid and the direct

$$CH_3—(CH_2)_7—CH_2—CH_2—(CH_2)_7—COCoA \xrightarrow[Fe^{2+},FAD]{NADPH,O_2} CH_3—(CH_2)_7—CH=CH—(CH_2)_7—COO^-$$

stearoyl CoA
(or palmitoyl CoA)

oleate
(or hexadecenoate)

FIGURE 4–12. "Anaerobic" pathway for synthesis of bacterial unsaturated fatty acids.

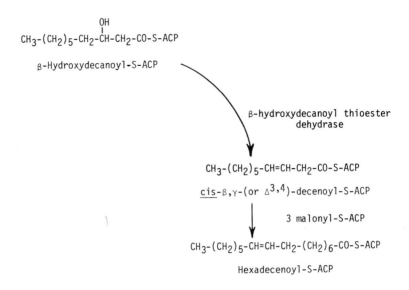

$$CH_3-(CH_2)_5-CH_2-\overset{\overset{\displaystyle OH}{|}}{CH}-CH_2-CO-S-ACP$$

β-Hydroxydecanoyl-S-ACP

β-hydroxydecanoyl thioester
dehydrase

$$CH_3-(CH_2)_5-CH=CH-CH_2-CO-S-ACP$$

<u>cis</u>-β,γ-(or $\Delta^{3,4}$)-decenoyl-S-ACP

3 malonyl-S-ACP

$$CH_3-(CH_2)_5-CH=CH-CH_2-(CH_2)_6-CO-S-ACP$$

Hexadecenoyl-S-ACP

substrate may be stearoyl-ACP, as in other systems.[107] Although the requirements of the *M. phlei* desaturase system are similar to those in other organisms, the exact mechanism of the reaction is not known.

The long-standing notion that mycobacteria do not produce polyenoic acids was found incorrect by Asselineau and her colleagues.[18, 20] From *M. phlei,* they isolated fatty acids with the general formula shown at the bottom of the page.

These "phleic acids" constitute a surprisingly high percentage (5 percent) of the total lipids and are found esterified to trehalose; therefore, they comprise their own series of acyltrehaloses. No related structures were recognized among the lipids of *M. tuberculosis* H37Rv or *M. bovis* BCG.

Recently Asselineau[21] addressed the problem of the biosynthesis of the phleic acids, since it was evident that none of the known pathways could

readily account for synthesis of a series of *cis* unsaturated bonds in 4-carbon units. The incorporation of specifically labeled fatty acids into the phleic acid skeleton revealed that palmitate is the precursor of phleic acids in which m = 14, and myristic acid is the direct precursor of phleic acids in which m = 12. Quite surprisingly, the unsaturated portion of the molecule derives from acetate. This probably is accomplished through preliminary condensation of two molecules into a 4-carbon unit (very likely crotonate), which would then be utilized in the elongation process (since crotonate is a vinylog of acetate), as shown in Figure 4–13.

Branched Acids

Mycobacteria produce a large variety of branched fatty acids.[66, 69] Studies by Campbell and Naworal revealed 24 nor-

---

$$CH_3-(CH_2)_m-(CH=CH-CH_2-CH_2)_n-COOH, \text{ where } m = 12 \text{ or } \underline{14}; \ n = 4, \underline{5} \text{ or } 6.$$

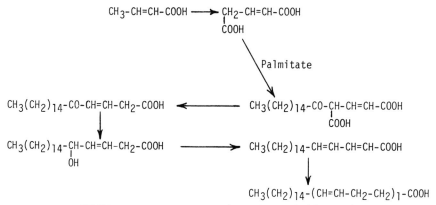

$CH_3-CH=CH-COOH \longrightarrow CH_2-CH=CH-COOH$
$\qquad\qquad\qquad\qquad\qquad\quad |$
$\qquad\qquad\qquad\qquad\qquad\;\; COOH$

Palmitate

$CH_3(CH_2)_{14}-CO-CH=CH-CH_2-COOH \longleftarrow CH_3(CH_2)_{14}-CO-CH-CH=CH-COOH$
$\qquad\qquad\qquad\qquad\qquad\qquad\qquad\qquad\qquad\qquad\qquad\qquad\qquad\qquad\quad |$
$\qquad\qquad\qquad\qquad\qquad\qquad\qquad\qquad\qquad\qquad\qquad\qquad\qquad\quad COOH$

$CH_3(CH_2)_{14}-CH-CH=CH-CH_2-COOH \longrightarrow CH_3(CH_2)_{14}-CH=CH-CH=CH-COOH$
$\qquad\qquad\qquad\quad |$
$\qquad\qquad\qquad\; OH$

$CH_3(CH_2)_{14}-(CH=CH-CH_2-CH_2)_1-COOH$

FIGURE 4–13. Biosynthesis of mycobacterial phleic acids.

mal and methyl-branched saturated acids in *M. phlei*. Iso- and ante-*iso*configurations were established by combined gas-liquid chromatography–mass spectrometry. From Campbell's analysis, the variety of iso- and ante-*iso*structures indicate that *M. phlei* has the ability to utilize leucine and isoleucine as "starters" in fatty acid biosynthesis; but *iso*butyrate is not incorporated into the fatty acids of *M. tuberculosis*

H37Rv. Biosynthesis probably proceeds by the mechanism outlined by Lennarz[229] for the synthesis of 12-methyltetradecanoic acid in *Micrococcus lysodeikticus* (Fig. 4–14). Other branched fatty acids in mycobacteria have one or more internal methyl branches. The principal members are tuberculostearic acid and the multi-branched phthienoic, mycocerosic, and phthioceranic acids (Fig. 4–15).

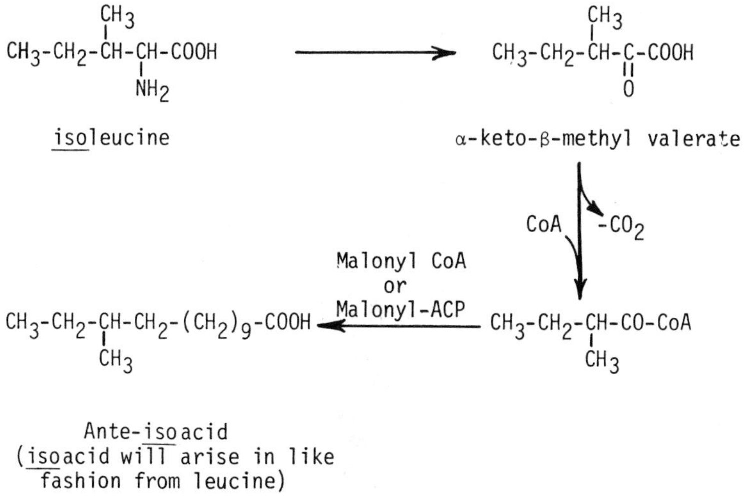

$$CH_3-CH_2-\overset{\overset{\textstyle CH_3}{|}}{CH}-\underset{\underset{\textstyle NH_2}{|}}{CH}-COOH \longrightarrow CH_3-CH_2-\overset{\overset{\textstyle CH_3}{|}}{CH}-\underset{\underset{\textstyle O}{\|}}{C}-COOH$$

isoleucine

α-keto-β-methyl valerate

CoA $\quad$ $-CO_2$

Malonyl CoA
or
$$CH_3-CH_2-\underset{\underset{\textstyle CH_3}{|}}{CH}-CH_2-(CH_2)_9-COOH \xleftarrow{\text{Malonyl-ACP}} CH_3-CH_2-\underset{\underset{\textstyle CH_3}{|}}{CH}-CO-CoA$$

Ante-iso acid
(iso acid will arise in like
fashion from leucine)

FIGURE 4–14. Possible route for synthesis of iso- and ante-*iso*fatty acids in mycobacteria.

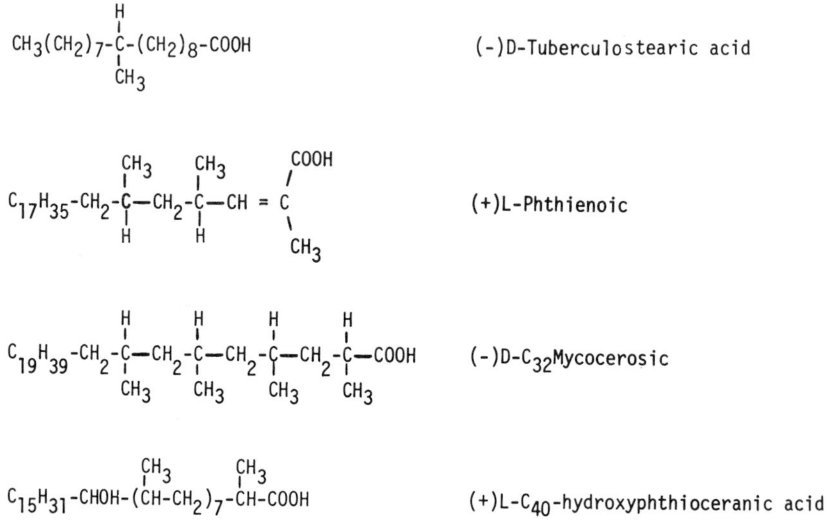

$$CH_3(CH_2)_7\text{-}\overset{\overset{\displaystyle H}{|}}{\underset{\underset{\displaystyle CH_3}{|}}{C}}\text{-}(CH_2)_8\text{-}COOH \qquad\qquad (-)D\text{-Tuberculostearic acid}$$

$$C_{17}H_{35}\text{-}CH_2\text{-}\overset{\overset{\displaystyle CH_3}{|}}{\underset{\underset{\displaystyle H}{|}}{C}}\text{-}CH_2\text{-}\overset{\overset{\displaystyle CH_3}{|}}{\underset{\underset{\displaystyle H}{|}}{C}}\text{-}CH=\overset{\overset{\displaystyle COOH}{\diagup}}{\underset{\underset{\displaystyle CH_3}{\diagdown}}{C}} \qquad\qquad (+)L\text{-Phthienoic}$$

$$C_{19}H_{39}\text{-}CH_2\text{-}\overset{\overset{\displaystyle H}{|}}{\underset{\underset{\displaystyle CH_3}{|}}{C}}\text{-}CH_2\text{-}\overset{\overset{\displaystyle H}{|}}{\underset{\underset{\displaystyle CH_3}{|}}{C}}\text{-}CH_2\text{-}\overset{\overset{\displaystyle H}{|}}{\underset{\underset{\displaystyle CH_3}{|}}{C}}\text{-}CH_2\text{-}\overset{\overset{\displaystyle H}{|}}{\underset{\underset{\displaystyle CH_3}{|}}{C}}\text{-}COOH \qquad (-)D\text{-}C_{32}\text{Mycocerosic}$$

$$C_{15}H_{31}\text{-}CHOH\text{-}(\overset{\overset{\displaystyle CH_3}{|}}{CH}\text{-}CH_2)_7\text{-}\overset{\overset{\displaystyle CH_3}{|}}{CH}\text{-}COOH \qquad\qquad (+)L\text{-}C_{40}\text{-hydroxyphthioceranic acid}$$

FIGURE 4–15.   Branched fatty acids of mycobacteria.

Chemistry and Biosynthesis of the O-Methylhexose-Containing Polysaccharides

Table 4–1 summarizes the elegant studies of Ballou and his associates on the O-methylhexose-containing poly-saccharides of mycobacteria. Most of these studies preceded recognition of the functions of the polysaccharides as regulators of fatty acid synthesis. The structures are presented in Figures 4–16 and 4–17, and the metabolic interrelations between the various forms of MGLP are depicted in Figure 4–18. According to Smith and Ballou,[327] a model of the 6-O-methylglucose lipopolysaccharide (MGLP) in a helical configuration reveals a hydrophilic side, with a high concentration of hydroxyl groups from the sugar moieties, and a lipophilic surface containing the acyl residues

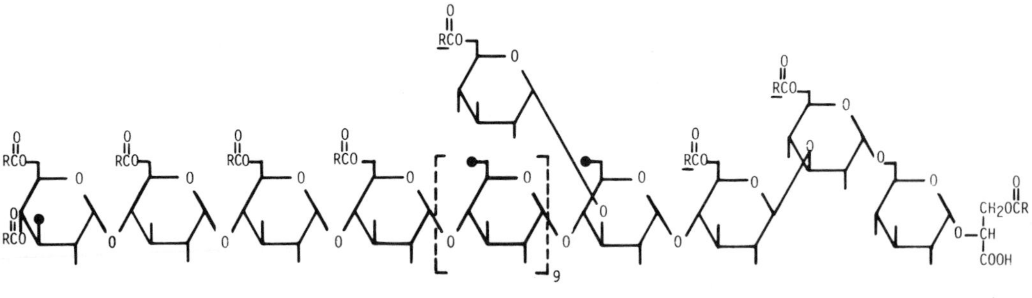

FIGURE 4–16.   Structure of MGLP-IV with six neutral acyl groups (R) and three succinyl groups (R). ●, Methyl ether substituents. (From Tung, K. K., and Ballou, C. E.: Biosynthesis of a mycobacterial lipopolysaccharide. Properties of a polysaccharide acyl CoA acyltransferase reaction. J. Biol. Chem. *248*:7126, 1973.)

TABLE 4–1.   The O-Methylhexose-Containing Polysaccharides of *Mycobacterium* sp.

Polysaccharide	Reference
6-O-Methylglucose-Containing Lipopolysaccharide (MGLP)	
First report of natural 6-O-methylglucose (6MeGlc). Saponification of MGLP from *M. phlei* (now identified as *M. smegmatis*) gave the polysaccharide (MPG), with a chain of at least seven 6MeGlc linked to 18 glucoses (Glc).	Lee and Ballou (1964)[225] Lee (1966)[224]
3-O-methylglucose (3MeGlc) recognized at nonreducing terminal and Glc(1 → 2) glyceric acid (GlyCOOH) at the reducing end. Reducing end identified as −Glc(α1 → 3)6MeGlc(α1 → 4)Glc(β1 → 3)Glc(α1 → 6)Glc(α1 → 2) GlyCOOH	Saier and Ballou (1968)[301] Saier and Ballou (1968)[302]
Complete structure for MGP.	Saier and Ballou (1968)[303] Ballou (1968)[35]
Intact MGLP from *M. smegmatis* resolved into four components. MGLP-I has no succinate; MGLP-II, -III, and -IV contain 1, 2, and 3 succinates, respectively. All MGLPs contain 3 acetates and 1 each of propionate, *iso*butyrate and octanoate.	Keller and Ballou (1968)[191]
Identical substances obtained from the cytosol of *M. tuberculosis*.	Lornitzo and Goldman (1968)[234] Saier and Ballou (1968)[301]
Some of the positions of acylation on MGP established by methyl replacement.	Gray and Ballou (1972)[151] Smith and Ballou (1973)[327]
6 MeGlc-nucleotides not involved in biosynthesis of MGLP; methylation probably occurs at polymer level via S-adenosyl-methionine. Partially acetylated oligosaccharides required for methylation. The degree of acetylation of oligosaccharides determines the amount and position of methylation.	Ferguson and Ballou (1970),[101] Grellert and Ballou (1972)[152]
A particulate enzyme transfers acyl groups to MGP or MGLP.	Tung and Ballou (1973)[361]
Metabolic turnover of acyl fragments examined: Monocarboxylic acids added before succinylation, and some of the former are added or exchanged after succinylation. See Figure 4–18 for the postulated exchange between the various MGLPs.	Narumi et al. (1973)[267]
3-O-Methylmannose-Containing Lipopolysaccharide (MMP)	
Discovered in *M. phlei* (now identified as *M. smegmatis*). 3-O-Methylmannose and mannose present. No acidic or basic functions.	Gray and Ballou (1971)[150]
Polysaccharide (PS) from the crude stimulating factor (SF) of *M. smegmatis* fatty acid synthetase recognized as having the same broad compositional features as MMP.	Ilton et al. (1971)[158]
MMP shown to be a mixture of at least four isomers (I–IV) with MW ranging from 2040 to 2480. All linear unbranched oligosaccharides with 11–14 3MeGlc units. For an example see Figure 4–17.	Maitra and Ballou (1977)[241]

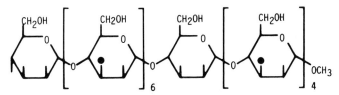

FIGURE 4–17.   Structure of MMP III, the member of the family of MMP molecules from *M. smegmatis* that possesses two unmethylated mannose units — one at the nonreducing end and the other at the middle of the chain. ●, methyl ether group. (From Maitra, S. K., and Ballou, C. E.: Heterogeneity and refined structures of 3-O-methyl-D-mannose polysaccharides from *Mycobacterium smegmatis*. J. Biol. Chem. 252:2459, 1977.)

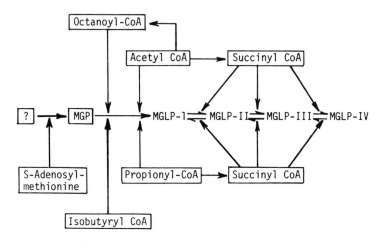

FIGURE 4–18. Possible metabolic interrelationships of the various mycobacterial MGLPs. (From Narumi, K., Keller, J. M., and Ballou, C. E.: Biosynthesis of a mycobacterial lipopolysaccharide: Incorporation of [14C]-acyl groups by whole cells *in vivo.* Biochem. J. *132*:329, 1973.)

and the methyl substituents from the 6-O-methyl sugars (Fig. 4–10). Apparently, this lipophilic surface complexes with the paraffin chains of the fatty acid analogs.[238] Smith and Ballou also inferred that the MGLPs may have a function in calcium ion transport, owing to the ability of the carboxylic groups of the glyceric acid and succinate to chelate metals.

Recently, Maitra and Ballou[241] proposed a conformation for the methylmannose lipopolysaccharide (MMP). The methyl groups of the 3-O-methylmannose moieties are arranged on one side of the molecule, thus providing a hydrophobic pocket that complexes with the fatty acid fragments; the other side presents a hydrophilic surface suitable for complexing with CoA. This type of arrangement would account for the fact that MMP readily complexes with palmitoyl CoA but not with palmitic acid. An alternative interpretation[48] is that MMP in solution assumes a helical conformation, which is analogous to the one for MGLP, with a hydrophobic channel that measures about 6 Å in diameter and approximately 29 Å long — dimensions appropriate for accommodating the paraffin chains of palmitoyl CoA in the form of

an inclusion complex. In order to explain the greater attraction of MMP for palmitoyl CoA as compared with palmitic acid, Bergeron and coworkers further postulate that ionized groups of the CoA moiety hydrogen bond to the hydrophilic exterior of the helical MMP. It is hoped that further study will clarify the mechanisms of these fascinating interactions.

ACYLGLYCEROLS AND ACYLHEXOSES

Lipids have several major functions to perform in mycobacterial physiology. They form an essential part of the cell wall and confer on mycobacteria their typical hydrophobic characteristics. Some may act as immunogens and antigens; they also can provide protective capsules and behave as phage receptor sites. The phosphoglycerides, in particular, are implicated in membrane structure and function; the acylglycerols act as storage compounds.

High levels of acylglycerols have long been recognized in mycobacteria,[23] but only recently have the effects of culture conditions on their synthesis, composition, and subcellular distribution been studied. Antoine and Tepper[12] confirmed earlier reports that glycerol-grown mycobacteria contained up to 23 percent lipid, as compared with about 14 percent for glucose-grown cells. Winder and Rooney[389] and Brennan and colleagues[59] drew attention to the vast amounts of triglyceride produced by glycerol-grown *M. tuberculosis* — up to 1 g of triglyceride per gram of cell N; i.e., perhaps 5 to 10 percent of the cell mass, when grown on Sauton medium containing 75 g of glycerol per liter. In a medium containing 0.5 percent glycerol and 0.5 percent glucose, about 5 percent of the dry cell weight is triglyceride.[247] Tween 80, which also is a common constituent of growth media, enhances the triglyceride content by providing metabolizable oleic acid.[378] The limiting of nitrogen in glycerol-grown *M. tuberculosis* enhances the production of lipid;[13] the majority of lipid that accumulates is probably triglyceride.

Walker and his colleagues[376] studied the identity and location of acyl substituents in mycobacterial triglycerides. In *M. bovis* BCG, position 1 of the triglyceride is occupied principally by C_{18}-related (stearic and oleic) fatty acids; in *M. smegmatis*, this position also contains more tuberculostearic acid. Position 2 is mostly esterified with C_{16}-related fatty acids, whereas the third position bears the higher C_{20} to C_{33} fatty acids.

Fat bodies (lipid vacuoles), which have been described in various mycobacteria, are probably the major repositories of cellular triglyceride (see Barksdale and Kim[40] for beautiful micrographs of these inclusions). Stimulation of the growth of *M. kansasii*, *M. marinum*, and *M. avium* with Tween 80, triolein, or other lipids induced the appearance of inclusion bodies,[312] resembling those described for *M. tuberculosis*[65] and *Corynebacterium*.[39] McCarthy[247] examined the uptake by *M. avium* of [^{14}C]-palmitate and reported that incorporation (largely into triglyceride) and degradation were very rapid. She concluded that triglyceride acted as a

source of energy for the actively growing cells as well as a means by *which free fatty acids were detoxified*. The high rate of triglyceride turnover described by Brennan and coworkers[59] also suggested that triglycerides were not simply metabolically stable storage compounds, a conclusion broadly compatible with McCarthy's observation.

In glucose-grown mycobacteria, fat bodies and triglycerides are virtually absent. Whereas triglycerides are ubiquitous in all lipid fractions of mycobacteria grown in glycerol medium, they are hardly detectable in the neutral lipids of glucose-grown *M. bovis* BCG, *M. smegmatis*, and *Corynebacterium diphtheriae*.[58, 59] Instead they were replaced to some degree by acylated glucoses (*iii*). For *M. bovis* the acyl group is a typical mycolic acid (see p. 94).

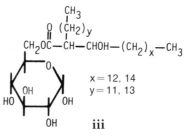

M. smegmatis x = 14 (70 percent) and 12 (30 percent); y = 13
M. diphtheriae x = 14; y = 13 (80 percent) and 11 (20 percent)
M. bovis has a large (C_{80}-type) mycoloyl substituent at the 6-position of glucose.

Conversely, when the medium glucose was replaced with glycerol, acylglucoses were meager. Owing to this reciprocity, analogous roles for both lipid classes may be implied. Indeed, Winder and coworkers[388] reported that acylated forms of glucose and the dimycoloyltrehalose of *M. smegmatis* turned over about 10 times per bacterial generation under conditions of active growth. Therefore, they are not very likely to be storage compounds. Still, despite their turnover rates, the relative paucity of the acyl sugars indicates that their metabolic role is, quantitatively, not a major one in the bacterial economy. Although the turnover of the fatty acid residues was not examined, it could have proved most informative since it now seems that 6-mycoloyl-6'-acetyltrehalose transfers mycolic acids to the cell wall of M. tuberculosis[337] (see p. 103).

Following reports of the effects of glucose on the lipids of mycobacteria, Suzuki and colleagues studied the influence of other sugars on the glycolipids of various Actinomycetales and other bacteria. With sucrose as a carbon source, two arthrobacteria, a corynebacterium, three nocardiae, and one brevibacterium (but not M. avium), produced characteristic mycoloyl glucosyl-β-fructosides.[334] When these bacteria as well as M. avium, "M. kode," and M. tuberculosis were grown on fructose, all produced a 6-O-mycoloylfructose and a 1,6-O-dimycoloylfructose.[163] The acyl substituents incorporated into the lipids characteristically reflected the genus; for example, the mycobacterial glycolipids showed pyrolysis patterns characteristic of the larger mycolic acids. Little physiologic import can be gleaned from these rather novel observations, but they demonstrate that the sugar or polyol component of neutral glycolipids may exhibit wide variability, depending on the major carbon source in the medium. This may be equally relevant when considering the influence of nutrients provided in the intracellular milieu in infection.

PHOSPHOLIPIDS
General Description

Besides the phosphatidylinositol mannosides, the principal mycobacterial phospholipids are cardiolipin (CL or bis-phosphatidylglycerol) (iv), phosphatidylethanolamine (PE) (v), and phosphatidylinositol (PI) (vi). See bottom of this page and top of opposite page.

Phosphatidylcholine (lecithin) is absent, and phosphatidylglycerol, phosphatidylserine, and lysophosphatidylethanolamine occur in small amounts. The phosphonic analogue of PE presumably exists in M. tuberculosis, since 2-aminoethylphosphonic acid has been identified.[306]

Palmitic ($C_{16:0}$), hexadecenoic ($C_{16:1}$), octadecenoic (or oleic, $C_{18:1}$) and tuberculostearic ($C_{19,br}$) are the major fatty acid constituents of mycobacterial phospholipids.[278] Table 4–2 summarizes the positional distribution of specific acyl functions in both phosphoglycerides and triacylglycerides.[376] Palmitic and tuberculostearic acids compromise about 90 percent of the phosphoinositide fatty acids,[54, 279] with tuberculostearic acid occurring only at the 1 position.[376] Cardiolipin is distinguished by considerable amounts of $C_{16:1}$ at the 2 position, and $C_{18:1}$ at the 1 position. In fatty acid composition, similarities between phospholipids and neutral lipids are not unexpected since

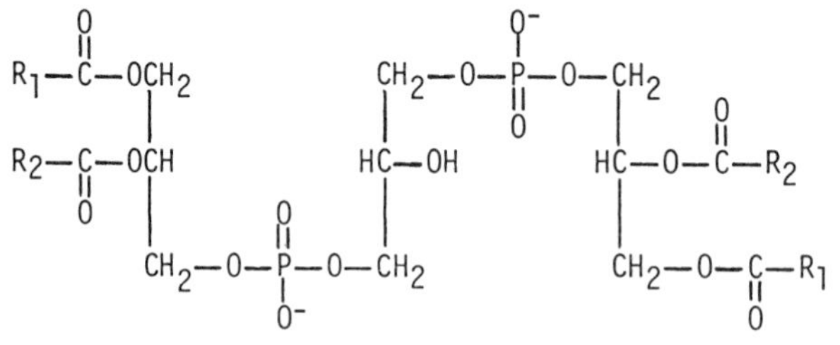

Cardiolipin (CL)

iv

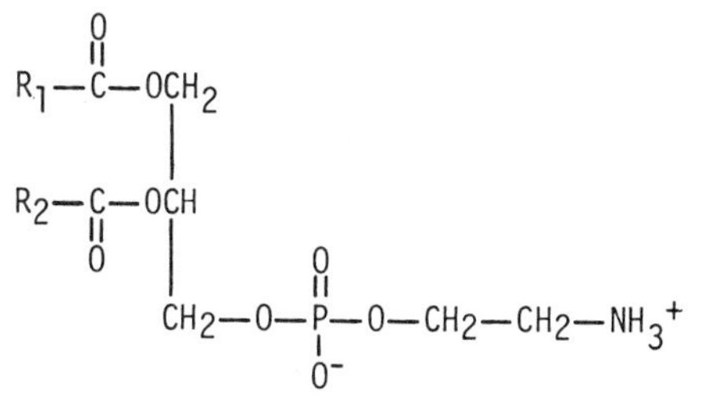

Phosphatidylethanolamine (PE)

v

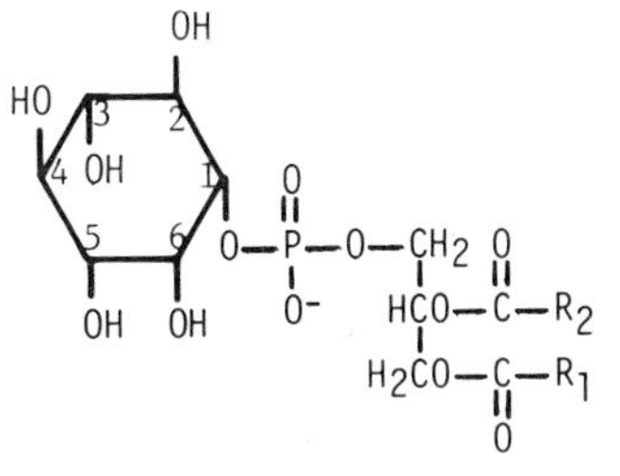

Phosphatidylinositol (PI)

vi

they are synthesized through the common precursor, phosphatidic acid. Table 4-3 summarizes the subcellular distribution of the phospholipids in mycobacteria.[8] These results are generally in accord with other data obtained by several investigators.[264, 275]

Transalkylation

Intact phospholipids of mycobacteria play an essential role in enzymatic transalkylation reactions. Tuberculostearic acid is synthesized from oleic acid.[231] According to Akamatsu and Law,[6, 7] the oleic acid must be esterified to a phospholipid (Fig. 4-19). The first step involves transfer of a methyl group from S-adenosylmethionine to the double bond of oleylphosphatidylethanolamine, apparently mediated through a membrane-associated enzyme. An intricate sequence of events embracing the reacting centers is then involved in the transformation of oleic to tuberculostearic acid.[61, 164, 228]

To accommodate the synthesis of the great variety of internally methyl-branched fatty acid homologues related to tuberculostearic acid, Campbell and Naworal[67] invoked a methyl transferase, operating principally at oleic acid but handling a few closely related materials in a limited fashion. The higher homologs of tuberculostearic acid very likely arise from chain elongation of the 10-methyloctadecanoate.

Structures of the Phosphatidylinositol Mannosides (Mannophosphoinositides)

Anderson in 1938 isolated from human tubercle bacilli a "phosphatide" fraction, which on hydrolysis with dilute acid yielded glycerophosphoric acid, mannose, and the hexahydric alcohol, "inosite." Alkaline saponification of the phosphatides yielded a

TABLE 4-2. Fatty Acid Location in Mycobacterial Phosphoglycerides and Triacylglycerides

	M. bovis BCG		M. smegmatis	
Position	TRIGLYCERIDES	PHOSPHOLIPIDS	TRIGLYCERIDES	PHOSPHOLIPIDS
1	18:1, 18:0, 16:0	18:0, 18:1, 19 Br	18:0, 18:1, 19 Br	18:0, 18:1, 19 Br
2	16:0, 18:0	16:1, 16:0	16:0, 16:1[a]	16:0, 16:1[a]
3[b]	20–33		20–26	

[a] In CL, 16:1 is the major component.
[b] Compare with Brennan et al.[59]

TABLE 4–3   Subcellular Phospholipid Composition

Fraction	Probable Identity	Phospholipid Composition (Percent of total PL)		
		CL	PIM_x	PE
A	Wall	33.5	59.5	7.0
B	Wall	37.3	53.3	9.4
C	Membrane	52.6	36.8	10.4
D	Membrane	51.7	38.6	9.8
E	Ribosome/membrane	52.9	37.9	9.2
Whole cells		50.8	40.2	9.0

Key to abbreviations: PL, phospholipid; CL, cardiolipin; PIM_x, phosphatidylinositol monomannosides and oligomannosides; and PE, phosphatidylethanolamine.

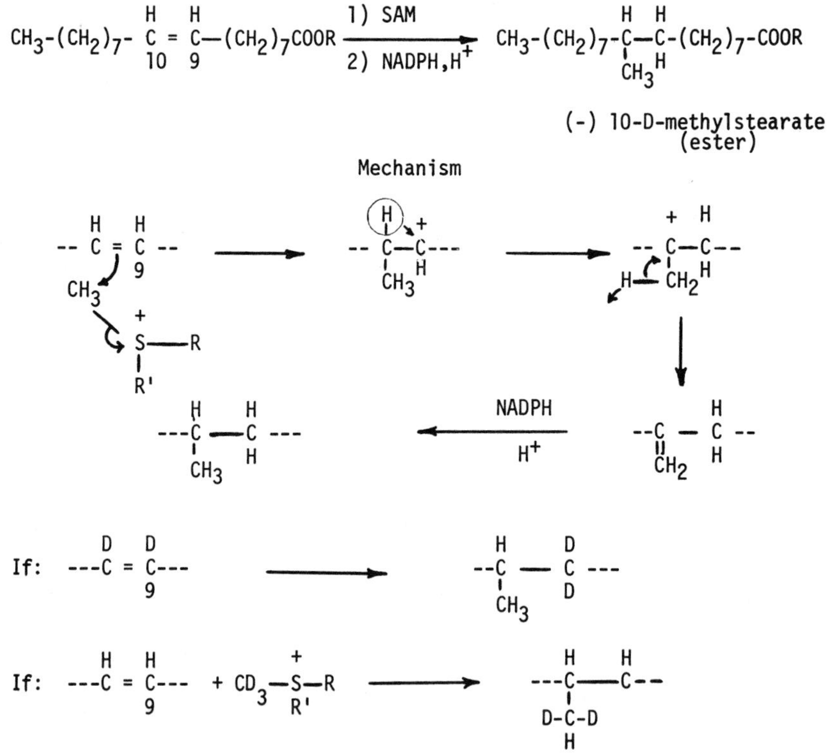

FIGURE 4–19.   Tuberculostearic acid, showing methylation of oleic acid. (From Goren, M. B.: Mycobacterial lipids. Selected topics. Bacteriol. Rev. *36*:33, 1972.)

"phosphorus-containing glycoside," which on dephosphorylation with dilute ammonia at 170 to 180° produced a "mannoinositose," containing mannose and inositol in the proportion of 2:1. Using the same approach 25 years later, Lee and Ballou[226] arrived at the complete structure (*vii*) of phosphatidylinositol dimannoside (PIM$_2$) from *M. tuberculosis* and *M. phlei*.

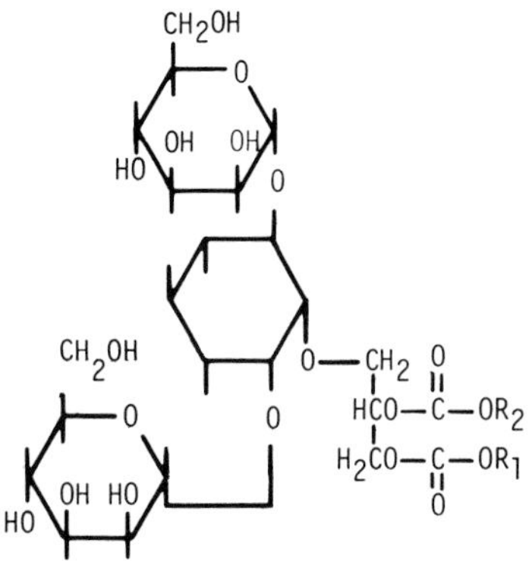

Phosphatidylinositol dimannoside (PIM$_2$)

vii

They showed in an elegant demonstration of the utility and sophistication of NMR spectrometry that the mannoses were attached glycosidically to positions 2 and 6 of the myoinositol ring.

The glycolipid was named 1-phosphatidyl-L-myoinositol 2, 6-di-O-α-D-mannopyranoside, which we shall abbreviate as:

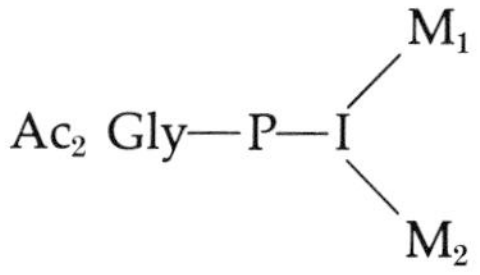

$$\text{Ac}_2\ \text{Gly—P—I}\begin{array}{c} \diagup\ M_1 \\ \diagdown\ M_2 \end{array}$$

Previously, Ballou and coworkers[38] had shown that the glycerol phosphate moiety was attached to the L-1 position of the myoinositol ring, thereby establishing the stereochemical identity of the phosphatidylinositol (PI) with corresponding substances from plant and animal sources.

Direct evidence for the existence of a phosphatidylmyoinositol pentamannoside (PIM$_5$) had been reported by Nojima[269] and by Ballou and colleagues.[38] Its structure (*viii*), shown below, was elucidated in a classic series of studies by Lee and Ballou.[227] Tetra- and trimannosides (PIM$_4$ and PIM$_3$) are also known and differ from the pentamannoside in lacking, respectively, one and two terminal mannoses in the tetrasaccharide chain. In addition, an inositol hexamannoside was isolated from *M. phlei* phospholipids. This has an addi-

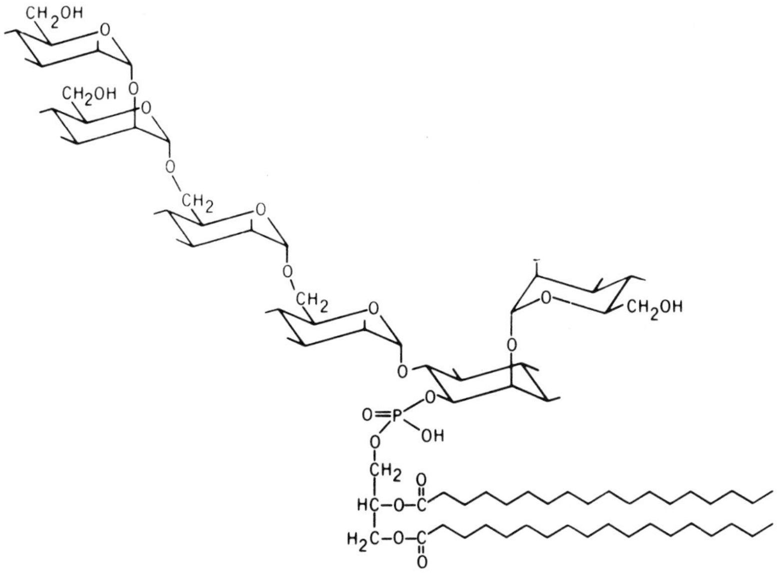

viii

tional α-1,2'-linked mannose at the end of the tetrasaccharide chain.

The status of phosphatidylmyoinositol monomannoside (abbreviated PIM$_1$

or Ac$_2$Gly—P—I$\overset{\diagup M_1}{}$) in Mycobacterium and in related actinomycetes has been controversial; however, its presence in these is certain.[38, 364] Ballou and Lee[37] proved that the mannose was attached to the 2-hydroxyl group of the myoinositol ring (ix).

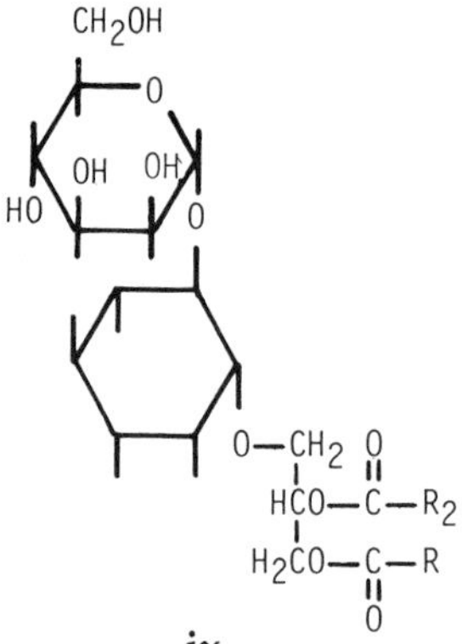

CH$_2$OH

ix

Phosphatidyl inositol monomannoside (PIM$_1$)

However, there is obviously little present in the majority of mycobacteria. (For a summary of evidence for the monomannoside distribution in mycobacteria and other genera, see Khuller and Brennan[195].)

The extensive structural studies of Ballou and colleagues were conducted on the deacylated glycophospholipids,

(abbreviated Gly—P—I$\overset{\diagup M_1}{\underset{\diagdown M_x}{}}$). It was assumed that the parent lipids were simple phosphatidyl derivatives with no acyl substituents beyond those on the glyceryl moiety. The parent substance, phosphatidylinositol, has the structure, Ac$_2$—Gly—P—I. It was surprising, therefore, when Pangborn and McKinney[279] isolated from M. tuberculo-

sis a series of phosphatidylinositol dimannosides (PIM$_2$s) containing a total of two, three, and four acyl residues. Brennan and Ballou[54] also found that ^{14}C-mannose from GDP-[^{14}C]-mannose was incorporated by cell-free extracts of M. phlei into three mannophospholipids that all yielded, upon saponification, the deacylated dimannoside,

Gly—P—I$\overset{\diagup M_1}{\underset{\diagdown M_1}{}}$. The intact lipids were isolated, characterized, and shown to be similar to three of the products described by Pangborn and McKinney.[279] They are almost certainly a diacyl- and a monoacyl-PIM$_2$—i.e., products with a total of four and three acyl groups respectively, as well as the simpler phosphatidylinositol dimannoside. The positions of the "extra" acyl groups are not known, but one is probably on the 6 position of a mannose residue.[55] Pangborn and McKinney[279] also described presumed mono- and diacyl phosphatidylinositol pentamannosides:

$$\left[Ac_2\text{—Gly—P—I}\overset{\diagup M_1}{\underset{\diagdown M_4}{}} \right\} Ac_{1\ or\ 2} \right]$$

Biosynthesis of Phosphatidylinositol Mannosides

Considerable effort has been devoted to the study of biosynthesis of phosphatidylinositol mannosides, but a number of major unresolved questions still remain. Ballou[36] has summarized the work accomplished in his laboratory. The probable biosynthesis of the various acylated phosphatidylinositol dimannosides is summarized in Figure 4–20.

Of several possible nucleoside diphosphate-mannoses, the guanosine analog, GDP-mannose, was the most effective donor of mannose for the synthesis of PIM$_x$ by a particulate fraction

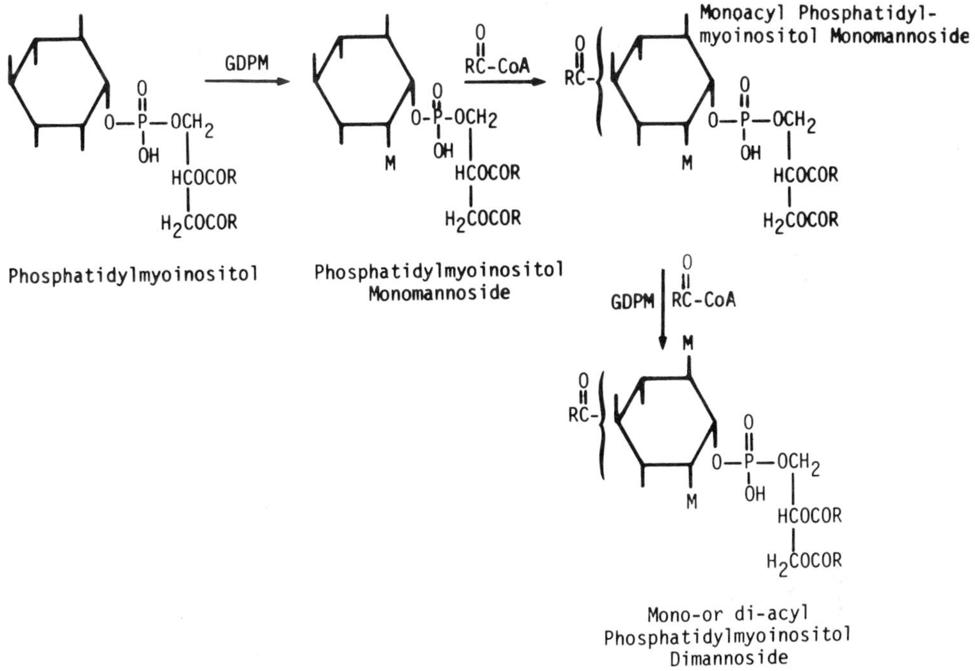

FIGURE 4–20. Proposed biosynthesis of mycobacterial dimannophosphoinositides. (Adapted from Brennan, P. J., and Ballou, C. E.: Biosynthesis of mannophosphoinositides by *Mycobacterium phlei*–enzymatic acylation of the dimannophosphoinositides. J. Biol. Chem. 242:3246, 1967.)

of *M. phlei*.[155] The major products of the reaction were PIM$_2$ and its mono- and diacylated forms, abbreviated[54]:

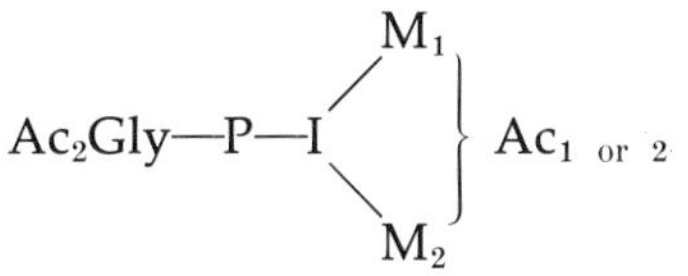

$$\text{Ac}_2\text{Gly—P—I} \begin{cases} \text{M}_1 \\ \text{M}_2 \end{cases} \text{Ac}_{1 \text{ or } 2}$$

Although the first mannosylation step was not demonstrable, it was presumed for several reasons that phosphatidyl inositol is nevertheless the primary receptor of mannose: exogenous PI greatly stimulated the reaction in *M. phlei*; in *P. shermanii*, where only PIM$_1$ is synthesized, added PI enhanced its synthesis by a factor of five;[56] in *C. aquaticum*, where a PIM$_1$ is the only obvious mannophospholipid in stationary phase cells, pulse chase experiments with ^{32}P$_i$ supported the sequence PI → PIM$_1$.[153]

Takayama and Goldman[340] noted that in a cell-free system from *M. tuberculo-*

sis, in which *endogenous* lipid acceptors and GDP-^{14}C-mannose were used, both PIM$_1$ and PIM$_2$ were synthesized. However, enzymatic degradation of the PIM$_2$ showed that only the mannose attached to the *6 position* of the inositol ring was radioactive. The data were interpreted to indicate that two reactions were taking place — one for the synthesis of PIM$_1$* from PI, the other for the independent synthesis of PIM$_2$; however, the monomannoside product of the first reaction does not serve as a substrate for the second mannosylation step:

$$\text{GDPM* + PI} \longrightarrow \text{P—I}^{(2 \rightarrow 1)} \text{M*}$$

$$\text{GDPM* + (endogenous} \rightarrow \text{P—I}^{(2 \rightarrow 1)} \text{M}$$
$$\text{acceptor)}$$

$$\text{M*} = [1\text{-}^{14}\text{C}]\text{mannose}$$

$$\begin{array}{c} 6 \\ \downarrow \\ 1 \\ \text{M*} \end{array}$$

The simplest explanation for this behavior is that some preformed PIM_1 must be endogenous in the cell-free extract. This PIM_1 is structurally distinct from the PIM_1* arising in the first reaction, since it is a more efficient substrate for the second mannosylation step. The disparate activities of the two PIMs may be due to differences in degree of acylation (refer to Figure 4–20). It is probable that de novo PIM_1* corresponds to the $Ac_2Gly—P—I \overset{M_1^*}{\diagup}$, and endogenous PIM_1 corresponds to the *monacyl* phosphatidylinositol monomannoside, $Ac_2Gly—P—I \overset{M_1—Ac}{\diagup}$, as shown in Figure 4–20.

The deluge of papers on the distribution of individual phosphatidylinositol mannosides in species of *Mycobacterium* and in other genera reveals the conflicting notions on the nature of the mannosides prominent in a given organism. Hackett and Brennan[153] have demonstrated (in *Corynebacterium*) how strikingly the mannophosphoinositide composition changes during the course of growth. They reported that dimannosides and trimannosides together constituted about 70 percent of the very early-phase products, and in later exponential phase, they were the only ones present. In early stationary phase, *tetramannosides* increased to comprise about 50 percent of the phosphoinositides; PI, present in only low amounts until this point, increased to comprise the other 50 percent. Finally, in late stationary phase, PIM_1 (meager throughout the earlier processes) became the major component (88 percent).

To account for some of the dynamic fluctuations, the authors suggest that in the final stages, the bulk of PIM_1 is achieved by catabolism at the expense of higher mannophosphoinositides. The unique structure of PIM_1 (mannose at the 2 position of the inositol) may make it the likely end-product of a series of degradative steps; except for

PIM_1, all of the higher mannophosphoinositides have the extra mannosyl groups attached to the 6 position. The structure of PIM_1 may therefore ensure stability to further degradation, and this might account for its prominence during the stationary phase.

Mannosyl - Phosphoryl - Polyisoprenols. Evidently stimulated by the surge of interest during the late 1960s concerning the role of glycosyl-phosphoryl-polyisoprenols as carriers for carbohydrates in bacterial polymer biosynthesis, Takayama and Goldman[341] sought such substances in mycobacteria. Thus, in *M. tuberculosis* H37Ra, a surprising 60 percent of lipid-bound ^{14}C-mannose from a cell-free synthesis system was found in the form of two mannosyl-phosphoryl-polyprenols. Similar products were shown to accumulate in the cell-free system of *M. smegmatis*.[336] In a most impressive paper, Takayama and coworkers[344] described the structures of these substances as obtained from *M. smegmatis*. Mass spectral analysis of one of the lipids, and the products of its reduction, ozonolysis, and epoxidation revealed the structure to be a mannosyl-1-phosphoryl-octahydroheptaprenol. The second lipid was characterized as the ubiquitous mannosyl-1-phosphoryl-decaprenol (x). Mycobacteria

$$[\text{Mannose}]-0-\text{PO}_3-[\text{CH}_2-\text{CH}=\overset{\overset{\displaystyle CH_3}{|}}{\text{C}}-\text{CH}_2]_9-\text{CH}_2-\text{CH}=\overset{\overset{\displaystyle CH_3}{|}}{\text{C}}-\text{CH}_3$$

x

are apparently unique in containing these two different polyisoprenol lipids.

Schultz and Elbein[315] essentially corroborated Takayama's findings; they also discerned a glucose-containing analog in *M. smegmatis*. Significantly, they found that a particulate enzyme system can synthesize mannose-containing oligosaccharides linked (presumably) to polyisoprenol and speculated that these lipopolysaccharides may be involved in

$$x \text{ GDP-Mannose} + \text{Phosphorylpolyprenol} \longrightarrow (\text{Mannose})_x\text{-Phosphoryl-Polyprenol}$$

$$(\text{Mannose})_x\text{-Phosphoryl-Polyprenol} \xrightarrow{\text{Protein}} \text{Glycoprotein}$$

$$(\text{Arabinomannan-protein?})$$

FIGURE 4–21. Postulated role of mycobacterial mannosylpolyprenols in cell wall proteoglycan synthesis.

the synthesis of mycobacterial cell wall arabinomannans.

Takayama and Armstrong[336] correctly pointed out that the scheme proposed by Brennan and Ballou[55] for phosphatidylinositol mannoside biosynthesis accounted for only the multiacylated PIM$_2$ and did not explain the synthesis of the higher homologs. Based on the surprising abundance of mannosyl polyprenols, Takayama and colleagues suggested that they may be implicated in mannoinositide synthesis — a view that has also been embraced by Ratledge.[290] However, K. Takayama has kindly informed us that so far his efforts to implicate polyprenol mannose in PIM$_x$ synthesis have been fruitless. Perhaps a more fascinating role that has been postulated for mycobacterial glycosylpolyprenols is in the biosynthesis of cell wall proteoglycan material (Fig. 4–21), since polyprenol carriers are now well recognized as essential in the biosynthesis of certain types of eukaryotic glycoproteins.[230]

Phospholipids — Functions and Activities

In experiments in which the subcellular fractions were carefully characterized, Akamatsu and colleagues[8] showed the protoplasmic fraction of *M. phlei* to have the highest content of phospholipids. The composition clearly resembled that found in whole cells. Thus, these lipids presumably fulfill the usual structural and functional roles shared by most bacterial protoplasmic phosphoglycerides. The phosphatidylinositol mannosides may be an exception in this respect, since they were concentrated mostly in cell wall fragments.[8, 130] Although no specific cellular function has been attributed to the phosphatidylinositol mannosides, their peripheral location and structural similarity to other bacterial glycophospholipids may provide some clues.

In membrane-associated teichoic acids of several gram-positive bacteria, the glycerophosphate backbone is covalently linked to either membranous glycolipid or to a phosphoglycolipid, e.g., to the phosphatidyldiglucosyl diglyceride (*xi*).[322]

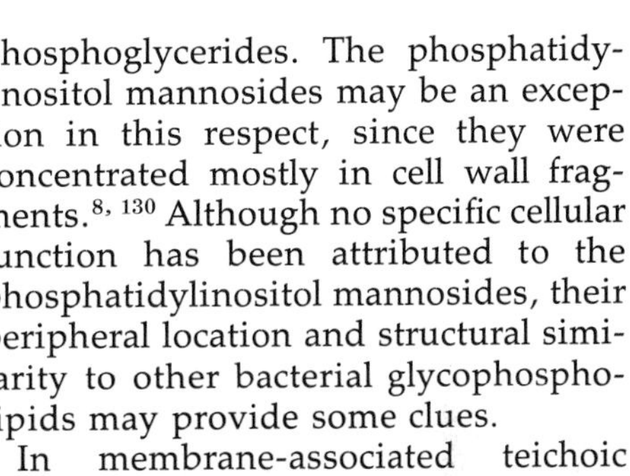

Phosphatidyldiglucosyl diglyceride from *Streptococcus faecalis*

xi

They may therefore serve to anchor the teichoic acid polymer to the membrane. The possibility that some of the phosphatidylinositol mannosides may be similarly attached to mycobacterial cell wall polymers and share a related function has not been explored, but this theory seems attractive. A role in which the mannophosphoinositides act as linkages (mostly noncovalent) between the cytoplasmic membrane and the cell wall could help explain their dual location and the greater concentration of the higher homologs in the cell wall.

Biologic Activities

The phospholipids are alleged to be among the most active antigenic substances elaborated by tubercle bacilli. Some 50 years ago, Boquet and Nègre prepared a methanol extract of *M. tuberculosis* designated "antigène méthylique." The somewhat modest protective and salutary effects of immunization with this antigen have been documented in several studies (for an early review, see Crowle[81]). The rigorously purified phospholipids have been judged to act merely as haptens, retaining serologic activity but not stimulating antibody formation. Pigretti and colleagues[282] found an immunologically active preparation to be separable into at least five components. Cord factor and several PIM_x species were identified among those components. None of these individually was active in protecting mice against challenge with virulent tubercle bacilli, but the activity seen in the original extract was largely restored on recombining the fractions. According to Khuller and Subrahmanyam,[196] PIM_x stimulates humoral antibodies in rabbits when administered in Freund's incomplete adjuvant either alone or in complex with methylated bovine serum albumin (MBSA). Precipitating, agglutinating, and complement-fixing antibody, resembling that recognized in human tuberculosis serum, was characterized.

Practical utilization of the antigenic properties of the phospholipids seems to rest for the present in their application to serologic diagnosis. Pangborn and McKinney[279] showed that certain combinations of dimannosides, with the pentamannosides, fixed-complement with human sera from cases

of tuberculosis. The higher phosphatidylinositol mannosides (including the hexamannoside) are also probably the most active sensitizing components of the Takahashi antigen.[307]

Motomiya and coworkers[264] found that the cardiolipin that is recoverable from various strains of mycobacteria behaves like beef heart CL in reacting with the Wasserman antibody "reagin" of syphilitic serum.

The haptenic qualities of other phosphatides are enhanced to antigenicity by combining them with lecithin and cholesterol and complexing the whole with methylated BSA.[270] With a phosphatidylinositol complex, the antiserum produced in rabbits was specific for inositol. Although lecithin was essential, digestion of the complex with phospholipase-C did not destroy the antigenicity until more than 97 percent of the phosphoryl choline had been lysed. The diglyceride so formed maintained the complex in its appropriate immunogenic conformation; nevertheless, diglyceride itself was incapable of combining with phosphatide and cholesterol to generate the complex de novo.

MYCOLIC ACIDS

No other group of substances isolated from mycobacteria has stimulated so much work as the mycolic acids; an extensive literature relating to the structural studies has been critically reviewed. (For appropriate references, see Lederer[220] and Goren[136].)

The mycolic acids are β-hydroxy acids substituted at the α-position with a moderately long aliphatic chain. Substances of this type are elaborated by all mycobacteria and by *Nocardia* and *Corynebacterium* as well, each producing several characteristic types. The structure of the simplest — corynomycolic acid — was established by Lederer and Pudles, and it was synthesized by a simple series of reactions,

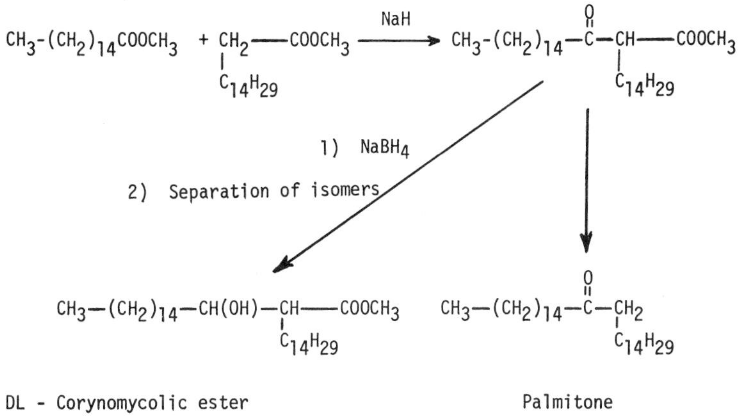

FIGURE 4–22. Synthesis of corynomycolic ester.

which in fact anticipated the biosynthetic sequences (Fig. 4–22).

The mycolic acids (and their esters) undergo a characteristic cleavage reaction on pyrolysis, essentially a reversal of a Claisen-type condensation reaction (Fig. 4–23); as a typical example, a methyl mycolate from human strains would give a nonvolatile "meroaldehyde" and *n*-hexacosanoic acid methyl ester. (The term meromycolic acid — "part mycolic acid" — was proposed by Polgar, and the corresponding aldehydes were designated meroaldehydes by Etemadi.) Mycolic acids of avian and saprophytic strains have a C_{22} side chain and yield tetracosanoic acid as the pyrolysis product.

From the estimated empirical formulas of the mycolic acids of *M. tuberculosis* (about 88 carbons) and the prominence of palmitic, stearic, and hexacosanoic acids in the species, the persuasive thesis was advanced that mycolic acid biosynthesis may proceed by appropriate Claisen-type condensations and reductions, of 2 moles each of stearic and hexacosanoic acids to give a C_{88} condensation product (*xii*, Fig. 4–24). Indeed, much experimental evidence could be marshalled in support of this very attractive biosynthetic scheme that appeared capable of embracing essentially all of the known types of mycolic acids (containing ketonic, hydroxyl, methoxy, or unsaturated functions). However, contradictory evidence from physical and chemical studies could not be reconciled with these proposed structures, and they were ultimately abandoned.

Mycolic Acid Structures

Essentially the entire structural spectrum of mycolic acids was resolved in a brilliant series of investigations by A. Etemadi (in Lederer's group), N. Pol-

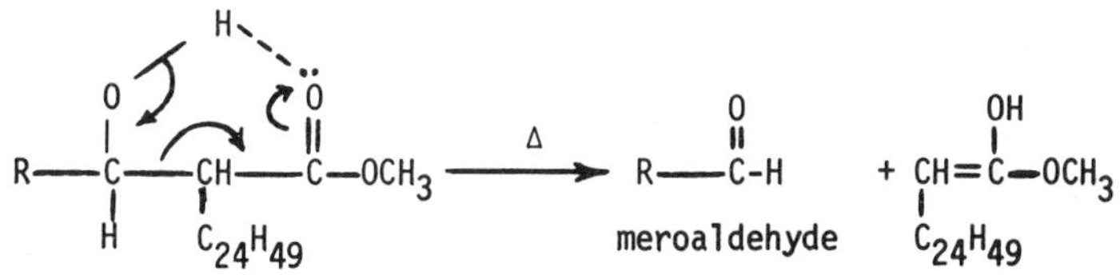

FIGURE 4–23. Pyrolysis of a methyl mycolate.

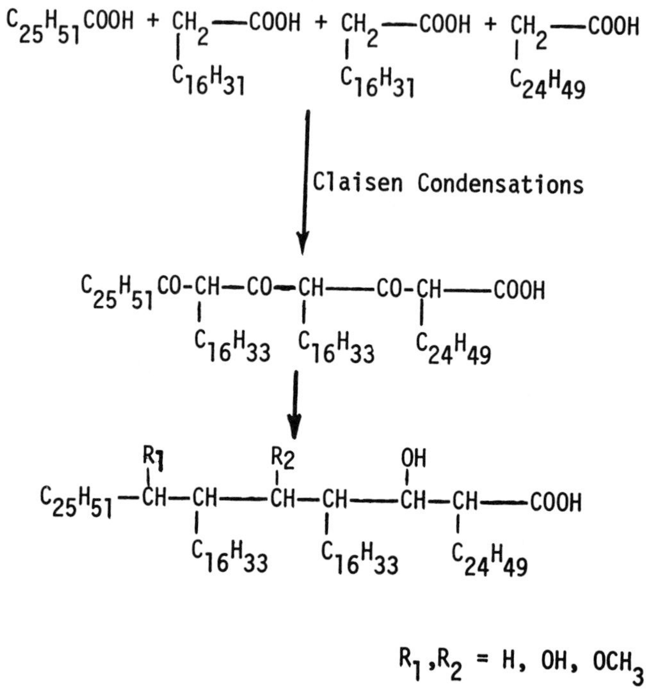

$$C_{25}H_{51}COOH + \underset{\underset{C_{16}H_{31}}{|}}{CH_2}—COOH + \underset{\underset{C_{16}H_{31}}{|}}{CH_2}—COOH + \underset{\underset{C_{24}H_{49}}{|}}{CH_2}—COOH$$

Claisen Condensations

$$C_{25}H_{51}CO-\underset{\underset{C_{16}H_{33}}{|}}{CH}—CO—\underset{\underset{C_{16}H_{33}}{|}}{CH}——CO-\underset{\underset{C_{24}H_{49}}{|}}{CH}——COOH$$

$$C_{25}H_{51}—\underset{\underset{C_{16}H_{33}}{|}}{\overset{\overset{R_1}{|}}{CH}}—CH——\underset{\underset{C_{16}H_{33}}{|}}{\overset{\overset{R_2}{|}}{CH}}—CH——\underset{\underset{C_{24}H_{49}}{|}}{\overset{\overset{OH}{|}}{CH}}—CH——COOH \qquad xii$$

$$R_1, R_2 = H, OH, OCH_3$$

FIGURE 4–24.   Mycolic acids—early postulates of structure and biogenesis. (From Goren, M. B.: Myco-bacterial lipids: Selected topics. Bacteriol. Rev. *36*:33, 1972.)

gar's group, and the Asselineaus' group through utilization of the most discriminating features of instrumentation: IR, NMR, and mass spectrometry. Preparative pyrolysis of the "homogeneous" samples of mycolates obtained from column and preparative thin-layer chromatography provided the meroaldehydes in whose structural elucidation resided the entire key to the structures of the mycolic acids. The α-branch, except for length, is essentially invariant in any group of mycolic acids. Any interesting functional changes are almost always found in the *mero* portion: methoxyl, keto, lone methyl branches, ethylenic, and cyclopropanoid groups.

Structural Features Clarified with NMR Spectrometry

An early resolution was achieved regarding the (controversial) multi-branched structure (*xii*) inherent in the biogenetic scheme shown in Figure 4–24. The meroaldehyde (*xiii*) generated from a pyrolysis of such a compound would have a C_{16} alkyl branch α to the aldehyde function. This possibility was eliminated from an examination of the NMR spectrum of the meroaldehyde: the single aldehyde proton (solid arrow) gave a resonance peak at 585 hertz (Hz). This was clearly a *triplet*, indicating the adjacent carbon to have

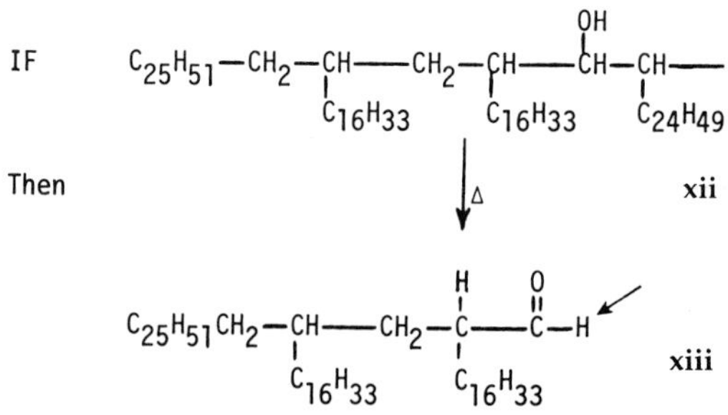

IF $$C_{25}H_{51}—CH_2—\underset{\underset{C_{16}H_{33}}{|}}{CH}——CH_2—\underset{\underset{C_{16}H_{33}}{|}}{CH}——\underset{\underset{C_{24}H_{49}}{|}}{\overset{\overset{OH}{|}}{CH}}—CH——$$

Then   xii

$$C_{25}H_{51}CH_2—\underset{\underset{C_{16}H_{33}}{|}}{CH}——CH_2—\underset{\underset{C_{16}H_{33}}{|}}{\overset{\overset{H}{|}}{C}}——\overset{\overset{O}{||}}{C}—H$$

xiii

two hydrogens. A doublet would have been obtained if a branch and a lone hydrogen (broken arrow) were present. (The splitting of the band arises from coupling interactions with protons on adjacent atoms; the multiplicity is $n + 1$, where n is the number of such protons. Chemical shifts throughout this section are described relative to tetramethyl silane for an instrument operating at 60 mHz.) A triplet signal at 395 to 409 Hz in the NMR spectrum of anhydromycolic acid (*xiv*), attributed to the single hydrogen on the β carbon, similarly proved the γ carbon as bearing two hydrogens rather than being branched.

from in vivo-grown tubercle bacilli is depicted in Figure 4–25. The relevant absorption bands are indicated by arrows.

The carbonyl ester absorption band, ordinarily located at about 1740 cm^{-1}, is seen in the mycolic esters as a split band whose principal peak is at about 1720 cm^{-1} — an effect attributable to intramolecular hydrogen bonding between the carbonyl group and the β-hydroxyl. In high-resolution IR spectrometry, this interaction is also revealed in the relative contributions of free and bonded OH imposed by the stereochemistry at the α- and β-carbons and reflected in the IR absorptions at 3626 cm^{-1} and 3534 cm^{-1}, respectively. C. Asselineau and coworkers[17] concluded from a study of six mycolic acids (a nocardomycolic, a corynomycolic, and four derived from mycobacteria) that these are all 2R, 3R configurations. Newman and "saw horse" projections are depicted in Figure 4–26; in the 2R, 3R configuration, the long alkyl chains eclipse only hydrogen atoms when the ester carbonyl and β-hydroxyl are H-bonded.

Cyclopropane substituents are correlated with the absorption band in the region 1,025 cm^{-1}. A band at 3,060 cm^{-1} has been assigned to the cyclopropane methylene group whose intensity accords with the number (one or two) of cyclopropane rings. These are also indi-

$$\text{\Large$\wedge\!\wedge\!\wedge$}\!-\!\overset{\gamma}{C}H_2\!-\!\overset{\beta}{C}H\!=\!C\!\!\begin{array}{l}\nearrow COOH \\ \\ \searrow C_{24}H_{49}\end{array}$$

xiv

Combined IR-NMR Spectrometry: Structure and Stereochemistry

A representative IR spectrum of partially purified methyl mycolates

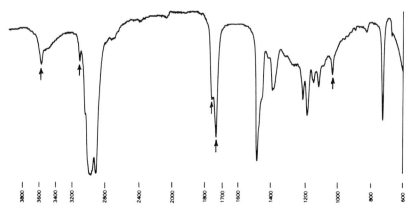

FIGURE 4–25. Infrared spectrum of methyl mycolates obtained from *M. tuberculosis* that was harvested from lungs of infected mice. (From Goren, M. B.: Mycobacterial lipids: Selected topics. Bacteriol. Rev. 36:33, 1972.)

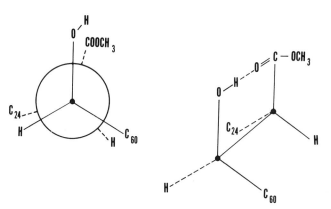

FIGURE 4–26. Newman and "saw-horse" projection of methyl mycolate, indicating the stereochemistry at the α and β carbons and the intramolecular hydrogen bonding. (From Goren, M. B.: Mycobacterial lipids: Selected topics. Bacteriol. Rev. 36:33, 1972.)

cated by NMR signals at +35 and −18 Hz.[117]

Structures of α-Smegmamycolic Acids

Mycolic acids of *M. smegmatis* were among the first to be most nearly characterized as a result of structural features (unsaturation), which simplified a direct chemical attack. This laid the groundwork for subsequent mass spectrometric investigations, leading to formulation (*xv*) for α-smegmamycolic methyl ester.[99]

The unsaturation (*trans-*) was recognized in IR and NMR spectrometry; absence of UV absorption indicated the double bonds to be isolated. The α-branch, β-hydroxyl character was revealed by smooth pyrolytic degradation of the methyl ester. The volatile product recovered was identified as methyl tetracosanoate, fixing the α-branch as C_{22}. Acetylation of α-smegmamycolic methyl ester gave a product characterized by NMR as containing only one acetyl function. In the NMR spectrum of a methyl ester, the three protons of the methoxyl give rise, at about 200 Hz, to a unique singlet whose integration serves as an internal standard. When a methyl mycolate of unknown hydroxyl content is acetylated, comparing the integral of the signal given by the newly introduced acetyl methyl group(s) with that of the calibrating methoxyl integral reveals the number of acetyl groups introduced and, therefore, the number of hydroxyl functions. Olefinic groups, methyl branches, cyclopropane rings, and so forth can also be recognized, and their numbers estimated.

Dehydration of the α-smegmamycolate gave the anhydro product, whose NMR spectrum revealed (by the triplet nature of the newly generated band at 395 to 409 Hz) that the γ carbon was unsubstituted. Ozonolysis of the β-acetate allowed recovery and identification by gas chromatography and mass spectrometry of fragments (*xv–a*) and (*xv–b*), whereas ozonolysis of the *mero*mycolic acid yielded these and an additional fragment, (*xv–c*).

From these data, the structure can be readily constructed. Mass spectrometry of α-smegma*mero*mycolic acid derivatives gave confirmatory data in regard to structure and homology.

In quick succession, structural and biosynthesis studies appeared on representatives of a host of mycolic acids — *M. kansasii*,[100] *M. tuberculosis*,[19, 98, 257] *Corynebacterium*, *M. avium*,[258, 375] *Nocardia*,[52] and *M. paratuberculosis*[215] — from which emerged unifying prin-

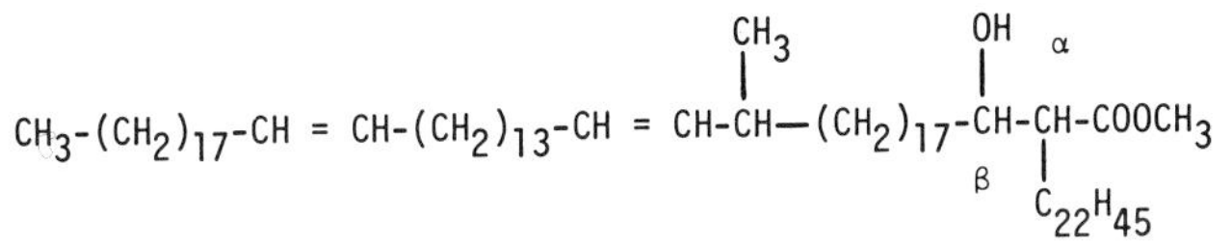

$$CH_3-(CH_2)_{17}-CH = CH-(CH_2)_{13}-CH = CH-\overset{\overset{\displaystyle CH_3}{|}}{CH}-(CH_2)_{17}-\overset{\overset{\displaystyle OH}{|}}{CH}-\underset{\underset{\displaystyle C_{22}H_{45}}{|}}{\overset{\displaystyle \alpha}{CH}}-COOCH_3$$

$$\overset{\beta}{}$$

xv

methyl α-smegmamycolate--$C_{80}H_{156}O_3$

$$CH_3-(CH_2)_{15-18}COOH$$

$$HOOC-(CH_2)_{12-16}COOH$$

$$HOOC-\overset{\overset{\displaystyle }{|}}{CH}-(CH_2)_{17}COOH$$
$$\underset{CH_3}{|}$$

xv–a   **xv–b**   **xv–c**

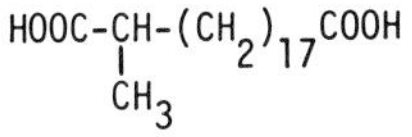

ciples concerning biogenetic and phylogenetic relationships. Several representative mycolic acid structures are given in Table 4–4 (after Lederer[220]). These include a variety of unsaturated, cyclopropanoid, methoxylated, and ketonic acids.

Total synthesis of the cyclopropanoid type (α) of mycolic acid is currently under investigation in the laboratory of W.J. Gensler. The stimulus for such efforts stems from the need to confirm the structural assignments that have been made and to prepare from synthetic products the glycolipids (e.g., cord factor) and other derivatives that are endowed with biologic properties of interest. Certainly these activities, if the synthetic products exhibit them, are intrinsic rather than a result of unrecognized or unsuspected levels of bacterial contaminants.

As an appropriate target for synthesis, Gensler and colleagues[127] selected the meromycolic acid shown below:

This is a principal meromycolate recognized in α-kansamycolic acid. To assemble the pieces that gave the meromycolic acid, the group chose the alkylation of metalated 1,3 dithianes. Figure 4–27, taken from Gensler and coworkers, depicts moieties A and B, which were constructed separately and then joined to give the complete carbon skeleton. Dotted lines indicate the points of bonding that were involved first in building A and B and then in combining the two halves of the molecule. One pathway for construction of the cyclopropanoid segments (Fig. 4–28) involved the conversion of cyclohexadiene to norcarene, ozonolysis to *cis*-1,2 cyclopropane diacetic acid, and then conversion to the tetrahydropyranyl bromo derivative used in building up the carbon skeleton. The product shown in Figure 4–27 contains all of the asymmetric centers of the meromycolic acid. The 1,3 dithianes were eliminated by Raney nickel desul-

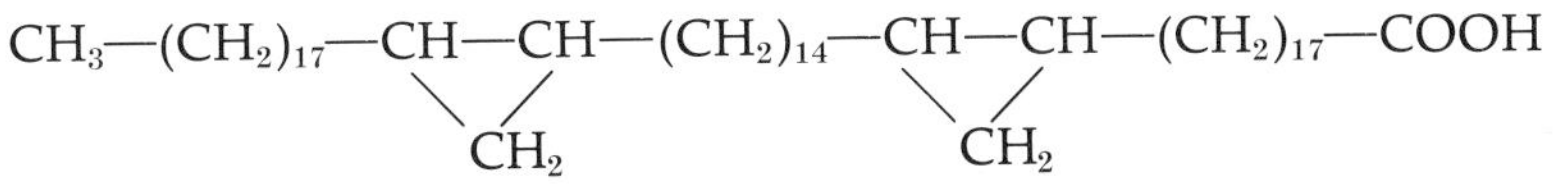

$$CH_3-(CH_2)_{17}-\overset{}{CH}-\overset{}{CH}-(CH_2)_{14}-\overset{}{CH}-\overset{}{CH}-(CH_2)_{17}-COOH$$
$$\underset{\displaystyle CH_2}{\diagdown\diagup} \qquad\qquad \underset{\displaystyle CH_2}{\diagdown\diagup}$$

TABLE 4-4.   Structures of Some Mycolic Acids

Mycolic Acid	Strain	Reference
Corynomycolenic acid	*Corynebacterium diphtheriae*	

$$CH_3(CH_2)_5CH\text{=}CH\text{—}(CH_2)_7\overset{\displaystyle OH}{\underset{\displaystyle\underset{C_{14}H_{29}}{H}}{C}}\text{—}CH\text{—}CO_2H$$

Ioneda et al. (1963) [162]

| Smegmamycolic acid | *M. smegmatis* | |

$$CH_3\text{—}(CH_2)_{17}\text{—}CH\text{=}CH\text{—}(CH_2)_{13}\text{—}\underset{\displaystyle CH_3}{CH}\text{=}CH\text{—}CH\text{—}(CH_2)_{17}\text{—}\overset{\displaystyle OH}{\underset{\displaystyle C_{22}H_{45}}{CH}}\text{—}CH\text{—}COOH$$

Etemadi et al. (1964) [99]

| Kansamycolic acid | *M. kansasii* | |

$$CH_3\text{—}(CH_2)_{17}\text{—}\underset{\displaystyle CH_2}{CH\text{—}CH}\text{—}(CH_2)_{14}\text{—}\underset{\displaystyle CH_2}{CH\text{—}CH}\text{—}(CH_2)_{17}\text{—}\overset{\displaystyle OH}{\underset{\displaystyle C_{22}H_{45}}{CH}}\text{—}CH\text{—}COOH$$

Etemadi et al. (1964) [100]

| Methoxylated mycolic acid | *M. tuberculosis,* var. *hominis,* (strain Test) | |

$$CH_3\text{—}(CH_2)_{17}\text{—}\underset{\displaystyle CH_3}{\overset{\displaystyle OCH_3}{CH\text{—}CH}}\text{—}(CH_2)_{16}\text{—}\underset{\displaystyle CH_2}{CH\text{—}CH}\text{—}(CH_2)_{17}\text{—}\overset{\displaystyle OH}{\underset{\displaystyle C_{24}H_{49}}{CH}}\text{—}CH\text{—}COOH$$

Etemadi (1966) [94]

| β-Mycolic acid | *M. bovis* BCG | |

$$CH_3\text{—}(CH_2)_{17}\text{—}\underset{\displaystyle CH_3}{\overset{}{CH}}\text{—}\underset{\displaystyle O}{\overset{}{C}}\text{—}(CH_2)_x\text{—}\underset{\displaystyle CH_2}{CH\text{—}CH}\text{—}(CH_2)_y\text{—}\overset{\displaystyle OH}{\underset{\displaystyle C_{24}H_{49}}{CH}}\text{—}CH\text{—}CO_2H$$

Adam et al. (1967) [4]

x = 11 to 21   max. x + y = 39: $C_{90}H_{176}O_4$

y = 28 to 18   min. x + y = 29: $C_{80}H_{156}O_4$

| Dicarboxylic mycolic acid | *M. phlei* | |

$$HOOC\text{—}(CH_2)_{14}\text{—}\underset{\displaystyle CH_3}{CH}\text{—}CH\text{=}CH\text{—}(CH_2)_{16}\text{—}\overset{\displaystyle OH}{\underset{\displaystyle C_{22}H_{45}}{CH}}\text{—}CH\text{—}COOH$$

Markovits et al. (1966) [242]

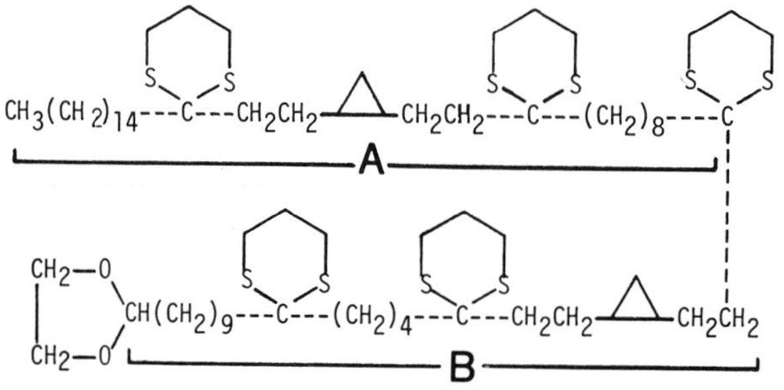

FIGURE 4-27.   Intermediate components utilized in construction of synthetic meromycolic acid. (From Gensler, W. J., Marshall, P. L., Langone, J. J., and Chen, J. C.: Synthesis of DL-methylmeromycolate. J. Org. Chem. 42:118, 1977.)

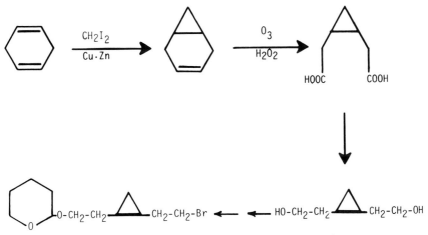

FIGURE 4–28. Intermediates in meromycolate synthesis.

furization to leave the hydrocarbon portions of the molecule intact.

Mass Spectrometry

Although mass spectrometry played only a subordinate role in establishing the α-smegmamycolic acid structures, the most sophisticated applications of this technique were required for determining other structures shown in Table 4–4. (For an illustrative, analytic discussion of representative mass spectrometric analysis as applied to a mixture of mycolic acids recovered from lung bacilli of infected mice, refer to Goren.[136])

Gensler's synthesis of an α-kansameromycolate makes available a structurally defined model compound as a reference standard for examination in mass spectrometry in order to either confirm or refute the deductions reached in the earlier examinations of the natural products. Gensler and Marshall[126] found that the mass spectrum of the synthetic meromycolic acid (methyl ester), and even of a simpler analog with one cyclopropane ring, was *not* informative for locating the *cyclopropane rings* — an important feature of earlier interpretations with the natural mycolic acid esters. This agrees with earlier evidence from Minnikin and Polgar[259] and from Lamonica and Etemadi.[212] These two studies did demonstrate, however, that the *meroaldehydes* (xvi) formed from pyrolytic cleavage of the mycolate esters yielded fragmentation patterns that were much more informative and, specifically, involved cleavages adjacent to the cyclopropane groups. See below.

It is regrettable that the final steps of the Gensler synthesis as originally envisaged were unsuccessful; they would have yielded the *meromycolaldehyde* (xvi) as the penultimate intermediate for conversion to meromycolic acid. This would have been the ideal syn-

$$CH_3-(CH_2)_x-CH-CH-(CH_2)_y-CH-CH-(CH_2)_z-\overset{\overset{\displaystyle O}{\parallel}}{C}-H$$
$$\qquad\qquad \underset{CH_2}{\diagdown\diagup} \qquad\qquad \underset{CH_2}{\diagdown\diagup}$$

xvi

$$CH_3-(CH_2)_{16}-CH_2-\overset{\overset{\displaystyle CH_2}{\diagup\diagdown}}{CH-CH}-CH_2-(CH_2)_{12}-CH_2-\overset{\overset{\displaystyle CH_2}{\diagup\diagdown}}{CH-CH}-CH_2-(CH_2)_{16}-COOCH$$

thetic model for comparison with those of natural origin derived from mycolic acids by pyrolysis.

As an alternative model for studying the natural products, chromic oxidation of molecules that contain cyclopropanes fused on a straight chain converts the adjacent methylene groups to ketones, which facilitate the generation of important fragments in mass spectrometry.[126, 286] In the study by Gensler and Marshall, chromium trioxide oxidation of the synthetic methyl α-kansameromycolate afforded four isomeric monoketones, which were separated by preparative thin-layer chromatography (the positions of oxidation are indicated by solid arrows. See above.) In mass spectrometry, these undergo facile characteristic cleavages on either side of the carbonyl group. The fragments generated by cleavage between the oxocarbon and cyclopropane rings (broken arrows) furnish more than sufficient information to fix

the positions of both the proximate (to the carboxyl) and distal cyclopropanes. It is probable that any remaining ambiguities involving mycolic acid structures containing cyclopropane substituents will be resolved through techniques such as those just discussed, in conjunction with sophisticated NMR spectroscopy.

Biosynthesis: Biogenetic Implications

Etemadi proposed a biosynthetic scheme embracing *Corynebacterium*, *Nocardia*, and *Mycobacterium* and including a complementary phylogenetic correlation based on the complexity of "mycolic" acids produced (Fig. 4–29).[95] The identification of a mycolic acid structure can therefore be exploited in taxonomic classification of both genera and species. Thus, the mass spectrometric identification of a typical mycolic acid fragmentation pattern, which was

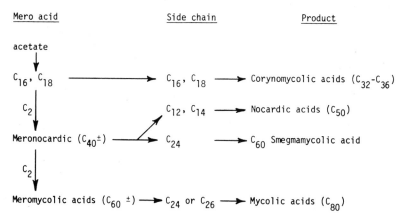

FIGURE 4–29. Proposed genesis of mycolic acids in corynebacteria, nocardia, and mycobacteria. (Adapted from Etemadi, A. H.: Correlations structurales et biogénétiques des acides mycoliques en rapport avec la phylogènese de quelques genres d'Actinomycetales. Bull. Soc. Chim. Biol. *49*:695, 1967.)

obtained from examining extracts of bacilli recovered from lepromatous tissue, was offered in evidence to support the mycobacterial etiology of this disease.[96] Ratledge alludes to the definitive distinction between true *Mycobacterium* and *Nocardia* organisms and those of the "rhodochrous" complex, based on the specific types of mycolic acids elaborated.

Implicit as a final stage in the biosynthesis scheme shown in Figure 4–29 is the Claisen condensation between a carboxylic acid (of low to intermediate molecular weight) and a meromycolate (as acceptor) — as indicated for the synthesis of corynomycolic acid (Fig. 4–22) and designated the "mycolic condensation." Gastambide-Odier and Lederer[119] had in fact demonstrated that *C. diphtheriae* grown in culture incorporated 1-^{14}C-palmitic acid into corynomycolic acid; and in accord with the anticipated Claisen condensation, the label was restricted to carbons 1 and 3 of the product.

$$CH_3-(CH_2)_{14}-\overset{\displaystyle OH}{\underset{\displaystyle *}{CH}}-CH-\overset{\displaystyle *}{COOH}$$
$$\underset{\displaystyle C_{14}H_{29}}{|}$$

In a re-examination of the system nearly two decades later, Walker and colleagues[377] and Promé and his associates[288] found that a cell-free extract of *C. diphtheriae* condensed two molecules of labeled palmitate, not into corynomycolate, but into the C_{32} β-keto ester of 2-tetradecyl 3-keto octadecanoic acid (a probable intermediate).

$$CH_3(CH_2)_4-\overset{\displaystyle O}{\overset{\displaystyle \|}{C}}-\underset{\displaystyle *}{CH}-\overset{\displaystyle *}{COOR}$$
$$\underset{\displaystyle C_{14}H_{29}}{|}$$

In this product, the *degree* of labeling of carbons 1 and 3 (starred) was identical.

Still, the palmitate molecule that contributed the side chain and terminal carboxyl was evidently carboxylated to an alkyl malonate through an activation step prior to the condensation. This cell-free system did not provide corynomycolate. With exponentially growing *C. diphtheriae*,[288] the β-keto intermediate was at once incorporated into a monoester of *trehalose*, a derivative unequivocally identified in field desorption mass spectrometry of the peracetate, as well as by appropriate chemical transformations. The degree of labeling of carbons 1 and 3 was unequal — more label being incorporated into carbon 3. The time course of ^{14}C incorporation showed that the peak of labeled trehalose keto ester was produced during the first seconds of incubation and that labeled corynomycolate was then produced at the expense of the keto ester.

Since mycolic acids in mycobacteria are found principally esterified to the cell wall arabinogalactan (see p. 68), the immediate appearance of the precursor Claisen condensation product as a derivative of *trehalose* raises the intriguing possibility that trehalose mycolates (such as cord factor, see p. 119) may play a role in transferring newly synthesized mycolic acids to cell wall. If all mycolate synthesized accumulated as trehalose derivatives, the steady state levels of these glycolipids would be enormous, whereas in fact they are quite meager. Important evidence in support of this postulated anabolic function derives from studies of Takayama and Armstrong,[337] which showed that *M. tuberculosis* strain H37Ra incorporates labeled acetate into trehalose 6-acetate, 6'- (labeled) mycolate and that following a chase with cold acetate the mycolate radiolabel of this glycolipid declines with time and appears instead in cell wall-associated mycolate. The peculiar toxicity of the trehalose mycolates and their implication in pathogenesis (see cord factor, p. 129) may therefore be (for the pathogen) a fortuitous expression of a biologic activity that is unrelated to the principal anabolic role which the glycolipid may have in intermediary metabolism.

With respect to the higher molecular weight mycolic acids as found in mycobacteria, the α-branch and its contiguous α-carbon and carboxyl derive from the condensation of the appropriate C_{24} or C_{26} carboxylic acid onto the mero acid. When $C_{23}H_{47} - {}^{14}COOH$ was incorporated by growing M. smegmatis, the label was entirely restricted to the terminal carboxyl of the mycolic acids.[97] When labeled palmitate or stearate was incorporated, radioactivity was distributed selectively in both the mero acid and in the pyrolysis-generated ester; this suggests that palmitate and stearate may function as initiators for synthesis of the long hydrocarbon chain and of the tetra- and hexacosanoic acids participating in the Claisen condensation. As depicted in Figure 4–30, the oriented, C_{18}-initiated C_2 condensations — augmented by desaturation, intervention of methyl donors, and side-chain condensation — can hypothetically give rise to the whole spectrum of mycolic acids. This scheme divides the biosynthesis into three stages involving a primary

and secondary sequence of 8 and 10 acetate incorporations, respectively, to build the high molecular weight meromycolate carbon skeleton with two unsaturated functions (the "doubly unsaturated precursor"). Indeed, this scheme is in accord with the distribution of unsaturation as seen in α-smegmamycolic acid and as reflected in the structures determined for the cyclopropanoid α-kansamycolic or α-mycolic acid Test (see Table 4–4 on p. 100), where the methylene groups bridge these same formerly unsaturated positions. In these products, as in the doubly unsaturated "precursor," the number of methylene groups distal and proximate to the carboxyl are odd, while those between the cyclopropanes (or between the two double bonds) are even. The double bonds are the sites for subsequent transformations: methylenation by S-adenosylmethionine provides the cyclopropanoid α-mycolates, or methylation yields various smegmamycolates. Combinations of these transformations with oxidations yield the methoxylated and ketonic α'- and β-mycolates shown in Table 4–4. Finally, the third stage involves the

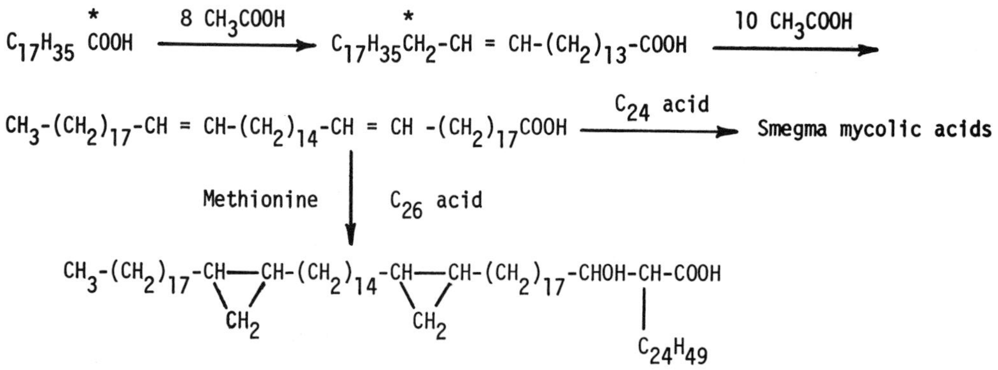

$$C_{17}H_{35} \overset{*}{-}COOH \xrightarrow{\text{8 CH}_3\text{COOH}} C_{17}H_{35}CH_2\text{-}CH \overset{*}{=} CH\text{-}(CH_2)_{13}\text{-}COOH \xrightarrow{\text{10 CH}_3\text{COOH}}$$

$$CH_3\text{-}(CH_2)_{17}\text{-}CH = CH\text{-}(CH_2)_{14}\text{-}CH = CH\text{-}(CH_2)_{17}COOH \xrightarrow{\text{C}_{24}\text{ acid}} \text{Smegma mycolic acids}$$

Methionine $\downarrow$ C_{26} acid

C_{26} acid

$$CH_3\text{-}(CH_2)_{17}\text{-}CH\underset{CH_2}{\overset{}{\diagup\!\!\diagdown}}CH\text{-}(CH_2)_{14}\text{-}CH\underset{CH_2}{\overset{}{\diagup\!\!\diagdown}}CH\text{-}(CH_2)_{17}\text{-}CHOH\text{-}CH\text{-}COOH$$

$C_{24}H_{49}$

FIGURE 4–30. Proposed biosynthetic sequences for mycobacterial mycolic acids: Two stages of acetate incorporation lead to a "doubly unsaturated precursor." Claisen condensation of the "precursor" with tetracosanoate leads to the smegmamycolate carbon skeleton. Alternatively, modification by methylenation, methylation, oxidation and so forth followed by Claisen condensation with C_{24} or C_{26} acids leads to the various mycobacterial mycolates. (Adapted from Etemadi, A. H.: Correlations structurales et biogénetiques des acides mycoliques en rapport avec la phylogènese de quelques genres d'Actinomycetales. Bull. Soc. Chim. Biol. 49:695, 1967.)

$$R-CH_2-\overset{*}{C}OOH + CH_3COOH \longrightarrow RCH{=}\overset{*}{C}H-CH_2-COOH$$

Claisen condensation with a preformed C_{24} or C_{26} acid to provide the α-branch and the β-hydroxyl function.

The specific positions of the double bonds in the meromycolate skeleton are accounted for by Etemadi on the basis of the mechanisms advanced by Konrad Bloch (see Scheuerbrandt et al.[313]) for unsaturated fatty acid biosynthesis in anaerobes. Following chain elongation through incorporation of acetate and through reduction, the β-hydroxy acid dehydrates to give a β,γ-unsaturated product (rather than the preferred α,β-isomer). (See above.)

This scheme of Etemadi's, vigorously defended in a number of publications, recommends itself especially because of its consistency and for the structural predictions to which it leads. On the other hand, until very recently, the construction of the meromycolic acids was nevertheless largely shrouded in conjecture. Ratledge suggests that formation of the mero fatty acid chain to the required molecular weight by successive additions of C_2 units seems, biosynthetically, "highly improbable."[290] C. Asselineau and colleagues consider an alternative hypothesis, which "is entirely consistent with all the results found in the literature."[17] At least for *Mycobacterium phlei* and possibly for *M. smegmatis,* they propose that unsaturated precursors of the meromycolate need not be formed exclusively in the manner proposed by Etemadi but instead might derive from saturated fatty acids of the same number of carbon atoms by the aerobic desaturase pathway (see Lennarz, Scheuerbrandt, and Bloch[231]). Thus, identical part structures are shared by the unsaturated phlei mycolic acids and (ordinary) lower molecular weight (C_{22} to C_{26}) phlei Δ^5-unsaturated acids — some of which are *branched* rather than normal. Analogous series of di- and tri-ethylenic compounds were also characterized.

Asselineau and collaborators as well as Bordet and Michel[52] consider that completion of the mero portions may also proceed in the *reverse* direction from that implicit in Etemadi's scheme — for example, by "head-to-tail" condensations of preformed sections as an alternative to chain elongation by 2-carbon units. This pathway for palmitic and tetracosanoic acid biosynthesis in *M. tuberculosis* strain H37Ra was originally described by Kanemasa and Goldman[176] (see p. 79) and would require an ω-oxidation of one or more components prior to the condensation step.

The data from the very informative, analytic study of lipids from *Nocardia asteroides* by Bordet and Michel[52] provide the basis for some of these hypotheses. This organism synthesizes nocardic acids, along with the closely related nocardanols (alcohols) and nocardones (ketones), all of which contain a total of about 50 carbon atoms. Structure (*xvii*) represents three of these lipids and shows their obvious relatedness and the more-or-less restricted position of ethylenic linkages recognized in all species. Here the mero portion contains about 32 to 36 carbons.

$$R'-CH{=}CH-(CH_2)_{13,\,15}-\overset{\overset{\textstyle X}{(\,)}}{C}-CH-R$$
$$\underset{\underset{\textstyle CH_3}{(CH_2)_{11,\,13}}}{}$$

xvii

where $X = H$, OH in the alcohols and acids; $X = O$ in the ketones; $R = H$ in the alcohols and ketones; $R = COOH$ in the acids; and $R' = C_{14}H_{29}$ to $C_{17}H_{35}$

According to data of Bordet and Michel, $1\text{-}^{14}C$-palmitate from the medium was incorporated into all three classes of compounds preceding, but in a fashion that made it quite evident that much of the labeled palmitate was participating in both roles in the "condensation mycolique." In this Claisen condensation a radiolabeled (and therefore palmitate-derived) *carboxyl* function in the C_{32-36} mero acid served as "acceptor" for $1\text{-}^{14}C$-palmitate as the "donor" species. This was indicated by the localization of radiolabel in carbon atoms 1 and 3 of the nocardomycolic acid (*xvii*) (both arrows) and in the ketone and carbinol carbons of the other analogs (broken arrow). The ketone and carbinol very likely arise from decarboxylation of a common keto acid intermediate. Although in the acid, carbon 3 (broken arrow) was not as heavily labeled as carbon 1 (solid arrow), it was unequivocally enriched in the isotope, as compared with a fairly uniform level of random labeling. Therefore, in the nocardomycolate, the $1\text{-}^{14}C$-labeled palmitate provided the "carboxy terminal" of a 34-carbon mero acid chain and has participated in a "condensation mycolique" at this labeled carboxyl. The remainder of the mero chain must have been constructed from $1\text{-}^{14}C$-labeled palmitate in the direction *away* from the labeled carboxyl. It is tempting to view the mero carbon skeleton of these specific substances as constructed from two molecules of palmitate or stearate, possibly by a head-to-tail condensation and a required desaturation. If the postulated "elongation" takes place following the mycolic condensation, it is possible that the preformed keto acid, which is also produced by *Corynebacterium diphtheriae,* may be converted by *Nocardia* species in culture to nocardomycolic acids. Such a demonstration would seem to provide unassailable evidence in support of a head-to-tail condensation process and, at the same time, confirm the conclusion of Bordet and Michel: "It seems reasonable that many processes are implicated in the biosynthesis of high molecular weight compounds..."[52]

Recent studies of Takayama and colleagues on the mode of action of isoniazid have shed important light on pathways of mycolic acid synthesis in *M. tuberculosis* strain H37Ra.[345] Careful column chromatography on Sephadex LH20 was applied to mixtures of intermediate-to-long-chain fatty acids obtained from alkaline saponification of harvested H37Ra. Characterization of components in specific fractions by preparative TLC and GLC and augmented by mass spectrometry disclosed, in several series of fatty acids, groups containing substances in the range C_{27} to C_{40} and C_{39} to C_{56}—saturated, unsaturated, and cyclopropanoid—which were suspected to be intermediate in mycolic acid biosynthesis. In a recent report of Takayama and colleagues,[342] most of the fatty acids of chain length C_{15} to C_{56} were isolated, purified, and generally characterized by Fourier-transform-NMR and by combined gas chromatography–mass spectrometry. Based on the results, the authors propose a five-stage primary pathway to the synthesis of meromycolic acids. In the first stage, a fatty acid synthetase system condenses 12 molecules of acetate to stearate, then to the saturated (C_{24}) tetracosanoic acid. The second stage involves a Δ^5 desaturase, which operates on tetracosanoic acid, converting it into Δ^5 tetracosenoic acid. This product is then elongated by condensation with 4 acetates to yield Δ^{13} dotriacontenoic acid (*xviii*).

$$CH_3\text{—}(CH_2)_{17}\text{—}CH\text{=}CH\text{—}(CH_2)_{11}\text{—}COOH$$

xviii

In the third stage, Δ^{13} dotriacontenoic acid is methylenated at the double bond (probably with S-adenosylmethionine as CH_2-donor) and again elongated by condensation with acetate to yield *cis*-15,16 methylene tetracontanoic acid (*xix*).

$$CH_3\text{—}(CH_2)_{17}\text{—}CH\text{—}CH\text{—}(CH_2)_{13}\text{—}COOH$$
$$\diagdown\diagup$$
$$CH_2$$

xix

$$CH_3-(CH_2)_{17}-CH-CH-(CH_2)_{10}-CH-CH-(CH_2)_{17}-COOH$$

with CH_2 bridging the two CH—CH groups.

xx

At the fourth stage, *cis*-15,16 methylene tetracontanoic acid is again desaturated (by a Δ^3-desaturase) and methylenated, and in the fifth stage, it is further elongated to the meromycolate characteristics of H37Ra. [See above (*xx*).] Essentially all of these products as well as intermediates were isolated and characterized, at least in part.

This elegant study provides experimental proof for several of the features that have been independently advanced by A. H. Etemadi and by C. Asselineau concerning mycolic acid syntheses. In a recent finding[335a] keto- and methoxyl-containing *mero*mycolates have been recognized in H37Ra, and this serves as yet another unifying principle in providing additional evidence that the mero acids are evidently synthesized in their entirety before undergoing the final "mycolic condensation."

Isoniazid and Mycolic Acid Biosynthesis

For about two decades following the recognition of isonicotinic acid hydrazide (INH) as a potent antitubercular drug, its mechanism of action remained an enigma. The prodigious efforts to seek evidence for the primary events following exposure of susceptible species to the drug are shown by the lengths of review articles dealing with the subject.[386, 396] Evidence from our Institution[112, 248] appeared to implicate a selective inhibition of DNA synthesis with all of its subsequent consequences on RNA and on protein synthesis.

A series of studies from the groups of Winder and, later, of Takayama provide compelling evidence that the primary immediate lesion may be "somewhere in the biosynthetic pathway to the mycolic acids."[387] In this seminal study, exposure of growing *M. bovis* BCG to 0.5 μg INH/ml and of *M. tuberculosis* H37Ra to 0.1 μg drug/ml produced complete or almost complete inhibition of mycolic acid synthesis in one hour or less, as judged from incorporation of label from ^{14}C glycerol into these products and cell wall. In the controls, total incorporation of carbon into the cell as a whole was almost unaltered for much longer periods. A block to mycolic acid synthesis occurred in both sensitive BCG and H37Ra at INH concentrations close to the minimal inhibitory ones, but it did not occur in INH-resistant BCG — an observation consistent with the argument that the effect on mycolic acids is related to the bactericidal action of the drug.[346] The resultant formation of a defective cell wall, deficient in mycolic acid, may lead to the loss of further material (e.g., polysaccharide) from the boundary layers, then ultimately to loss of acid-fastness and death. The loss of acid-fastness under the influence of INH has long been recognized and is consistent with a diminished content of cell wall mycolic acids, which are implicated as both a reactant for the dyes and a necessary lipid barrier to prevent the destaining by acid alcohol.

Takayama's studies adopted ^{14}C-acetate as an evidently more suitable and sensitive label for incorporation into mycolate, and his studies early confirmed the report of Winder and Collins that INH effects an immediate inhibition of mycolate synthesis in H37Ra. All three mycolates — α, α' (methoxylated), and β (keto) — are inhibited to a similar degree,[346] and the 60 min. required for establishing complete loss of mycolate synthesis coincided with the apparent beginning of decline in cell viability. The damage to cell wall, which evidently arises from a depletion of available mycolic acid, results in a wrinkling of the mycobacterial cell surface that gives way to a rough, ragged aspect with eventual extrusion of cytoplasmic material and then fragmentation occurs. It is of interest that if low level INH incubation is not too prolonged, then mycolate synthetase activity can be slowly recovered after thorough washing of the cells. However, after 10 hr incubation with 0.5 μg INH/ml, mycolic acid synthesis is irreversibly inhibited.[338]

Of course, these developments raise intriguing questions and equally fascinating prospects for specific investigations — principally, to answer how isoniazid inhibits mycolic acid synthesis. Are the targets specific enzymes involved in the elaboration of the meromycolates? Some evidence favoring this interpretation comes from Takayama and Schnoes[343] and from Takayama and colleagues.[345]

These studies provide strong evidence that either long- or short-term exposure of H37Ra to isoniazid inhibits the synthesis of saturated fatty acids greater than C_{26} and unsaturated acids greater than C_{24}. Elongation of the C_{39} to C_{56} acids containing double bonds (or cyclopropane rings) was inhibited by INH to the same extent as mycolic acid synthesis. Although not yet entirely delineated, the site of the block induced by INH is suspected to be in the desaturation of tetracosanoic acid — thus, the Δ^5-desaturase enzyme may be the specific target of isoniazid.[342] (See also Chapter 20.)

MYCOBACTERIAL CELL WALL, WAX D, AND ADJUVANT ACTIVITY

It seems appropriate to introduce this section with a reproduction (slightly modified) from Kanetsuna and San Blas,[178] tentatively proposed for the structure of a portion of the cell wall of mycobacteria (Fig. 4–31). In the cell wall itself, all of these individual components are greatly multiplied so as to make up, in essence, a gigantic insoluble polymer, whose monomeric units are represented here. This structure also encompasses features of a composite wax D, with molecular weights in the region of 30,000 to 60,000 and of

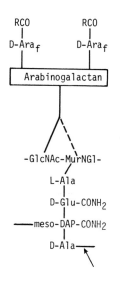 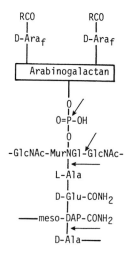

FIGURE 4–31. Oligomeric components of mycobacterial cell wall (and wax D) according to Kanetsuna and San Blas. Mycoloylated arabinogalactan is covalently linked to muramic acid of glycan chain by phosphodiester bridge. Arrows indicate linkages subject to enzymatic attack. (From Kanetsuna, F., and San Blas, G.: Chemical analysis of a mycolic acid-arabinogalactanmucopeptide complex of a mycobacterial cell wall. Biochim. Biophys. Acta *208*:434, 1970.)

certain soluble mycobacterial antigens.

The subjects have been elegantly reviewed in successive publications of Lederer[220, 222] and Lederer and coworkers,[223] and in the reviews by Barksdale and Kim[40] and by Ratledge.[290] Appropriate references for the succeeding section can be found in these sources as well as in Goren.[136]

Mycobacterial cell wall substance may be regarded as composed of two major components — a glycolipid and a peptidoglycan. Figure 4–31 illustrates (top) portions of the glycolipid as constituted of mycolic acid residues, esterified via an arabinose linkage to a complex arabinogalactan polymer. The evidence for this ubiquitous and substantially exclusive association of mycolic acid and arabinose in the cell wall derives from the initial studies of Azuma and Yamamura.[34] They found that mild HCl-catalyzed hydrolysis of firmly bound lipids of tubercle bacilli released 5-mycoloyl arabinose. Succeeding studies regularly demonstrated this glycolipid (and mycoloyl arabinobiose) from similar acid hydrolysis of cell walls, defatted cells, whole cells, wax D, and bound waxes of a variety of mycobacterial species and strains.

The arabinogalactan polymer is connected at intervals by a phosphodiester bridge, probably from an arabinose,[10, 177] to a glycan chain that consists of alternating and repeating units of N-acetyl glucosamine linked β 1→4 to N-glycolyl muramic acid. The evidence for the phosphodiester bridge stems from the recognition of muramic acid-6-phosphate in *M. butyricum*[233] and from its subsequent, almost routine, identification in cell wall and cell wall-derived preparations of other mycobacteria. Kanetsuna and San Blas[178] suggest that a second type of covalent linkage (glycosidic) may also bond the arabinogalactan to the peptidoglycan. In the usual fashion, the glycan, via the 3-lactyl group of muramic acid, connects to a peptide: *L*-Ala-*D*-Glu-*meso* DAP-*D*-Ala. The more detailed structure of

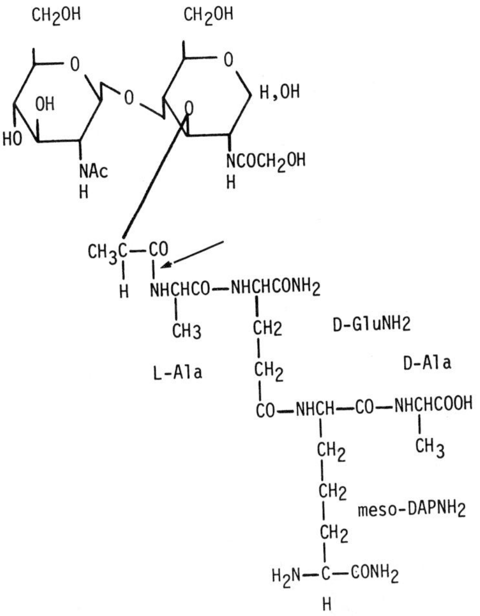

FIGURE 4–32. Detail of peptidoglycan "monomer" (disaccharide-tetrapeptide).

the peptidoglycan "monomer" in Figure 4–32[220] shows that in both the glutamic and diaminopimelic acid residues the "free" carboxyls are amidated. For cross-linking and insolubilizing the murein, the terminal *D*-Ala of the monomer provides a direct interpeptide linkage with the remaining amino group of DAP, probably on "parallel" peptidoglycan chains (a link to an adjacent peptide unit would not constitute a cross-link). In addition, Wietzerbin et al.,[385] using mass spectrometry, have described and characterized alternative links in *M. smegmatis*, mediated via *meso*-diaminopimelyl-to-proximate *meso*-diaminopimelic acid linkages.

In the hypothetical cell wall (Fig. 4–31), solid arrows delineate sites susceptible to specific enzymatic and autolytic attack; some have been exploited for degradative and structural studies of a great variety of cell wall preparations, as described in Ghuysen,[128] Lederer,[222] and Kotani and his coworkers.[206] Wietzerbin-Falszpan and colleagues[384] isolated the tetrapeptide from enzymatic hydrolysis of *M. smegmatis*, BCG, *M. phlei*, or *C. fermentans* cell walls (Fig. 4–32, solid arrow at the muramyl-to-peptide linkage), from which several important features were discerned: chemical analysis established the configuration of the N- and C-terminal alanines and of the diaminopimelic acids as L, D, and *meso*, respectively, and confirmed earlier conclusions of the γ-glutamyl to DAP linkage. Methodology of Das and his coworkers[83] was especially fruitful in defining the sequence of the amino acids by mass spectrometry. Acetylation of the tetrapeptide, followed by methylation in which the

$$\underset{}{\overset{O\quad H}{\overset{\|\quad\ |}{-C-N-R}}}$$

functions are converted to the more volatile N-methylated peptides (with less hydrogen bonding),

transforms the tetrapeptide into (*xxi*) which, in simplified form reduces to (*xxi–a*). (See below.)

In mass spectrometry, oligopeptides such as those just mentioned or even more complex will yield a peak corresponding to the molecular ion (in this instance, M$^+$ 683) and a group of principal peaks generated by successive fragmentation at the carbonyl-to-nitrogen linkages, beginning at the carboxy terminal and progressing stepwise toward the amino terminal in the reverse direction to that of Edman degradation. This yields successively smaller, recognizable fragments. Thus, in *xxi–a*, the molecular ion M$^+$ 683 generates the peaks, m/e 566 and 567, m/e 298, and m/e 128, following successive losses of (methylated) alanine, DAP, and glutamine — scissions a, b, and c. Fragmentation at a′ yields the major peak m/e 484,

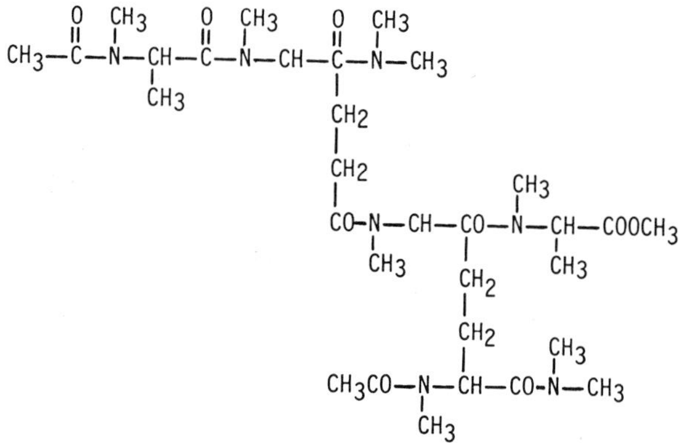

xxi

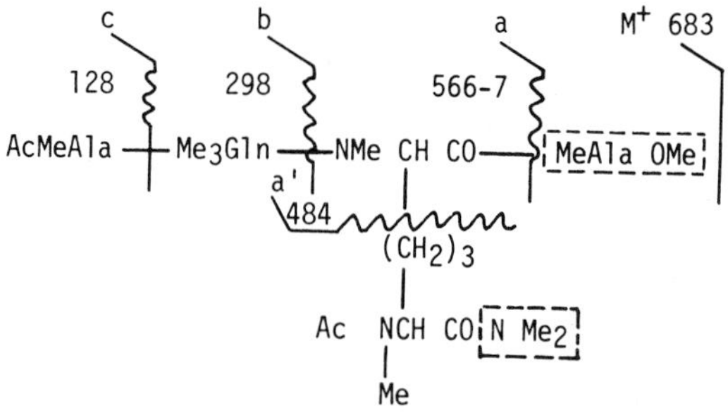

xxi–a

and this is definitive for the structure as written because it excludes a possible isomeric structure in which the residues within the broken lines are transposed.

Figure 4–32 shows the muramic acid moiety of the disaccharide to be N-glycolylated rather than N-acetylated, as is almost ubiquitous among other bacteria. This feature was first revealed by mass spectrometry and subsequently by chemical identification and synthesis.[33] The suggestion that biosynthesis of N-glycolyl muramic acid proceeds by the pathway UDP-N-acetylglucosamine → UDP-N-acetyl muramic acid → UDP-N-glycolyl muramic acid has been substantiated: Gateau and colleagues[124] have shown that cell-free extracts of *Nocardia asteroides* indeed oxygenate UDP N-acetyl muramic acid to the glycolyl derivative.

Since cycloserine inhibits bacterial cell wall synthesis by interfering with the formation and utilization of D-alanine, it is satisfying that H37Ra and *M. phlei* grown in the presence of this antibiotic accumulate the precursor of the cell wall glycolipid, UDP-N-glyc Mur-L-Ala-γ-D-Glu-*meso*-DAP.[339]

The Cell Wall Glycolipid: Mycoloyl Arabinogalactan

Culture filtrates of *M. tuberculosis* as well as other mycobacteria have been found rich in soluble antigenic "polysaccharides," specific components of which were originally described by Florence Seibert in 1949.[320] Takeya and coworkers[349] identified a serologically potent arabinogalactan "glycopeptide" in culture filtrates of tubercle bacilli and inferred (probably correctly) this to be a product split from cell wall. Birnbaum and Affronti[49] also found the polysaccharide from several mycobacterial species to be closely related to Seibert's polysaccharide I and very likely consisting of arabinogalactan derived from cell wall. Thus, abundant arabinogalactan, often associated with remnants of peptidoglycan, is shed into the medium during cultivation of mycobacteria. In a continuing series of investigations, Misaki and collaborators[260] prepared clean and relatively homogeneous examples of arabinogalactan, suitable for definitive structural analysis. By digestion of cell walls (from *M. tuberculosis, M. bovis* BCG, *M. phlei,* and *M. smegmatis,* among others), with 0.5 M NaOH at 70° for 8 hr under nitrogen, mycolic residues are cleaved, and polysaccharide is solubilized. This is separated into several fractions by ethanol precipitation, and the crude arabinogalactan, which is obtained with 65 to 85 percent ethanol, is purified by gel filtration. When tested with an antiserum raised against BCG cell wall, the products from the various species were serologically identical, giving the same single precipitin lines in Ouchterlony (immunodiffusion) tests.

Beautifully detailed chemical studies showed that arabinogalactans of various mycobacteria have essentially the same structures, and they act as common antigens of *Mycobacterium, Corynebacterium,* and *Nocardia* species. The polysaccharides appear to be constructed on a main chain of galactopyranose and arabinofuranose in a ratio of about 2.7:1, with multiple branches composed principally of arabinose oligosaccharides. Arabinose serves for the nonreducing terminal components (linked to mycolic acids) as well as for most of the points of branching. Although Misaki's data consistently suggested that galactose in the polymer is largely in pyranose form, Vilkas and her associates[366] provided evidence that some galactose is present in the furanose form. The exact distribution of sugars remains uncertain; however, Misaki proposed a tentative structure for the mycoloyl arabinogalactan that is in accord with most of the available evidence (Fig. 4–33). This structure also shows the mycoloyl ester functions, linked to terminal arabinose components.

$$5)\text{-}\alpha\text{-D-Ara}_f(1 \to 5)\text{-}\alpha\text{-D-Ara}_f(1 \to 4)\text{-}\beta\text{-D-Gal}_p(1 \to 4)\text{-}\beta\text{-D-Gal}_p(1 \to 4)\text{-}\beta\text{-D-Gal} \quad (\to$$

```
                    3
                    ↑
                    1

               α-D-Ara_f

                    2
                    ↑
                    1

               α-D-Ara_f
                         n
                    5
                    ↑
                    1
      R-CO → α-Ara_f
```

$$n > 3$$

$$D\text{-Ara}_f = D\text{-Arabinofuranose}$$

$$D\text{-Gal}_p = D\text{-Galactopyranose}$$

$$R\text{-CO} = \text{Mycolic acid residue}$$

FIGURE 4–33.   Structure of the mycolóylated arabinogalactan according to Misaki and colleagues. (From Misaki, A., Seto, N., and Azuma, I.: Structure and immunological properties of D-arabino-D-galactans isolated from *Mycobacterium* species. J. Biochem. 76:15, 1974.)

Wax D

It is appropriate to consider the waxes D, a group of important mycobacterial lipids, from the perspective of their relation to cell wall. The waxes D are chloroform-soluble but acetone-insoluble, heterogeneous glycolipids or peptidoglycolipids and are recovered from mycobacterial harvests, as summarized in Figure 4–2. The adjuvant-active waxes D, such as from human strains of *M. tuberculosis* or from *M. kansasii*, are ideally a heterogeneous (in molecular weights) group of peptidoglycolipids, having all of the components of the cell wall — i.e., mycoloyl arabinogalactan linked via a phosphodiester bridge to muramic acid of the glycan, then to the peptides. The portion of cell wall oligomer depicted in Figure 4–31 (at a high enough multiplicity, up to MW 30 to 60 × 10³) is a fairly acceptable structural representation of these idealized adjuvant-active waxes D. On the other hand, waxes D of most bovine, avian, atypical, and saprophytic mycobacteria (especially from older

cultures) have only a meager nitrogen content; they lack the peptidoglycan and are largely lipopolysaccharides. They could be depicted as a heterogeneous polymeric form of the mycoloylated arabinogalactan of Misaki shown in Figure 4–33. They are inactive as adjuvants because this activity is evidently conferred by the *peptidoglycan* and, therefore, have been of only marginal interest biologically.

The waxes D in human strains of *M. tuberculosis* have achieved prominence because of the remarkable and diverse biologic activities that they exhibit. (See especially the treatise of Jollès and Paraf[170] for a review on the chemical and biologic basis of adjuvant activity.) The origin of this complex spectrum of mycobacterial lipids, glycolipids, and peptidoglycolipids can be reconciled with an autolytic degradation of the mycobacterial cell wall at sites, such as those indicated by the arrows in Figure 4–32. Although an accumulation of an excess of appropriate cell wall precursor may also be contributory, there is now widespread agreement that the various waxes D are mainly solvent-soluble autolysis products of cell wall. Accordingly, the very difficult studies devoted to elucidating the structure of this heterogeneous material have contributed much to our understanding of mycobacterial cell wall structure (for review, see Goren[136]).

Indeed, much of the mystery surrounding wax D has been resolved, and the undeniable heterogeneity of wax D products somewhat clarified when considered in relation to the cell wall. In retrospect, this seems almost self-evident; and yet, the recognition of muramic acid[169, 331] as a constituent of waxes D that contained the specific peptides (Ala-Glu-DAP-Ala, and so forth) was almost tantamount to "revelation," for despite the seemingly obvious relation to cell wall, the manner in which the peptide and glycan of adjuvant-active wax D were linked remained an enigma for many years.

Adjuvant Activity

Barksdale and Kim[40] informatively recapitulated the concepts and experiments of Lewis and Loomis, of Dienes, and of Freund to probe the influence of tubercle bacilli (presented in various fashions) on the immune response to heterologous antigens. These led to the development of Freund's adjuvant: "dead *M. tuberculosis* in water-in-oil emulsions . . . behave like living *M. tuberculosis* in enhancing antibody production to cointroduced antigens, as well as inducing specific delayed hypersensitivity to tuberculin." These and other manifestations of a perturbation of the immune system by mycobacterial components are well documented and have been elicited with whole cells, with delipidated *M. tuberculosis*,[382] with cell walls of mycobacteria, nocardia, and corynebacteria,[29, 205] with deproteinized and delipidated cell walls (i.e., "cell wall skeleton") and with appropriate waxes D. With respect to an ad-

ministered antigen, adjuvant-active wax D will stimulate immunoglobulin production, (especially of IgG$_2$) and induction of delayed hypersensitivity. With a brain antigen, it will induce allergic encephalomyelitis; and it elicits adjuvant arthritis in susceptible rats as effectively, or more so, than whole, killed tubercle bacilli.

The waxes that are active contain both the mycoloyl arabinogalactan and peptidoglycan, while the waxes D of bovine, avian, saprophytic, and most atypical strains are inactive. By fractional ultracentrifugation of various wax D solutions in ether, Jollès, Samour, and Lederer[168] separated several sedimenting (Dp) and nonsedimenting (Ds) fractions. The early Dp fractions invariably had the greatest content of peptidoglycan, and these were most potent as adjuvants. The Ds fractions (prominent in inactive waxes D) ordinarily lack the nitrogenous constituents and are inactive. Stewart-Tull and White,[332] however, found that the wax D of *young* cultures of saprophytic strains closely resembled that of human strains of *M. tuberculosis* in both *chemical* and *biologic* properties. With prolonged cultivation, however, the wax derived from the relatively rapid-growing strain assumed the glycolipid form — deficient in peptidoglycan and, accordingly, biologically inactive. In the interpretation of Stewart-Tull and White, when materials are abundant, even saprophytic strains produce adjuvant-active wax D, but when nutrients — especially nitrogenous ones — are exhausted, mycobacterial growth is maintained by autonutrition from peptidoglycolipid.

Purification of Wax D; Correlation of Structures With Specific Activities

Wax D prepared according to classical methods contains variable amounts of heterogeneous contaminants: tuberculoproteins, free mycolic acids, cord factor, trehalose monomycolate, and glyceryl mycolates.[30] Some of these undoubtedly influence the biologic activities. Chemical changes induced by extensive acetylation of wax D facilitated a subsequent chromatographic separation of nitrogen-free components from peptidated ones.[350] The latter retained adjuvant activity, albeit diminished, but had lost the arthritogenic properties. Instead, peptidated acetyl wax D is protective against the arthritogenic property of ordinary wax D and of mycobacterial cell wall. The structural features of cell walls, waxes, and enzymatic cleavage products, which are implicated in the elicitation of adjuvant arthritis, continue to receive intensive probing. Recently Koga and colleagues[201] reported that a wide range of bacterial purified cell walls have arthritogenic activity in the rat. Water-soluble components obtained by digestion of the cell wall with a peptidoglycan-degrading enzyme (*Flavobacterium* L-11 enzyme) retained this activity. (The L-11 enzyme solubilizes the cell wall by cleaving the *peptides* but leaves the glycan and the arabinogalactan intact.) Digestion of the arabinogalactan (AG) portion by means of M-2 enzyme (an AG-degrading enzyme) did not significantly affect the arthritogenic activity. However, analogous water-soluble components in which the glycan was degraded by mutanolysin were not arthritogenic. The accumulated evidence is quite persuasive for supporting the theory that the arthritogenic activity resides in an intact (and evidently appropriately structured) glycan chain. It would be informative to determine whether *acetylation* of such an active product would effect the kinds of transformation seen with wax D — i.e., render it protective and palliative as well as nonarthritogenic.

Adjuvant Activity and Chemical Structure: The Least Common Denominator

Although the property of adjuvanticity is by no means restricted to struc-tures related to specific bacterial cell walls, a principal thrust in efforts to define a structural common denominator for activity has nevertheless involved this mycobacterial organelle. Perhaps the recognition of such impressive adjuvant activity in the much smaller (albeit complex) wax D molecules magnified the propinquity of achieving the desired resolution. Still, some of the convictions that were held based on wax D studies have been found erroneous: the stringency with which the apparent requirement for mycolic acid substituents and the arabinogalactan has been cloaked is apparently without substance. Instead, the activity seems to be almost exclusively associated with components of the peptidoglycan.

The abandonment of chemical degradations (with their accompanying but unrecognized deep-seated transformations), which diminished or destroyed biologic activities, in favor of more gentle and specific enzymatic attack on cell wall is largely responsible for the dramatic progress in delineating the structural features associated with adjuvancy. Parallel investigations of Migliore-Samour and Jollès[256] and of Stewart-Tull and coworkers[330] revealed hitherto unrecognized, water-soluble "native" mycobacterial glycopeptides with potent adjuvant activity. These are obtained directly from *M. tuberculosis* (12 weeks old) culture filtrates (Stewart-Tull), or by vigorous physical solubilization (homogenization), or by solvent extraction of delipidated *M. tuberculosis* cells followed by chromatography (Migliore-Samour and Jollès). These products are almost lipid-free and contain arabinogalactan, mannose, and some peptidoglycan.

Contemporaneous studies in the groups of Petit, Lederer, and colleagues at Orsay and of Kotani and colleagues in Osaka, utilizing enzymatic solubilization processes, defined the least common denominator of bacterial cell wall structure in which adjuvant activity resides. (For the most comprehensive re-

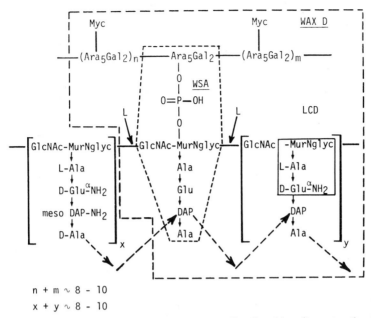

$n + m \sim 8 - 10$

$x + y \sim 8 - 10$

FIGURE 4-34. A simplified scheme of the mycobacterial cell wall and its adjuvant-active derivatives, as obtained by 1) enzymatic digestion: wax D (by autolysis) and WSA (with lysozyme); and by 2) synthesis: muramyl dipeptide — the least common denominator (LCD) of adjuvant activity. (Adapted from Lederer, E.: Natural and synthetic immunostimulants relative to the mycobacterial cell wall. Med. Chem. 5:257, 1977.)

view of these studies, see Lederer[222].) The French group[1, 2] prepared water-soluble adjuvants (WSA) by lysozyme digestion of purified cell walls of *M. smegmatis* and gel filtration of the water-soluble components to separate an active, substantially lipid-free arabino-galactan-peptidoglycan (WSA — about 20,000 daltons). These are likely closely related to the products of Stewart-Tull and of Migliore-Samour. Figure 4-34[222] is a simplified rendering of the myco-bacterial cell wall structure and its adjuvant derivatives, somewhat expanded from the scheme given in Figure 4-31. The "monomer" of lipid-free WSA is shown outlined (dotted line) and consists principally of arabinogalac-tan linked to peptidoglycan. Lower molecular weight fragments obtained in the gel filtration and lacking *neutral sugars* were at least as active as WSA in replac-ing whole mycobacterial cells, wax D, or cell walls in Freund's adjuvant. Since

these are constituted therefore only of peptidoglycan, it raises the exciting pos-sibility that adjuvant-active oligomers may be common to a great variety of bacterial cell walls and thus not re-stricted to the *Corynebacterium-Myco-bacterium-Nocardia* (CMN) group. Treat-ment of WSA fractions with *Myx-obacter* AL_1 amidase[3] allowed recovery by preparative high-voltage electro-phoresis of the pure disaccharide tetra-peptide (i.e., the "monomeric unit") of *M. smegmatis* peptidoglycan (Fig. 4-34, in large brackets; also shown in Fig. 4-32). As an adjuvant for stimulating humoral antibody production and de-layed type hypersensitivity, this prod-uct can replace killed mycobacteria in complete Freund's adjuvant; quite simi-lar species prepared from purified *E. coli* cell walls, in which muramic acid is N-acetylated and *D* Glu and *meso* DAP are *not* amidated, have similar activity. But neither the disaccharide GNAc $\beta(1$

→ 4) Mur-NGly nor the tetrapeptide L-Ala-D-isoGluNH₂-DAP-*D*-Ala are adjuvant active.

Kotani's parallel studies continued a long series that had its origin in the illuminating study of BCG cell wall, in which the crucial importance of the extraordinary levels of cell wall-associated lipids (60 percent) became evident. The variety of biologic, pathologic, and immunologic activities possessed by bacterial cell walls in general seemed to Kotani to be:

... A natural consequence of the fact that the cell wall together with the capsule, forms the outermost layer that is in contact with environmental factors (and it) probably contains compounds which enable these organisms to survive and evolve a variety of responses in the cells and tissues, including the immune response.[206]

The isolation from mycobacteria of water soluble principles (free of mycolates), with adjuvant activity vis-à-vis humoral and cellular responses, sharpened the likelihood that bacterial cell walls *in general* might have immunologic adjuvant activity. We should suggest parenthetically that, in retrospect, surely it seems not surprising that the ubiquitous bacterial peptidoglycan should elicit in the parasitized host the primal, but by no means primitive, cellular immune response and cellular sensitization. However, the exquisite degree to which the latter has been amplified (almost exclusively) in some CMN preparations may, nevertheless, bespeak an influence of the specific lipids and their mode of attachment, which is still poorly understood.

Kotani sought and demonstrated immunoadjuvant activity in cell walls from a variety of gram-positive bacteria — *Staphylococcus aureus, Streptococcus pyogenes, S. salivarius, S. faecalis, S. mutans, Lactobacillus plantarum, N. asteroides* — and in walls of various fungi.[206-208] Many of these share similarities in the molecular pattern of their peptidoglycan portion with that of mycobacteria.[314] Products of cell wall diges-

tion obtained by enzyme treatments (e.g., with L-11, L-3, Chalaropsis-β enzymes, mutanolysin, and lysozyme) that solubilize cell walls by attacking sites of the peptidoglycan[206] also demonstrate the expected adjuvant activity. Nonpeptidoglycan portions of the cell wall were unnecessary. Where tested for in these and in the products of the Petit-Lederer group, of Migliore-Samour and Jollès, and of Stewart-Tull and coworkers, the relatively simple, water-soluble peptidoglycan preparations were free of the detrimental immunologically-mediated qualities of whole mycobacteria, cell wall, or wax D — for example, induction of adjuvant arthritis, inordinate sensitization to endotoxin, and hepatomegaly or splenomegaly;[77] of course, these do not induce tuberculin hypersensitivity. However, Kotani and colleagues[210] found that even the synthetic N-acetylmuramyl peptides are pyrogenic and correlated the order of pyrogenicity with order of adjuvant activity.

With the activity pinpointed as residing within the disaccharide tetrapeptide, the direction of the remaining studies was clearly defined. In degradation and synthesis studies, both groups delineated N-acylmuramyl dipeptides as the required least common denominator of activity, specifically, N-acylmuramyl-L-alanyl-D-isoglutamine (Fig. 4–34 — LCD, enclosed in small square frame).[93, 209, 252] Essentially, no simpler, derived products are active; an intact N-acylmuramyl structure seems to be stringently required, and the glutamic moiety must be amidated. The influence of a variety of chemical transformations was examined by the groups at Orsay and Osaka; these transformations ordinarily result in loss or decrease in activity. Although replacement of L-Ala by L-Ser is tolerated, substitution of D-Ala for L-Ala leads to an *antiadjuvant effect.*[222]

Equally subtle modifications examined by Kotani and coworkers[209] yielded only inactive substances: N-acetylmuramyl-L-alanyl-*L-isoglutamine,* N-acetyl-muramyl-L-alanyl-*D-glutamine,* and N-acetylmuramyl-L-alanyl-D-*isoaspara-gine.*

The route of presenting the "candidate" adjuvants influences the activity. Audibert and associates[28] showed that N-acetylmuramyl-*L*-Ala-D-*glutamic acid* is only a weak adjuvant vis-à-vis eliciting humoral antibody and is without effect on delayed hypersensitivity when it is presented with ovalbumin in Freund's incomplete adjuvant. However Chedid and colleagues[76] made the important observation that this substance, as well as LCD, is active in both responses when injected with antigens subcutaneously *in saline.* Moreover the (natural) amidated form (LCD), at somewhat higher dosage, can be given orally while the antigen (BSA) is injected, to elicit high levels of humoral anti-BSA. The nonamidated counterpart is much less effective. Accordingly, Chedid and his fellow workers suggest that the expression of activity by the orally administered muramyl-alanyl-isoglutamine may reflect a resistance to degradation conferred by the D-isoglutamine moiety. It may also be inferred that the influence of the muramyl dipeptide is at least partly systemic, since the antigen and adjuvant need not be given at the same site.

Mechanism of Action of WSA (Water-Soluble Adjuvant). Modolell and coworkers[262] found that WSA did not affect the viability and survival of mouse lymphoid cells in culture, nor was there any measurable influence on cellular respiration or disturbance of membrane phospholipid metabolism. It was therefore possible, in the absence of any demonstrable toxicity, to study the in vitro adjuvant effect of WSA on antibody formation by mouse lymphoid cells in response to various antigens. WSA significantly increased the numbers of antibody-forming cells to sheep red blood cells (SRBC), to DNP (dinitrophenyl)-edestin (a thymus cell-dependent antigen), and to DNP-dextran (T cell-independent). Depletion of the T-cell population with anti-θ serum did not significantly alter the response; moreover, the effect of WSA was demonstrable with lymphoid cells from Nu/nu mice. It seems clear, therefore, that the adjuvant properties of WSA do not require participation of T-cells. B-cells also are not affected by WSA; no evidence of splenic mouse lymphocyte stimulation was found on incubation with even relatively large amounts (50 μg/ml) of WSA. Instead, the activity seems to depend upon the participation of adherent cells — macrophages. When the lymphoid cells were depleted of the adherent population, the number of cells producing antibody to DNP-dextran was *unaffected* by WSA. Reconstitution of the depleted population with even a small percentage of macrophages, however, restored the activity. The effect of WSA on macrophages was demonstrable as well when these cells were first preincubated with very low levels (.01 μg/ml) of the adjuvant, washed, reconstituted with the nonadherent cell population, and then incubated with antigen (either SRBC or DNP-dextran). Thus, at the cellular level, WSA may stimulate macrophages to secrete a lymphocyte-activating factor, or influence subsequent processing of the antigen to increase production of "super-antigen," or by binding to the macrophage surface, "somehow influence collaborative processes between macrophages and lymphocytes."[262]

Adjuvants, Antitumor Activity, and the Influence of Lipids

The utility of mycobacteria and mycobacterial fractions in experimental tumor immunotherapy has stimulated an ever-increasing number of studies devoted to the recognition of components in which activity resides and to the mechanism of action.* The simple

---

*See Bast et al.,[41] Chapter 9, and this chapter's section on trehalose glycolipids.

adjuvants discussed in this section are among the substances under scrutiny, since the demonstrable antitumor activities of viable BCG and of the nonviable vaccines, like MER (methanol-extraction residue) of BCG[379] and the cell wall vaccines of E. Ribi and coworkers[291] are believed to depend, at least in part, upon their adjuvant properties.[41, 53, 172]

It seems astonishing that the common denominator of adjuvant activity of mycobacterial cell walls appears to reside in simple N-acylmuramyl dipeptides, which are almost monotonously common among a host of microorganisms. These are free of lipids (mycolates), which were long believed to have a role in conferring the exquisite levels of hypersensitization and systemic immunostimulant properties peculiar to the CMN (*Corynebacterium-Mycobacterium-Nocardia*) genera. Why were these activities also not recognized amongst the other bacteria in infection, or were only weakly expressed when they were tested as substitutes for mycobacteria in Freund's incomplete adjuvant? Lederer suggests that in these " 'other bacteria' the peptidoglycan may be covered by other constituents (lipopolysaccharide, teichoic acids, etc.), and therefore cannot react with the receptor on the macrophage membrane."[222]

On the other hand, there is evidence of an often unexpressed reluctance on the part of investigators to abandon completely the conviction that the lipids of CMN cell walls, or lipids in general, have a role in eliciting at least some of the immunologically mediated phenomena that have been documented over the years. There can be no doubt that this is so! Studies of Parish[280] have shown how the immune response to flagellin changes from a humoral to a cellular one (establishment of delayed-type hypersensitivity-DTH) if the antigen is first conjugated with ketene dimer to introduce somewhat lipophilic acetoacetyl groups. Coon and Hunter[80] conjugated the ϵ-amino groups of lysine residues in bovine serum albumin

(BSA) with dodecanoic anhydride, to produce dodecanoyl BSA. This antigen, when injected in saline into guinea pigs, elicits a pure DTH response to native BSA, with essentially no evidence of a humoral component. The ordinary haptene-directed humoral response to DNP-BSA is likewise converted into a haptene-specific *cellular* response if the carrier protein is lipidated either by conjugation with dodecanoic anhydride or by a simple but powerful physical "coating" of DNP-BSA with the quaternary dimethyl dioctadecyl ammonium bromide.[82] In the interpretation of Dailey and Hunter, the potent cellular response seemed to result from a specific localization and long retention of the lipidated antigen in the paracortical area of lymph nodes — a major site of thymus-derived cell localization. This seemed directly attributable to the influence of the lipid moieties; native BSA remains free in the medullary sinuses, is rapidly cleared from the lymph node, and does not detectably enter the paracorticol area.

Juy and Chedid[172] reported that WSA and the muramyl dipeptide activate macrophages in vitro to a state of cytotoxicity for mastocytoma cells, but only WSA (which is not completely free of mycolic acid!), injected intraperitoneally, would activate macrophages in vivo to a similar cytotoxicity. Goren, Yarkoni, and Rapp have found an adjuvant-active disaccharide-tetrapeptide-tripeptide-disaccharide isolated from *Lactobacillus plantarum* (provided by Dr. S. Kotani) to be ineffective in regression of line 10 tumors in strain 2 guinea pigs, even when the adjuvant was pretreated with cord factor and mineral oil and injected intralesionally (in the form of Ribi-type emulsions).

As discussed in the succeeding section, in the Ribi systems this physical treatment with cord factor, in part, serves to promote an evidently *necessary* association of the antitumor agents (e.g., BCG cell wall skeleton, certain mutant-derived endotoxins) with the oily phase of the emulsion, and this association may also be effected by chemical alteration of the agent — specifically, by acylation to introduce intermediate (palmitate, stearate)-to-high molecular weight (mycolate) ester or amide functions.

Azuma and coworkers[31, 32, 32a] are conducting a systematic study to determine the effect of such acylations on the adjuvant and potential antitumor activities of the simple muramyl peptides. In their products, the 6-primary hydroxyl substituent of the N-acylmuramyl group in the dipeptide is esterified to various carboxylic acids, so as to give the structure (*xxii*).

R-COOCH$_2$

HO

NHCOCH$_3$

CH$_3$-CH-CO-L-Ala-D iso Gln

xxii

In the first studies,[31] the 6-O-stearoyl product was found to be somewhat poorer than the nonacylated parent compound in inducing good levels of DTH to azobenzene-arsonate-N-acetyltyrosine (ABA-tyrosine) but essentially equal in enhancing the humoral response of mice to the T-independent antigen DNP-Ficoll. Both substances were inactive as mitogens for mouse spleen cells and ineffective in stimulating in vivo spleen effector cell cytotoxicity for P815-X2 mastocytoma cells. Neither did these two exhibit antitumor activity for E14 and melanoma B16 transplantable murine tumors. Since in these tumor systems and in mitogenic activity, BCG cell wall skeleton is demonstrably active, the results suggest that the simple muramyl peptide can represent only a part of the immunologic activity of the CMN cell walls and that mycolic acids and arabinogalactan may indeed modify and potentiate the activities of the peptidoglycan.

These concepts gain affirmation in the results of more recent studies.[32] Higher molecular weight analogs of (*xxii*) were prepared with mycolic acids of *M. tuberculosis* and with the analogs of intermediate molecular weight, corynomycolic and nocardomycolic acids (for methodology, see Kusumoto et al.[211]). All of these "mycoloyl" derivatives were active in inducing DTH to ABA-N-acetyltyrosine. The effect on in vivo induction of cell-mediated cytotoxicity was striking; in contrast to the inactivity of the parent compound or the 6-O-stearoyl derivative, the three "mycolates" effectively activated spleen cells to in vitro cytotoxicity when the donor animals were preimmunized intraperitoneally with the adjuvants and mastocytoma cells. The peak of activity was reached with the nocardomycolate. The mycobacterial mycolic acid ester was also a mitogen for spleen cells from several strains of mice and exhibited significant suppression of the MH-134 hepatoma in syngeneic mice. It is, therefore, evident that reintroduction of mycolate components into the naked N-Ac-Mur-dipeptide may begin a restoration of activities that are easily demonstrated with intact cell wall skeleton but that appear to be lost by the simple muramyl dipeptides.

TREHALOSE GLYCOLIPIDS: CORD FACTOR AND THE SULFATIDES

We referred to the dynamic metabolic role of the nonreducing disaccharide *trehalose* as betrayed by its turnover rate. After the Anderson group identified this sugar as a component of the "neutral fats," some 40 years elapsed before a ubiquitous distribution and probable anabolic role for trehalose was recognized in *Corynebacterium*, *Nocardia*, and *Mycobacterium*. In addition to their anabolic function, certain trehalose end-

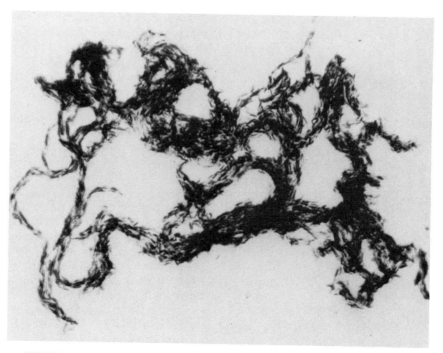

FIGURE 4–35. Serpentine cords of *Mycobacterium tuberculosis,* from veil growth.

products as well as compounds of presumed intermediary metabolism have assumed a primary importance as putative agents of virulence in tubercle bacilli. Following earlier morphologic descriptions by Koch and by Maximow, Middlebrook, Dubos, and Pierce[255] recognized that virulent tubercle bacilli appear to be distinguished from avirulent and attenuated forms and from most saprophytic mycobacteria through an unusual growth in the form of "serpentine cords" (Fig. 4–35). They are also distinguished cytochemically from

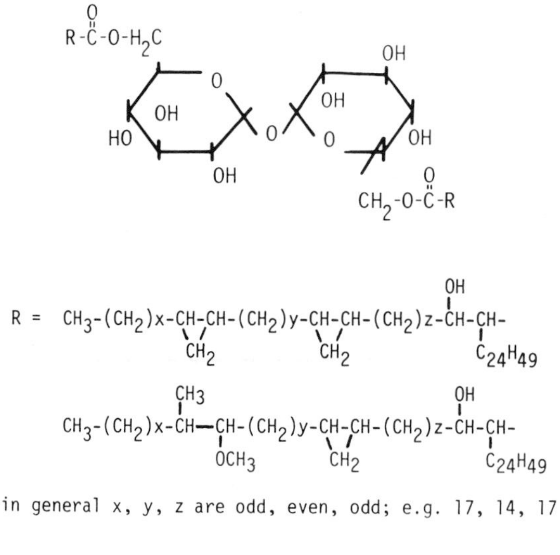

FIGURE 4–36. Trehalose 6,6'-dimycolate (cord factor) from *M. tuberculosis.* Heterogeneity in structures is provided by differences in mycolic acid structures and homology.

$$R = CH_3-(CH_2)x-CH-CH-(CH_2)y-CH-CH-(CH_2)z-CH-CH-$$

with $\overset{\backslash}{C}H_2$, $\overset{\backslash}{C}H_2$, and OH, $C_{24}H_{49}$

$$CH_3-(CH_2)x-CH—CH-(CH_2)y-CH-CH-(CH_2)z-CH-CH-$$

with CH_3, OCH_3, CH_2, OH, $C_{24}H_{49}$

in general x, y, z are odd, even, odd; e.g. 17, 14, 17

avirulent and saprophytic species by an ability to absorb the cationic phenazine dyestuff "neutral red." Dubos' derived, heuristic hypothesis[92] — i.e., that some peripherally located substance or substances of virulent tubercle bacilli might be responsible for cord formation and neutral red fixation and, therefore, might be related to virulence — stimulated a search for such substances and led Hubert Bloch to the trehalose glycolipid(s), which he named "cord factor," i.e., trehalose-6,6'-dimycolate (Fig. 4–36). A more accurate conformation of 6,6' diesters of trehalose as developed by Kato and Asselineau[188] is also

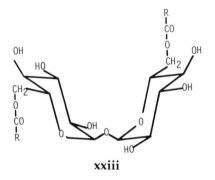

xxiii

shown (*xxiii*). (For reviews, see Lederer,[221] Lederer,[222] and Goren.[137])

Middlebrook's studies, on the other hand, led to the neutral red-reactive sulfolipids or sulfatides of *M. tuberculosis*, which are also derivatives of trehalose. Indeed, these two classes of compounds have assumed a significance that equals or surpasses that envisaged for them at their discovery.

Cord Factor

As originally described by Bloch, a gentle extraction of cord-forming *M. tuberculosis* cells with petroleum ether disrupted the cords and yielded an extract that, when coated onto dried *Bacillus subtilis* (or H37Ra) and ingested by peripheral blood leukocytes, inhibited

their migration in the same manner as Bloch had previously described for intact tubercle bacilli. Hence, as stated by Bloch, "Disrupting the bacillary cords . . . removed a material which by itself simulated the migration-inhibitory effect of the untreated virulent organisms; whereas the virulent bacilli — lost their inhibitory action by removal of this material . . . (This) therefore will be referred to hereafter as 'cord factor'. "[50]

It is unfortunate that this imaginative and clever sobriquet (which, owing to convenience and widespread usage, should not now be abandoned) conveys the notion of an activity for the substance that has never been documented, even some 25 years after isolation of the glycolipid. Indeed "cord factors" and closely related analogs have been isolated from noncording saprophytic mycobacterial species and from *Nocardia* and *Corynebacterium*. Thus, the mechanism of or any chemical participants in cord formation remain unresolved.

Bloch also found that some component(s) of the extract had a peculiar and characteristic toxicity for mice, a property that led to the recognition of much richer sources of the substance — principally, the waxes C and D of the classical Anderson and Asselineau lipid fractions. With the collaboration of Hans Noll, and later with Asselineau and Lederer as well, the chemical structure of cord factor was elucidated and elegantly detailed in a succession of classical papers.[271, 273]

In brief, highly purified samples of cord factor* were characterized as containing two molecules of mycolic acid (or acids) esterified to a molecule of trehalose. The position of esterification

---

*The inordinate skill and care of these investigators enabled them to secure highly purified cord factor. In our examination,[139] of an original sample from H. Bloch, we found it to be about as free of extraneous contaminants as products that have been prepared (with much greater ease) by the more sophisticated techniques currently available.

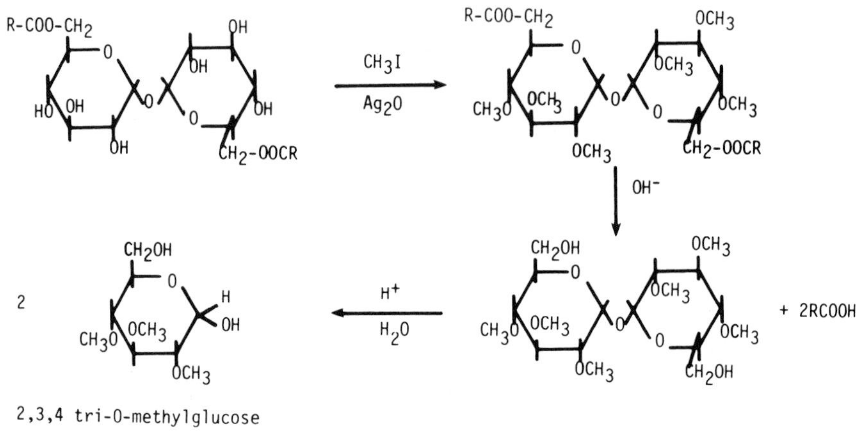

FIGURE 4–37. Symmetry of cord factor structure as determined by permethylation analysis.

was revealed by a difficult permethylation (Fig. 4–37), which blocks the free hydroxyl groups, and alkaline saponification (to release a hexa-O-methyl trehalose, followed by acidic hydrolysis, which yielded only 2, 3, 4, tri-O-methyl glucose and thus revealed that in cord factor, trehalose is symmetrically substituted with mycolic acid in the 6,6' positions.

Cord factors of *M. tuberculosis*, of *M. bovis* BCG, and, more recently, of *M. phlei*, *M. avium*, *M. tuberculosis* strains "Peurois" and "Aoyama B," and of *M. lepraemurium* have all been identified as trehalose 6,6' dimycolates. In short, trehalose 6,6' dimycolate and the trivial name, "cord factor," have become synonymous through accepted and widespread usage.

The resolution of the structural problems in 1956 occurred at a time when the intimate details of mycolic acids structures were unknown. These have, of course, been largely clarified (as described in the section on mycolic acids). Because of this structural heterogeneity in *types* and in *homology*, it seemed likely that all types and distributions would be represented in any sample of natural cord factor. Indeed, available evidence already supports this interpretation. Thus, as stated by Goren in a recent review,[137] "it is not yet feasible to assign single unique structures to cord factor or even to decide *whether any individual molecule of cord factor is entirely symmetrical*, (and therefore) it is unlikely that an entirely homogeneous example of natural cord factor will be isolated in the near future." Nevertheless, improvements in chromatographic techniques and methodology are bringing that goal much closer — despite the sophistry of the restriction, "entirely homogeneous."

In 1973 to 1974, Toubiana[357a] demonstrated that multiple thin-layer chromatographic developments with quite pure cord factor "Peurois" samples effected a separation of otherwise unresolved components into a form of nested "hats," or spear points, which were interpreted to represent different species (or homologies) of trehalose 6,6' dimycolates. Recently, a facilitated resolution applicable to preparative scale was achieved by conversion of cord factor preparations to the per-trimethylsilylated derivatives, in which all of the polar, dominant contributions of the multiple hydroxyl functions are masked; thus, the chromatographic mobilities of the various components depend upon the properties conferred by the subtle differences in mycolate structures. The technique has been exploited for cord factor of *M. phlei* by Promé and colleagues[287]; with cord factor "Peurois" and *M. bovis* AN5[357a]; and for the highly purified glycolipids from *M. tuberculosis* strain Aoyama B, *M. avium,* and *M. bovis* by Strain, Toubiana, and coworkers.[333] In the terminology of Ribi and collaborators, these have been designated "P3." By accepted usage the term "P3" is now understood to describe highly purified cord factor products, ordinarily obtained from somewhat impure cord factor concentrates by preparative centrifugal or high-pressure-liquid chromatography on microparticulate silica gel,[296] followed by elimination of residual traces of mycolic acids on diethylamino ethyl cellulose.[139] As indicated by centrifugal or thin-layer chromatography, these products are demonstrably free of polar polymeric material, trehalose monomycolates, free mycolic acids, or other detectable contaminants. Still, like all cord factor samples, they exhibit the same intrinsic heterogeneity attributable to the differences in mycolate components. In the studies of Promé and coworkers,[287] cord factor of *M. phlei* was pertrimethylsilylated, separated by preparative TLC into three principal fractions, the glycolipids regenerated with dilute acid, and the mycolate components recovered by alkaline methanolysis and identified. In this fashion, cord factor *M. phlei* was seen to consist of three species — the symmetric α,α dimycolate; γ,γ dimycolate; and the mixed unsymmetric α,γ dimycolates. In this series, the dicarboxylic acids (see Table 4–4) esterified to 2-eicosanol at the ω-carboxyl were designated "γ mycolic acids" (*xxiv*). Shown below.

In the studies of Strain and colleagues[333] a quite similar resolution of P3 samples from virulent human and bovine tubercle bacilli revealed six separable mycolate components: symmetric α,α (dicyclopropane), symmetric methoxy (designated $\beta\beta$), and symmetric keto mycolic acids (designated γ,γ) (see Table 4–4). In addition, the unsymmetric α,β; α,γ; and β,γ trehalose dimycolates were identified. In contrast, cord factor of *M. bovis* BCG lacked the methoxy-substituted mycolic acids. The authors speculated that the virulence of pathogenic mycobacteria may be related to the presence or absence of a given mycolate component.

Miscellaneous Trehalose Esters of Mycobacteria, Nocardia, and Corynebacteria

In addition to the symmetric dimycolates, a 6-monomycolate of trehalose was recovered from both the firmly bound lipids and wax D of strain H37Rv by Kato and Maeda;[190] and Takayama and Armstrong[337] recognized a dissymmetric 6-acetate, 6'mycolate of trehalose in extracts of the attenuated H37Ra strain. Dissymmetry of yet another sort was recognized in a trehalose diester of *M. fortuitum*[367] in which the acyl substituents (palmitic and tuberculostearic acids) were located on the same glucose moiety (see p. 125). This is uniquely recognizable from the mass spectrum of the peracetylated material, in which a prominent peak associated with the unsubstituted glucose is evident. Unusual fully acylated trehalose esters have been recognized in *M. phlei* and *M. smegmatis.* In the studies of C. Asselineau and coworkers[20] the former have been characterized as substituted with unusual polyunsaturated "phleic" acids, the

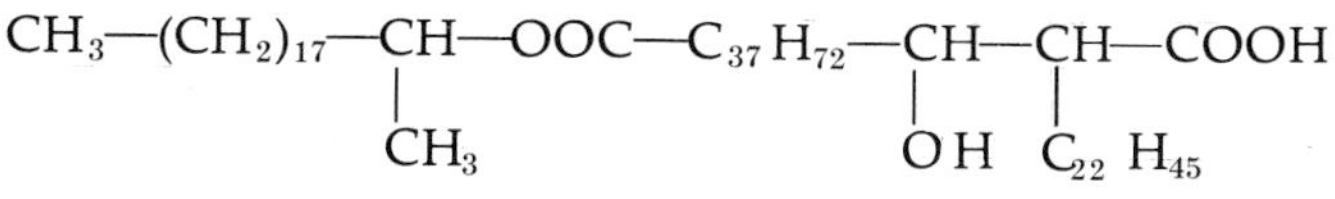

$$CH_3—(CH_2)_{17}—\underset{\underset{CH_3}{|}}{CH}—OOC—C_{37}H_{72}—\underset{\underset{OH}{|}}{CH}—\underset{\underset{C_{22}H_{45}}{|}}{CH}—COOH$$

xxiv

principal homolog being a hexa-
triaconta-4, 8, 12, 16, 20-pentaenoic
acid (see Fig. 4–13, p. 81).

Corynebacterium and *Nocardia* also
elaborate α-branched β-hydroxy acids
of intermediate-to-low molecular
weight, which are included in the spectrum of "mycolic acids" and these, too,
are incorporated into trehalose derivatives, some biologic activities of which
are quite similar to those of the mycobacterial cord factors. Trehalose 6,6'
diesters containing corynomycolic acids
and corynomycolenic acids were identified in extracts of C. *diphtheriae*,
whereas C. *hofmanii* contains a trehalose
diester of the more unsaturated cory-
nomycoladienoic acid.[221]

Determination of Structure

Owing to the dominant position cord
factors have assumed amongst the mycobacterial lipids because of their remarkable and exploitable biologic activities, a variety of efforts have been
devoted to their structural analyses.

Permethylation. The classical methodology of Noll and coworkers[273] of
Ag_2O-CH_3I permethylation analysis has
only rarely been repeated with other
cord factor samples or closely related
analogs.[337] Variants for achieving the
permethylation of lower molecular
weight species[161] have utilized CH_3I and
NaH in dimethyl formamide (DMF) and
BF_3-catalyzed permethylation of trehalose monomycolate with diazometh-
ane.[190] However, these latter methods
have met with indifferent success in attempts to permethylate the mycobacterial cord factors, especially on a very
small scale. A variant developed by
Goren and Toubiana[147b] has been extremely fruitful. The glycolipid is dissolved in a mixture of anhydrous ether-
DMF-methyl iodide in the presence of
beads of molecular sieve and treated directly with an oil-dispersion of NaH,
in considerable excess to achieve a facile
and almost quantitative permethylation. The contaminating mineral oil is

later separated from the product by simple microchromatography. Cord factors
Peurois, Aoyama B (P3), and of M. *lepraemurium*[142] have been identified as
6,6' dimycolates in this way; i.e., by
saponifying the permethylated product,
then identifying the methylated carbohydrate. The method has been applied
to quantities as small as 200 μg.

Except for the diazomethane-BF_3 procedure, all of these methods (depending
as they do upon methylation) can induce
acyl migrations in the presence of strong
bases; thus, bases promote the rearrangement of 4-acylglucoses (and probably of comparable trehaloses) to 6-acyl
carbohydrates. Accordingly, if a cord
factor were actually either a 4,4', 4,6',
or 6,6' diacyltrehalose, or a mixture of
these, the products of permethylation
could conceivably be the same in all
cases. The disadvantage appears to be
circumvented by recently applied
methodology of Promé and coworkers.[287]
(See Fig. 4–38.) The free hydroxyl functions of cord factor are blocked by transformation into alkali-stable tetrahydropyranyl ethers, and the product is
deacylated with sodium methylsulfinyl
methide ("dimsyl sodium") to free the
hydroxyl functions, which were originally involved in the ester linkage.
These OH groups are now distinguished by methylation with CH_3I
in the same alkaline medium; the pyran-
yl ethers are then hydrolyzed by weak
acid to regenerate the hydroxyl groups,
which were originally free in the glycolipid. The resulting sugars contain O-
methyl ethers located solely *at the position where the acyl groups were initially
present.* All of these steps are carried out
under nonisomerizing conditions and
evidently without a need to isolate any
of the intermediate products.

Mass Spectrometry. As reviewed by
Lederer,[221] mass spectrometry of low-to-
intermediate molecular weight cord factors, such as the peracetylated derivatives, can give meaningful information,
but permethylated derivatives have received much less attention. In mass

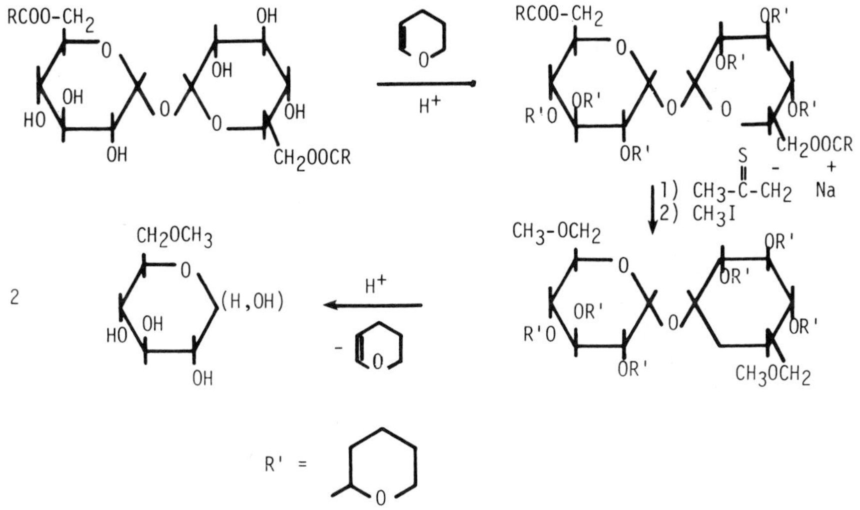

FIGURE 4–38. Structural analysis of cord factor by methyl replacement: The methyl ethers appear at the positions originally bearing the acyl substituents.

spectrometry, the peracetylated "cord factor" from *C. diphtheriae* was recognized as a mixture of a symmetric saturated diester, symmetric unsaturated diesters, and an unsymmetric diester (*xxv*) containing both examples as discernible from the weak molecular ion peaks. Shown below.

A well-known primary cleavage at the anomeric oxygen generates important oxonium fragments corresponding to about half the original molecule, in this case recognized from strong peaks at *m/e* 807 and 809. These contain the unsaturated and saturated corynomycolates, respectively. The analogous and very specific fragments (*xxvi*) from another peracetylated glycolipid allowed Vilkas et al.[367] to characterize the unsymmetric trehalose diester of *M. fortuitum* (p. 123) as having one glucose moiety entirely unsubstituted.

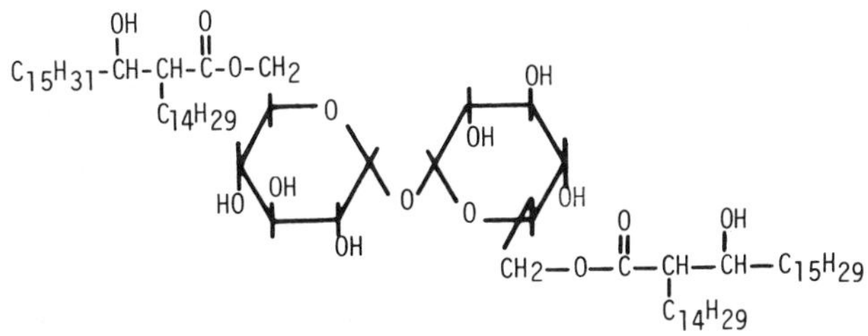

xxv

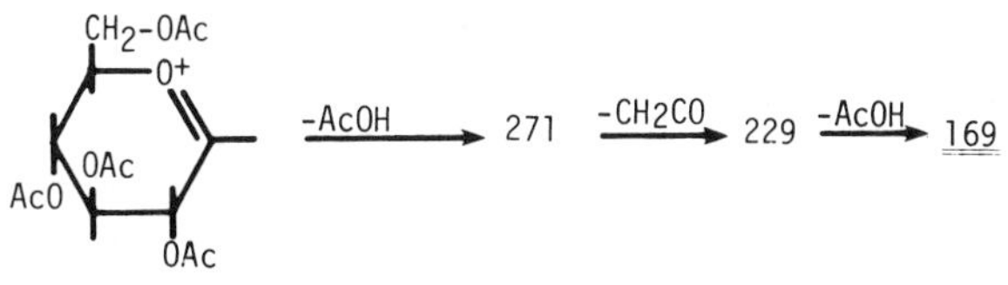

xxvi (m/e 331)

A very prominent peak m/e 331 is attributable to the oxonium ion (*xxvi*) derived from the unsubstituted glucose moiety of the trehalose core. Successive losses of molecules of acetic acid (and/or ketene) lead to the series m/e 271, 229, and 169, with the latter providing the base peak in the spectrum. Molecular ions are not seen in the mass spectra of peracetylated cord factors from mycobacteria (MW above 3000), but the oxonium fragments from the primary cleavage at the glycosidic oxygen (or more often, after subsequent loss of molecules of acetic acid) may afford peaks useful in structure determination. Some of these have been extensively detailed by Adam and coworkers.[4] Relevant examples (shown later in the Chapter), chosen from structural studies on mycobacterial sulfatides, were especially selected to illustrate further some of the intimate details of structure that this powerful tool can reveal.

Proton and ^{13}C Magnetic Resonance. Although NMR can provide important and useful structural information, ^{13}CMR spectra obtained (nondestructively) with sufficient sample can be interpreted to provide most structural details of a purified cord factor sample. Thus the symmetric 6,6'-

disposition of the mycolate residues as well as their internal structures have recently been determined for cord factor "Peurois" and a P3 from *M. phlei* (Wenkert, personal communication). This technique requires from 50 to 100 mg of a cord factor sample. For scarce products (e.g., cord factor from *M. lepraemurium*), one must still resort to chemical methods.

Synthesis of Cord Factor and Analogs

Early on, as the structure of cord factor was being established, initial efforts at synthesis were already undertaken in anticipation of confirming the inferred structure-biologic function relationships. These, as well as more recent syntheses, are "partial" rather than "total" inasmuch as the molecule was assembled from the naturally occurring components (trehalose and mycolic acids). The limitations of the early synthesis schemes have been reviewed by Tocanne[353] and by Toubiana and coworkers.[358] Considerably more elegant methodology has evolved recently for the synthesis of trehalose dimycolates as well as of diesters of much lower molecular weight.

In Figure 4–39, 6,6'-didesoxydibromo

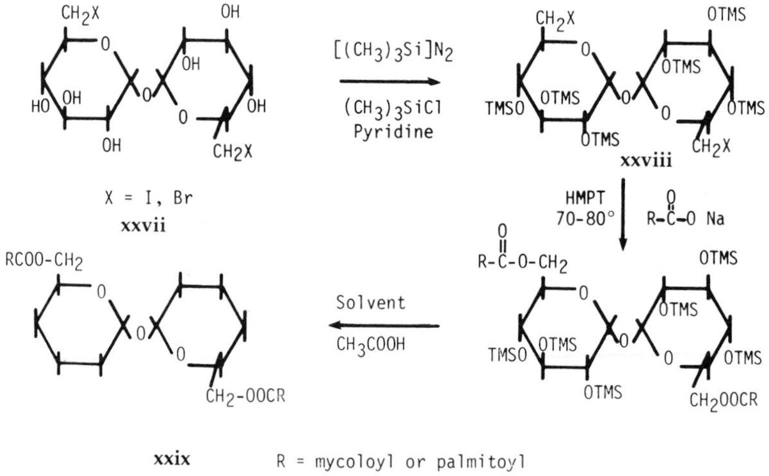

FIGURE 4–39. Improved cord factor synthesis.

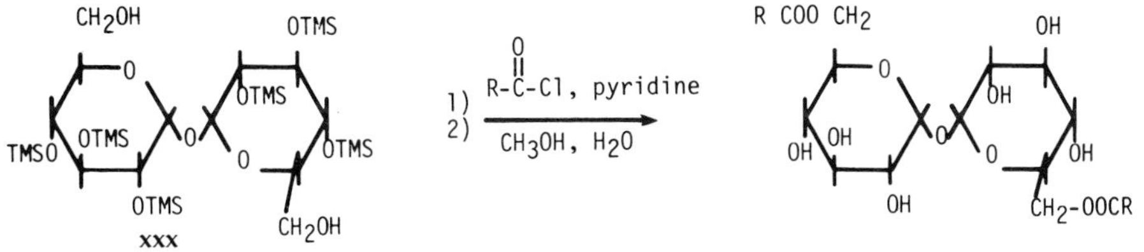

FIGURE 4–40. Synthesis of simple cord factor analogs by acylation of hexa-O-trimethylsilyl trehalose.

(or iodo) trehalose (*xxvii,* as shown on opposite page) is converted to the hexa-trimethylsilyl (TMS) derivative (*xxviii*), for protecting the hydroxyl functions and promoting the solubility of the carbohydrate in the reaction solvent (hexamethylphosphoric triamide). At a moderately elevated temperature (70 to 80°) this intermediate condenses readily with carboxylic acid salts to yield the hexa-TMS derivative of cord factor (or analog). The protecting groups are then easily removed by heating in solvents containing water or small amounts of acetic acid and the (cord factor) products (*xxix*) are purified by chromatography. Trehalose 6,6′ dimycolate synthesized in this manner has the physical and spectroscopic properties of the natural products, as well as those biologic activities that have been tested.

An extremely useful variant (Fig. 4–40) for synthesis of the lower molecular weight analogs involves esterification of 2, 3, 4, 2′3′4′ hexa-O-trimethylsilyl trehalose (*xxx*) with an acid chloride, followed by detrimethylsilylation. The intermediate (*xxx*) is readily obtainable from octa-TMS-trehalose by a selective detrimethylsilylation of the 6,6′ hydroxyl functions with alcoholic potassium carbonate.[125, 139a, 358] In this fashion, trehalose 6,6′ dipalmitate, dibehenate, dibehenoyl behenoate (Toubiana), di-*p* nitro-(and amino) benzoate (Gensler), and dihemisuccinate (Goren and Brokl) have been prepared. The diesters of Toubiana and colleagues[359] have been examined for antitumor activity while the hemisuccinate and the *p* aminobenzoate were used to prepare protein conjugates of trehalose. The hemisuccinate conjugate elicits antibodies in rabbits with trehalose specificity.

Synthetic Pseudo-Cord Factors

In addition to the simpler 6,6′-diesters of trehalose of Toubiana, other pseudo-(ψ) cord factors based on sucrose, glucose, or mannose have been synthesized by J. Asselineau's group; biologic activities of these compounds have been assessed in an extensive collaborative program with the late Masahiko Kato of Osaka. The thrust of these investigations has been to gain insight into structure-biologic activity relationships — and they revealed a surprising stringency that is imposed by the stereochemical disposition of the hydroxyl functions in the carbohydrate moiety.

Our own studies (in progress) concern ψ-cord factors in which we alter the functional role of the trehalose core in its covalent bonding to a variety of simple lipid substituents and assess the influence of these alterations on biologic activities.[142, 146] The synthesis studies are concerned with three types of ψ-cord factors, depicted in abbreviated form in Figure 4–41. This shows: a) the true cord factor structure; b) "mirror" ψCF, in which the functionality of the ester linkage is reversed so that trehalose is behaving as a carboxylic compound esterified to a lipid alcohol; c) "amide" ψ-cord factors of 6,6′-dideoxydiamino trehalose (suggested to us by Dr. B. C. Das); and d) "mirror amide" ψCF in

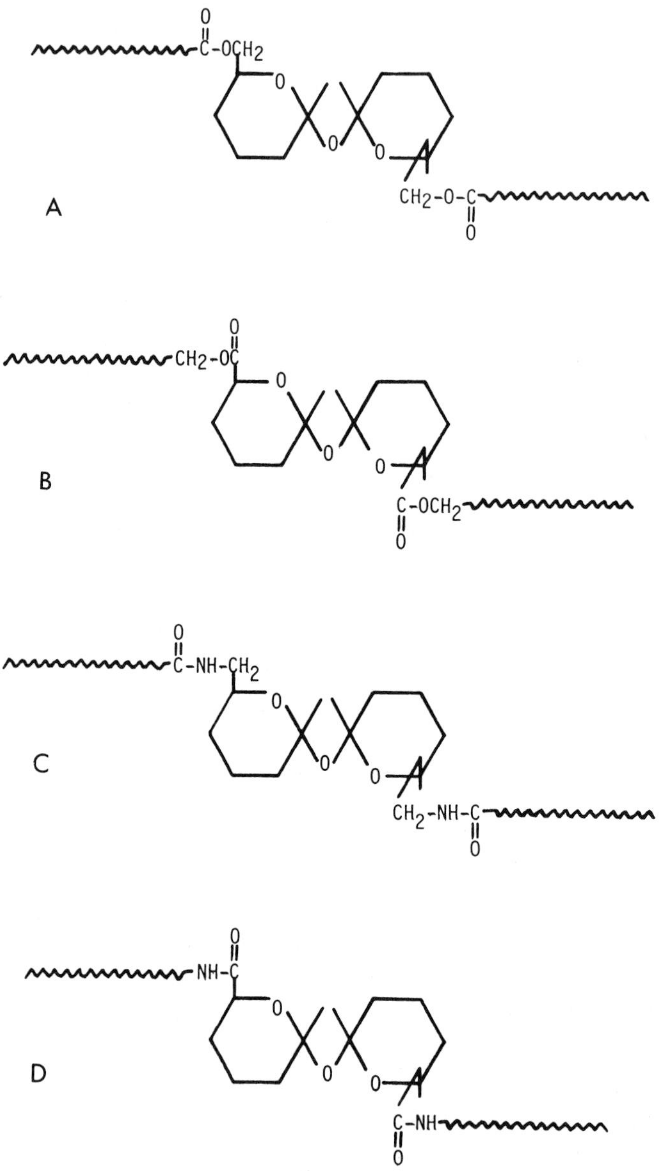

FIGURE 4–41. Various pseudo-cord factor (ψ CF) structures obtainable by synthesis. The variants are based on alterations in the covalent linkages between the carbohydrate core and the lipid substituents.

A, trehalose 6,6′ diesters (true cord factor); B, esters of trehalose 6,6′ dicarboxylic acid ("mirror" pseudo-CF); C, amides of -6,6′-diamino trehalose (amide pseudo-CF); and D, amides of trehalose 6,6′ dicarboxylic acid ("mirror" amide pseudo-cord factors).

which the functionality of the components in the latter group is reversed.

The "mirror" types of ψCF are based upon α-D-glucopyranuronosyl $(1\rightarrow1)$ α-D-glucopyranuronoside — "trehalose-6,6'-dicarboxylic acid" (TDA), which is prepared by a catalytic oxidation of trehalose, as shown in Figure 4–42. This also depicts the conversion of TDA (*xxxi*) into the bis *n*-octadecylamide (*xxxii*). Figure 4–43 depicts alternate synthesis pathways leading from TDA to the higher molecular weight bis-di-*n*-octadecylamide (BDA–TDA) (*xxxiii*) and to a "mirror" ψCF (*xxxiv*) in which trehalose dicarboxylic acid has been esterified with p-hexadecyloxyphenyl butanol. These products and analogs have been tested for cord-factorlike toxicity in mice and for antitumor activity in strain 2 guinea pigs.

Biologic Activities

In addition to the immobilizing effect of cord factor on polymorphonuclear leukocytes, which Bloch described, he recognized a peculiar and characteristic toxicity that purified cord factor and even impure concentrates of the glycolipid exerted in mice: a few repeated intraperitoneal injections of small amounts of the material dissolved in paraffin oil killed a majority of the animals — particularly C57Bl and Dba mice. We have abundantly confirmed Bloch's observation that in young (12 to 14 g) C57 Bl mice, some 10 μg of highly purified material injected at 2 to 3 day intervals elicits a precipitous weight loss, and the mice begin to die after about a week. Yet a much larger dose (50 to 100 μg) is rarely lethal. Figure 4–44 compares the toxicity of the cord factor P3 (Aoyama B) with that of TDA bis-*n*-octadecylamide (*xxxii*) in C57Bl mice. Four intraperitoneal injections of 10 μg P3 or 100 μg of the ψ cord factor were lethal to all the mice; however, they survived four 50 μg doses of the latter. The bis-octadecylamide, nevertheless, sensitized the mice to cord factor; a single injection of 10 μg P3 was lethal for the survivors. The aromatic diester of TDA [(*xxxiv*) in Fig. 4–43]

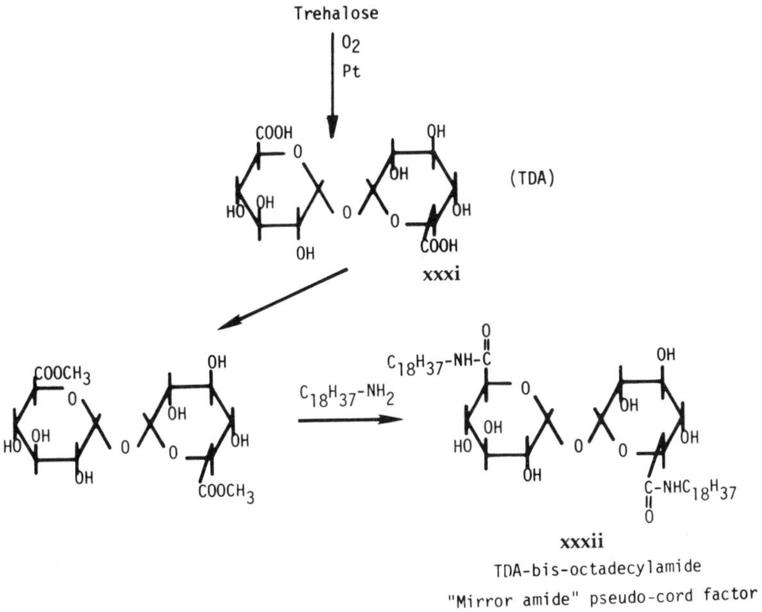

FIGURE 4–42. Synthesis of a simple "mirror-amide" pseudo-cord factor.

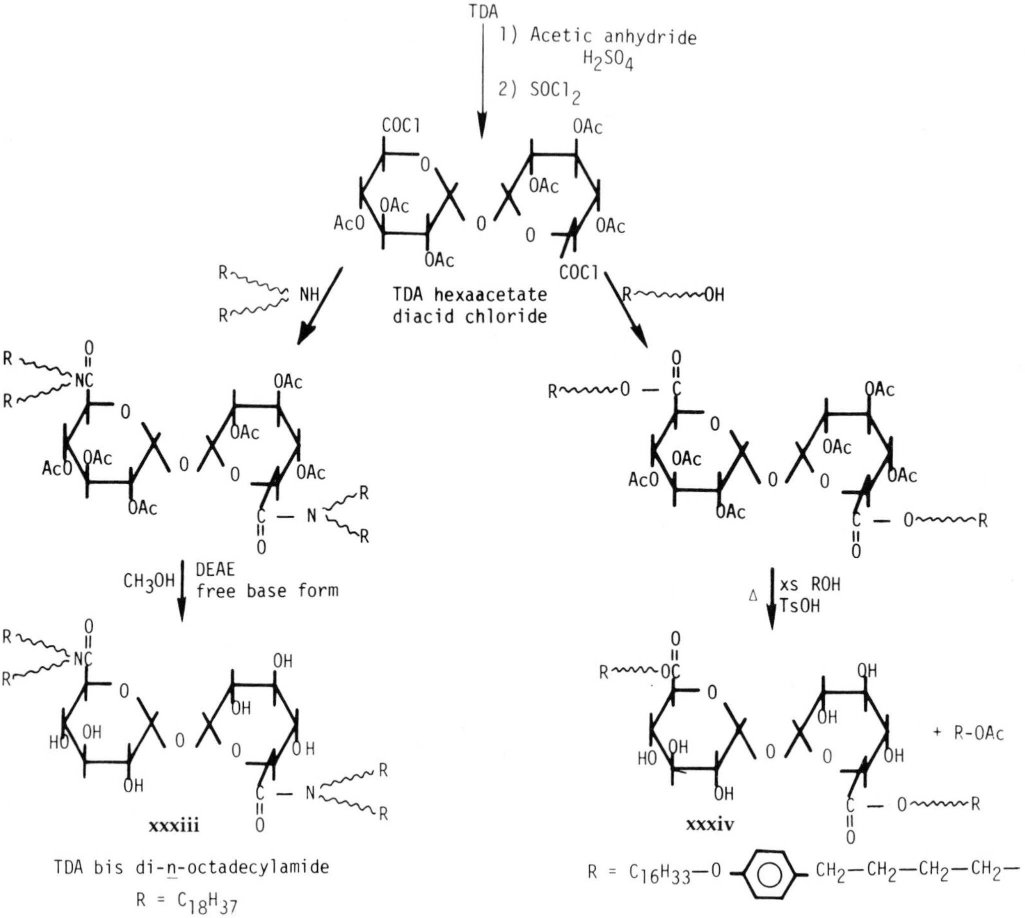

R = $C_{18}H_{37}$

"Mirror amide" pseudo-cord factor — "Mirror" pseudo-cord factor

FIGURE 4–43. Synthesis of (1) a more complex "mirror amide" and (2) a "mirror" ψCF.

is slightly more toxic than *xxxii.* But the ψ-cord factor (*xxxiii*), of higher molecular weight and "branched" so as to more nearly resemble a mycolate, is surprisingly of very low toxicity.

Aside from an intense peritonitis, the most striking feature to be seen at necropsy of mice dying from cord factor intoxication is acute pulmonary hemorrhage. The ψ-cord factors elicit the same behavior. To an immunologist the terms "anaphylaxis" and "Shwartzman reaction" come to mind, but no evidence in support of either phenomenon has been forthcoming and the evolution of the pathology remains unknown. Very early in the history of cord factor it was speculated that the unusual toxicity might be associated with the rather bizarre and extraordinary detergent-like structure of the lipid. The behavior of several ψCF seems to support this notion. Most detergents (and natural lipids) do not have such an abundance of lipophilic relative to hydrophilic structures. Still, Bloch[50] found similar gross toxic activity in simple extracts of ox lungs — an improbable source of cord factor.

Biochemical Mechanisms in Cord Factor Toxicity. In the interpretations of Bekierkunst and collaborators, cord factor (and tuberculosis infection) stim-

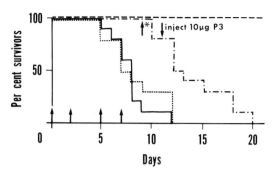

FIGURE 4–44. Toxicity of cord factor ("Aoyama B" P3) and of the bisoctadecyl amide of trehalose dicarboxylic acid [(*xxii*) of Fig. 4–42] in C57 black mice. Oil solutions of the lipids were injected intraperitoneally on days indicated by arrows.

Key:
    — — —   oil control
    ————   P3 (Aoyama B) 10 μg
    - - - - - -   TDA diamide 100 μg
    —.—.—.   TDA diamide 50 μg
    *   fifth injection of TDA diamide 50 μg

ulate mammalian nicotinamide adenine dinucleotidase activity, leading to depressed levels of host-NAD, especially in lung, liver, and spleen tissues and an associated depression in activities of NAD-linked microsomal enzymes.[16] These observations were largely confirmed by Shankaran and Venkitasubramanian,[321] who noted yet additional aberrations in depression of muscle and liver glycogen synthesis and deranged pyruvate metabolism. In studies of both groups, cord factor intoxication was in part relieved by administration either of NAD (Bekierkunst) or nicotinamide (Venkitasubramanian).

In a prodigious series of studies, Masahiko Kato described other biochemical lesions induced in cord factor intoxication and in tuberculosis, which were ultimately traced to a direct physical attack by the agents on mitochondrial membranes and mitochondria, especially of lung, liver, and spleen.[181-184] This is demonstrable, both in vivo and in vitro, with isolated mitochondrial preparations, and the attack results in a pathologic, irreversible mitochondrial swelling with fragmentation of cristae. A comparable disruption of liver micro-

somes by the membrane-active glycolipid may account for the depression by cord factor of microsomal enzyme activities reported by I. Toida.[354, 355] The biochemical consequences of the mitochondrial attack translate into a severe disturbance in electron flow along the mitochondrial respiratory chain and disruption of oxidative phosphorylation. This activity and its toxic manifestation in vivo are surprisingly sensitive to structural changes in the glycolipid molecule: they are destroyed by acetylation or permethylation. In synthetic analogs, studied abundantly in a fruitful collaboration between M. Kato and J. Asselineau, substitution of sucrose or glucose for trehalose results in a marked attenuation but not in total abrogation of the activity.[188] Substitution at the 6 position of the carbohydrate is stringently required; 1- and 2-mycoloyl glucose are devoid of toxicity. The stereochemical disposition of the hydroxyl groups at positions 2, 3, and 4 (of 6-mycoloyl methyl glycosides) critically affects the biologic activity.[24] Thus, the association between substantially spatial orientations and expression of at least these activities bespeaks not simply the random attack of a detergent molecule but rather a more specific interaction between the cord factor hydroxyl functions and presumed sites of attack on the membrane surface. Invariably those substances found to be inactive in vivo did not derange mitochondrial structure or function in vitro.

Immunogenic, Granulomagenic, and Adjuvant Activity. Cord factor is not in itself immunogenic, but Ohara and colleagues[274] demonstrated its haptenic properties in stimulating antibody formation when injected into animals, with swine serum as a carrier protein. According to Kato,[185-187] complexes of cord factor with methylated bovine serum albumin (MBSA) stimulated production of 19S IgM precipitins with cord factor (and trehalose) specificity when given in Freund's incomplete adjuvant to mice and rabbits. Mice immunized in this fashion or passively protected with rabbit antiserum were evidently highly resistant to toxic doses of cord factor and to intravenous challenge with virulent tubercle bacilli. In infection, however, cord factor is evidently not presented to the host's immune system in an immunogenic fashion: antibody against cord factor is not detectable in sera of either active, convalescent, or pneumonectomized human tuberculosis patients.[186]

Bekierkunst and coworkers[44] found that when dilute cord factor solutions in mineral oil are emulsified in Tween-saline and injected intravenously into mice, the oil solution of glycolipid (both are required) stimulates formation of pulmonary granulomas. In the interpretation of Barksdale and Kim,[40] these would appear to be "foreign body type granulomas" rather than "infectious agent granulomas," although in mice they appear to exhibit at least some of the characteristics of the latter; thus, the pulmonary granulomatous response to cord factor is evidently much greater in mice that have been infected intraperitoneally with BCG. Guinea pigs as well as rabbits seem to be relatively insensitive to intravenous oily-cord factor

aqueous emulsions.[263] Rabbits sensitized with BCG do not respond vigorously to cord factor nor does cord factor act to inhibit macrophage migration from either cord-factor-injected or BCG-sensitized rabbits. Still, in mice the cord factor granuloma confers some protection against an intravenous challenge with virulent tubercle bacilli.[44, 249]

Oil solutions of cord factor emulsified in Tween-saline are adjuvant active. Bekierkunst and colleagues[47] described a curious reversal of activities in which cord factor but not wax D elicited an enhanced humoral response in mice to sheep erythrocytes (Compare with White et al.[382, 383]). The observation was subsequently confirmed by Saito and associates[304] who showed that in mice, cord factor as a substitute for killed mycobacteria in Freund's complete adjuvant was more active than an equal weight of killed tubercle bacilli; it elicited delayed hypersensitivity to protein antigens in rats but when presented in this fashion to guinea pigs was inactive. Independently, Granger, Yamamoto, and Ribi[149] recognized this inactivity in guinea pigs. However, when presented in another fashion, cord factor also induces delayed hypersensitivity to protein antigens in this animal species. P_3 in $CHCl_3$-CH_3OH was mixed with either tuberculoprotein or bovine serum albumin, the solvent evaporated, the protein-cord factor wet with a little mineral oil, and the whole emulsified in Tween-saline. The emulsion injected into footpads of guinea pigs elicited a powerful delayed-type hypersensitivity to the proteins.

Antitumor Activity. Based upon mechanisms that are not entirely understood but that probably implicate detergent-like activity and adjuvant behavior, trehalose dimycolates have emerged as a principal factor or cofactor in contributing to antitumor activity of a variety of preparations. Following upon recognition of the granulomagenic and adjuvant activity, Bekierkunst and colleagues reported that mice given CF emulsions intravenously resisted the induction of pulmonary adenomas, which are elicited by an injection of urethane. An intraperitoneal injection of cord factor or even of much simpler analogs, such as trehalose 6,6' dipalmitate, also suppressed the proliferation of Ehrlich ascites cells.[45, 393]

With only few exceptions, cord factor when used alone has been largely ineffective in suppression or regression of various experimental tumors. However, it has shown marked antitumor activity against a syngeneic murine leukemia[217] and the 1023 syngeneic murine fibrosarcoma.[392] In the latter study, aqueous emulsions of cord factor solutions in mineral oil were injected directly into 7-day-old established tumors and induced complete regression in a number of animals. An amplified granulomagenic activity of cord factor with increase in the oil content of the emulsion is reflected in an enhanced antitumor activity. Thus, .05 ml of emulsions containing 9 percent oil (and 150 μg cord factor) were more than twice as effective as those containing only 1 percent oil, curing all of the mice. Leclerc's system examined the suppression of growth of L1210 lymphocytic leukemia cells injected intraperitoneally into (C57 Bl/6 $\times$ DBA/2) F_1 hybrids. Intraperitoneal injection of an oil or peanut oil solution of cord factor as an aqueous emulsion 14 days prior to challenge prevented growth of the tumor cells in over 80 percent of the animals. In these studies, WSA and muramyl dipeptides were entirely inactive.

For several years, cord factor has played a dominant and almost exclusive role in the very impressive antitumor activity of experimental vaccines based upon the oil solutions-aqueous emulsions (alluded to earlier), which found their basis in the "cell wall" vaccines of E. Ribi and colleagues. These were the subject of a prodigious series of investigations targeted at the development of a nonviable and effective immunogen against tuberculosis.[291, 292] The cell wall vaccines were prepared by grinding lyophilized mycobacterial cell walls (of BCG, *M. tuberculosis* H37Ra, or virulent strains) in a small but stringently required amount of mineral oil and emulsifying the paste in Tween-saline. The lipophilic mycobacterial cell walls evidently associate and remain with the oil phase in the final emulsion, giving the oil droplets the appearance of being "coated" with cell wall particles. (Hydrophilic cell walls, such as those from *Listeria monocytogenes*, do not behave in a similar fashion.) The oil-cell wall vaccines, injected intravenously into mice or subhuman primates, elicit extensive pulmonary and splenic granulomas; at the same time, they confer high levels of protection against aerosol challenge with virulent tubercle bacilli. (See Chapters 8 and 11 and Youmans and Youmans[397] for full discussion.) If oil emulsions and aqueous suspensions of BCG cell wall are simply mixed together without the prior association, the mixture is virtually inactive. Efforts to dissociate the granulomagenic properties from the immunogenic have been unsuccessful; deproteinized and delipidated cell wall ("cell wall skeleton"), or chemically degraded cell wall, lost these activities; however, both were essentially completely restored in parallel if the inactive cell walls were combined with a small amount of tuberculoprotein and cord factor (P3) or cord factor-containing mycobacterial lipids. Indeed, an effective but nonspecific and short-lived resistance to tuberculosis challenge can be elicited with vaccines containing P3, oil, and *heterologous* antigens (such as BSA, acylated [dodecanoyl] BSA, and lipopolysaccharides of *E. coli* or *S. typhimurium*).[293] The degree of resistance was consistent with the level and duration of pulmonary granuloma stimulated by these agents.

Many of these combinations just mentioned evolved following recognition of the antitumor activity of the oil-BCG cell wall vaccine in the model strain 2 guinea pig-line 10 tumor system of H. J. Rapp and colleagues.[289] This tumor line, originally established as a hepatocarcinoma by feeding guinea pigs diethylnitrosamine, is carried in an ascites form for successive transplant generations. Intradermal inoculation of 10^6 cells into a recipient establishes a growing-tumor nodule, which metastasizes by the sixth day to the regional lymph nodes, continues to grow, and kills the recipient in about 10 weeks. Intralesional injection of 7-day-old tumor nodules with viable BCG cured about 50 percent or more of the animals and rendered them immune to a subsequent rechallenge with line 10 cells. Indeed, this second challenge is briskly rejected with a typical delayed hypersensitivity response.[398]

When the oil-BCG cell wall "vaccine" is substituted for viable BCG, the results obtained are equally as good or even better.[253, 399] Degraded cell wall ("cell wall skeleton," or CWS) is less effective, but full activity is essentially restored if the CWS is "coated" with cord factor (P3) before the oil is added. In quite similar studies, Bekierkunst and colleagues[46] showed that the limited antitumor activity of delipidated and deproteinized cell wall of H37Ra (oil/Tween-saline emulsion) was notably increased if the cell walls were first treated with cord factor. Only rarely has an aqueous emulsion of cord factor-in-oil — in the absence of a second component — shown tumor regression activity; invariably, both components are required.

With cord factor as a common denominator several additional interesting natural products were discerned. These ordinarily exhibited either no significant or only transient tumor regression activity, but when cord factor was present, impressive activity was elicited. Included are cell wall of *M. smegmatis*, cell wall and endotoxin of *E. coli*, phenol-water extracts ("endotoxin-like") of *Coxiella burnetii*[193] or from mycobacteria,[251] and especially endotoxins of rough (Re) mutants of *Salmonella typhimurium*.[294, 295] The latter, in combination with cord fac-

tor, have been among the most potent agents in stimulating (on intravenous injection) massive and prolonged pulmonary granulomas in mice, in protecting *nonspecifically* against airborne *M. tuberculosis* challenge, and in tumor regression. On the other hand, wild-type Salmonella endotoxins, which have a more abundant or even a complete adornment of carbohydrates (as in the "O" antigens) are notably inactive.

Role of Cord Factor in Experimental Tuberculosis Immunization and Tumor Regression

It seems logical that the granulomagenic and adjuvant properties of cord factor probably contribute to the spectrum of activities within the granulomatous pulmonary environment during challenge with *M. tuberculosis* and in the tumor environment during its regression under attack by the host-immune system. For eliciting a considerable degree of resistance to *M. tuberculosis* challenge, the granulomagenic and adjuvant behavior alone seems sufficient, although undeniably the resistance may be enhanced considerably, specifically when mycobacterial cell wall or associated protein antigens have been used in the "immunization." On the other hand, cord factor type of toxicity and adjuvant activity coupled with even extensive granuloma are in themselves not sufficient in the tumor system. Other qualities of cord factor that may be invoked in these phenomena might reside in its demonstrable behavior as a chemotaxigen (with fresh plasma), which was recognized by Kelly,[192] and in a stimulating effect on macrophages. Yarkoni, Wang, and Bekierkunst[394] found that intraperitoneal injection of cord factor oil emulsions into mice stimulates the peritoneal macrophages harvested after several days, as recognized in their content of lysosomal acid phosphatase and by increased phagocytic capability for *L. monocytogenes*. Viable or killed BCG, injected intraperitoneally, stimulated the adherent cell population in a like manner. However, attempts at a similar stimulation of prepared macrophage monolayers in vitro were unsuccessful.

The eloquent review of Bast and colleagues[41] provides a logical scenario of immunologic events that are triggered in the tumor environment on treatment with, for example, viable BCG. Successful immunotherapy requires a small tumor burden, contact between tumor cells and the immunostimulant (most effectively achieved by intralesional injection), an appropriate dose of viable BCG organisms, an adequate ability of the host to respond to the stimulus (i.e., an intact thymus-dependent response), certainly functional macrophages and histiocytes, and preferably, an ability of the host to develop an immune response to tumor-associated antigens.

Two mechanisms to account for the antitumor activity of immunostimulants have been proposed.

In the first, tumor cells are killed nonspecifically as "innocent bystanders" at sites of inflammation that contain leukocytes that have been activated by local or systemic administration of immunostimulants. In the other mechanism, immunostimulants act as adjuvants to augment immunity against tumor-specific antigens.[41]

Viable BCG would seem to be adequately endowed with both qualities, in the absence of any direct toxic activity of BCG demonstrable against tumor cells in vitro. In brief, the site of BCG infection is one of intense chronic granulomatous inflammation characterized by an abundant influx of lymphocytes, macrophages, and activated histiocytes. Lymphocytes under the stimulus of mycobacterial antigens (sustained in these circumstances) have been shown to kill or inhibit growth of tumor cells by direct contact or by release of lymphokines. The latter embrace factors that activate macrophages nonspecifi-

cally to either a cytotoxic or cystostatic level for bacteria and neoplastic cells but not normal cells. Macrophage processing of tumor antigens in the site, amplified by the adjuvant qualities of the mycobacterial component, adds a *specific* dimension to the immunologic events; under the circumstances of an effective therapy, it provides the systemic tumor-specific immunity in which tumor cells in metastatic foci are destroyed. In the main, cord factor may have the ability to stimulate what would appear superficially to be the same series of events; nevertheless, it is manifestly insufficient.

In Ribi's recent analysis of the endotoxin-P3-oil system, early tumor-damaging effects are likely attributable to microvascular damage and the activation of macrophages mediated by endotoxin. The concomitant development of a (persistent) cellular hypersensitization to protein contaminants of the endotoxin (or of BCG cell walls) appears to be an essential part of the mechanism — to sustain an intense granulomatous reaction at the site. This development of DTH occurs over 4 to 5 days and requires an association of the antigen with the oil droplet component of the vaccine. The same stringent requirement applies to the BCG cell wall-oil droplet vaccine. As reviewed by Bast, and fellow researchers, radiolabeled ". . . cell walls attached to oil droplets localize in paracortical areas of regional lymph nodes (see for example dodecanoyl BSA, p. 118) where a brisk granulomatous reaction is elicited. Cell walls that are not attached to oil droplets pass through the same nodes, producing little change in their architecture."[41]

This requirement for association of endotoxin with the oil droplets is evidently met by incorporating P3 into the system — very likely owing to the surface-active detergentlike properties of cord factor. It is demonstrable with labeled protein antigens such as PPD or BSA (see p. 132).[149]

We have reached similar conclusions, which are supported by the biologic activities of the synthetic pseudo-cord factors as well as by those of certain natural lipids, of which some are related to trehalose dimycolate while others are not.[142, 146]

None of the synthetic ψCF has a toxicity matching that of natural cord factor, nor do the natural products such as croton oil, retinol (vitamin A alcohol), or the sulfolipids of *M. tuberculosis* exhibit significant "cord-factorlike" toxicity. In line 10 tumor studies, the entirely nontoxic mycobacterial sulfolipids and the *least toxic* of the pseudo-cord factors (BDA-TDA) are completely effective substitutes for cord factor in combination with the mutant Re endotoxin.[146] Neither the sulfatides nor BDA-TDA have the granulomagenic qualities of cord factor.[391a] The sulfatides are not adjuvant active,[304] nor do these substances alone possess antitumor activity. Croton oil, retinol, several of the other more toxic ψ-cord factors, and even *di-n-octadecylamine*[132a] are effective when combined with endotoxin in regressing established line 10 tumors, although less so than the previously mentioned substances. McLaughlin and coresearchers[249-251] found in parallel studies that the very weakly toxic arabinose monomycolate, trehalose monomycolate, and the entirely nontoxic mycolic acid can also effectively substitute for cord factor in this system.

The antitumor activity of any of these substances, in combination with mutant endotoxin, denies an important role for cord-factorlike toxicity in this behavior and possibly for adjuvant activity; both of these may be adequately provided by the endotoxin. All of them share — in common with trehalose dimycolate — amphipathic, surface-active character. Simplistically, they would all seem capable of associating with polar functional groups on the endotoxin molecules via their individual concentrated polar areas, which are highly variable, and therefore orient hydrophobic "tails" outward from the surface into the oil phase. This would ensure the stringently required association of endotoxin with the oil vehicle.

It seems likely that a vast number of other agents — even simple-structured ones exist or can be synthesized — will be able to provide this behavior in an adequate degree. Although the emergence of these agents may ultimately abolish the need for cord factor as a required component in these preparations, it does not diminish the importance of this still-fascinating glycolipid. Its serendipitous utilization with various cofactors revealed the extraordinary potentiation of cryptic antitumor (and antitubercular) activities of the "cofactors" — activities that otherwise would probably have long remained unrecognized.

SULFATIDES OF *M. TUBERCULOSIS*

The sulfolipids, or sulfatides, of *M. tuberculosis* are the second group of trehalose esters that were discovered in the search for substances that could be implicated in cord formation or in neutral red reactivity. The reactivity, it was reasoned, was quite likely the property of a peripherally located and probably (strongly) acidic substance that complexed the dye. According to Middlebrook, Coleman, and Schaefer,[254] treatment of virulent tubercle bacilli cells with hexane that contained small amounts of an aliphatic amine (to facilitate the solubilization of *acidic* materials) extracted lipid substances that complexed and solubilized neutral red into the organic phase — a property consistent with the behavior of a strongly acidic, fairly high molecular weight lipid. Solvent separations showed the activity to concentrate in fractions enriched, not in phosphorus, but in sulfur — i.e., a "sulfolipid." In unpublished studies of Middlebrook and Coleman, the sulfolipid was recognized to be an ester of trehalose sulfate, probably substituted with methyl-branched acids.

In the succeeding investigations of Goren and colleagues (originally begun in collaboration with Middlebrook), the "sulfolipid" (SL) of H37Rv was recognized to consist of several distinct "families" of closely related sulfatides. The separation of the various sulfatide families from neutral and acidic components and from those as yet uncharacterized is achieved by multiple column chromatographies on diethylaminoethyl cellulose (DEAE).[133] After neutral and weakly acidic contaminants are separated, ammoniated solvents elute the various sulfatides individually and as mixtures to yield, in succession, tetraacylated components SL-II', SL-II, SL-I (principal), and SL-I' and finally a triacylated product designated SL-III. Individual sulfatides are purified from these fractions by additional chromatographies.

Structural Studies

The principal efforts involved elucidation of the SL-I structure, since it is by far the most abundant sulfatide — about 0.7 percent based on dry bacillary harvest — elaborated by *M. tuberculosis*. The infrared spectrum of NH₄SL-I taken as a smear on a KBr plate (Fig. 4–45) is most informatively interpreted on the basis of its structure, now known — a tetraacyl trehalose 2-sulfate. Peaks at 3220 cm⁻¹ and the broadened band between 1400–1450 cm⁻¹ are attributable to NH absorption; abundant H-bonded hydroxyl functions are evident from the broad band in the 3300 cm⁻¹ region. The carbonyl region (1660 to 1745 cm⁻¹) exhibits shouldering and band broadening that is associated with a multiplicity of ester functions and with carbonyl-to-OH interactions in the "smear."[133] The sulfate ester is characterized by peaks at 1250 and 824 cm⁻¹; the latter is attributable to a sulfate group occupying a secondary equatorial position. This band disappears when NH₄SL-I is desulfated. A weak band at about 808 cm⁻¹ is specifically associated with a "Type 3" absorption of α,α trehalose. As established by permethylation analysis, all of the SL families are structured on trehalose-2-sulfate. The deep absorption band at 1370 is due to a mul-

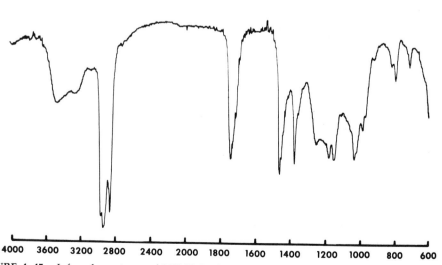

4000	3600	3200	2800	2400	2000	1800	1600	1400	1200	1000	800	600

FIGURE 4–45. Infrared spectrum of NH₄SL-I taken as a "smear" on KBr plate. Absorption bands confirm the structure as a sulfated trehalose esterified with multibranched acyl substituents.

tiplicity of methyl branches, which characterize phthioceranic and hydroxyphthioceranic acyl substituents on the trehalose core; these are apparently unique to the mycobacterial sulfatides.

With the exception of SL-III, the ammonium forms of the remaining sulfatide families are remarkably sensitive to desulfation; complete loss of (radiolabeled) sulfate and of neutral red reactivity occurs spontaneously and fairly rapidly at room temperature when the sulfatide is merely dissolved in reagent grade "anhydrous" ether. The sodium salt is quite stable except in the presence of even traces of acid. (For a mechanistic interpretation of this behavior, see Goren.[135]) Practically, the spontaneous desulfation was employed as a rather precise method for deter-

mining the molecular weight (about 2400) of the principal sulfatide NH$_4$SL-I and for preparing desulfated lipid for the structural studies.[134]

Distribution of the Acyl Functions

Permethylation under nonisomerizing conditions (see Fig. 4–46) of desulfated SL-I, designated SL I-CF, and alkaline hydrolysis of the product yielded a methylated carbohydrate that was identified as 2,3,4,4' tetra-O-methyl trehalose; acid cleavage yielded two fragments: 2,3,4 tri-O-methylglucose (xxxv) and 4-O-methylglucose (xxxvi). In these products, methyl groups indicate positions on the carbohydrate that were unoccupied (free) during the permethylation; OH groups represent positions

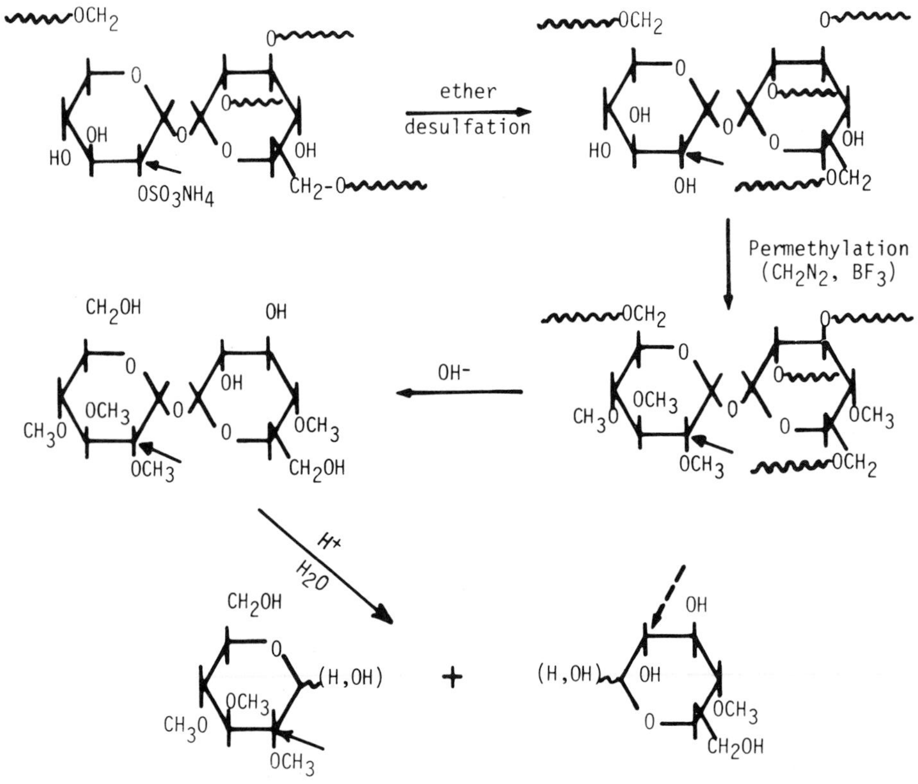

FIGURE 4–46. Location of acylated positions in SL-I.

that were blocked by some substituents. Since the sulfate ester in SL-I is located at a 2 position (Fig. 4–46, arrows), at least one 2 position is *vacant* after desulfation and would be *methylated* in the succeeding permethylation reaction. In (*xxxvi*), the 2 position (broken arrow) is unmethylated; therefore, it must have been occupied (by an acyl group) during the permethylation reaction. Accordingly, (*xxxvi*) cannot represent the glucose moiety originally bearing the sulfate. Instead, the sulfate was originally present in fragment (*xxxv*) (arrow). This glucose originally was also substituted by an acyl function at the 6 position. Fragment (*xxxvi*) derives from a glucose moiety acylated at the 2, 3, and 6 positions, with the 4 position vacant. Accordingly, SL-I is a 2,3,6,6' tetraacyl trehalose-2'-sulfate. The locations of the acyl functions in the remaining SL families were derived in a similar fashion and are summarized in Table 4–5.[141]

Identification of the Acyl Substituents[140]

From alkaline solvolysis of either SL-I or the desulfated analog, methyl esters of the substituent carboxylic acids were prepared and separated into three principal series: *A, B,* and *C*. Component *B* was easily identified by gas chromatography and mass spectrometry as a mixture of nearly equal amounts of methyl palmitate and stearate, with minor quantities of lower homologs. Component *C* was composed of a series of closely related homologs partly separable by silicic acid chromatography. The infrared patterns of the individual *C* fractions indicated these to be hydroxylated esters, heavily substituted with methyl branches. From mass spectrometry and NMR spectra of *C* and of derived products (for example, O-methyl ether and the corresponding ketone) the structure of the *C*-series acids was established as shown below (*xxxvii*).

In the principal member, n equals 7, but homologs with up to 10 methyl branches have been identified. The *C* series have been given the trivial name, *hydroxyphthioceranic acids.* The *A* components are almost identical with those of the *C* series except that they lack a hydroxylic function. By mass spectrometry and NMR, *A* was seen to be the completely reduced analog of *C*, viz., (*xxxviii*) with a similar homology. By dehydration and catalytic hydrogenation, *C* components are converted into corresponding members of the *A* series. In the principal homolog of *A*, n = 6. Both lower and higher homologs have been recognized. Members of this series are designated phthioceranic acids.

In both series, the individual components that have been separated are all dextrorotatory. Therefore, like the phthienoic acids (see p. 149), they have the L-configuration. The phthioceranic homologs of lower molecular weight would be the enantiomers of the mycocerosic acids (see p. 151). Their biosynthesis is judged to occur in the same fashion (but probably with different enzymes) by condensations of palmitate with successive molecules of methyl malonate. Thus, when H37Rv is culti-

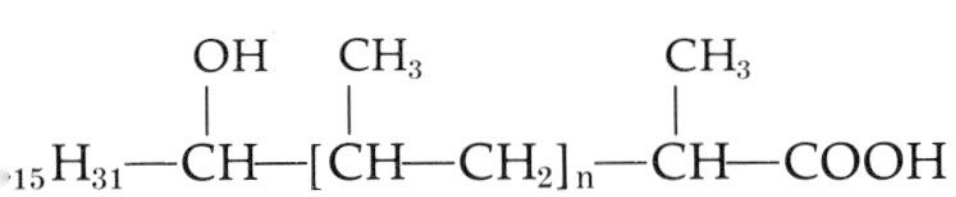

$$\underset{15}{H_{31}}-\overset{\overset{\displaystyle OH}{|}}{CH}-[\overset{\overset{\displaystyle CH_3}{|}}{CH}-CH_2]_n-\overset{\overset{\displaystyle CH_3}{|}}{CH}-COOH$$

hydroxyphthioceranic acid
xxxvii

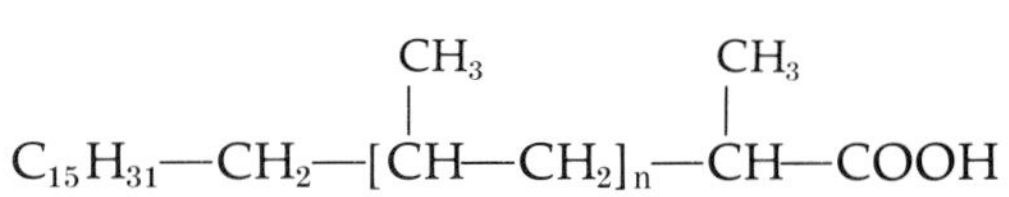

$$C_{15}H_{31}-CH_2-[\overset{\overset{\displaystyle CH_3}{|}}{CH}-CH_2]_n-\overset{\overset{\displaystyle CH_3}{|}}{CH}-COOH$$

phthioceranic acid
xxxviii

TABLE 4–5.   Gross Structures of Five SL Families

Sulfatide[a]	Trehalose positions substituted	Palmitate/ stearate	Phthio-ceranate[b]	Hydroxy-phthio-ceranate[c]
		Mols Acyl Substituent		
SL-II'	2,4,6,6'	1	0	3
SL-II	2,3,6,6'	1	0	3
SL-I (principal)	2,3,6,6'	1	1	2
SL-I'	2,3,6,6'	1	2	1
SL-III	2,3,6	1	0	2

[a] Sulfate in 2'-position.

[b] Phthioceranate: $C_{16}H_{33}$—$[\overset{\overset{\text{CH}_3}{|}}{C}H$—$CH_2]_n$—$\overset{\overset{\text{CH}_3}{|}}{C}H$—COOH *where* n = 2–9; 6 principal.

[c] Hydroxyphthioceranate: $C_{15}H_{31}$—$\overset{\overset{\text{OH}}{|}}{C}H$—$[\overset{\overset{\text{CH}_3}{|}}{C}H$—$CH_2]_n$—$\overset{\overset{\text{CH}_3}{|}}{C}H$—COOH *where* n = 2–10; 7 principal.

vated with 1-^{14}C-propionate, the radiolabel is heavily incorporated into both the phthioceranic and hydroxyphthioceranic acids of all SL families. The B components (principally palmitate and stearate) are essentially free of radiolabel.

Quantitative separation of the ester mixture derived from SL-I indicates the molar ratios of A:B:C in this principal

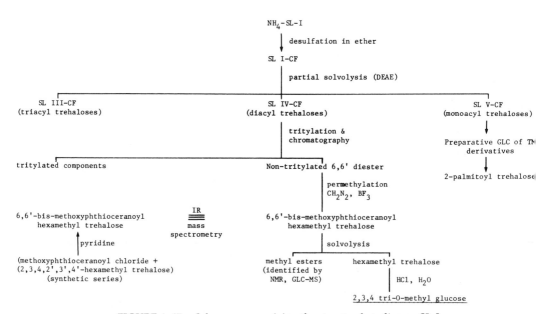

FIGURE 4–47.   Scheme summarizing the structural studies on SL-I.

sulfatide to be 1:1:2. The molar ratios of the substituents in the remainder of the SL families are given in Table 4–5.

Location of the Individual Acyl Substituents[141]

The final task in deriving the complete structure of SL-I lay in assigning the specific locations of the single *A, B,* and of the two *C* substituents on the trehalose core. This was achieved as summarized in Figure 4–47.

Desulfated SL-I (designated SL I-CF) was gently and partially methanolyzed in ether-methanol solution on a column of DEAE cellulose in the free base form, yielding a triacyl trehalose mixture (mixed SL III-CF), diacyl trehaloses (mixed SL IV-CF), and monoacyl trehaloses (mixed SL V-CF). These are readily separable by column chromatography on DEAE acetate. The principal component of mixed SL IV-CF is the symmetric 6,6'-bis-hydroxyphthioceranoyl trehalose, which is a pseudocord factor, slightly toxic and having antitumor activity. This accounts for the two *C* substituents. The assignment was confirmed by synthesis. Since only two more substituents are present in SL-I, positional assignment (2 or 3)

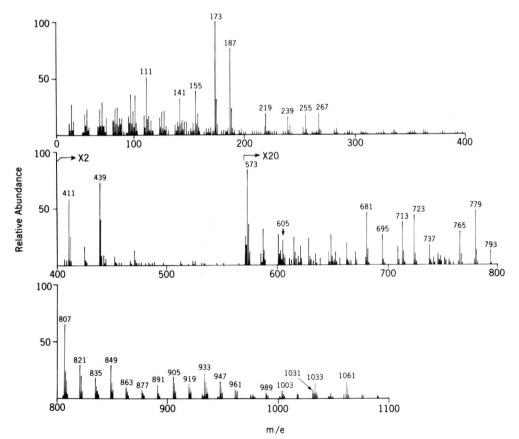

FIGURE 4–48. Mass spectrum of permethylated SL IV′-CF. Definitive peaks due to the unacylated carbohydrate moiety (*xxxix*) are at *m/e* 219, 187, 155. The diacylated oxonium ions (*xL*) or (*xli*) are associated with peaks *m/e* 1031, 1003; 989, 961; 947, 919; 905, 877. By loss of phthioceranic acids, all of these generate the peaks *m/e* 439 and 411, containing stearate or palmitate at a 2 position. Expulsion of the substituents as ketenes generates the *base peak* in the spectrum, *m/e* 173. (From Goren, M. B., Brokl, O., Roller, P., Fales, H. M., and Das, B. C.: Sulfatides of *Mycobacterium tuberculosis:* The structure of the principal sulfatide (SL-I). Biochemistry 15:2728, 1976.)

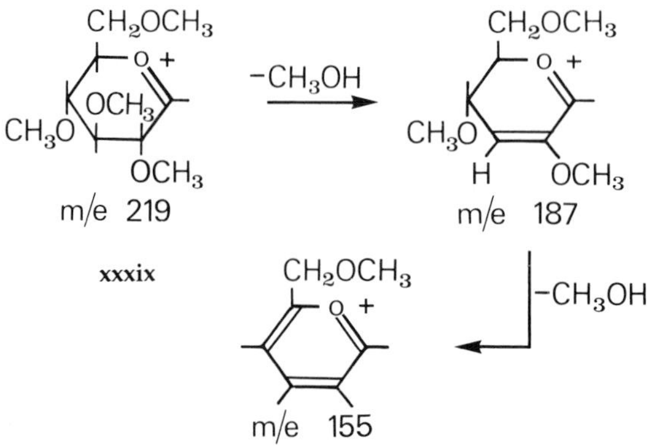

FIGURE 4-49. Fragmentation of the unacylated moiety of permethylated SL IV'-CF in mass spectrometry.

to either one (phthioceranate or palmitate/stearate) defines the complete structure. This was achieved at first by isolating and identifying trehalose-2-palmitate from the SL V-CF (monoacyl) mixture by preparative gas chromatography.

An independent confirmation of this structural feature was sought and realized among the products from partial *acidic* solvolysis of SL I-CF. This procedure yielded a diacyltrehalose (SL IV'-CF), different from that obtained in the methanolysis on DEAE, and uniquely confirmed the disposition of both the palmitate and phthioceranate substituents. The methodology exemplifies a particularly fortuitous utilization of mass spectrometry. SL IV'-CF, obtained in the partial acidic solvolysis is a 2,3 diacyl trehalose, instead of the symmetric 6,6' compound obtained in the alkaline methanolysis. It contains one unacylated glucose moiety, and the second is substituted with *A* and *B*. In mass spectrometry of the *permethylated* derivative (spectrum is reproduced in Fig. 4-48), a primary cleavage at the anomeric oxygen yields two oxonium fragments. The first one [(*xxxix*) in Fig. 4-49], *m/e* 219, is attributable to the unacylated glucose moiety, and it subsequently undergoes successive losses of CH$_3$OH (32 mass units, or m.u.) to generate the fragments *m/e* 187 and *m/e* 155 (Fig. 4-49) — a prominent series in the mass spectrum.

Concerning the second principal oxonium fragment, earlier definitive studies of Kochetkov and Chizov, as well as unpublished studies of B. C. Das and Goren, showed that with a permethylated 2,3-diacyl hexose, the primary oxonium fragment formed [(*xl*) or (*xli*) in Fig. 4-50] undergoes the following cleavages: the acyl function in the 3 position is eliminated as the carboxylic acid, after which, the acyl group in the 2 position is expelled as a *ketene* [Fig. 4-50, (*xl*)].

The fragmentation pattern of SL IV'CF followed this sequence and unequivocally showed that palmitate-stearate occupies the 2 position. Referring to the mass spectrum and (*xli*) in Figure 4-50, peaks in the higher mass region — *m/e* *1031 & 1003; 989 & 961; 947 & 919; 905 & 877* — are attributable to oxonium fragments containing palmitate or stearate (paired, italicized — 28 m.u. homology) and homologs of *A* with n=7, 6, 5, 4. By loss of the *A* components (from the 3 position) as the carboxylic acids — i.e.,

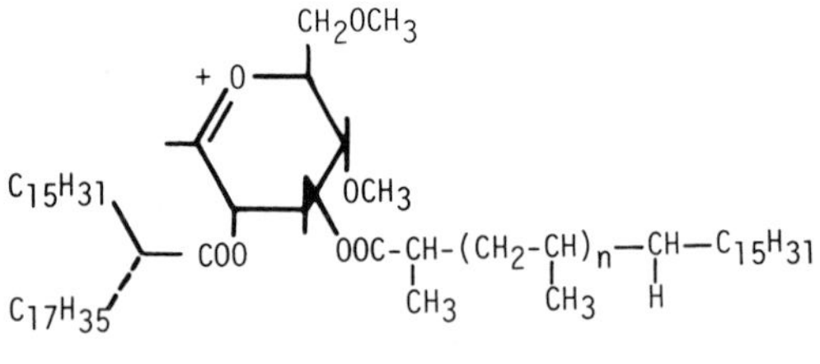

xl

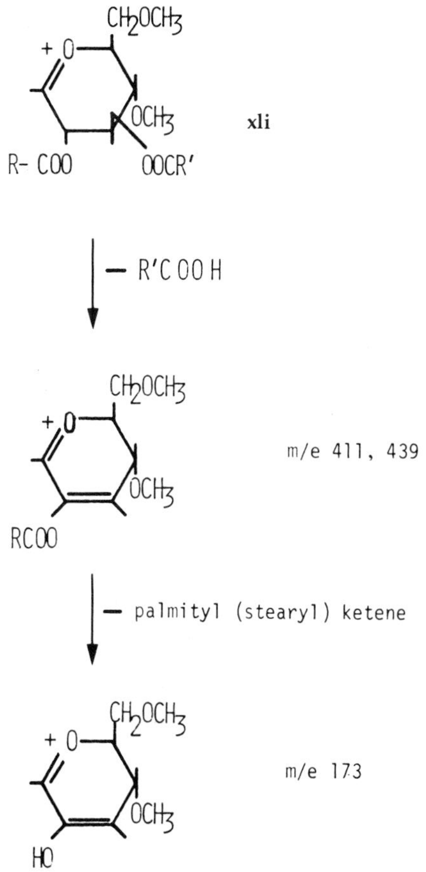

FIGURE 4–50. Fragmentation of the diacylated moiety of permethylated SL IV'-CF in mass spectrometry.

Biologic Activities

Cord-factorlike Toxicity

Neither SL-I nor SL-III exhibits overt cord-factorlike toxicity when oil solutions of these lipids are administered intraperitoneally to mice (multiple 100 μg doses). However, preliminary studies of Goren and C. Tihon[147a] indicated that several spaced injections of SL-I (in oil), though not toxic of themselves, inordinately sensitized the mice to a subsequent single injection of cord factor (10 μg); furthermore, combinations of the apparently nontoxic SL-I with cord factor were much more toxic than the latter alone. A collaborative study[189] subsequently defined a synergistic toxicity of the two trehalose glycolipids. In addition, nontoxic desulfated SL-I also exhibited a synergistic potentiation of the toxicity of cord factor administered simultaneously. In vitro studies established that aqueous dispersions of SL-I attacked liver mitochondrial membranes more vigorously than even cord factor; however, the activity was antagonized by bovine serum albumin (BSA) and, therefore, by serum proteins. On the other hand, in the presence of cord factor, the detoxifying influence of BSA was abrogated.

Antitumor Activity

Until recently, cord factor has been considered as a seemingly required component of the tumor-regressing oil, cell-wall or endotoxin preparations described by Ribi and by Bekierkunst. However, the amphipathic glycolipid probably functions merely to bring about the required association between the oil phase and the second component, e.g., the endotoxin. It is not surprising that the sulfatides can effectively replace cord factor in some of the preparations. In the line 10 systems, intralesional injection of tumors with "Ribi"-type preparations containing

losses of 592, 550, 508 and 466 m.u. (42 m.u. homology) — all of the pairs generate two important fragments (m/e 439 and 411), in which the stearate or palmitate component is retained. Their expulsion as stearyl (palmityl) ketene yields the fragment m/e 173, which is, in fact, the base peak in this spectrum. This sequence uniquely confirms the positional assignments. The complete structure of SL-I is 2-palmitoyl (stearoyl)-3-phthioceranoyl-6,6'-bis-hydroxyphthioceranoyl trehalose-2'-sulfate (Fig. 4–51). (For comparison, the structure of SL-III is also given.)

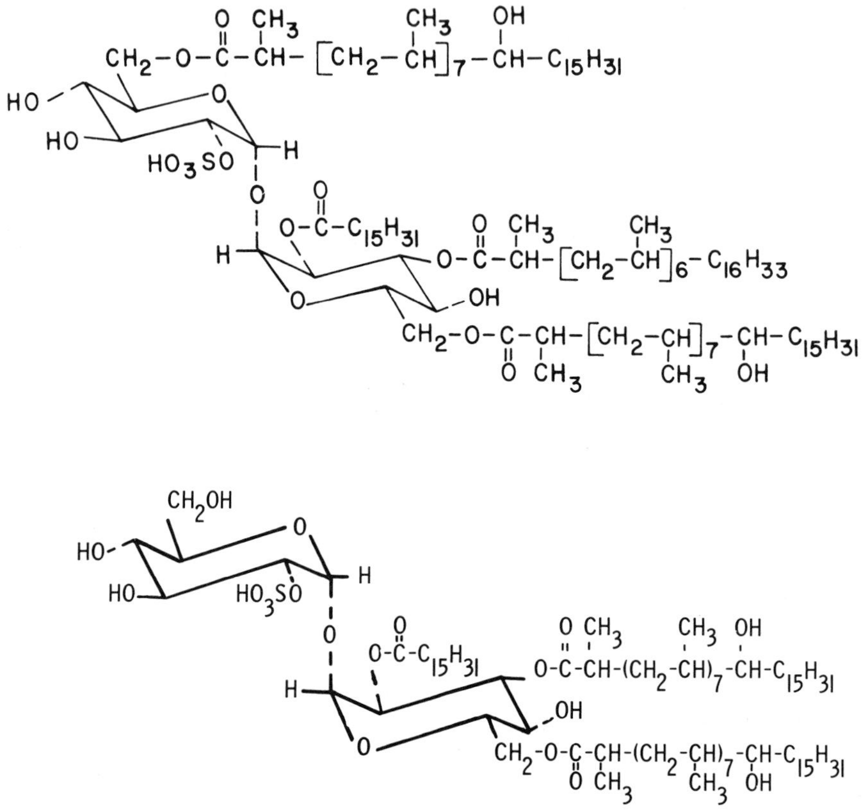

FIGURE 4–51. Structures of SL-I (principal sulfatide; top) and SL-III (a minor sulfatide, lower) of *M. tuberculosis* H37Rv.

300 μg Re endotoxin admixed with 150 to 250 μg of SL-I or SL-III has given very high cure rates.[146, 392a] Neither SL-I nor SL-III in the absence of endotoxin is effective. Higher levels of the sulfatides, however, may antagonize the activity either by an unfavorable influence on the emulsion or because of dysfunctions, which the sulfatides can induce in macrophages.

Assocation of Sulfatides with Virulence

Because much of the neutral red reactivity of virulent *M. tuberculosis* strains was attributable to their sulfolipid content, Middlebrook soon inferred this lipid to be a factor in the pathogenesis of tuberculosis. Indeed, studies by Gangadharam and colleagues[111] and Goren and his coworkers[143] established a significant correlation between the elaboration of sulfatides in culture and the rank order of virulence for the guinea pig ("infectivity," according to Gangadharam and coworkers)[111] among a series of British, Indian, and East African strains of *M. tuberculosis* spanning a broad spectrum of virulence as assessed by Mitchison.[261] With only modest exceptions, the most virulent strains were prolific in elaborating strongly acidic lipids (principally SL), whereas the attenuated ones were notably deficient in these components. Figure 4–52 demonstrates the distribution of acidic lipids for this series of *M. tuberculosis*

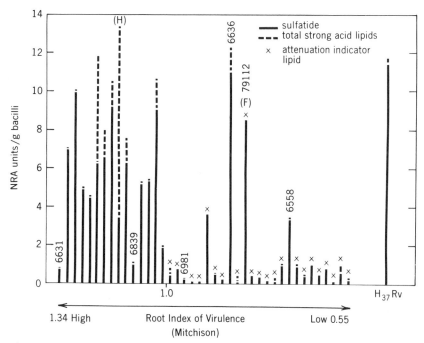

FIGURE 4–52. Distribution of acidic lipids and of the Attenuation Indicator Lipid in 40 strains of *M. tuberculosis*. (From Goren, M. B., Brokl, O., and Schaefer, W. B.: Lipids of putative relevance to virulence in *Mycobacterium tuberculosis*: Correlation of virulence with elaboration of sulfatides and strongly acidic lipids. Infect. Immun. 9:142, 1974.)

strains. In related studies,[144] an Attenuation Indicator (AI) lipid was also recognized, significantly restricted in distribution to the strains of virulence "root index" below 1.0, considered attenuated by Mitchison. The distribution of AI lipid (crosses in Fig. 4–52) clearly divides the strains into two populations separated (fortuitously!) at this same root index. (See also Chapter 5.)

Putative Functions of the Acidic Lipids in Pathogenesis

The significant distribution of relatively high levels of strongly acidic lipids (principally the sulfatides) among the more virulent of the Mitchison strains suggests that these may be a necessary (though not sufficient) requirement for the virulent state in *Mycobacterium tuberculosis*—perhaps in supporting the intracellular survival of the pathogen. Indeed, plausible roles which the sulfalipids might assume in this environment may be invoked from their chemical structures. Thus, the demonstrable surface-active properties might be directed against and disrupt lysosomal membranes, just as mitochondrial membranes are attacked.[189] Within the phagosomal environment, the anionic SL distributed at the surface of the tubercle bacilli might also function to adsorb, immobilize, and possibly distort lysosomal enzymes so as to render them nonfunctional. Indeed, Kanai[173] has shown that tubercle bacilli recovered from lungs of infected mice are coated with host lysosomal *acid phosphatase*. In a more cryptic fashion — by orientation of the sulfatide within the lipid bilayer membrane or by distortion of membrane structure — the functional properties of phagosomal or lysosomal membranes might be disturbed.

In studies on the lysosomal response of mouse peritoneal macrophages grown in culture and infected with various mycobacteria, Armstrong and Hart[14] observed the rather surprising phenomenon that phagosomes containing viable virulent tubercle bacilli are resistant to fusion with the secondary lysosomes or dense granules that characterize these phagocytes, especially in serum-rich culture medium. In the ordinary course of events following phagocytosis of a host of foreign bodies, these dense granules, readily labeled by ferritin or colloidal thorium oxide, fuse with and discharge their contents of lysosomal enzymes and the electron opaque marker into the phagosome. (For reviews, see Cohn and Fedorko[79] and Goren.[138]) In the study by Armstrong and Hart, using ferritin-prelabeled macrophages, virtually all phagosomes containing damaged tubercle bacilli showed signs of fusion, as indicated by the presence of the marker within the phagolysosome, but with phagosomes containing intact organisms, signs of phagosomal-lysosomal fusion were infrequent. A quite similar behavior has been recognized with *Chlamydiae* species and with *Toxoplasma gondii.*[138] From their results, Armstrong and Hart concluded that "intracellular survival of *M. tuberculosis* in cultured macrophages is associated with a tendency to non-fusion of dense granules with the phagosome and that fusion leading to digestion is determined by recognition of the bacillus as nonviable." In their elegant study, Jones and Hirsch[171] also found that lysosomal constituents are not delivered to phagocytic vacuoles harbouring live toxoplasma and suggested that "this was almost certainly due to effects exerted by the parasite locally, *probably as a result of secretion of some substance that*

altered the vacuolar membrane (authors' italics)." For *M. tuberculosis,* we speculated that the sulfatides may induce this kind of dysfunction.[143]

Lysosomotropism of Sulfatides and Antagonism of Fusion

Studies dedicated to exploring this hypothesis[145] showed that SL, in the form of fine aqueous dispersions, is readily endocytosed by normal (nonelicited) mouse pertioneal macrophages in culture. It accumulates abundantly in the secondary lysosomes, where it is recognized in the form of discrete lipid droplets. Levels from 10^{-3} to 10^{-1} ng per cell are well tolerated and are distinctly *protubercular*. SL-exposed cells, unlike control monolayers, are intensely stained by neutral red, suggesting that at least some SL is adsorbed at the surface of the macrophage membrane, where it mimics the adsorption of the dye by tubercle bacilli.

Accumulation of even very low levels of either SL-I or SL-III (but *not of desulfated SL*) in macrophage secondary lysosomes renders them almost entirely incompetent for fusing with phagosomes containing suitable target particles. However, the effect is strain-related; peritoneal macrophages of some strains of mice (Swiss-Webster, for example) resist the effect of the sulfatides and other antagonists to fusion (Goren and Swendsen, unpublished data). The specific antifusion behavior of the sulfatides can be confirmed at the ultrastructural level with ferritin-labeled cells and by darkfield vital fluorescence microscopy. In this technique, developed by Hart and Young,[154] macrophage monolayers are briefly exposed to dilute acridine orange (AO), which accumulates almost exclusively in lysosomes. The monolayer is then allowed to phagocytose viable baker's yeast cells. Under blue-violet irradiation, phagolysosome formation in normal cells is discerned as a

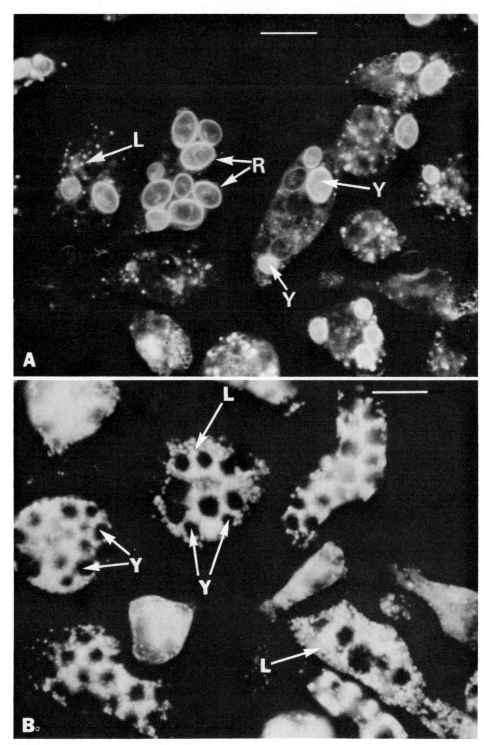

FIGURE 4–53. *A,* Living macrophages (controls) with acridine-stained lysosomes (L) after incubation with live yeasts. Some yeasts are surrounded by a bright intraphagosomal rim (R), and others show over-all fluorescence (Y) from diffusion of marker into the phagosome. Bar represents 10 μm. *B,* Living macrophages pretreated with sulfatide (SL-I) before acridine staining and yeast uptake. Dark spaces (Y) are unstained yeast in nonfused phagosomes. (From Goren, M. B., Hart, P. D., Young, M. R., and Armstrong, J. A.: Prevention of phagosome-lysosome fusion in cultured macrophages by sulfatides of *Mycobacterium tuberculosis.* Proc. Nat. Acad. Sci. U.S.A. 73:2510, 1976.)

progressive and colorful influx of AO marker into yeast-containing phagosomes, as shown in Figure 4–53, *A*. In susceptible cells previously exposed to mycobacterial SL, this behavior is completely abolished (*B*). In these, the phagosomes appear as dark spaces amid a background of fluorescent lysosomes. Although this dysfunction seems to be caused by the lysosomal sequestration of SL, adsorbed lipid at the macrophage membrane surface and subsequently internalized with the yeasts may also contribute to the effect from within the phagosome. As a putative demonstration of such an influence from within this domain, antagonism to fusion was achieved to a significant extent by attaching microdroplets of SL to the yeast cells before they were phagocytosed by normal macrophages.

The results in toto seem to incriminate the mycobacterial sulfatides as putative agents in virulence, and to demonstrate that a natural product elaborated by an intracellular pathogen may indeed induce the fusion dysfunction and thus favor the pathogen's intracellular survival. The mechanism is as yet uncertain. Simplistically, the effect may depend upon a distortion of limiting membranes as the micellar, and therefore polyanionic, sulfatide adsorbs to cationic protein sites. This interpretation may be supported by the earlier finding[154] that the polysulfonated aromatic derivative suramin also induces a similar dysfunction after sequestration in lysosomes. The analogy allows the extrapolation that polyanionic character may be at least one structural common denominator capable of conferring this kind of activity. The demonstrations of this behavior by dextran sulfate 500 and certain carageenans reinforce this conviction.[138] However, the polyanions may function via additional mediators. Lowrie, Jackett, and Ratcliffe[235] found that the intracellular level of cyclic adenosine monophosphate (cAMP) is raised in mouse peritoneal macro-

phages following phagocytosis of a species virulent for the mouse, *Mycobacterium microti*, which (like *M. tuberculosis*) interferes with the phagosome-lysosome fusion process. Ingestion of *M. lepraemurium* or of latex beads, both of which elicit a prompt fusion response, did not alter the intracellular cAMP level. Lowrie and his collaborators favored the interpretation that the pathogen itself may generate and secrete cyclic AMP from within the phagosome. If the cyclic nucleotide is the true mediator, then it seems probable that the polyanionic agents may stimulate cAMP production within the macrophage — a possibility that is, of course, subject to testing.

It seems plausible that the role of the sulfatides in fusion dysfunction might be abrogated by humoral antibodies with specificity for SL, especially for the trehalose sulfate core. According to Middlebrook,[253a] there is no evidence that even haptenic sensitization to the sulfatides occurs either in tuberculous animals or in response to injections of SL. Studies with this direction, using complexes of SL with methylated bovine serum albumin and SL-protein conjugates, are currently in progress in Goren's laboratory.

[NOTE: Recent studies (M. Goren, C.L. Swendsen, and Janet Henson; in preparation) suggest that the acridine-orange technique described in the preceding is subject to artifacts that are (disturbingly) most prominently expressed in the presence of polyanionic substances. Despite the impressive visual evidence from vital fluorescence microscopy of fusion inhibition by polyanionics (as documented in Fig. 4–53, *A* and *B*), the interpretation given this evidence *may* not be secure. Because current data obtained from electron microscopy studies are also not unequivocal, the role of polyanionics (including SL) in inducing fusion dysfunction is therefore at present uncertain.]

MISCELLANEOUS LIPIDS OF POSSIBLE RELEVANCE IN PATHOGENICITY

From time to time, a relationship has been inferred between virulence in *M. tuberculosis* and the ability to elaborate specific multimethyl-branched carboxylic acids, e.g., phthienoic[68] or mycolipenic[283] acids, the glycol ester phthiocerol dimycocerosate, and possibly the branched phthioceranic acids found in the sulfatides of *M. tuberculosis*. However, it is our opinion that any inferred relationships to virulence, with some exceptions, are still tenuous.

"Phthioic" and mycocerosic acids were among the earliest mycobacterial lipid constituents of exciting biologic interest to be described by the Anderson group. The efforts to resolve the structural problems almost rival those devoted to the mycolic acids in magnitude. These efforts were extremely painstaking since they were, of course, not facilitated, by such tools as GLC, PMR and mass spectrometry until some 30 years after their discovery. The fascinating history of these acids is given in careful detail by Asselineau,[23] and for appropriate references, that admirable treatise should be consulted.

Phthienoic and Mycolipenic Acids

When originally isolated from phosphatide fractions of tubercle bacilli by Anderson, the dextrorotatory-branched acid, designated "phthioic acid," was thought to be a saturated substance with the empirical formula $C_{26}H_{52}O_2$. Early on, Chargaff synthesized a series of α-branched acids for comparison with the natural product. The *unsaturation* of phthioic acid was not realized for some 20 years, when independently, Chanley and Polgar[73] and Cason and Sumrell[70] recognized phthioic acid as a mixture of α,β unsaturated acids — a structural feature that had escaped detection owing to the sluggish reactivity of the acids with halogens and was only discerned years later from ultraviolet spectrophotometry (absorption at 218 nm).

Separate studies by Cason (working with samples of phthioic acid from Anderson), by Polgar (with other samples isolated independently from harvests of tubercle bacilli and designated "mycolipenic" acids), and by Asselineau established the structures and the identity for some of these examples. By fractional distillation, Cason and Sumrell[79] isolated a dozen acids, six of them unsaturated, from a 24 g sample of Anderson's methyl phthioate. Among these, C_{27} and C_{29} members are prominent. The C_{27} phthienoic acid was found to be identical with Polgar's C_{27} mycolipenic acid, for which the structure (*xlii*) shown below was established. Homologs from C_{25} to C_{31} have also been recognized.

The natural acids (many synthetic analogs also have been prepared) have the *trans* structure, and the methyl branches are all of the *L* configuration.

Several years ago, Professor Cason was kind enough to provide us a sample of the original C_{27}-phthienoic acid isolated from the Anderson methyl phthioate. In his correspondence, Professor Cason included several historical vignettes concerning this substance.

I do not have the tare on this vial, so do not know how much is there; however

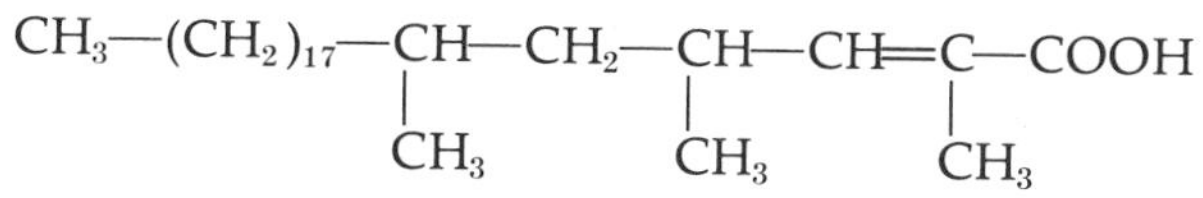

$$CH_3-(CH_2)_{17}-\underset{\underset{CH_3}{|}}{CH}-CH_2-\underset{\underset{CH_3}{|}}{CH}-CH=\underset{\underset{CH_3}{|}}{C}-COOH$$

xlii

when Hans-Reudi Urschler removed the remainder of the sample for work on the structure (*Alas! before availability of mass spectrometry*) . . . The first mixture (phthioic acid, that is) which we obtained from Prof. Anderson was examined in the above noted paper[70] where we stated that the phthioic acid contained "at least 12 compounds." Of course, subsequent work by us after the availability of gas chromatography revealed that this number should be multiplied by about three. The multiplicity of compounds, and especially the demonstrated α,β-unsaturation were quite a blow to Prof. Anderson, so much so that I made a special trip to New Haven . . . to convince him that no-one could have done better work than he, but that he had been fortunate enough to live to see the introduction of revolutionary new methods in separation processes.

Biologic Activities

The phthienoic acids were amongst the first lipids of tubercle bacilli in which biologic activities associated with the inflammatory characteristics of a tuberculosis lesion were discerned. In Florence Sabin's studies with admittedly less-than-refined products from the Anderson group, phosphatide fractions injected intraperitoneally in rabbits elicited formation of "tubercular" lesions with characteristic epithelioid and giant cell forms.[300] Still, a course of 12 injections each of 80 mg of phosphatides was necessary to produce an intense reaction. On the other hand, Husseini and Elberg,[157] in studying purified natural or synthetic analogs, found that 1 mg of purified C27-phthienoic acid produced a significant reaction. These and other studies (reviewed by J. Ungar[362]) examined the influence on biologic activities of unsaturation and of various alkyl substituents, especially methyl branches, along the fatty acid chain. The variety of results are somewhat difficult to interpret and are now largely of academic interest, since many of the synthetic active acids are only remotely related to identified compo-

nents of mycobacteria. Broadly, given a sufficiently long fatty acid chain of about 20 to 30 carbons, then $\alpha,\ \beta$-unsaturation, α-methyl groups or alkyl groups, methyl substituents at about the tenth carbon, or multiple methyl groups at select positions (as in 3, 12, 15-trimethyl docosanoic acid) promote the inflammatory activity. The influence of the α,β-unsaturation is quite remarkable; the hydrogenated analog of phthienoic acid has about 1/50 the biologic activity. In Ungar's interpretation, the active fatty acids produced small foci of necrosis, recognizable shortly after injection of the substance; therefore, the response is quite different from the necrosis and caseation seen as much later phenomena in tuberculosis. The lesions in Ungar's assessment are "foreign body reactions," and, as described by Husseini and Elberg,[157] "similar to that seen in the more nonspecific aspects of tuberculosis pathology."

The chemically poorly defined PmKo of Choucroun, extracted by liquid paraffin from mycobacteria and evidently containing wax D[23], as well as purified wax D preparations, are superior in respect to these kinds of biologic activities. According to White,[380] injections of 40 μg wax D (in oil-in-water emulsions) into guinea pig footpads elicit an almost tumorlike proliferation of cells, appearing like the epithelioid cells of a tuberculosis granuloma. In the popliteal gland, a similar proliferation was clearly recognizable as due to transformed macrophages.

Objections have been voiced that although the effects in the instance of the acidic substances may be provoked by milligram quantities of purified lipids, the amounts nevertheless are orders of magnitude greater than could be provided by a few tubercle bacilli. Perhaps in the infectious process, an immune sensitization to these mycobacterial constituents can dramatically alter the response. In Ungar's hands, the active acids were no more effective in tuberculous animals than in controls — observations that would deny a role for these as haptens in inducing a specific allergy. Still, it has been countered that Catel and Schmidt[72] reported much greater sensitivity of infected animals (and children) to small challenge doses, especially of "phthioic" acid dissolved in Nujol. In some of the few children tested, 0.1 to 1 mg of "phthioic" acids elicited an extraordinarily strong response, which superficially resembled a (somewhat strange) tuberculin reaction. It sometimes was delayed for a week before it appeared, and in some subjects, gave a prolonged sustained reaction for three weeks or longer. Regrettably, earlier reviews of this study have failed to mention Catel's conclusion: in not a single instance were epithelioid cells at all prominent in biopsy specimens; instead, only a perivascular proliferation of vacuolated fibroblasts, accompanied by small numbers of leukocytes and lymphocytes, could be seen. In this study, "only tuberculoprotein elicited the specific tissue reaction from the (tuberculo) allergic organism."[72]

As yet another measure of a potential contribution to virulence, the influence of cells and of specific lipids on leukocytic linear migration has been assessed. Bloch[50] described the inhibitory effect of both phagocytosed virulent tubercle bacilli and cord factor on leukocytes, and Choucroun and coworkers[78] showed that the inhibitory capacity of virulent cells is quantitatively greater than that of avirulent *M. tuberculosis*. According to Husseini and Elberg,[157] of the spectrum of substances they examined, C_{27}-phthienoic acid exhibited the most dramatic influence on leukocytes, even at quite low concentrations (2.5 × 10^{-4} M).

For an interpretive opinion, the following is quoted from J. Cason.[67a]

I have always felt that their (Husseini and Elberg) observed activity of inhibiting leukocytic migration is of fundamental significance in connection with virulence. This led us to examine three lots of H37Ra and one lot of BCG, with the result that we could find no significant amounts of the phthienoic acids. Subsequent work, with GC and mass spectrometry (unpublished) has confirmed that only minimal amounts of the phthienoic type acids are present, and acids were present of types never detected in the virulent strains.

The apparent restriction in distribution of phthienoic acids to virulent strains is also addressed by Asselineau,[23] and, indeed, the distribution of these acids and their influence on leukocytes may be a more valid criterion for correlation with pathogenicity and "aggressiveness" than is the tissue response.

Mycocerosic Acids

From the various waxes of tubercle bacilli, the Anderson group isolated several presumed C_{30} and C_{31} methyl-branched levorotatory "mycocerosic" acids. Analogous or entirely similar substances were independently studied by Polgar ("mycoceranic" acids), Cason ("phthianoic" acids), and Asselineau, who retained Anderson's designation. In Polgar's studies,[284] the positions of methyl branches were established as summarized below, and led to a tentative C_{31} mycoceranic acid structure.

Alpha-bromination and dehydrobromination of this material affords an α,β-unsaturated acid, which (excluding the stereochemistry of the methyl

$$CH_3(CH_2)_{21}-\underset{\underset{CH_3}{|}}{CH}-CH_2-\underset{\underset{CH_3}{|}}{CH}-CH_2-\underset{\underset{CH_3}{|}}{CH}-COOH$$

proposed C_{31} mycocerosic acid structure

branches) would resemble phthienoic acid.

$$R-\underset{\underset{CH_3}{|}}{CH}-CH_2-\underset{\underset{CH_3}{|}}{CH}-CH=\underset{\underset{CH_3}{|}}{C}-COOH$$

On ozonolysis of this substance, pyruvic acid is obtained as one product and thus establishes the position of the first methyl branch. On the other hand, permanganate oxidation of the α,β-unsaturated product affords a carboxylic acid in which the terminal 3-carbon unit has been eliminated. (See below.) By repetition of these sequences, the position of three methyl substituents was recognized. The starting substance and all of the derived methyl-branched acids are levorotatory; they have been related to D-glyceraldehyde and are thus of the D-configuration.

In an early application of mass spectrometry to the study of the mycobacterial lipids, Asselineau and colleagues[27] examined a sample of methyl mycocerosate from Anderson. This gave a parent molecular ion peak, M^+ 494, corresponding to a methyl ester of a C_{32} carboxylic acid — and, therefore, to revision of the tentative structure suggested by Polgar to accommodate an additional methylene group (to n = 22). A synthetic compound corresponding to this structure [(methyl) 2D,4D,6D-trimethyl nonacosanoate] was different, however, from Anderson's methyl ester. By gas chromatography combined with mass spectrometry, the latter was found to consist of some 6 substances, with the principal component again being recognized as the ester of a C_{32} acid (M^+ 494). A comparison of carbon numbers in the acids (from mass spectrometry) with the (log) retention

time in gas chromatography as well as additional mass spectrometric analysis showed that the principal component (C_{32}), along with a C_{30} and a C_{34} acid, very likely contained four methyl branches rather than three — in positions 2,4,6 and 8. The revised (and now accepted) structure of C_{32} mycocerosic acid is 2,4,6,8 tetramethyl octacosanoate. (See top of opposite page.)

In our own studies of the substance designated the AI lipid (see Table 4–6), a series of complex mycocerosic acids (as methyl esters) were recognized in combined gas chromatography-mass spectrometry (in collaboration with Henry Fales). This study revealed, by their characteristic mass spectra, five homologs of mycocerosic acid: C_{29} and C_{30} were most abundant, with lesser amounts of C_{27}, C_{32}, and an apparent C_{28}.

The mycocerosic acids are evidently not found in mycobacterium species that do not contain phthiocerol or related alcohols, e.g., the phenol glycol of mycosides A and B. Because of their branched configurations (*resemblance* to phthienoic acids), mycocerosic acids would be expected to elicit quite similar tissue responses, as described earlier (compare with Ungar[362]). Studies in our laboratory [240a] indicate that guinea pigs infected with H37Rv respond much more vigorously than controls to intradermal challenge with 50μg of mycocerosic acids as a fine aqueous suspension (compare with Catel and Schmidt).

Biosynthesis

The three classes of multibranched mycobacterial acids — phthienoic, mycocerosic, and phthioceranic (from the

---

$$R-\underset{\underset{CH_3}{|}}{CH}-CH_2-\underset{\underset{CH_3}{|}}{CH}-CH=\underset{\underset{CH_3}{|}}{C}-COOH \xrightarrow{\text{KMnO}_4} R-\underset{\underset{CH_3}{|}}{CH}-CH_2-\underset{\underset{CH_3}{|}}{CH}-COOH$$

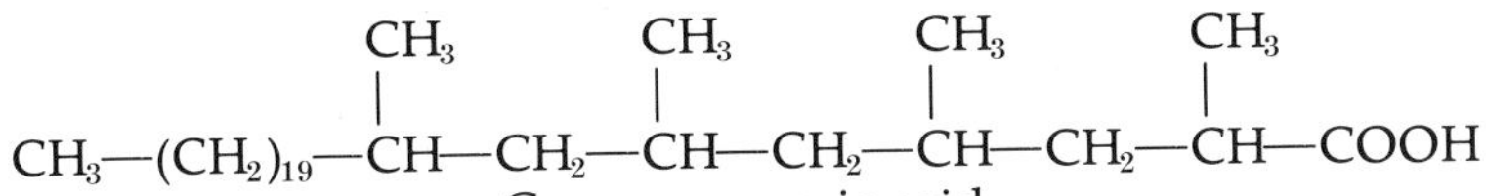

$$
\begin{array}{cccc}
CH_3 & CH_3 & CH_3 & CH_3 \\
| & | & | & | \\
CH_3-(CH_2)_{19}-CH-CH_2-CH-CH_2-CH-CH_2-CH-COOH
\end{array}
$$

C_{32} mycocerosic acid

sulfatides) — are all very likely elaborated by a similar biosynthetic scheme, which in the mycocerosic groups generates the D-series and generates the L-series of stereoisomers in the remaining two. The publications Chemistry and Industry and Angewandte Chemie are often the vehicles for the launching of a "trial balloon" in areas of chemistry much more esoteric than their names would imply. In the former, Polgar and Robinson[285] suggested that the methyl branches in C_{27} phthienoic acid might be generated by the Claisen-like successive condensation of three propionate units to a stearic acid receptor. In Woodward's "propionate rule,"[391] *propionate* may replace *acetate* in the building of a number of macrolide antibiotics and thus provide the methyl branches. The hypothesis with respect to mycobacterial lipids was beautifully confirmed by Gastambide-Odier and colleagues.[115] Radiolabeled (1-^{14}C, 3-^{3}H) propionic acid was abundantly incorporated into the mycocerosic acid fraction of *M. tuberculosis* strain H37Ra; the

tritium was found almost entirely in the methyl branches, as determined by a modified Kuhn-Roth oxidation and by recovery of the radiolabeled acetate generated by these methyl branches. See below.

The pathway very likely involves methyl malonyl CoA; for a C_{27} mycocerosic acid, stearoyl ACP may be invoked as a receptor. See below.

When *M. tuberculosis* H37Rv is cultured in the presence of ^{14}C-labeled propionate, the label is freely incorporated into the multimethyl-branched phthioceranic and hydroxyphthioceranic acid substituents of the sulfatides but only minimally into the stearate/palmitate components. Thus, these methyl branches are generated in a similar fashion.

Phthiocerol Dimycocerosate

From the chloroform-soluble waxes of *M. tuberculosis*, Stodola and Anderson isolated a methoxyglycol, which was named "phthiocerol." The diester

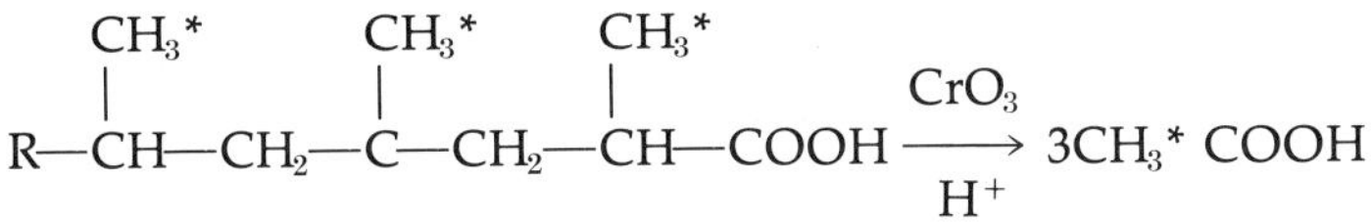

$$
\begin{array}{ccc}
CH_3{}^* & CH_3{}^* & CH_3{}^* \\
| & | & | \\
R-CH-CH_2-C-CH_2-CH-COOH & \xrightarrow[H^+]{CrO_3} & 3CH_3{}^*\ COOH
\end{array}
$$

oxidative degradation of mycocerosate

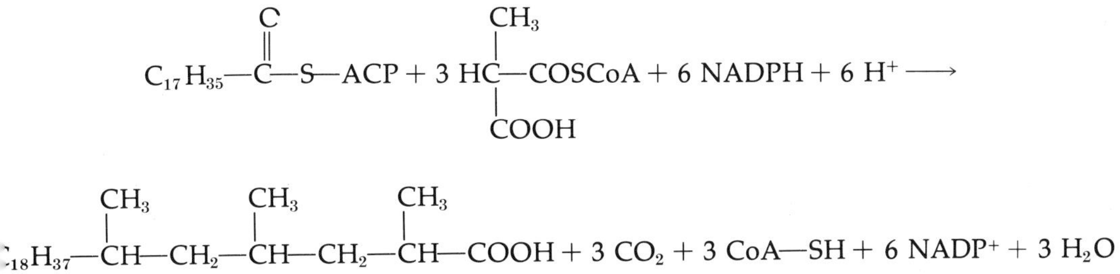

$$
\begin{array}{cc}
C & CH_3 \\
\| & | \\
C_{17}H_{35}-C-S-ACP + 3\ HC-COSCoA + 6\ NADPH + 6\ H^+ \longrightarrow \\
& | \\
& COOH
\end{array}
$$

$$
\begin{array}{ccc}
CH_3 & CH_3 & CH_3 \\
| & | & | \\
C_{18}H_{37}-CH-CH_2-CH-CH_2-CH-COOH + 3\ CO_2 + 3\ CoA-SH + 6\ NADP^+ + 3\ H_2O
\end{array}
$$

possible pathway for mycocerosate biosynthesis

(DIM) formed with the mycocerosic acids is readily recoverable from wax C and was prominent in a number of mycoside-related studies.[324] The structure of some representatives is given below.

In phthiocerol, as well as in the related phenol glycols of the mycosides A and B, the methyl branch and the terminal-CH_2-CH_3 are derived from incorporation of two molecules of propionate, whereas the methyl of the methoxyl group is derived from methionine (Fig. 4–54). The dihydroxy acid derives from tetracosanoic acid.

In our laboratory, DIM was found to be a ubiquitous constituent in more than 40 patient isolates of *M. tuberculosis* of a wide spectrum of virulence and was apparently as prominent in highly attenuated strains as in the most virulent ones. We also identified it in H37Ra. However, a notably attenuated mutant of H37Rv, accidentally selected for under undefined culture conditions, lost the capacity for synthesis of DIM and does not produce the Attenuation Indicator Lipid (AI).[144] It is not known whether the attenuation and loss of DIM were related or were independently expressed. The biochemical lesion might rest in an inability of the mutant to synthesize mycocerosic acids, phthiocerol, and phthiocerol-like alcohols (as in AI) or to esterify these if they are synthesized. A limited number of other *M. tuberculosis* strains with DIM deficiency have also been recognized by Smith and colleagues.[326] They include the widely studied *M. tuberculosis*, Brévannes — a strain that was highly virulent but now is considerably attenuated. Our examination of the lipids from a lyophilized harvest of this strain (kindly provided by Dr. Merrill Chase) showed them to be devoid of both DIM and AI.

Iron-Chelating Agents

To provide for iron transport and assimilation, mycobacteria have evidently developed a much more elaborate and complex system than that characterizing most other microorganisms. This is, in large measure, due to the barrier to transport that is imposed by the abundance of cellular lipid. The rationale for considering the components of this complex as putative agents in virulence was summarized by Ratledge.[290] An enhanced availability of iron can exacerbate mycobacterial infections, while iron deprivation affords some protection. Furthermore, as Kochan and coworkers have shown, in serum-rich medium, growth of *M. tuberculosis* is limited by the availability of iron because of its powerful chelation

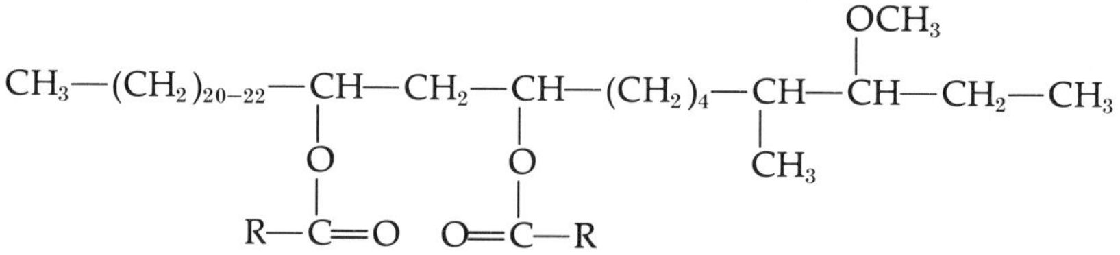

$$CH_3-(CH_2)_{20-22}-\underset{\underset{R-C=O}{O}}{CH}-CH_2-\underset{\underset{O=C-R}{O}}{CH}-(CH_2)_4-\underset{\underset{CH_3}{|}}{CH}-\overset{\overset{OCH_3}{|}}{CH}-CH_2-CH_3$$

phthiocerol dimycocerosate (DIM)

R = mycocerosic acids

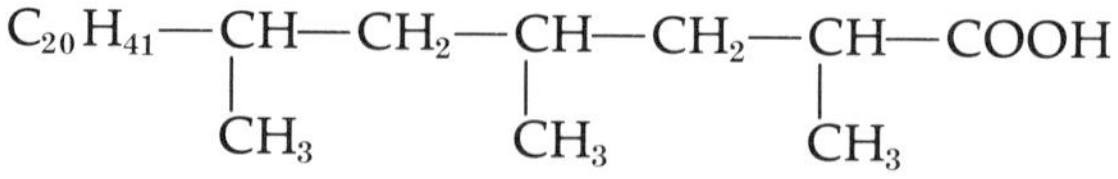

$$C_{20}H_{41}-\underset{\underset{CH_3}{|}}{CH}-CH_2-\underset{\underset{CH_3}{|}}{CH}-CH_2-\underset{\underset{CH_3}{|}}{CH}-COOH$$

xliii

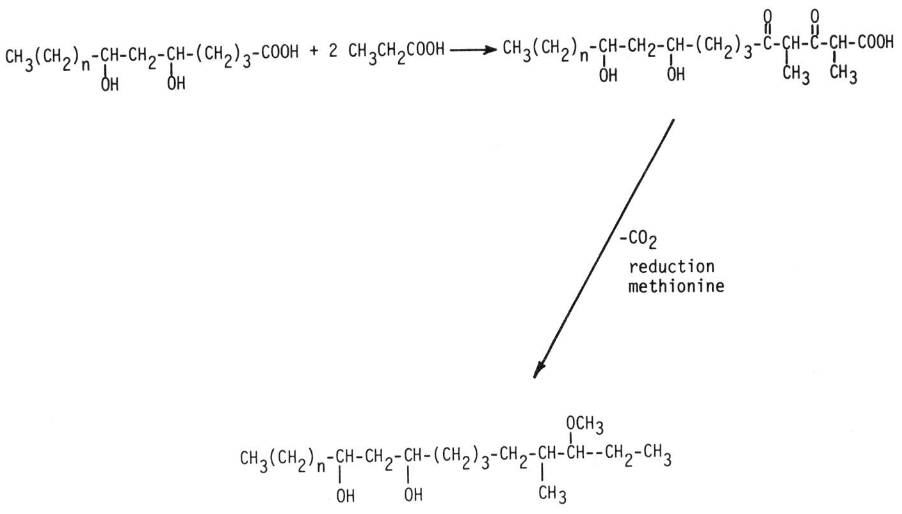

$$CH_3(CH_2)_n\text{-}CH\text{-}CH_2\text{-}CH\text{-}(CH_2)_3\text{-}COOH + 2\ CH_3CH_2COOH \longrightarrow CH_3(CH_2)_n\text{-}CH\text{-}CH_2\text{-}CH\text{-}(CH_2)_3\text{-}\overset{O}{\overset{\|}{C}}\text{-}CH\text{-}\overset{O}{\overset{\|}{C}}\text{-}CH\text{-}COOH$$

$-CO_2$
reduction
methionine

$$CH_3(CH_2)_n\text{-}CH\text{-}CH_2\text{-}CH\text{-}(CH_2)_3\text{-}CH_2\text{-}CH\text{-}\overset{OCH_3}{CH}\text{-}\text{-}CH_2\text{-}CH_3$$

phthiocerol

FIGURE 4–54.   Biosynthesis of phthiocerol.

by transferrin (see Kochan[200]). To successfully compete with transferrin, mycobacteria must elaborate an agent (or agents) that can "rob" the iron from its complex in serum. The mycobactins — required growth factor(s) for in vitro cultivation of *M. paratuberculosis* (*M. johnei*) — have a powerful iron-chelating ability and have been proposed for just such a function. Before their isolation by solvent extraction from *M. phlei*,[105] the unknown factors were supplied to *M. paratuberculosis* in the form of dried killed mycobacteria or their extracts. Most of the intriguing structural work on these substances is from the laboratory of G. A. Snow, Pharmaceuticals Division of Imperial Chemical Industries, Ltd., and is summarized in a thorough review.[328]

The mycobactins comprise some nine families of related lipids whose synthesis is highly stimulated by iron deprivation. The general structure of the mycobactins is given in Figure 4–55.[328] In 7 of these ("P"-type), R_1 is a lipid substituent of some 17 to 20 carbons, while in the remaining two ("M"-type), R_1 is a small radical (C_1–C_2) and the large lipid

moiety is on the "bridge" at R_4. The functional properties and the cooperative interaction with yet other iron chelates were delineated by Ratledge.[290]

The structural features that confer the remarkable iron-chelating activity are the N^6-hydroxylysines at A (Fig. 4–55) (in the form of a cyclic structure), at A', where the hydroxy amino group is acylated to give a secondary hydrox-

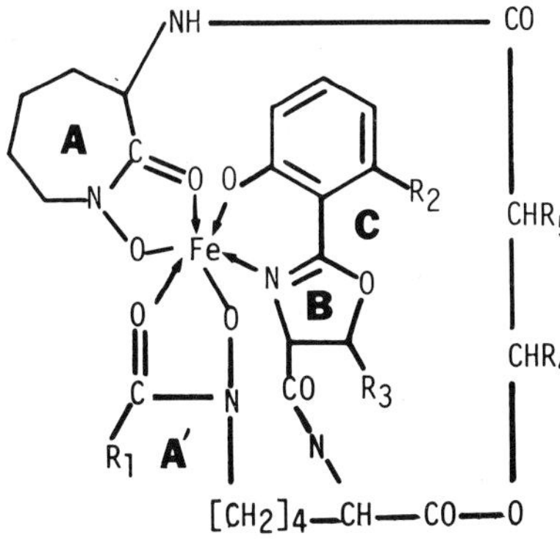

FIGURE 4–55. Mycobactin structure. (Adapted from Snow, G. A.: Mycobactins: Iron-chelating growth factors from mycobacteria. Bacteriol. Rev. 34:99, 1970.)

amic acid, and at B—an oxazoline structure, which can derive from either serine or threonine by a ring closure with an aromatic acid unit (either salicylic or 6-methyl salicylic acid) at C. The combination and correct stereochemical disposition of the two hydroxamic acids, the phenolic hydroxyl and the proximate nitrogen atom of the oxazoline ring, results in a formidable ability to chelate almost selectively with ferric iron; a stability constant in excess of 10^{30} has been calculated. X-ray crystallography of ferrimycobactin P shows that the iron atom is exposed in a "splayed V-shaped cleft in the chelating lipid." The release of the "exposed" iron is by reduction (via an NAD^+-linked reductase) to Fe^{II} mycobactin; the reduced iron has little or no affinity for the agent.

Although this would seem to be a uniquely designed and functional system, Ratledge has adroitly inferred and revealed it limitations; because of its lipid nature, mycobactin is found almost exclusively within the cell envelope and not in the culture medium. It is grossly limited (by solubility) in its ability to chelate and transport insoluble or colloidal iron and essentially can bind only soluble iron. The apparent solutions to the dilemma were resolved in an elegant series of studies (reviewed by Ratledge[290]) in which the deficiency is seen to be relieved by two other soluble ferric-chelating substances, whose synthesis is also stimulated in iron deprivation: salicylic acid (or the 6-methyl analog) and "exochelins."[236, 237] One of the latter, an oligopeptide containing ϵ-N-hydroxylysine, allothreonine, and β-alanine solubilizes and chelates insoluble Fe^{3+} and transfers it to mycobactin at the cell boundary. The iron-mycobactin complex moves through the cell envelope where the iron is reduced, released, and (inferentially) accepted by salicylate for final transfer to porphyrins. Although salicylate had at one time been a choice candidate for the initial solubilization

of extracellular iron for transfer to mycobactin, this role was contraindicated when salicylate was found nonfunctional in the presence of phosphate. The role of salicylate as presently postulated is inferred from its stimulated synthesis when iron limits growth and in probable inhibition of its function by *p*-amino-salicylic acid.

Carotenoids

Although the contribution of carotenoids to virulence is equivocal, the polyisoprenoids appear to protect mycobacteria against photodynamic killing and therefore contribute to survival of pathogenic species during growth or exposure in an open environment. Aside from its undeniable intellectual stimulation, the encyclopedic review article of Barksdale and Kim[40] is embellished by remarkably striking color photographs of a crystal of β-carotene and of lucent orange colonies of a constitutively chromogenic mycobacterium (supplied by George P. Kubica). In our opinion, and uninfluenced by color photographs, the section on carotenoids is one of the most excellent and informative in the review.

From the previous restriction, it may be correctly inferred that some mycobacteria are not at all chromogenic, or perhaps only marginally so (*M. bovis, M. smegmatis, M. marinum, M. fortuitum,* for example). Others are *constitutively* chromogenic and produce polyunsaturated pigments under essentially all conditions of growth whether in light or darkness — i.e., scotochromogenic (*M. phlei, M. gordonae, M. scrofulaceum*). In other species (e.g., *M. vaccae, M. avium, M. kansasii*), carotenoid synthesis may be dramatically induced or enhanced by exposure to light, although not all strains may respond. Thus, many *M. avium,* almost all of *M. kansasii* and *M. marinum,* and all of *M. vaccae* strains that have been examined are photochromogenic. These processes of pigmentation are therefore of value in mycobacterial taxonomy. (See also Chapter 18.)

Runyon,[299] on very practical grounds, rejects the criticisms raised in the past on the use of pigmentation in classification.

In clinical laboratories, if a dark-grown culture is distinctly golden or orange-yellow, it is a warning that the strain is probably a saprophyte, not significant in disease. Human and bovine tubercle bacilli are never really golden . . . on media used in clinical laboratories; neither are *M. fortuitum* nor *M. ulcerans*. . . . The photochromogenicity of *M. kansasii* and *M. marinum* is an especially useful characteristic for species identification. . . . *Crystals* (of carotene) in colonies of Group II scotochromogens should alert one to the possiblity that the strain in question is *M. kansasii*.

Biosynthesis

Excellent reviews of Goodwin,[131] of Batra,[42] and of Liaaen-Jensen and Andrewes[232] deal with the chemistry and biosynthesis of carotenoids in microorganisms and in higher plants. The accompanying Figure 4–56 (kindly provided by Drs. Barksdale and Kim)[40] illustrates the probable biosynthetic pathway for β-carotene in *M. marinum*. Head-to-head condensation of two molecules of geranylgeranyl pyrophosphate yields the complete carotenoid carbon skeleton (C_{40}) in the form of the acyclic prephytoene pyrophosphate, and thence phytoene. Successive desaturations, which can be inhibited by diphenylamine, lead to the still acyclic lycopene (identical with the pigment of tomatoes), which possesses the full complement of double bonds. Two successive ring closures then lead to the fully conjugated β-carotene. The alternate (dotted) route of cyclization leads to α-carotene, in which one terminal cyclohexene has the nonconjugated (α-ring) configuration but the second (β-ring) is conjugated.

Photoinduction of Carotenoids Synthesis

Although scotochromogens may be indifferent to, or only slightly stimulated to carotenoids production by light, cultures of *M. kansasii* and *M. marinum* elaborate many times their basal level of carotenoids (principally β-carotene) following photoinduction.[351] Batra and Storms[43] reported that dark-grown *M. marinum* does not form carotenoids because the carotenogenic enzymes are in a genetically repressed state. Derepression of the genetic sites in this organism and in other mycobacteria ordinarily requires *both* light and oxygen.

Teleologically, the function of the carotenoids would seem to be protection of the microorganism against photo-induced cell death. Indeed Tsukamura[360] and David[84] provide evidence that in mycobacteria there is, in fact, a correlation between the presence of carotenoid pigment and decreased sensitivity to ultraviolet irradiation.

Photo-induced injury and cell death have been ascribed to the specific intervention of singlet molecular oxygen,[180] a form in which the spins of the valence electrons are paired, but in a higher energy state than the *unpaired* triplet ground state of ordinary oxygen. The electrons in singlet oxygen may occupy the same or different orbitals, as shown below.

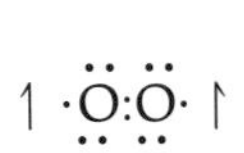

↑ ·O:O· ↑

triplet, ground state
spins unpaired
different orbitals

↓ ·O:O· ↑

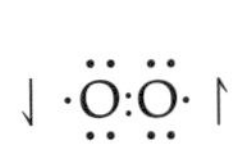

sigma singlet O_2
spins paired
different orbitals

O:O: ↓↑

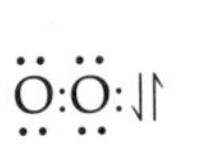

delta singlet O_2
spins paired
same orbital

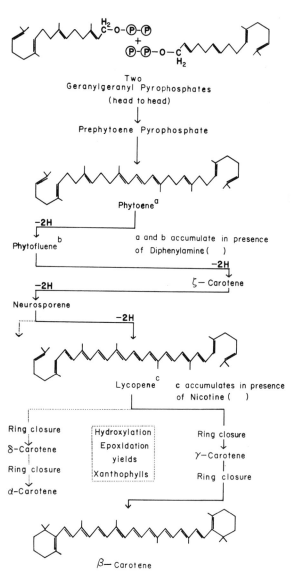

FIGURE 4–56. Probable biosynthetic pathway for β-carotene in *Mycobacterium marinum*. (From Barksdale, L., and Kim, K.-S.: *Mycobacterium*. Bacteriol. Rev. *41*:217, 1977.)

Singlet oxygen can dissipate its energy and thus revert to the ground state by emission of light or by participating in oxygenating reactions with suitable electron dense targets, usually unsaturated linkages in organic molecules.

The killing potential of singlet oxygen within or at the surface of a microorganism is recognized from its implication as the mediator in the photodynamic action of certain dyes on a variety of substrates.[9, 329] These dyes (eosin is an example) are toxic only in the presence of light and oxygen. As shown in Figure 4–57, from its ground state (singlet), the dye is activated by light to form an *excited* singlet state and then, by a change in spin multiplicity, to an excited *triplet* state. In the presence of oxygen, the dye reverts to the singlet ground state, with the concomitant generation of singlet molecular oxygen.

Probably by behaving as singlet oxygen scavengers, the carotenoid pigments can exert a protective effect against photodynamic killing. Accord-

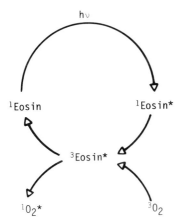

$h\nu$

$^1\text{Eosin}$ $^1\text{Eosin*}$

$^3\text{Eosin*}$

$^1\text{O}_2\text{*}$ $^3\text{O}_2$

FIGURE 4–57. Photodynamic activation of eosin and generation of singlet molecular oxygen. (Asterisks indicate excited states.)

ing to Burchard and Dworkin,[63] and Burchard and Hendricks,[64] an endogenous photosensitizer may be functional both in photodynamic killing (as a counterpart of eosin) and in the induction of carotenoid synthesis as competing processes. In mycobacteria, porphyrins and flavins appear to be implicated as these mediators, as interpreted from the action spectra.

In H. L. David's comprehensive studies of carotenoids in *M. kansasii*,[85, 86] some dozen polyisoprenoids were separated, nine of which were identified. Carotenogenesis was induced in the presence of oxygen by incident light of wavelengths 420, 540, and 650 nm, with minima at 360, 470, 600, and 700 nm. By following incorporation of radiolabeled acetate into lipid products, David found that within two minutes of exposure to light, polyisoprenoid precursors were detectable. The profiles of these precursors changed in a manner suggestive of a sequential synthesis of protein enzymes in the pathway leading to β-carotene; this was synthesized and began to accumulate within eight minutes. After 10 minutes, the putative intermediates were detectable only in trace amounts, indicating their rapid conversion to the end-product by the battery of enzymes.

Synthesis of messenger-RNA began almost immediately after illumination and continued for nearly an hour after a shift to dark conditions, but in the dark, carotenoids synthesis continued for several hours, in accordance with the longer survival of the individual enzymes.

MYCOSIDES

Historically, mycoside studies had their origin in the efforts of Smith and colleagues[323] to associate immunizing properties of fractions from tubercle bacilli with their infrared spectra. Later, the emphasis shifted to correlating the IR spectra of specific lipids with individual mycobacterial species.[324] The mycosides have been defined as "glycolipids or glycolipid peptides limited in distribution to a single species of mycobacteria,"[325] but this restriction is no longer valid. The substances were originally designated by the letters G and J; soon afterwards, the term "mycoside" was coined: "mycoside A" to describe particular substances characteristic of photochromogenic strains of mycobacteria, "mycoside B" for certain lipids that typified bovine strains, and "mycoside G" for the specific lipid isolated from *M. marinum*.[268] Indeed, these are structurally related. Mycoside C, originally recognized in avian strains, is chemically unrelated to the preceding groups of mycosides except for similarities in carbohydrate components. The three substances are *not* ubiquitous among mycobacteria; the name has become so loosely used that almost any glycolipid or peptidoglycolipid of mycobacteria could be called (*incorrectly*) a "mycoside."

Mycosides A, B, and G

Mycosides A, B, and G are quite similar phenolic glycolipids (Table 4–6)

TABLE 4-6. Structures of Mycosides A-, B-, and G-Related Phthiocerol Dimycocerosates (DIM) and Phenolic Phthiocerol Diesters

Name	Structure	Reference
DIM (Phthiocerol dimycocerosate)	$CH_3—(CH_2)_n—CH—CH_2—CH—(CH_2)_4—CH—CH_2—CH_3$ (with OCH_3 on terminal CH, OR' substituents) n = 20–22	Noll (1975)[272] Smith et al. (1960)[326] Goren et al. (1974)[143]
Generalized structure for AI lipid and Mycoside A, B, and G	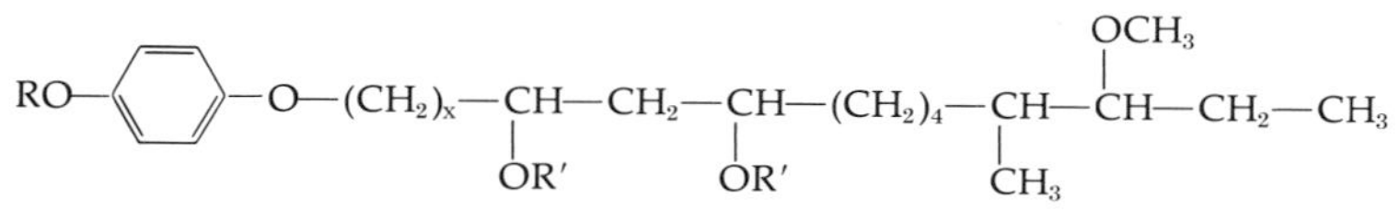	Goren et al. (1974)[144]
Phenolic phthiocerol Diesters (AI) lipid of Goren et al. (1974)[144]	$RO—⟨C_6H_4⟩—O—(CH_2)_x—CH—CH_2—CH—(CH_2)_4—CH—CH_2—CH_3$ (with OCH_3, CH_3, OR' substituents) R = CH_3; x = 16, 18	
Mycosides A and A'	R = Trisaccharide (?) composed of 2-O-methylfucopyranoside, 3-O-methylfucofuranoside, 2-O-methylrhamnofuranoside, 3-O-methylrhamnofuranoside,2,4-di-O-methylrhamnopyranoside. The trisaccharide may or may not be mycolated. x = 16, 17, 18, 19, 20	MacLennan et al. (1961)[240] Gastambide-Odier et al. (1965, 1967)[121, 122] Gastambide-Odier and Sarda (1970)[120] Gastambide-Odier and Ville (1970)[123] Gastambide-Odier (1972)[113]
Mycoside B	R = 2-O-methylrhamnose x = 14, 15, 16, 17, 18	MacLennan et al. (1961)[240] Gastambide-Odier et al. (1965, 1967)[121, 122] Gastambide-Odier and Sarda (1970)[120] Demarteau-Ginsburg and Lederer (1963)[88]
Mycosides G and G'	R = An α-linked 3-O-methylrhamnopyranoside x = 18, 19, 20, 21, 22 R' = Acyl functions of palmitic acid or mycocerosic acids, with chain length C_{24} to C_{32}, e.g., $C_{20}H_{41}—CH—CH_2—CH—CH_2—CH—CH—CH—COOH$ (with CH_3, CH_3, CH_3 branches)	Sarda and Gastambide-Odier (1967)[305] Ville and Gastambide-Odier (1970)[372] Gastambide-Odier (1972, 1973)[113, 114]

whose structures have been determined largely by Gastambide-Odier. (For an absorbing account of the earlier work on mycosides A and B, see Gastambide-Odier and Sarda[120].) These share a similar "backbone," which is related to the β-glycol, *phthiocerol*. The two aliphatic hydroxyl groups are esterified by two acyl radicals, principally palmitate/stearate and the multimethyl-branched mycocerosate (see p. 153).

The major difference between mycosides A, B, and G is in the nature of sugar substituents glycosidically attached to the aromatic hydroxyl groups, as shown in Table 4–6. Mycoside G from *M. marinum* has a larger aliphatic chain on its phenolic glycol, and its major sugar is 3-O-methyl-L-rhamnopyranoside (acofriose).[305, 372]

Recently, Gastambide-Odier[114] discovered variants of mycosides A and G

(A' and G') in which the carbohydrate moieties are clearly esterified with mycolic acids. Mass spectrometry showed these to be methoxylated (α') mycolic acids, with a C_{22} α-branch. Whether all other examples of A, B, and G mycosides may be acylated in a similar fashion is not yet clear.

Biosynthesis

Figure 4–58 summarizes the likely sequence for the synthesis of the mycoside A, B, and G series. The aromatic portion of the phenol glycols probably arises from tyrosine (not phenylalanine), since radioactivity from tyrosine-3-^{14}C is incorporated into the lipid.[122] Alternatively, propionate entering the shikimic acid pathway by way of pyruvate may also give rise to the phenolic segment. The methyl branches on the

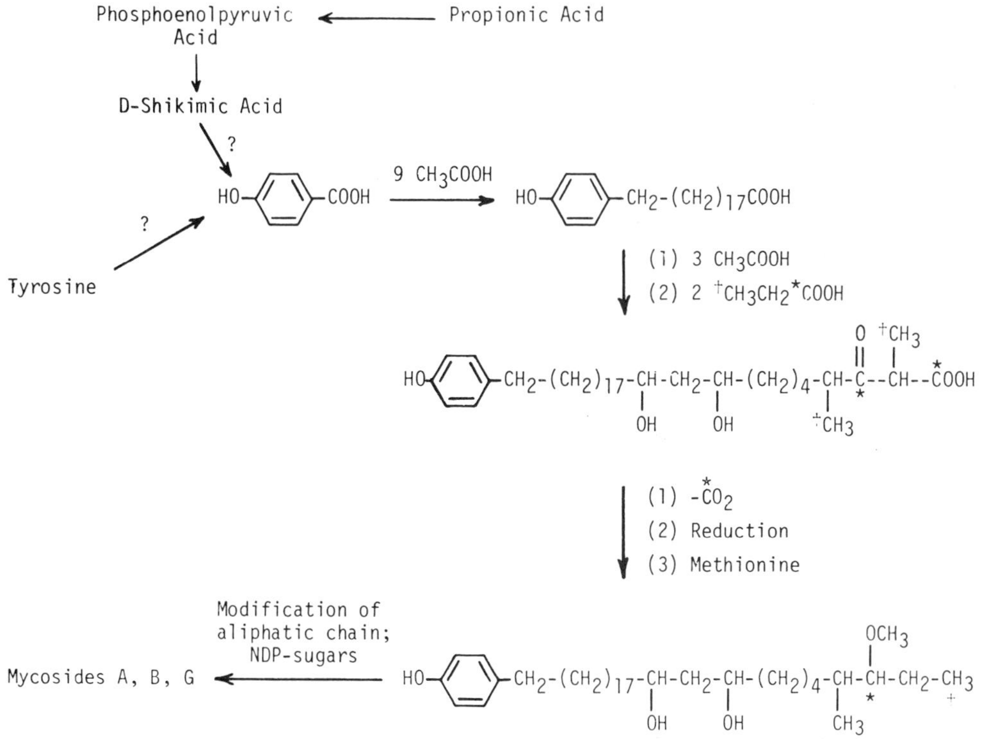

FIGURE 4–58. Proposed biosynthesis of mycosides A, B, and G. Daggers and stars represent ^{14}C. (Adapted from Gastambide-Odier, M., Sarda, P., and Lederer, E.: Biosynthese des aglycones des mycosides A et B. Bull. Soc. Chim. Biol. 49:849, 1967.)

aliphatic chain come from incorporation of propionic acid, as in phthiocerol (see p. 155).[116]

Biologic Roles

From the evidence that showed the A and G variants to be mycoloylated, Gastambide-Odier[114] suggested that they may play a role in some form of transport from the cell surface, owing to their amphipathic construction, with polar sugars bound through an aromatic nucleus to an apolar aglycone. Alternatively, they may function in anabolic processes, although none have been demonstrated. For the C-mycosides, Barksdale and Kim[40] have also considered possible functions in transporting and in contributing to prevention of water loss from the cell during periods of excessive drying. The mycoloylated G mycosides may provide a similar function.

Mycosides A, B, and G have not been discerned in human strains of tubercle bacilli and, as shown in Table 4–6, are restricted to certain Group I photochromogens and to bovine strains. However, Goren, Brokl, and Schaefer[143] found that certain lipids closely related to these mycosides serve as a phenotypic marker of attenuation in some wild-type strains of *M. tuberculosis*. From the lipid composition of 40 patient isolates derived from Madras, Burma, Rangoon, and East Africa, two major populations were distinguished. Nearly all of the attenuated strains[261] were characterized by the same nonpolar lipid, identified as the phenolic methyl ether of the aglycone moiety of mycosides A, B, and G. This lipid (the "Attenuation Indicator," or AI lipid) was absent from the virulent strains. Presence of AI lipids was found to be definitive for attenuation, irrespective of other phenotypic characteristics. A companion substance, phthiocerol dimycocerosate (DIM), is present among all members of the series; nevertheless, it may have some relevance to the virulent state (see p.

154). Clearly, the ability to synthesize the aromatic-substituted phthiocerol is common to the Group I photochromogens, bovine strains, and the attenuated human strains, and it may be the product of a similar biosynthetic pathway not found in more virulent *M. tuberculosis*. Possibly, genetic modification of fully virulent strains — as by lysogenization or transduction — may have provided the determinants for attenuation and for phenolic phthiocerol diester synthesis. The ubiquity of the phthiocerol backbone also prompted the supposition that if it has phage receptor function, it could provide (via specific phages) the interspecies means of access to genetic information. In recent collaborative studies of J. Grange and colleagues,[148a] a relationship has been discerned between phage type and the presence or absence of mycobacterial sulfatides (see p. 145) and of the attenuation indicator lipid. Of 9 phage-type A and 3 phage-type B strains, most were rich in sulfatide (SL), and only one had the AI lipid; 12 out of 14 intermediate (I) phage type were characterized by the AI lipid and elaborated only meager levels of SL in culture.

There seems little doubt that mycosides A, B, and G are externally located on the mycobacterial cell surface, and it has been noted (Lederer[218]) that there are distinct differences in the morphology of colonies of mycoside-containing and mycoside-free strains. However, the evidence is more convincing with the C-type mycosides.

C-Mycosides

The C-mycosides have received much more structural attention than the preceding ones, to which they are chemically only marginally related. This chemical emphasis is in keeping with the emergence of their fascinating biologic roles. In their classical paper, Smith and colleagues[326] described isola-

TABLE 4-7. C-Mycosides of *Mycobacterium* sp.

Organism	Structure*	Mycoside Designation	Reference
A nonphotochromogenic			
Mycobacterium 1217	R—CO—NH—Phe—*a*Thr—Ala—Alol—O—(di or tri—O—Me—Rha)	C$_{1217}$	Lanéelle and Asselineau (1968)[214]
M. scrofulaceum	(Ac—6—deoxytal) with O	C$_s$	Vilkas et al. (1968)[368]
M. butyricum		C$_{b1}$	Vilkas and Lederer (1968)[369]
A rapid grower (Group IV)	R—CO—NH—Phe—*a*Thr—Ala—Alol—O—(di or mono—O—Me—Rha), with OH	C′	Lanéelle et al. (1971)[216]
M. butyricum	R—CO—NH—Phe—*a*Thr—Ala—X—(di or tri—O—Me—Rha)	C$_b$	Vilkas et al. (1966)[370]
M. kansasii		—	Nacash and Vilkas (1967)[266]
M. avium 802	(di—Ac—6—deoxytal) *or* (di—Ac—3—O—Me—6—deoxytal)	C$_2$	Vilkas (1966)[385]
M. avium 802	R—CO—NH—Phe—*a*Thr—Ala—Alol—O—(Ac—3,4 di—O—Me—Rha), with OH; (di—Ac—6—deoxytal) *or* (di—Ac—3—O—Me—6—deoxytal)	C$_2$	Voiland et al. (1971)[373]
M. marianum	R—CO—NH—Phe—*a*Thr—Ala—X—(di—Ac—6—deoxytal), with O OH O; (Ac—di—O—Me—Rha) (Ac—di—O—Me—Rha)	C$_m$	Chaput et al. (1962)[74]

*The amino acids, including *allo*-threonine (*a*Thr), are of the unnatural D-configuration. Alaninol (Alol) has the L-configuration. X may be —N—Ser—CO—, alaninyl, ethanolaminyl, or CO— of the preceding alanine. Ac = acetyl; Rha = L-rhamnose; 6–deoxytal = 6–deoxy–L–talose, R = fatty acyl CH$_3$ OCH$_3$ (usually a β-oxygenated carboxyl—about C$_{28}$). Noteworthy structural exceptions are the principal lipid substituents in mycoside C$_s$ of *M. scrofulaceum*, which are C$_{32}$ and C$_{35}$ unsaturated acids methoxylated in the α-position.

tion by column chromatography of lipids (called "J" substances) common to some scotochromogens, nonphotochromogens and *M. marinum* (*M. scrofulaceum* in current nomenclature). Since the strains examined spanned the accepted classification of atypical mycobacteria based on pigment formation,[298] Smith and his coworkers were unsure of their grounds for attributing group specificity to the J substances. It is satisfying now to note that all the strains examined almost certainly belong to the distinct *M. avium/M. intracellulare/M. scrofulaceum* (MAIS) immunologic sub-group. The J substances all showed previously unrecognized infrared spectra, characterized by absorption bands attributable to peptide bonds and ester linkages. The general name "mycoside C", or C-mycoside, was later coined for those substances.[325] Table 4–7 is a compilation of the structures proposed for C-mycosides from various sources (with some modifications of our own conception, for which supportive evidence is reviewed).

The gross structural features of the C-mycosides may be broadly described as follows:

1. A β-oxygenated carboxylic acid (usually about C_{28}), amide-linked to the amino group of D-phenylalanine, which is the N-terminal amino acid of an oligopeptide.
2. The peptide moiety has the structure:

    D-Phe—(D-*allo*Thr—D-Ala)$_n$,

    xliv

    where n may be 1, 2, or 3, and all amino acids have the unnatural D-configuration.
3. The C-terminal end of the peptide may be the carboxyl group of *D*-alanine, it may be amidated with an amino alcohol, L-alaninol, or with the extremely rare N-methyl-O-methylserine, or possibly with an ethanolamine substituent.[214]

4. The terminal group of the oligopeptide is bound to the reducing hydroxy function of a 6-deoxy-sugar.
5. Single 6-deoxysugars are usually linked O-glycosidically to the β-hydroxyl of *allo*-threonine.

The 6-deoxysugars that can occupy these positions were originally identified by MacLennan[239] in an ambitious effort. With simple classical techniques such as demethylation to determine the composition of the parent sugar and a variety of colorimetric reactions, he showed that glucose, arabinose, rhamnose, 3-O-methylrhamnose, 2,3- and 3,4-di-O-methylrhamnose, 6-deoxy-talose, and 3-O-methyl-6-deoxytalose were associated with his C-mycoside preparations. Although glucose and arabinose are no longer regarded as constituents of C-mycosides, MacLennan's other assignments have been sufficiently confirmed, and his simple procedures are still adequate for identifying the sugar components of C-mycosides.

The structures summarized in Table 4–7 derive from the exemplary individual and collaborative efforts of three groups of French investigators during the period 1961 to 1971. Nevertheless, several structural features still require some resolution.

The first members of the C-group to receive detailed attention were mycosides C_1 and C_2 from *M. avium*, No. 802.[75, 167] Mild acid hydrolysis of C_1 or C_2 yielded a number of peptides, and from these the pentapeptide structure shown below was proposed. In addition, the D-phenylalanine was determined to be amide-linked to monohydroxy fatty acids. An inference that the C-terminal D-alanine was esterified to a trisaccharide was ultimately revised to provide the proposed structure (opposite page) for mycosides. Thus, two moles of carbohydrate are attached to the peptide chain, specifically

D-Phe—D-*allo*Thr—D-Ala—D-*allo*Thr—D-Ala—

$$C_x H_y (OH)\text{—}CO\text{—}D\text{-}Phe\text{—}D\text{-}alloThr\text{—}D\text{-}Ala\text{—}D\text{-}alloThr\text{—}D\text{-}Ala\text{—}COOR$$

$$\underset{\underset{\text{3,4-di-O—methylrhamnose}}{|}}{O}$$

where

x = 45 or 42; y = 88 or 84; R = 6-deoxytalose or 3-O—methyl-6-deoxytalose

xlv

---

to *allo*-threonine and (inferentially) to the suspected C-terminal amino acid.

It was not realized then that the alkaline degradative conditions, which purported to show that sugars were ester-linked to the terminal alanine, were instead cleaving those sugars attached to *allo*-threonine by a β-elimination process. Moreover, other evidence showed that a terminal *alaninol* mediates a glycosidic (not ester) linkage between the oligopeptide and the second deoxysugar. In the light of these later developments, Voiland and colleagues[373] clarified the earlier controversial details, so that the most recent structural expression for mycoside C_2 (Table 4–7) is indeed based on hard evidence. Just as the proposed structures for mycoside C_2 have undergone modification, so the one suggested for mycoside C_m may also require re-examination; most likely it also contains a linkage alaninol, and the positions of the substituent sugars may need revision.

With respect to some of the other C-mycosides (Table 4–7), other areas of uncertainty that may now be addressed concern the length of the oligopeptide chains and the possible distribution of N-methyl-O-methylserine, which is not yet unequivocal.

The lengths of the oligopeptide chains have been points of controversy that stemmed from the resistance to acid hydrolysis of the N-acyl substituted D-phenylalanine, as Vilkas and her coworkers recognized.[370] Phenylalanine is therefore underestimated; apparent

ratios of 1:2:2 for D-Phe:D-*allo* Thr:D-Ala were repeatedly obtained (after 6 to 24 hours of hydrolysis). More correct ratios, approximating 1:1:1, are derived when the hydrolysis is prolonged to 48 hours. Accordingly, Lanèelle and Asselineau[214] were constrained to revise their earlier pentapeptide structure for mycoside C_{1217} in favor of the tripeptide expression. The former had been derived on the basis of a 16-hour acid hydrolysis and, by revision, was brought into closer agreement with both nitrogen content and estimated molecular weight. It is important to note that the structure proposed by Voiland and colleagues[373] for mycoside C_2 is based on extensive hydrolysis (48 hr) and also on the recognition of several peptide fragments. There are no doubts, therefore, about the validity of its pentapeptide structure. On the other hand, a re-examination of the oligopeptide moiety of mycoside C_m may be warranted, since its peptide structure was inferred from products of rather brief hydrolysis (6 hr).

We alluded earlier to the equivocal state of N-methyl-O-methyl-serine as a constituent of C-mycosides. This amino acid was first isolated from mycoside C_b of *M. butyricum*.[370, 371] However, the amount relative to other amino acids was not established. Voiland and coworkers[373] searched unsuccessfully for N-methyl-O-methyl serine in their mycoside C_2 preparation and among its by-products. One explanation for the conflicting reports may be that the substituted amino acid is a component of only a minor mycoside in the preparation.

A most impressive aspect of the extensive work on C-mycoside structures is in the sophisticated mass spectrometric methods that have been utilized in sequencing of the peptides. As applicable mass spectrometric methods were developed,[83, 219, 352] they were at first invoked to provide confirmatory evidence for the earlier elegant classical structural studies on peptides. They were also utilized by Vilkas and colleagues[370] to confirm the point of attachment of the long chain acyl substituents on the peptide

moiety and to identify the fatty acyl fragments. Later, the methodology provided evidence from which essentially the complete structure of a C-mycoside could be derived. Excellent examples are those in which Vilkas and colleagues derived a partial structure for mycoside C_b and a complete structure for mycoside C_{b1}.

A consideration of how a portion of the cleavage pattern for the native mycoside C_{b1} was interpreted illustrates the utility of the mass spectrometric method. Figure 4–59 is taken from Vilkas and Lederer[369] and was used by

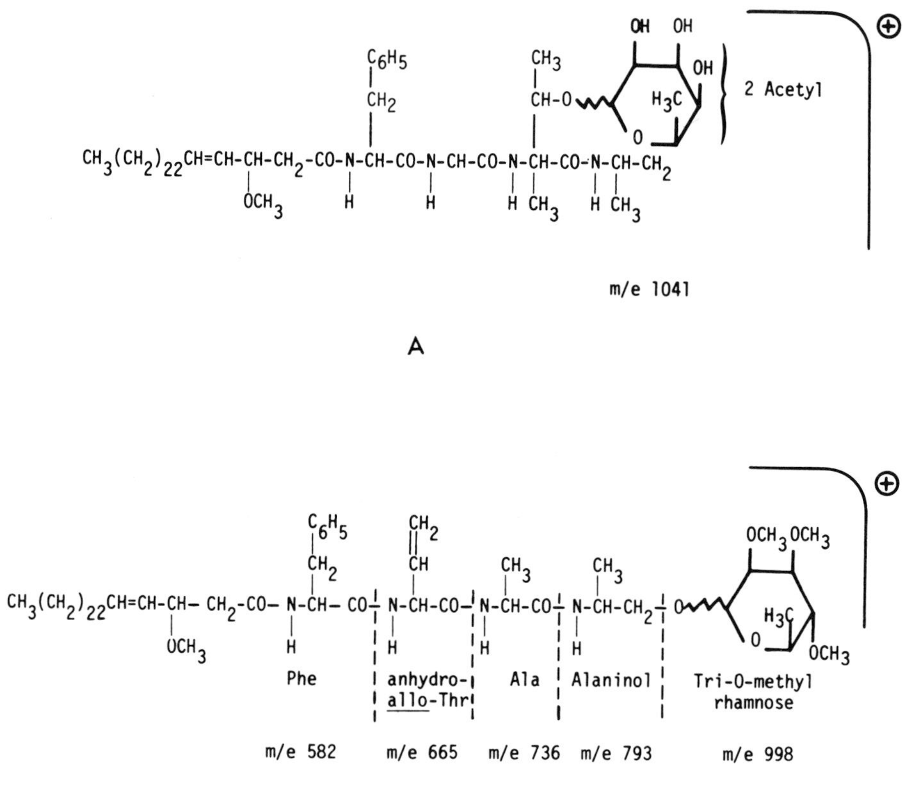

FIGURE 4–59.   Mass fragmentation of the native mycoside C_{b1} from *M. butyricum. A,* Structural definition of one of the major fragments (*m/e* 1041), i.e., the fragment arising due to loss of the terminal tri-O-methylrhamnose (minus H) from the native C-mycoside. *B,* Structural interpretation of the second major fragment (*m/e* 998; owing to loss of diacetyl-6-deoxytalose from the β-hydroxy of *allo*-threonine) and other smaller fragments. (From Vilkas, E., and Lederer, E.: N-methylation de peptides par la methode de Hakomori. Structure du mycoside C_{b1}. Tetrahedron Lett. 26:3089, 1968).

Goren[136] (unintentionally but regrettably, without acknowledgement) to illustrate the remarkable versatility of this method. As shown in Figure 4–59, *A*, the molecular ion, M$^+$ = 1,246 was not in evidence; instead, the major observed fragments were at *m/e* 1041 due to loss of the terminal tri-O-methyl-rhamnose minus H (205 mass units), and at *m/e* 998 (Fig. 4–59, *B*) owing to loss from the intact molecule of the *allo*-threonine-linked diacetyl-6-deoxytalose (248 mass units). This intermediate then fragments according to the sequence shown. The principle peaks reflect the fortuitous manner in which amino acid residues are sequentially lost after initial cleavage of the sugar fragments. The technique has been applied to mycoside C$_{1217}$ to confirm the revised (tripeptide) structure[213], and by M. Goren, B.C. Das, and O. Brokl[144b] to establish an almost identical structure for mycoside C$_{sm}$ of *M. smegmatis* (see also Furuchi and Tokunaga[110]).

Biosynthesis of Mycobacteria

The biosynthesis of the C-mycosides (as yet unexplored) must be complex. Of several conceivable pathways, two seem the most feasible to us (Fig. 4–60). In one, amino acids or small peptides are added sequentially to an activated fatty acid, and the other mirrors some features of peptidoglycan synthesis — in particular, the steps leading to the formation of a nucleotide-6-

deoxysugar-L-alaninol-tripeptide. As in cell wall peptidoglycan synthesis, amino-acyl-tRNAs and a polyprenol phosphate carrier may be involved.

Nucleotide-6-deoxysugars would seem to be the most likely precursors of 6-deoxy-O-*methyl* sugars. Thus, Okuda and colleagues[276, 277] isolated CDP-vinelose from *Azotobacter vinelandii* and proposed that a CDP-linked 6-deoxy-4-ketohexose may undergo rearrangement to provide the site to which the methyl group of methionine (or *S*-adenosylmethionine) is transferred (Fig. 4–61). Indeed, the latter are the methyl donors in the biosynthesis of 3-O-methyl-6-deoxytalose and 3,4 di-O-methylrhamnose of mycoside C$_2$ (*M. avium*).[62]

D-cycloserine, O-carbamyl-D-cycloserine, or D-norvaline — all known to be antagonists of alanine metabolism — could be utilized to test for the speculative pathways of Figure 4–60. In *M. tuberculosis* H37Ra and in *M. phlei*, D-ala-D-ala synthetase and probably the D-alanine racemase are susceptible to D-cycloserine. Consequently, it inhibits the synthesis of the cell wall peptidoglycan (see p. 109).[87, 281, 339] Similarly, it is quite likely that D-cycloserine and probably O-carbamyl-D-cycloserine would inhibit the synthesis of C-mycosides, perhaps resulting in the accumulation of a fragment whose structure might illuminate steps in the biosynthetic pathway. D-norvaline or other structural analogues

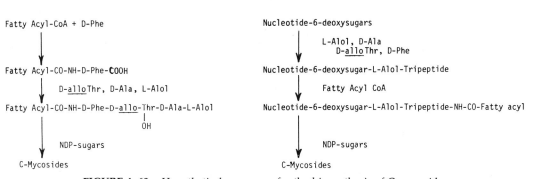

FIGURE 4–60. Hypothetical sequences for the biosynthesis of C-mycosides.

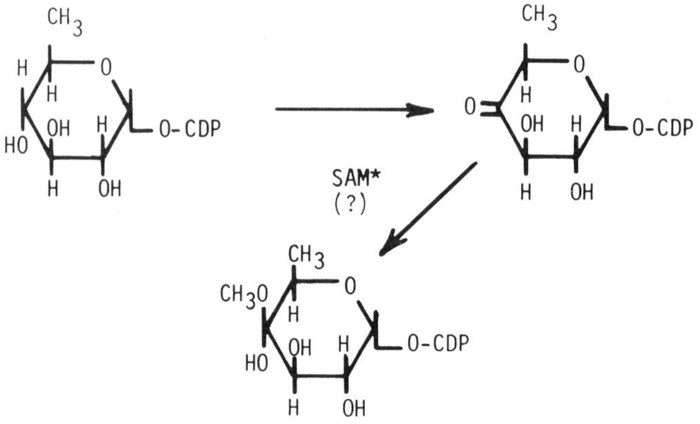

*S-adenosylmethionine

FIGURE 4–61. Possible route for biosynthesis of 6-deoxy-O-*methyl* sugars.

of D-alanine might be incorporated into oligomers, which are unable to participate in the final synthesis of C-mycosides.

C-Mycosides and Identification of Atypical Mycobacterial Strains

The C-mycosides described by Smith and colleagues were long regarded as species- or type-specific lipids. However, their distributional limitation was called into question by the observation[266] that *M. kansasii* contains both a C-mycoside and an A-mycoside. However, recent developments from this and other laboratories demonstrate that the C-mycosides can be used to achieve a reliable identification of individual strains of atypical mycobacteria.

The majority of atypical mycobacteria are smooth-colony-forming and are endowed with species or type-specific antigens not shared by the rough-colony-forming mycobacteria such as *M. tuberculosis* or *M. bovis*. Schaefer utilized these surface antigens to devise a seroagglutination procedure for the identification and classification of atypical mycobacteria. When it was applied to strains in Runyon's four groups, 31 distinct but related serotypes were recognized, comprising the *Mycobacterium avium/M. intracellulare/M. scrofulaceum* (MAIS) complex.[148, 290a, 309, 310, 390]

Schaefer[308] also recognized that serologically active specific lipids could be extracted from lyophilized cells of the bacteria with boiling methanol. These crude lipids were active in complement fixation and in Ouchterlony precipitation tests, when examined with the specific antisera. Exploratory studies of Brokl, Schaefer, and Goren[61a] yielded a partial separation of these "antigens" from extracts of *M. intracellulare*, serotype 8 (Davis). A gross preliminary chemical characterization revealed that they contained lipid, carbohydrate, and peptide components, and among the latter, phenylalanine and threonine (or *allo*-threonine) were prominent. These observations led to the inference that the serologically active lipids might be structured on the C-mycosides, and serologic specificity might reside in the type and abundance of carbohydrates that adorn a more or less common lipopeptide "core."

Marks, Jenkins, and their colleagues from Cardiff, in a search for other easily identifiable features characteristic of atypical mycobacteria, recognized an array of closely related polar and apolar lipids shared by most smooth colony strains in the MAIS complex. It was possible to identify many of these serotypes on the basis of the thin-layer chromatographic profiles, which these select lipids exhibited; and their distinct color reactions with orcinol in sulfuric acid suggested them to be glycolipids. Until recently, this was the extent of their characterization; nevertheless, it allowed a reliable (albeit empirical) identification of some individual serotypes. Six serotypes of organisms classified as *M. intracellulare* or *M. avium* and several *M. scrofulaceum* serotypes were distinguished in this way.[165, 166, 243] Sehrt and coworkers[319] and Brennan and his fellow workers[53a] essentially confirmed these observations. Thus, species in the MAIS complex could be readily identified by this procedure, provided that reference strains are examined in parallel. We recently initiated studies to identify these characteristic lipids and described our results in a preliminary report.[57]

A feature of the specific lipids of *M. intracellulare* serotypes isolated by the extraction procedure of Marks and colleagues[243] is the presence of both apolar and polar definitive components. Individually, these groups can be satisfactorily separated by first treating the bacteria with acetone to solubilize the apolar variety, then extracting with refluxing methanol to recover the polar type.[57] I.R. spectrometry of the two classes showed absorption bands at 3300, 1640, and 1540 cm^{-1}, which is characteristic of peptide linkages, and at 1740 cm^{-1} owing to ester absorption. In fact, gross features of all the spectra were identical with those of the C-mycosides.

Our parallel studies of the Schaefer antigens, on the one hand, and the Marks-Jenkins lipids, on the other, revealed the entirely unexpected feature that the Schaefer antigens were in fact the polar serotype-identifying components of the Marks-Jenkins extracts; and all of these, both polar and apolar,

are families of mycoside-C variants. In serotype 9 the former consist of two major members, whereas the apolar group contains at least six components. Individual lipids from each group have been isolated and their structures examined in some detail.[53b, 57] Examples from both groups contained alanine, *allo*-threonine, phenylalanine and alaninol, which were present in the approximate ratio of 1:1:1:1, suggesting a tripeptide-based structure similar to that described by Lanéelle and Asselineau.[214]

In the apolar family, three members contain 3,4-di-O-methylrhamnose attached to alaninol, with 3-O-methyl-6-deoxytalose linked to *allo*-threonine. These are therefore closely related to the C-mycosides already described. One other member of the apolar family has 3-O-methylrhamnose linked to alaninol with 6-deoxytalose at the *allo*-threonine position and yet another member retains the 6-deoxytalose but replaces the 3-O-methylrhamnose with the 3,4 di-O-methylrhamnose.

The polar definitive lipids (Schaefer antigens) contain substantially more carbohydrate (approximately 50 percent) than the apolar group. Most of it was released as oligosaccharides (from *allo*-threonine) by the β-elimination reaction (vide supra) and, in the case of the major antigen from serotype 9, this was characterized as an oligosaccharide containing 6-deoxytalose, rhamnose, 3,4-di-O-methylrhamnose, 2,3-di-O-methylrhamnose and an unidentified sugar. As in the majority of the apolar C-mycosides, a single 3,4 di-O-methylrhamnose is attached to alaninol. Our information on these various types of C-mycosides is summarized in Figure 4–62. Only the polar C-mycoside peptidoglycolipids were serologically active; all other cellular fractions, including the apolar C-mycosides, were not.[53b, 57] Thus our data show that Schaefer's serologically active lipids are structured on a C-mycoside core; moreover, they revealed that the Marks-Jenkins specific lipids comprise a similar, related group

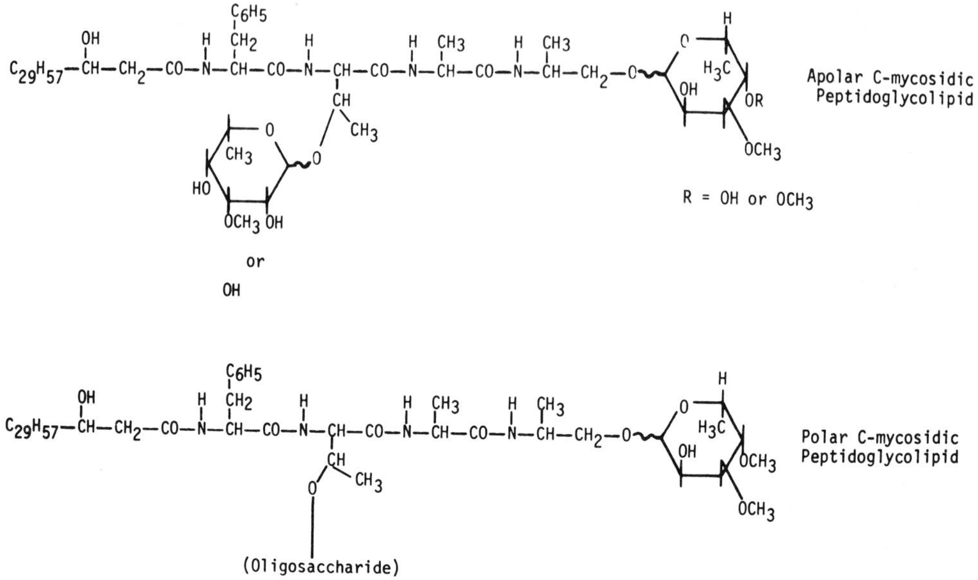

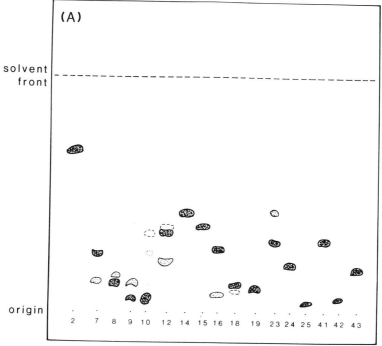

FIGURE 4–62. Tentative structures for the various C-mycosides from *Mycobacterium intracellulare* (serotype 9). (Brennan, P. J., and Goren, M. B., unpublished.)

FIGURE 4–63. Thin layer chromatography of the deacetylated Schaefer antigens from a variety of *M. avium/intracellulare/scrofulaceum* serotypes (serotype numbers are given below the line of origin). The solvent was chloroform-methanol-water (30:8:1, by volume), and lipids were located with a solution of orcinol in H_2SO_4. Each serotype exhibits its own characteristic pattern, which can be used to identify mycobacterial strains. (From Brennan, P. J., Souhrada, M., Ullom, B., McClatchy, J. K., and Goren, M. B.: Identification of atypical mycobacteria by thin-layer chromatography of their surface antigens. J. Clin. Microbiol. *8*:374, 1978.)

of C-mycoside variants. The Schaefer antigens are included among these as individual components, heretofore unrecognized.

Figure 4–63 depicts a thin layer chromatographic profile of the Schaefer antigens from a variety of MAIS serotypes. Whole lipids were deacetylated prior to chromatography, which by enhancing the polarity of the lipids, facilitated their resolution. This procedure is used in our laboratory to provide a facile means for identification of MAIS serotypes.[53a]

Identification of other atypical mycobacteria by the TLC procedures is not well documented. Marks and Szulga[244] examined extracts from 13 strains of *M. fortuitum*. All of these gave identical lipid patterns that were distinct from those of MAIS serotypes, since they yielded a purple color with acid orcinol. Other Group IV rapid growers, *M. chelonei* and *M. peregrinum*, produced related patterns, but the color had more of a gray or red texture. Specific lipid patterns have also been used to identify *M. szulgai, M. xenopi, M. gordonae,* and *M. kansasii* and its aberrant relative.[166, 243, 335]

The chemistry of the characteristic lipids and antigens of rapidly growing and other, more "anonymous," types has not been explored. It would be entirely fortuitous (but nevertheless fascinating) if the characteristic lipids of some of them are based on mycosides A, B, or G, with polar multiglycosyl variants as the serologically active determinants. The polar multiglycosyl variants idea may find support in the large variety of 6-deoxyhexoses associated with mycoside A[123] and the consequent anticipation of multiglycosylated versions. Gastambide-Odier and colleagues, who have described their interest in the biologic functions of mycoside G (and who will undoubtedly pursue the subject with the same enthusiasm that they earlier devoted to their chemistry and biosynthesis) have stated, "Les residus glycosidiques specifiques des mycosides A, B et G pour-

raient être les groupements determinants d'haptènes characterisant respectivement les bacilles atypiques photochromogènes, les souches bovines de *Mycobacterium tuberculosis* et *Mycobacterium marinum.*"

C-Mycosides — Physiologic Aspects

Though mycosides were long considered to occur near the surface of mycobacteria, until recently, they had no recognized biologic function or activity, apart from their influence on colony morphology. Our evidence (summarized in the previous section) — i.e., certain of the structurally more elaborate C-mycoside-peptidoglycolipids have serologic activity—fortifies the growing conviction that they have a distinct role to play in mycobacterial morphology and probably in pathogenicity.

Early on, Smith and colleagues observed distinct differences in the surface structure of C-mycoside-containing and C-mycoside-free strains.[106] Thus, a scotochromogenic strain failed to produce its associated C-mycoside as cultures developed a colony form that was predominantly rough. On replating the cultures at high density, a smooth colony could occasionally be detected; this colony on mass culture again yielded the specific mycoside. Moreover, the sero-agglutination test of Schaefer and the Marks-Jenkins TLC procedure apply only to smooth colony-forming mycobacteria; the type-specific, C-mycosidic antigens and lipids that are the bases of these tests are absent from rough colony variants.[53b, 311]

There is now ample evidence that C-mycosides are elaborated in the form of a protective capsule around certain pathogenic mycobacteria. This may serve to protect and insulate the pathogen within phagolysosomes of the host cells from the lysosomal enzymes. In liver and spleen tissue from mice infect-

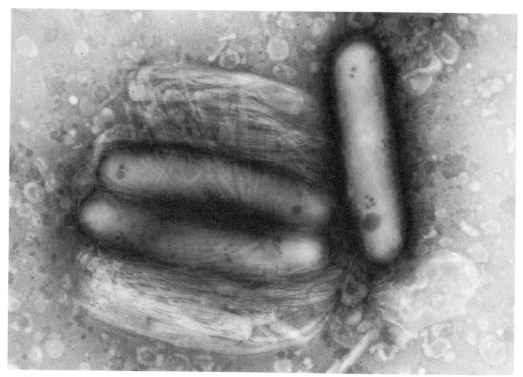

FIGURE 4–64.   Parallel fibrils of C-mycosides wrapped longitudinally around *M. lepraemurium*. Bacteria were removed from mouse liver with a needle and "spread" on water surface. Negatively stained with ammonium molybdate. × 41,000. (Figure provided by Dr. Philip Draper.)

ed with the obligate intracellular pathogen *M. lepraemurium*, the bacteria are contained within vacuoles in phagocytic cells. Separating the membrane of the vacuole and the bacterium is a conspicuous electron-transparent zone (Fig. 4–64), which is due to a collection of "parallel fibrils wrapped longitudinally around the bacteria."[91] The fibrils are composed almost entirely of simple C-mycoside-peptidoglycolipid material. This observation has assumed added importance since electron-transparent zones seem to be a characteristic feature of pathogenic mycobacteria within phagosomes. There is serologic evidence that both *M. lepraemurium* and *M. avium* are closely related. Since both are severe pathogens in their respective hosts, Draper[90] sought similarly constructed protective

capsules in *M. avium* 357. The organism was grown in liquid medium, and again a fibrillar C-mycoside capsule was discerned. Kim and colleagues found the following: "A superficial wrapper consisting of long parallel filaments measuring 5 nm in diameter,"[197] which surrounds *Mycobacterium* (sp. NQ) when grown in pellicle form. Apparently, this also contains components characteristic of C-mycoside. The material often fills the spaces between adjacent cells of the pellicle and can be readily removed by agitation of cells with glass beads.

Yet another role has been discerned for the simpler C-mycoside-peptidoglycolipids. It was independently found by three laboratories that phage-inhibiting substances could be extracted with organic solvents from *M.*

smegmatis,[160, 356] *M. phlei,*[71] *M. bovis* BCG, and atypical mycobacteria.[110] Tokunaga and coworkers[357] observed that minute quantities of a lipid extract from *M. smegmatis* dramatically inactivated mycobacteriophages D4 and D29 (both virulent for *M. smegmatis*) — apparently, by adsorption to the phage tails. These lipids did not affect mycobacteriophages that are specific for other strains of mycobacteria. Almost simultaneously, Goren and his collaborators[147] and Furuchi and Tokunaga[110] recognized that the receptor-site substance for mycobacteriophage D4 is a C-mycoside. Furuchi and Tokunaga demonstrated that it was a mixture of tripeptide-based C-mycosides, probably similar to mycoside-C_{1217} and mycoside-C_{b1} (Table 4–7). They also showed that a D4-resistant mutant of *M. smegmatis* was devoid of C-mycosides. Unfortunately, the morphology of the mutant was not examined; it would have been interesting to see if it displayed rough colony characteristics. Goren and colleagues found that the heterologous mycosides C_s and C_{1217}, elaborated respectively by *M. scrofulaceum* and *Mycobacterium (sp.) 1217*, are essentially indistinguishable from the *M. smegmatis* specific lipids in their behavior towards D4. Figure 4–65 illustrates the adsorption of D4 to fila-

mentous microcrystals of the *M. smegmatis* mycoside (C_{sm}), leaving little doubt that they are the receptors. Phage D4 was also found to be virulent for *Mycobacterium (sp.) 1217.*

In summary, the surface location of the C-mycosides and their elaboration as a capsular shield protective against the phagolysosomal environment is strongly suggestive of a role for these peptidoglycolipids in pathogenesis. The advantages that they provide to certain mycobacteria in the invasive process may be analogous to those conferred by the O-antigenic lipopolysaccharides to the more virulent strains of *Salmonella typhimurium.* The analogy between the C-mycosides and the O-antigenic lipopolysaccharides may be further extended. Our studies of the Schaefer antigens suggest that the antigenic specificity of a particular serotype is determined by oligosaccharide moieties, which modify a relatively invariant fatty acyl peptide core. More precisely, we believe that the attachment of several different 6-deoxyhexoses, either singly or in combination at the mid-chain *allo*-threonine and at the terminal alaninol of a common oligopeptide, offers an enormous potential for structural variability. These permutations would seem sufficient to explain the antigenic specificity of most of the

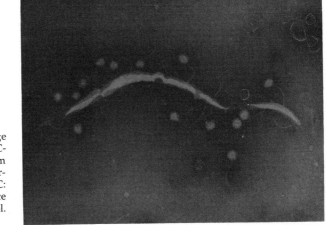

FIGURE 4–65. Mycobacteriophage D4 adsorbed to microcrystalline C-mycoside of *M. smegmatis.* (From Goren, M. B., McClatchy, J. K., Martens, B., and Brokl, O.: Mycosides C: Behaviour as receptor site substance for mycobacteriophage D4. J. Virol. 9:999, 1972.)

serotypes in the *M. avium*/*M. intra-cellulare*/*M. scrofulaceum* complex. Hence, these antigenic peptidoglycolipids may be the mycobacterial counterpart, in microcosm, of the enterobacterial O-antigenic lipopolysaccharides.

MYCOBACTERIAL LIPIDS AND THE IN VIVO ENVIRONMENT

Many of the studies reviewed in the preceding sections have demonstrated that individual lipids derived from in vitro harvests of mycobacteria are endowed with significant biologic activities. A principal interest must still be manifest in the special associations between the intracellular pathogen and its host. In the past, thoughtful scientists have expressed their genuine concern as to whether we have described authentic lipid components of mycobacteria as they may be produced in the in vivo environment, or instead, merely artifactual consequences of in vitro cultivation. Efforts at identifying any of these substances from in vivo-derived bacilli were for many decades entirely unrewarding. For Anderson it was a frustrating effort, for he and his colleagues were unable to detect in human tuberculous lung tissue phthiocol, tuberculostearic, or "phthioic" acids —all of which, he was convinced, were distinguishing lipids for virulent tubercle bacilli. Because of the increased sophistication of methodology, equipment, and instrumentation, more recent studies with such direction have been more fruitful. Elegant methodology for recovering cells of lung bacilli has been described by Segal and Bloch,[317] Artman and Bekierkunst,[15] and Kanai and Kondo.[174] Their individual studies assessed the metabolic, biochemical, pathogenic, immunogenic, lipid, and surface characteristics of in vitro tubercle bacilli as compared with those derived in vivo. Indeed, two distinct but interconvertible phenotypes are de-

termined by the respective cultural milieu. The results are reviewed extensively by Barksdale and Kim.[40]

With respect to mycobacterial lipids of interest, phthiocerol dimycocerosate (DIM), mycolic acids, and tuberculostearic acid were among the first to be recognized (by infrared spectrometry) in extracts of *M. bovis* recovered from lungs of infected mice.[175, 202, 203] This would have alleviated Anderson's apprehensions, to a degree. By infrared and mass spectrometry, Etemadi and Convit[96] identified typical mycolic acids in bacillary harvests from lepromatous tissues. In our laboratory,[61b, 136] we isolated and identified mycolic acids, DIM, trehalose, and hexacosanoic acid from lung bacilli of mice aerogenically infected with H37Rv. Draper and Rees[91] obtained abundant harvests of C-mycoside variants from liver lesions of mice infected with *M. lepraemurium* (MLM). From bacillary harvests obtained from similarly infected livers, Draper,[89] and L.A. Davidson and P. Draper[87a] prepared MLM cell walls and lipid extracts. Among the latter, they identified and characterized the mycolic acids of *M. lepraemurium.* From small samples of these cell wall-associated lipids, Goren, Brokl, and Jiang[142] isolated and purified C-type mycosides and identified the "cord factor" of this organism—a trehalose-6,6'-dimycolate. Thus, with the "abundant" bacillary and lipid harvests obtainable from these liver lesions, recovery and identification of lipid components is clearly facilitated.

Despite the elegant methodology, the problem is more difficult with *M. tuberculosis* recovered from infected mouse lungs. From such sources, Kondo and Kanai[202, 203] described an apparent arabinose mycolate and toxic lipids (insufficient for characterization), which may be presumed to contain cord factor. According to Segal,[316] the in vivo phenotype of H37Rv does not bind neutral red — suggesting, in Segal's interpretation, that the sulfatides may not be produced in the intracellular environment. However, in vivo-derived bacilli are notably hydrophilic owing to an avid coating with host-derived lysosomal constituents, and these may mask neutral red-reactive sites. Still, trypsinization merely abolished a weak, residual, neutral red activity that was believed to be associated with tissue contaminants. Paradoxically, the total lipids content of the hydrophilic lung bacilli is greater than that of its in vitro-derived counterpart.[318]

Gangadharam[110a] was unsuccessful in attempts to isolate sulfolipid from in vivo bacilli, and our efforts to obtain either cord factor or the sulfatides from lung bacilli (H37Rv) have also been fruitless. We have suggested from an interpretation of electron microscopy profiles and from observations in vital fluorescence microscopy[138, 145] that the lysosomotropic sulfatide within macrophage *phagosomes* may penetrate and traverse the phagosomal membrane to accumulate in neighboring lysosomes. It is possible that the sulfatide should be sought principally, not in the entrapped bacilli, but rather in the cytoplasmic organelles of the entrapping phagocytic cells.

We submit that the search for phosphatidylinositol mannosides, the sulfatides and cord factor of in vivo-derived bacillary harvests seems still to be justified. Because of the putative participation of specific trehalose esters as intermediates in the biosynthesis and transfer of mycolic acids to cell wall, the propinquity of identifying the trehalose mycolates would appear considerably enhanced, provided that a sufficient harvest of lipids is available. In a search for cord factor, our inference that *M. lepraemurium* would meet this requirement was gratifyingly correct. The unequivocal identification of cord factor in cells of lung bacilli will undoubtedly be successful, therefore, if the somewhat more prodigious effort that this requires is expended. For this purpose, the Moreau strain of BCG, relatively prolific in cord factor elaboration,[26] may

serve very well; at the same time, it would relieve the operational inconveniences and hazards that the search with fully virulent *M. tuberculosis* entails.

SUMMATION AND CONCLUSIONS

A principal objective of the earliest investigations on mycobacterial lipids was to seek and to identify specific components that might be implicated with biologic events in the pathogenesis of tuberculosis. Some of these goals, which were originally set as the task for the Anderson group, have been realized, although the anticipation that simple individual lipid substances might directly elicit such responses as the tubercle was, in retrospect, probably too naive in concept. Still, agents as diverse as the multiple methyl-branched phthienoic and mycocerosic acids, on the one hand, and cord factor, on the other, are nevertheless potent inducers of foreign body granulomas when presented in appropriate fashion. Cord factor is more effective by several orders of magnitude, and the response is apparently not enhanced by prior presensitization with BCG. But active infection evidently enhances the sensitivity to the branched-chain acids, and this may still be an area for continued investigations. The original observations of Catel and Schmidt have not, to our knowledge, been further pursued critically. Various studies may be rewarding — with sensitized animals, to examine not only responses to intradermal challenges but also effects on leukocytes, lymphocyte transformation, macrophage-migration inhibition, and stimulation of pulmonary granulomas by emulsions of oil solutions.

The trehalose mycolates and their biosynthetic intermediates have clearly emerged as among the most fascinating of the mycobacterial lipids for their toxicity, membrane-disruptive behavior, granulomagenic properties, adjuvant activity, and direct or "helper" antitumor properties. The sulfatides act synergistically with cord factor to potentiate membrane-disruptive activity and therefore toxicity. It is perhaps equally fascinating from the standpoint of the mycobacterium itself that at least some of these glycolipids appear to have a prominent role in mycolate and, therefore, cell wall biosynthesis. According to Barksdale and Kim,[40] owing to their amphipathic configurations, these glycolipids very likely have a role in facilitating the inward transport of polar nutrients from the cell surface.

The requirements for cord factor as a component of certain tumor-regressive preparations may decline, since the role appears to be essentially physical or related to the disposition of hydrophobic-hydrophilic components; nevertheless the glycolipid has not yet been supplanted by either natural or synthesized substitutes. In the mouse fibrosarcoma 1023, oil emulsions of cord factor alone are sufficiently active without requiring a second cofactor, and the activity cannot be attributed solely to physical or surface-active properties. No natural or synthesized cord factor analogs have yet been found to effectively substitute for the trehalose glycolipid in this system. And according to E. Yarkoni,[391a] neither the sulfatides nor the pseudocord factors that have been examined elicit pulmonary granulomas in mice (intravenous injection of emulsified oil solutions). Also, we found no pseudocord factors that exhibited the same high level of mouse toxicity. Cord factor, therefore, exhibits some almost unique biologic properties that may ultimately secure for this glycolipid the distinction that Ratledge proposes — that cord factor is likely to be the progenitor of the generalized nonspecific immunity induced by mycobacteria. However, because of the unnatural requirements (oily solutions or their aqueous emulsions) for expression of its biologic activities and the

emergence of some simpler substitutes for cord factor, our endorsement of this view is, at best, reserved.

The pathway of mycolic acid biosynthesis is, at least in *M. tuberculosis* H37Ra, on the threshold of final clarification through utilization of the elegant techniques in separation and structural probing that have developed over the last two decades. The antagonism of mycolate biosynthesis by INH has been a powerful tool in facilitating these studies, and the relationship of INH to assembling the huge meromycolate skeleton gives insight into the essentially unique and limited antibiotic spectrum of this chemotherapeutic agent. Perhaps the resistance of the atypical mycobacteria to INH will ultimately be explained in the behavior of the relevant enzyme system. (See also Chapter 20.)

Identification and synthesis of the molecular common denominator of adjuvant activity clearly stands as another triumph, whose genesis may be traced to the original studies with the mycobacterial waxes and to the recognition that peptide-containing waxes D are potently granulomagenic and adjuvant-active. The subsequent evolution implicated the mycobacterial cell wall and its solubilized products and ultimately identified the muramyl dipeptide as the smallest entity retaining adjuvant behavior. This is, of course, a structural common denominator characteristic of a vast host of bacteria. Some bacteria exhibit adjuvant activity when presented in sufficient amount in oil-in-water emulsion.[381] Still, why have mycobacteria played an almost unique role as the microbial component of Freund's complete adjuvant? We cannot offer an unequivocal answer. The special behavior of mycobacteria may be due to oil-soluble components (such as cord factor and wax D) that are immediately available to initiate the granulomatous response, which is then sustained, probably owing to the notable resistance to intraphagocytic degradation of the bacillary bodies.[179] There can be little doubt that this is attributable to their contents of unusual lipids, of which at least part (in the form of the mycoloyl arabinogalactan) is covalently bound to the adjuvant-active peptidoglycan. No simple "painting" of other bacterial genera with lipids is liable to confer this behavior.

After a latent period of more than a decade, the roles of some mycosides have assumed a much greater importance than Lederer once humorously ascribed to them — "Being in charge of mycobacterial public relations." Instead, the abundance of C-mycoside and its tapelike cocoon forms, as elaborated by *M. lepraemurium* in the intraphagosomal environment, bespeaks a prominent role for this relatively inert lipid in a passive defense of the organism against the onslaught of lysosomal hydrolases. Perhaps a similar function has evolved for the fibrillar analog seen in *M. avium*. C-mycosides have been identified as receptor-site substances for certain mycobacteriophages; more elaborate variants are endowed with antigenic and serologically active properties in *M. intracellulare*. The distribution of simpler variants in *M. intracellulare* and their associated lipid chromatography patterns serve to identify individual serotypes.

As trehalose multiesters, the sulfatides of *M. tuberculosis* are related (distantly) to cord factor and possess the most elaborate multimethyl-branched acyl substituents characterized in mycobacteria so far. Although essentially nontoxic, they synergistically potentiate the peculiar toxicity of cord factor; at low, but not at high doses, they can substitute for the dimycolate as the cofactor with *Salmonella* Re endotoxin in antitumor preparations. The dose limitation may be attributable to physicochemical properties of SL — it is much more polar in character than cord factor. Perhaps of more importance is the property of the lysosomotropic SL to induce dysfunction in phagosome-lysosome fusion in macrophages — and indeed in toxicity to macrophages. In this behavior, it is demonstrably protubercular. Therefore, the sulfatides may be principal mycobacterial components that are functional in promoting the intracellular survival and thus the pathogenic properties of *M. tuberculosis.*

As we stated earlier, in the history of mycobacterial lipids research, it is possible to define several "golden ages." We suggest that in the future, the last two decades will be considered among them.

ACKNOWLEDGMENTS

The authors gratefully acknowledge the assistance of Ethel Goren, Juanita Derry, Susan Walker, and Ervella Gentry in preparing the manuscript. We thank Nadia de Stackelburg for her careful collaboration with Ethel Goren in preparing the numerous schemes and figures of complex chemical structures, for additional art work, and for photography.

We are especially grateful to Dr. Lane Barksdale for providing us with some half dozen excellent illustrations and electron photomicrographs, and we thank Dr. Philip Draper for Figures 4–6 and 4–64 and Dr. A. L. Lehninger for permission to reproduce Figure 4–9. We thank the American Society for Microbiology and the American Chemical Society for permission to use numerous figures taken from ASM and ACS publications.

Mrs. Olga Brokl and Mrs. Beth Ullom have been valuable and faithful colleagues in our research efforts described herein.

As cited in this chapter, the work of the authors originating at National Jewish Hospital and Research Center was supported in part by Public Health Service grants and contracts from the U.S.-Japan Cooperative Medical Science Program, administered by the National Institute of Allergy and Infectious Diseases.

APPENDIX A.   Abbreviations

ABA	azobenzene-arsonate	3 MeGlc	3-O-methylglucose
Ac	acyl	6 MeGlc	6-O-methylglucose
Ac₂Gly-P-I-(M)	intact phosphatidylinositol mannosides	MER	methanol extraction residue
		MGLP	6-O-methylglucose-containing lipopolysaccharide
ACP	acyl carrier protein		
AG	arabinogalactan		
AI	attenuation indicator	MGP	6-O-methylglucose-containing polysaccharide
Ala	D-alanine		
Alol	L-alaninol	MMP	3-O-methylmannose-containing polysaccharide
Ara_f	D-arabinofuranoside		
BDA-TDA	Bis-di-n-octadecylamide of trehalose dicarboxylic acid	Mur	murein
		MurNglyc (MurNGl)	N-glycolylmuramyl
BSA	bovine serum albumin		
CF	cord factor	Myc	mycoloyl
CL	cardiolipin (diphosphatidyl glycerol)	NADH	reduced nicotinamide adenine dinucleotide
		NADPH	reduced nicotinamide adenine dinucleotide phosphate
CMN	*Corynebacterium-Mycobacterium-Nocardia* group		
CoA	coenzyme A		
CWS	cell wall skeleton	NMR	nuclear magnetic resonance
DAP	diaminopimelic acid	NDP	nucleotide diphosphate
DEAE	diethylaminoethyl-cellulose	P3	cord factor (trehalose 6,6' dimycolate)
6-Deoxytal	6-deoxy-L-talose		
DIM	phthiocerol dimycocerosate	PE	phosphatidylethanolamine
DMF	dimethylformamide	Phe	D-phenylalanine
DNP	dinitrophenyl	PI	phosphatidylinositol
DTH	delayed type hypersensitivity	PIM₁	phosphatidylinositol monomannoside
FAD	flavin adenine dinucleotide	PIM₂	phosphatidylinositol dimannoside
FMN	flavin mononucleotide		
Gal_p	galactopyranoside	PIM₃	phosphatidylinositol trimannoside
GDPM	guanosinediphosphomannose	PIM₄	phosphatidylinositol tetramannoside
GLC	gas-liquid chromatography	PIM₅	phosphatidylinositol pentamannoside
Glc	glucose		
GlcNAc(GNAc)	N-acetylglucosamine	PIM_x	families of phosphatidylinositol mannosides
Glu	D-glutamate		
Gly	glycerol	PMR	proton magnetic resonance
Glyc	glycolyl	PS	polysaccharide
GlyCOOH	glyceric acid	R_e	rough mutant
Gly-P-I-(M)	glycerylphosphorylinositol mannosides	Rha	L-rhamnose
		Ser	serine
HPLC	high-performance-liquid chromatography	SF	stimulatory factor
		SL	sulfolipid
Hz	hertz	SRBC	sheep red blood cells
I	inositol	TDA	trehalose-6,6'-dicarboxylic acid
IR	infrared		
Isoglu	*iso*glutamine	*a*Thr	*allo*-D-Threonine
LCD	least common denominator (of adjuvant activity)	TLC	thin layer chromatography
		TMS	trimethylsilyl
M	mannose	UDP	uridine diphosphate
MAIS	*Mycobacterium avium-intracellulare-scrofulaceum* complex	UV	ultraviolet
		WSA	water soluble antigen
MBSA	methylated bovine serum albumin		

REFERENCES

1. Adam, A., Ciorbaru, R., Petit, J.-F., and Lederer, E.: Isolation and properties of a macromolecular water-soluble immuno-adjuvant fraction from the cell wall of *Mycobacterium smegmatis*. Proc. Natl. Acad. Sci. USA *69*:851, 1972.

2. Adam, A., Ciorbaru, R., Petit, J.-F., Lederer, E., Chedid, L., Lamensans, A., Parant, F., Parant, M., Rosselet, J. P., and Berger, F. M.: Preparation and biological properties of water-soluble adjuvant fractions from delipidated cells of *Mycobacterium smegmatis* and *Nocardia opaca*. Infect. Immun. *7*:855, 1973.

3. Adam, A., Ciorbaru, R., Ellouz, F., Petit, J.-F., and Lederer, E.: Adjuvant activity of monomeric bacterial cell wall peptidoglycans. Biochem. Biophys. Res. Commun. *56*:561, 1974.

4. Adam, A., Senn, M., Vilkas, E., and Lederer, E.: Spectrométrie de masse de glycolipides 2. Diesters de tréhalose naturels et synthetiques. Eur. J. Biochem. *2*:460, 1967.

5. Aebi, A., Asselineau, J., and Lederer, E.: Sur les lipides de la souche humaine "Brévannes" de *Mycobacterium tuberculosis*. Bull. Soc. Chim. Biol. *35*:661, 1953.

6. Akamatsu, Y., and Law, J. H.: Enzymatic synthesis of 10-methylene stearic acid and tuberculostearic acid. Biochem. Biophys. Res. Commun. *33*:172, 1968.

7. Akamatsu, Y., and Law, J. H.: Enzymatic alkylenation of phospholipid fatty acid chains by extracts of *Mycobacterium phlei*. J. Biol. Chem. *245*:701, 1970.

8. Akamatsu, Y., Ono, Y., and Nojima, S.: Phospholipid patterns in subcellular fractions of *Mycobacterium phlei*. J. Biochem. (Tokyo) *59*:176, 1966.

9. Allen, R. C., Stjernholm, R. L., and Steele, R. H.: Evidence for the generation of an electronic excitation state(s) in human polymorphonuclear leukocytes and its participation in bactericidal activity. Biochem. Biophys. Res. Commun. *47*:679, 1972.

10. Amar, C., and Vilkas, E.: Isolement d'un phosphate d'arabinose à partir des parois de *Mycobacterium tuberculosis* H37Ra. C. R. Acad. Sci. Serie D *277*:1949, 1973.

11. Anderson, R. J.: The chemistry of the lipids of tubercle bacilli. The Harvey Lectures series. *35*:271, 1940.

12. Antoine, A. D., and Tepper, B. S.: Environmental control of glycogen and lipid content of *Mycobacterium tuberculosis*. J. Bacteriol. *100*:538, 1969.

13. Antoine, A. D., and Tepper, B. S.: Environmental control of glycogen and lipid content of *Mycobacterium phlei*. J. Gen. Microbiol. *55*:217, 1969.

14. Armstrong, J. A., and Hart, P. D.: Response of cultured macrophages to *Mycobacterium tuberculosis* with observations on fusion of lysosomes with phagosomes. J. Exp. Med. *134*:713, 1971.

15. Artman, M., and Bekierkunst, A.: Studies on *Mycobacterium tuberculosis* H37Rv grown *in vivo*. Am. Rev. Respir. Dis. *83*:100, 1961.

16. Artman, M., Bekierkunst, A., and Goldenberg, I.: Tissue metabolism in infection: biochemical changes in mice treated with cord factor. Arch. Biochem. Biophys. *105*:80, 1964.

17. Asselineau, C., Lacave, C. S., Montrozier, H. L., and Promé, J.-C.: Relations structurales entre les acides mycoliques insaturés et les acides inférieures insaturés synthétisés par *Mycobacterium phlei*. Implications metaboliques. Eur. J. Biochem. *14*:406, 1970.

18. Asselineau, C., Montrozier, H. L., and Promé, J.-C.: Presence d'acides polyinsaturés dans une bacterie: isolement, à partir des lipides de *Mycobacterium phlei*, d' acides hexatriacontapentaene 4, 8, 12, 16, 20 oique et d'acides analogues. Eur. J. Biochem. *10*:580, 1969.

19. Asselineau, C., Montrozier, H., and Promé, J.-C.: Structures des acides α-mycoliques isolés de la souche Canetti de *Mycobacterium tuberculosis*. Bull. Soc. Chim. Fr. 592, 1969.

20. Asselineau, C. P., Montrozier, H. L., Promé, J.-C., Savagnac, A. M., and Welby, M.: Étude d'un glycolipide polyinsaturé synthétisé par *Mycobacterium phlei*. Eur. J. Biochem. *28*:102, 1972.

21. Asselineau, C. P., and Montrozier, H. L.: Étude du processus de biosynthèses des acides phléiques, acides polyinsaturés synthetises par *Mycobacterium phlei*. Eur. J. Biochem. *63*:509, 1976.

22. Asselineau, J.: Lipides du bacille tuberculeux. Adv. Tuberc. Res. *5*:1, 1952.

23. Asselineau, J.: The Bacterial Lipids. San Francisco, Holden-Day, 1966.

24. Asselineau, J., and Kato, M.: Chemical structure and biochemical activity of cord factor analogs. II Relationships between activity and stereochemistry of the sugar moiety. Biochemie *55*:559, 1973.

25. Asselineau, J., and Lederer, E.: Chemistry and metabolism of bacterial lipids. *In* Bloch, K. (ed.): Lipide Metabolism. New York, John Wiley & Sons, 1960, p. 337.

26. Asselineau, J., and Portelance, V.: Comparative study of the free lipids of eight BCG daughter strains. Recent Results Cancer. Res. *47*:214, 1974.

27. Asselineau, J., Ryhage, R., and Stenhagen, E.: Mass spectrometric studies of long chain methylesters. A determination of the molecular weight and structure of my-

cocerosic acid. Acta Chem. Scand. *11*:196, 1957.

28. Audibert, F., Chedid, L., Lefrancier, P., and Choay, J.: Distinctive adjuvanticity of synthetic analogs of mycobacterial water-soluble components. Cell. Immunol. *21*:243, 1976.

29. Azuma, I., Kishimoto, S., Yamamura, Y., and Petit, J.-F.: Adjuvanticity of mycobacterial cell walls. Jpn. J. Microbiol. *15*:193, 1971.

30. Azuma, I., Ribi, E., Meyer, T. J., and Zbar, B.: Biologically active components from mycobacterial cell walls. I. Isolation and composition of cell wall skeleton and component P_3. J. Nat. Cancer Inst. *52*:95, 1974.

31. Azuma, I., Sugimura, K., Taniyama, T., Yamawaki, M., Yamamura, Y., et al.: Adjuvant activity of mycobacterial fractions: Adjuvant activity of synthetic N-acetyl-muramyl dipeptide and the related compounds. Infect. Immun. *14*:18, 1976.

32. Azuma, I., Sugimura, K., Yamawaki, M., Uemiya, M., Yoshimoto, T., Yamamura, Y., Kusumoto, S., Okada, S., and Shiba, T.: Adjuvant activity of mycobacterial fractions. VI. Adjuvant and anti-tumor activities of synthetic 6-O''mycoloyl''-N-acetyl-L-alanyl-D-isoglutamine. *In* Proceedings, Twelfth Joint Conference on Tuberculosis. U.S.-Japan Cooperative Medical Science Program. 1977, p. 398.

32a. Azuma, I., Sugimura, K., Yamawaki, M., Uemiya, M., Kusumoto, S., Okada, S., Shiba, T., and Yamamura, Y.: Adjuvant activity of synthetic 6-O-"mycoloyl"-N-acetyl-muramyl-L-alanyl-D-isoglutamine and related compounds. Infect. Immun. *20*:600 (1978).

33. Azuma, I., Thomas, D. W., Adam, A., Ghuysen, J. M., Bonaly, R., Petit, J.-F., and Lederer, E.: Occurrence of N-glycolylmuramic acid in bacterial cell walls. Biochim. Biophys. Acta *208*:444, 1970.

34. Azuma, I., and Yamamura, Y.: Studies on the firmly bound lipids of human tubercle bacillus. II. Isolation of arabinose mycolate and identification of its chemical structure. J. Biochem. *53*:275, 1963.

35. Ballou, C. E.: Structure of a lipopolysaccharide from *Mycobacterium* species. Accs. Chem. Res. *1*:366, 1968.

36. Ballou, C. E.: Biosynthesis of mannophosphoinositides in *Mycobacterium phlei*. Methods Ezymol. *28*:493, 1972.

37. Ballou, C. E., and Lee, Y. C.: The structure of a myoinositol mannoside from *Mycobacterium tuberculosis* glycolipid. Biochemistry *3*:682, 1964.

38. Ballou, C. E., Vilkas, E., and Lederer, E.: Structural studies on the myo-inositol phospholipids of *Mycobacterium tuberculosis*. J. Biol. Chem. *238*:69, 1963.

39. Barksdale, L.: *Corynebacterium diphtheriae* and its relatives. Bacteriol. Rev. *34*:378, 1970.

40. Barksdale, L., and Kim, K.-S.: *Mycobacterium*. Bacteriol. Rev. *41*:217, 1977.

41. Bast, R. C. Jr., Bast, B. S., and Rapp, H. J.: Critical review of previously reported animal studies of tumor immunotherapy with nonspecific immunostimulants. International Conference on Immunotherapy of Cancer. Ann. N.Y. Acad. Sci. *277*:60, 1976.

42. Batra, P. P.: Mechanism of light-induced carotenoid synthesis in nonphotosynthetic plants. *In* Griese, A. C.: Photophysiology. Vol. 6. Academic Press, New York, 1971, p. 47.

43. Batra, P. P., and Storms, L.: Mechanism of photoinduced and antimycin A-induced carotenoid synthesis in *Mycobacterium marinum*. Biochem. Biophys. Res. Commun. *33*:820, 1968.

44. Bekierkunst, A., Levij, I. S., Yarkoni, E., Vilkas, E., Adam, A., and Lederer, E.: Granuloma formation induced in mice by chemically defined mycobacterial fractions. J. Bacteriol. *100*:95, 1969.

45. Bekierkunst, A., Levij, I. S., Yarkoni, E., Vilkas, E., and Lederer, E.: Suppression of urethane-induced lung adenomas in mice treated with trehalose-6,6'-dimycolate (cord factor) and living bacillus Calmette-Guérin. Science *174*:1240, 1971.

46. Bekierkunst, A., Wang, L., Toubiana, R., and Lederer, E.: Immunotherapy of cancer with nonliving BCG and fractions derived from mycobacteria: role of cord factor (trehalose-6,6'-dimycolate) in tumor regression. Infect. Immun. *10*:1044, 1974.

47. Bekierkunst, A., Yarkoni, E., Flechner, I., Morecki, S., Vilkas, E., and Lederer, E.: Immune response to sheep red blood cells in mice pretreated with mycobacterial fractions. Infect. Immun. *4*:256, 1971.

48. Bergeron, R., Machida, Y., and Bloch, K.: Complex formation between mycobacterial polysaccharides or cyclodextrins and palmitoyl coenzyme A. J. Biol. Chem. *250*:1223, 1975.

49. Birnbaum, S. E., and Affronti, L. F.: Mycobacterial polysaccharides. II. Comparison of polysaccharides from strains of four species of mycobacteria. J. Bacteriol. *100*:58, 1969.

50. Bloch, H.: Studies on the virulence of tubercle bacilli. Isolation and biological properties of a constituent of virulent organisms. J. Exp. Med. *91*:197, 1950.

51. Bloch, K., and Vance, D.: Control mechanisms in the synthesis of saturated fatty acids. Ann. Rev. Biochem. *46*:263, 1977.

52. Bordet, C., and Michel, G.: Structure et biogènese des lipides a haut poids

moléculaire de *Nocardia asteroides*. Bull. Soc. Chim. Biol. *51*:527, 1969.

53. Borsos, T., and Rapp, H. J., eds: Conference on the use of BCG in therapy of cancer. National Cancer Institute Monograph *39*:1973.

53a. Brennan, P. J., Souhrada, M., Ullom, B., McClatchy, J. K., and Goren, M. B.: Identification of atypical mycobacteria by thin-layer chromatography of their surface antigens. J. Clin. Microbiol. *8*:374, 1978.

53b. Brennan, P. J., and Goren, M. B.: Structural studies on the type-specific antigens and lipids of smooth-colony mycobacteria: *Mycobacterium intracellulare* serotype 9. Submitted for publication.

54. Brennan, P. J., Ballou, C. E.: Biosynthesis of mannophosphoinositides by *Mycobacterium phlei*. The family of dimannophosphoinositides. J. Biol. Chem. *242*:3046, 1967.

55. Brennan, P. J., and Ballou, C. E.: Biosynthesis of mannophosphoinositides by *Mycobacterium phlei* — enzymatic acylation of the dimannophosphoinositides. J. Biol. Chem. *243*:2975, 1968.

56. Brennan, P. J., and Ballou, C. E.: Phosphatidylmyoinositol mannoside in *Propionibacterium shermanii*. Biochem. Biophys. Res. Commun. *30*:69, 1968.

57. Brennan, P. J., Brokl, O., and Goren, M. B.: Chemistry of the type specific antigens and lipids of *Mycobacterium intracellulare*. *In* Proceedings, Twelfth Joint Meeting Tuberculosis Panel: U.S.-Japan Cooperative Medical Science Program, 1977, p. 100.

58. Brennan, P. J., Lehane, D. P., and Thomas, D. W.: Acylglucoses of the corynebacteria and mycobacteria. Eur. J. Biochem. *13*:117, 1970.

59. Brennan, P. J., Rooney, S. A., and Winder, F. G.: The lipids of *Mycobacterium tuberculosis* BCG: Fractionation, composition, turnover and the effects of isoniazid. Ir. J. Med. Sci. *3*:371, 1970.

60. Brindley, D. N., Matsumura, S., and Bloch, K.: *Mycobacterium phlei* fatty acid synthetase — a bacterial multienzyme complex. Nature *224*:666, 1969.

61. Bristol, G., and Schroepfer, G. J., Jr.: Concerning the biosynthesis of tuberculostearic acid. Biochim. Biophys. Acta *125*:389, 1966.

61a. Brokl, O., Schaefer, W. B., and Goren, M. B.: Unpublished data.

61b. Brokl, O., Segal, W., Goren, M. B. and Das, B. C.: Unpublished observations.

62. Bruneteau, M., and Michel, G.: Biogenèse des O-methyl-6-déoxyhexoses présents dans le mycoside C₂. Biochem. Biophys. Acta *201*:493, 1970.

63. Burchard, R. P., and Dworkin, M.: Light-induced lysis and carotenogenesis in *Myxococcus xanthus*. J. Bacteriol. *91*:535, 1966.

64. Burchard, R. P., and Hendricks, S. G.: Action spectrum for carotenogenesis in *Myxococcus xanthus*. J. Bacteriol. *97*:1165, 1969.

65. Burdon, K. L.: Fatty material in bacteria and fungi revealed by staining dried, fixed slide preparations. J. Bacteriol. *52*:665, 1946.

66. Campbell, I. M., and Naworal, J.: Mass spectral discrimination between monoenoic and cyclopropanoid, and between normal, iso-, and anteiso-fatty acid methyl esters. J. Lipid Res. *10*:589, 1969.

67. Campbell, I. M., and Naworal, J.: Composition of the saturated and monounsaturated fatty acids of *Mycobacterium phlei*. J. Lipid Res. *10*:593, 1969.

67a. Cason, J.: Private communication, 1972.

68. Cason, J., Freeman, N. K., and Sumrell, G.: The principal structural features of C_{27} phthienoic acid. J. Biol. Chem. *192*:415, 1951.

69. Cason, J., and Miller, W. T.: Complexity of the mixture of fatty acids from tubercle bacillus. J. Biol. Chem. *238*:883, 1962.

70. Cason, J., and Sumrell, G.: Investigation of a fraction of acids of the phthioic type from the tubercle bacillus. J. Biol. Chem. *192*:405, 1951.

71. Castelnuovo, G., Bellezza, G., and Yamanaka, S.: Phage inhibiting substances of mycobacteria. I. The nature of phage inhibiting substances of *Mycobacterium phlei*. Ann. Inst. Pasteur *119*:302, 1970.

72. Catel, W., and Schmidt, W.: Klinische und experimentelle untersuchunge über das wesen der lokalen tuberkulin empfindlichkeit. Deut. Med. Wochenschr. *75*:1140, 1950.

73. Chanley, J. D., and Polgar, N.: Constituents of the lipids of tubercle bacilli. Part II. J. Chem. Soc. 1954:1003.

74. Chaput, M., Michel, G., and Lederer, E.: Structure du mycoside C_m, peptidoglycolipide de *Mycobacterium marianum*. Biochim. Biophys. Acta *63*:310, 1962.

75. Chaput, M., Michel, G., and Lederer, E.: Structure du mycoside C₂ de *Mycobacterium avium*. Biochim. Biophys. Acta *78*:329, 1963.

76. Chedid, L., Audibert, F., Lefrancier, P., Choay, J., and Lederer, E.: Modulation of the immune response by a synthetic adjuvant and analogs. Proc. Nat. Acad. Sci. U. S. A. *73*:2472, 1976.

77. Chedid, L., Parant, M., Parant, F., Gustafson, R. H., and Berger, F. M.: Biological study of a nontoxic, water-soluble immunoadjuvant from mycobacterial cell walls. Proc. Nat. Acad. Sci. U. S. A. *69*:855, 1972.

78. Choucroun, N., Delaunay, M., Bayinet, S., and Robineaux, R.: Effets produit par la phagocytose de bacilles Koch vivants ou

tués, et par une fraction lipopolysaccharidique isolée de ces bacilles, sur les phenomenes de migration leucocytaire *in vitro.* Ann. Inst. Pasteur. *80*:42, 1951.

79. Cohn, Z. A., and Fedorko, M.: The formation and fate of lysosomes. *In* Dingle, J. T., and Fell, H. B. (eds.): Lysosomes in Biology and Pathology. Vol. 1. Amsterdam, North-Holland, 1969, p. 43.

80. Coon, J., and Hunter, R.: Selective induction of delayed hypersensitivity by a lipid conjugated protein antigen which is localized in thymus dependent lymphoid tissue. J. Immunol. *110*:183, 1973.

81. Crowle, A. J.: Immunizing constituents of the tubercle bacillus. Bacteriol. Rev. *22*:183, 1958.

82. Dailey, M. O., and Hunter, R. L.: The role of lipid in the induction of hapten-specific delayed hypersensitivity and contact sensitivity. J. Immunol. *112*:1526, 1974.

83. Das, B. C., Géro, S. D., and Lederer, E.: N-methylation of N-acyl oligopeptides. Biochem. Biophys. Res. Commun. *29*:211, 1967.

84. David, H. L.: Response of mycobacteria to ultraviolet light irradiation. Am. Rev. Respir. Dis. *108*:1175, 1973.

85. David, H. L.: Carotenoid pigments of *Mycobacterium kansasii.* Appl. Microbiol. *28*:696, 1974.

86. David, H. L.: Biogenesis of β-carotene in *Mycobacterium kansasii.* J. Bacteriol. *119*:527, 1974.

87. David, H. L., Goldman, D. S., and Takayama, K.: Inhibition of the synthesis of wax D peptidoglycolipid of *Mycobacterium tuberculosis* by D-cycloserine. Infect. Immun. *1*:74, 1970.

87a. Davidson, L. A.: The surface structure of pathogenic mycobacteria Ph.D. thesis, University of London (1976).

88. Demarteau-Ginsburg, H., and Lederer, E.: Sur la structure chimique du mycoside B. Biochim. Biophys. Acta *70*:442, 1963.

89. Draper, P.: The walls of *Mycobacterium lepraemurium:* Chemistry and ultrastructure. J. Gen. Microbiol. *69*:313, 1971.

90. Draper, P.: The mycoside capsule of *Mycobacterium avium* 357. J. Gen. Microbiol. *83*:431, 1974.

91. Draper, P., and Rees, R. J. W.: The nature of the electron transparent zone that surrounds *Mycobacterium lepraemurium* inside host cells. J. Gen. Microbiol. *77*:79, 1973.

92. Dubos, R. J.: Cellular structures and functions concerned in parasitism. Bacteriol. Rev. *12*:173, 1948.

93. Ellouz, F., Adam, A., Ciorbaru, R., and Lederer, E.: Minimal structural requirements for adjuvant activity of bacterial peptidoglycan derivatives. Biochem. Biophys. Res. Commun. *59*:1317, 1974.

94. Etemadi, A. H.: Sur la structure des acides mycoliques methoxylés isolés de la souche humaine Test de *Mycobacterium tuberculosis.* C. R. Acad. Sci. (Paris) serie C *263*:1257, 1966.

95. Etemadi, A. H.: Correlations structurales et biogénétiques des acides mycoliques en rapport avec la phylogènese de quelques genres d'Actinomycetales. Bull. Soc. Chim. Biol. *49*:695, 1967.

96. Etemadi, A. H., and Convit, J.: Mycolic acids from "noncultivable" mycobacteria. Infect. Immun. *10*:236, 1974.

97. Etemadi, A. H., and Lederer, E.: Biosynthese de l'acide α-smegma-mycolique. Biochim. Biophys. Acta *98*:160, 1965.

98. Etemadi, A. H., and Lederer, E.: Sur la structure des acids α-mycoliques de la souche humaine Test de *Mycobacterium tuberculosis.* Bull. Soc. Chim. Fr. 1965:2640.

99. Etemadi, A. H., Okuda, R., and Lederer, E.: Sur la structure de l'acide α-smegma-mycolique. Bull. Soc. Chim. Fr. 1964:868.

100. Etemadi, A. H., Miquel, A. M., Lederer, E., and Barber, M.: Sur la structure des acides α-mycoliques de *Mycobacterium kansasii.* Spectrometrie de masse á haute résolution pour des masses de 750 à 1200. Bull. Soc. Chim. Fr. 1964:3274.

101. Ferguson, J. A., and Ballou, C. E.: Biosynthesis of a mycobacterial lipopolysaccharide. Properties of the polysaccharide methyltransferase. J. Biol. Chem. *245*:4213, 1970.

102. Fisher, C. A., and Barksdale, L.: Cytochemical reactions of human leprosy bacilli and mycobacteria: Ultrastructural implications. J. Bacteriol. *113*:1389, 1973.

103. Flick, P. K., and Bloch, K.: In vitro alterations of the product distribution of the fatty acid synthetase from *Mycobacterium phlei.* J. Biol. Chem. *249*:1031, 1974.

104. Flick, P. K., and Bloch, K.: Reversible inhibition of the fatty acid synthetase complex from *Mycobacterium smegmatis* by palmitoyl-coenzyme A. J. Biol. Chem. *250*:3348, 1975.

105. Francis, J., Macturk, H. M., Madinaveita, J., and Snow, G. A.: Mycobactin, a growth factor for *Mycobacterium johnei.* 1. Isolation from *Mycobacterium phlei.* Biochem. J. *55*:596, 1953.

106. Fregnan, G. B., Smith, D. W., and Randall, H. M.: A mutant of a scotochromogenic *Mycobacterium* detected by colony morphology and lipid studies. J. Bacteriol. *83*:828, 1962.

107. Fulco, A. J.: Metabolic alterations of fatty acids. Ann. Rev. Biochem. *43*:215, 1974.

108. Fulco, A. J., and Bloch, K.: Cofactor requirements for fatty acid desaturation in *Mycobacterium phlei.* Biochim. Biophys. Acta *63*:545, 1962.

109. Fulco, A. J., and Bloch, K.: Cofactor requirements for the formation of Δ^9-unsaturated fatty acids in *Mycobacterium phlei*. J. Biol. Chem. *239*:993, 1964.

110. Furuchi, A., and Tokunaga, T.: Nature of the receptor substance of *Mycobacterium smegmatis* for D_4 bacteriophage adsorption. J. Bacteriol. *111*:404, 1972.

110a. Gangadharam, P. R. J.: Unpublished data.

111. Gangadharam, P. R. J., Cohn, M. L., and Middlebrook, G.: Infectivity, pathogenicity, and sulpholipid fraction of some Indian and British strains of tubercle bacilli. Tubercle *44*:452, 1963.

112. Gangadharam, P. R. J., Harold, F. M., and Schaefer, W. B.: Selective inhibition of nucleic acid synthesis in *Mycobacterium tuberculosis* by isoniazid. Nature *198*:712, 1963.

113. Gastambide-Odier, M.: Variantes de mycosides characterisées par des residus glycosidiques substitues par des chaines acyles. I: Spectres de masse des mycosides G' et A' peracetyles. Org. Mass. Spectrom. *7*:845, 1972.

114. Gastambide-Odier, M.: Variantes de mycosides charactérisées par des résidus glycosidiques substitués par des châines acyles: Nature mycolique des mycosides G'. Europ. J. Biochem. *33*:81, 1973.

115. Gastambide-Odier, M., Delaumeny, J.-M., and Lederer, E.: Biosynthese de l'acide C_{32} mycocérosique: Incorporation d'acide propionique. Biochim. Biophys. Acta *70*:670, 1963.

116. Gastambide-Odier, M., Delaumeny, J.-M., and Lederer, E.: Biosynthesis of phthiocerol: Incorporation of methionine and propionic acid. Chem. & Ind. 1963: 1285.

117. Gastambide-Odier, M., Delaumeny, J.-M., and Lederer, E.: Mise en évidence de cycles propaniques dans divers acides mycoliques de souches humaines et bovines de *Mycobacterium tuberculosis*. C. R. Acad. Sci. *259*:3404, 1964.

118. Gastambide-Odier, M., Delaumeny, J.-M., and Kuntzel, H.: Biosynthèses des acides phthienoiques. Incorporation d'acide propionique. Biochim. Biophys. Acta *125*:33, 1966.

119. Gastambide-Odier, M., and Lederer, E.: Biosynthèse de l'acide corynomycolique à partir de deux molecules d'acide palmitique. Biochem. Z. *333*:285, 1960.

120. Gastambide-Odier, M., and Sarda, P.: Contributions à l'étude de la structure et de la biosynthèse de glycolipides specifiques isolés de mycobactéries. Les mycosides A et B. Pneumologie *142*:241, 1970.

121. Gastambide-Odier, M., Sarda, P., and Lederer, E.: Structure des aglycones des mycosides *A* et *B*. Tetrahedron Lett. *35*:3135, 1965.

122. Gastambide-Odier, M., Sarda, P., and Lederer, E.: Biosynthèse des aglycones des mycosides A et B. Bull. Soc. Chim. Biol. *49*:849, 1967.

123. Gastambide-Odier, M., and Ville, C.: Desoxysucres isolés du mycoside A. Identification des dérivés acetylés des méthyl 2,4-di-O-methylrhamnopyranoside, 2-O-methylrhamnofuranoside, 3-O-methylrhamnofuranoside, 2-O-methylfucopyranoside et 3-O-methylfucofuranoside. Bull. Soc. Chim. Biol. *52*:679, 1970.

124. Gateau, O., Bordet, C., and Michel, G.: Etude de la formation de l'acide N-glycolylmuramique du peptidoglycane de *Nocardia asteroides*. Biochim. Biophys. Acta *421*:395, 1976.

125. Gensler, W. J., and Alam, I.: Trehalose covalently conjugated to bovine serum albumin. J. Org. Chem. *42*:130, 1977.

126. Gensler, W. J., and Marshall, P. J.: Determination of cyclopropane-substituted acids by mass spectrometry. J. Org. Chem. *42*:126, 1977.

127. Gensler, W. J., Marshall, P. J., Langone, J. J., and Chen, J. C.: Synthesis of DL-methyl meromycolate. J. Org. Chem. *42*:118, 1977.

128. Ghuysen, J.-M.: Use of bacteriolytic enzymes in determination of wall structure and their role in cell metabolism. Bacteriol. Rev. *32*:425, 1968.

129. Gilleland, H. E., Jr., Stinnett, J. D., Roth, I. L., and Eagon, R. G.: Freeze-etch study of *Pseudomonas aeruginosa*: Localization within the cell wall of an ethylenediaminetetraacetate-extractable component. J. Bacteriol. *113*:417, 1973.

130. Goldman, D. S.: Subcellular localization of individual mannose-containing phospholipids in *Mycobacterium tuberculosis*. Amer. Rev. Respir. Dis. *102*:543, 1970.

131. Goodwin, T. W.: Biosynthesis of carotenoids and plant triterpenes. Biochem. J. *123*:293, 1971.

132. Goren, M. B.: Improved surface culturing of *Mycobacterium tuberculosis*. J. Bacteriol. *94*:1258, 1967.

132a. Goren, M. B.: Unpublished observations.

133. Goren, M. B.: Sulfolipid I of *Mycobacterium tuberculosis*, strain H37Rv. Purification and properties. Biochim. Biophys. Acta *210*:116, 1970.

134. Goren, M. B.: Sulfolipid I of *Mycobacterium tuberculosis*, strain H37Rv. II. Structural studies. Biochim. Biophys. Acta *210*:127, 1970.

135. Goren, M. B.: Mycobacterial sulfolipids: Spontaneous desulfation. Lipids *6*:40, 1971.

136. Goren, M. B.: Mycobacterial lipids: Selected topics. Bacteriol. Rev. *36*:33, 1972.

137. Goren, M. B.: Cord factor revisited: A trib-

ute to the late Dr. Hubert Bloch. Tubercle 56:65, 1975.

138. Goren, M. B.: Phagocyte lysosomes: Interactions with infectious agents, phagosomes, and experimental perturbations in function. Ann. Rev. Microbiol. 31:507, 1977.

139. Goren, M. B., and Brokl, O.: Separation and purification of cord factor (6,6'-dimycoloyl trehalose) from wax C or from mycolic acids. Recent Results Cancer Res. 47:251, 1974.

139a. Goren, M. B., and Brokl, O.: Unpublished material.

140. Goren, M. B., Brokl, O., Das, B. C., and Lederer, E.: Sulfolipid I of *Mycobacterium tuberculosis*, strain H37Rv. Nature of the acyl substituents. Biochemistry 10:72, 1971.

141. Goren, M. B., Brokl, O., Roller, P., Fales, H. M., and Das, B. C.: Sulfatides of *Mycobacterium tuberculosis*: The structure of the principal sulfatide (SL-I). Biochemistry 15:2728, 1976.

142. Goren, M. B., Brokl, O., Jiang, K.-S., and Roller, P.: Trehalose derivatives — cord factor and pseudo-cord factors: Structures and biological activities. *In* Proceedings, Eleventh Joint Meeting, Tuberculosis Panel. US-Japan Cooperative Medical Science Program 1976, p. 62.

143. Goren, M. B., Brokl, O., and Schaefer, W. B.: Lipids of putative relevance to virulence in *Mycobacterium tuberculosis*: Correlation of virulence with elaboration of sulfatides and strongly acidic lipids. Infect. Immun. 9:142, 1974.

144. Goren, M. B., Brokl, O., Schaefer, W. B.: Lipids of putative relevance to virulence in *Mycobacterium tuberculosis*: phthiocerol dimycocerosate and the attenuation indicator lipid. Infect. Immun. 9:150, 1974.

144a. Goren, M. B., Cernich, M. S., and Brokl, O.: Some observations on mycobacterial acid fastness. Amer. Rev. Respir. Dis. 118:151, 1978.

144b. Goren, M. B., Das, B. C., and Brokl, O.: Unpublished data.

145. Goren, M. B., Hart, P. D., Young, M. R., and Armstrong, J. A.: Prevention of phagosome-lysosome fusion in cultured macrophages by sulfatides of *Mycobacterium tuberculosis*. Proc. Nat. Acad. Sci. U.S.A. 73:2510, 1976.

146. Goren, M. B., Jiang, K.-S., and Moore, J.: Cord factors and pseudo cord factors II. Structures, syntheses, biological activities. *In* Proceedings, Twelfth Joint Conference on Tuberculosis. U. S.-Japan Cooperative Medical Science Program, 1977, p. 371.

147. Goren, M. B., McClatchy, J. K., Martens, B., and Brokl, O.: Mycosides C: Behaviour as receptor site substance for mycobacteriophage D4. J. Virol. 9:999, 1972.

147a. Goren, M. B., and Tihon, C.: Unpublished studies.

147b. Goren, M. B., and Toubiana, R.: In preparation.

148. Goslee, S., Rynearson, T. K., and Wolinsky, E.: Additional serotypes of *Mycobacterium scrofulaceum*, *Mycobacterium gordonae*, *Mycobacterium marinum*, and *Mycobacterium xenopi* determined by agglutination. Int. J. Syst. Bacteriol. 23:182, 1976.

148a. Grange, J. M., Aber, V. R., Allen, B. W., Mitchison, D. A., and Goren, M. B.: Correlation of bacteriophage types of *Mycobacterium tuberculosis* with guinea pig virulence and *in vitro* indicators of virulence. J. Gen. Microbiol. 108:1, 1978.

149. Granger, D. L., Yamamoto, K., and Ribi, E.: Delayed hypersensitivity and granulomatous response after immunization with protein antigens associated with a mycobacterial glycolipid and oil droplets. J. Immunol. 116:482, 1976.

150. Gray, G. R., and Ballou, C. E.: Isolation and characterization of a polysaccharide containing 3-O-methyl-D-mannose from *Mycobacterium phlei*. J. Biol. Chem. 246:6835, 1971.

151. Gray, G. R., and Ballou, C. E.: The 6-O-methylglucose-containing lipopolysaccharides of *Mycobacterium phlei*. Locations of the acyl groups. J. Biol. Chem. 247:8129, 1972.

152. Grellert, E., and Ballou, C. E.: Biosynthesis of a mycobacterial lipopolysaccharide. Evidence for an acylpolysaccharide methyltransferase. J. Biol. Chem. 247:3236, 1972.

153. Hackett, J. A., and Brennan, P. J.: Biosynthesis of the mannophosphoinositides of *Corynebacterium aquaticum*. Biochem. J. 148:253, 1975.

154. Hart, P. D., and Young, M. R.: Interference with normal phagosome-lysosome fusion in macrophages, using ingested yeast cells and suramin. Nature 256:47, 1975.

155. Hill, D. L., and Ballou, C. E.: Biosynthesis of mannophospholipids by *Mycobacterium phlei*. J. Biol. Chem. 241:895, 1966.

156. Hung, J. G. C., and Walker, R. W.: Unsaturated fatty acids of mycobacteria. Lipids 5:720, 1970.

157. Husseini, H., and Elberg, S.: Cellular reactions to phthienoic acid and related branched chain fatty acids. Am. Rev. Tuberc. 65:655, 1952.

158. Ilton, M., Jevans, A. W., McCarthy, E. D., Vance, D., White, H. B., III, and Bloch, K.: Fatty acid synthetase activity in *Mycobacterium phlei*: Regulation by polysaccharides. Proc. Natl. Acad. Sci. U. S. A. 68:87, 1971.

159. Imaeda, T., Kanetsuna, F., and Galindo, B.: Ultrastructure of cell walls of genus *Mycobacterium*. J. Ultrastruct. Res. 25:46, 1968.

160. Imaeda, T., and San-Blas, F.: Adsorption of mycobacteriophage on cell wall components. J. Gen. Virol. 5:493, 1969.

161. Ioneda, T., Lederer, E., and Rozanis, J.: Sur la structure des diesters de trehalose ("cord factors") produits par *Nocardia asteroides* et *Nocardia rhodochrous*. Chem. Phys. Lipids. 4:375, 1970.

162. Ioneda, T., Lenz, M., and Pudles, J.: Chemical constitution of a glycolipid from *C. diphtheriae*. Biochem. Biophys. Res. Commun. 13:110, 1963.

163. Itoh, S., and Suzuki, T.: Fructose lipids of Arthrobacter, Nocardia, and Mycobacteria grown on fructose. Agr. Biol. Chem. (Tokyo) 38:1443, 1974.

164. Jaureguiberry, G., Lenfant, M., Toubiana, R., Azerad, R., and Lederer, E.: Biosynthesis of tuberculostearic acid in a cell-free extract. Identification of 10-methylenestearic acid as an intermediate. Chem. Commun. 23:855, 1966.

165. Jenkins, P. A., Marks, J. Schaefer, W. B.: Lipid chromatography and seroagglutination in the classification of rapidly growing mycobacteria. Am. Rev. Respir. Dis. 103:179, 1971.

166. Jenkins, P. A., Marks, J., and Schaefer, W. B.: Thin layer chromatography of mycobacterial lipids as an aid to classification: The scotochromogenic mycobacteria, including *Mycobacterium scrofulaceum, M. xenopi, M. aquae, M. gordonae, M. flavescens*. Tubercle 53:118, 1972.

167. Jollès, P., Bigler, F., Gendre, T., and Lederer, E.: Sur la structure chimique du mycoside C peptideglycolipide de *Mycobacterium avium*. Bull. Soc. Chim. Biol. 43:177, 1961.

168. Jollès, P., Samour, D., and Lederer, E.: Analytical studies on wax D, a macromolecular peptidoglycolipid fraction from human strains of *Mycobacterium tuberculosis*. Arch. Biochem. Biophys. Suppl. 1:283, 1962.

169. Jollès, P., Samour-Migliore, D., DeWijs, H., and Lederer, E.: Correlation of adjuvant activity and chemical structure of mycobacterial wax D fractions: The importance of amino sugars. Biochim. Biophys. Acta 83:361, 1964.

170. Jollès, P., and Paraf, A.: Chemical and biological basis of adjuvants. New York, Springer-Verlag, 1973.

171. Jones, T. C., and Hirsch, J. G.: The interaction between *Toxoplasma gondii* and mammalian cells. II. The absence of lysosomal fusion with phagocytic vacuoles containing living parasites. J. Exp. Med. 136:1173, 1972.

172. Juy, D., and Chedid, L.: Comparison between macrophage activation and enhancement of nonspecific resistance to tumors by mycobacterial immunoadjuvants. Proc. Nat. Acad. Sci. U. S. A. 72:4105, 1975.

173. Kanai, K.: Detection of host-originated acid phosphatase on the surface of "*in vivo* grown tubercle bacilli." Jpn. J. Med. Sci. Biol. 20:73, 1967.

174. Kanai, K., and Kondo, K.: Separation and properties of "*in vivo* grown tubercle bacilli" associated with the lysosomal membrane. Jpn. J. Med. Sci. Biol. 23:303, 1970.

175. Kanai, K., Wiegeshaus, E., and Smith, D. W.: Demonstration of mycolic acid and phthiocerol dimycocerosate in "*in vivo* grown tubercle bacilli." Jpn. J. Med. Sci. Biol. 23:327, 1970.

176. Kanemasa, Y., and Goldman, D. S.: Direct incorporation of octanoate into long chain fatty acids by soluble enzymes of *Mycobacterium tuberculosis*. Biochim. Biophys. Acta 98:476, 1965.

177. Kanetsuna, F.: Chemical analyses of mycobacterial cell walls. Biochim. Biophys. Acta 158:130, 1968.

178. Kanetsuna, F., and SanBlas, G.: Chemical analysis of a mycolic acid-arabinogalactan-mucopeptide complex of mycobacterial cell wall. Biochim. Biophys. Acta 208:434, 1970.

179. Karnovsky, M. L.: In "Discussion" *in* van Furth, R. (ed.): Mononuclear Phagocytes in Immunity, Infection, and Pathology. Blackwell, Oxford, 1975, p. 594.

180. Kasha, M., and Khan, A. U.: The physics, chemistry and biology of singlet molecular oxygen. Ann. N. Y. Acad. Sci. 171:5, 1970.

181. Kato, M.: Studies of a biochemical lesion in experimental tuberculosis in mice. III. Site of lesion in electron transport chain. Am. Rev. Respir. Dis. 94:388, 1966.

182. Kato, M.: Studies of a biochemical lesion in experimental tuberculosis in mice. VI. Effect of toxic bacterial constituents of tubercle bacilli on oxidative phosphorylation in host cell. Am. Rev. Respir. Dis. 96:998, 1966.

183. Kato, M.: Studies of a biochemical lesion in experimental tuberculosis in mice. XI. Mitochondrial swelling induced by cord factor *in vitro*. Am. Rev. Resp. Dis. 100:47, 1969.

184. Kato, M.: Site II — specific inhibition of mitochondrial oxidative phosphorylation by trehalose-6,6'-dimycolate (cord factor) of *Mycobacterium tuberculosis*. Arch. Biochem. Biophys. 140:379, 1970.

185. Kato, M.: Antibody formation to trehalose-6,6'-dimycolate (cord factor) of *Mycobacterium tuberculosis*. Infect. Immun. 5:203, 1972.

186. Kato, M.: Immunochemical properties of anti-cord factor antibody. Infect. Immun. 7:9, 1973.

187. Kato, M.: Effect of anti-cord factor antibody on experimental tuberculosis in mice. Infect. Immun. 7:14, 1973.

188. Kato, M., and Asselineau, J.: Chemical structure and biological activity of cord factor analogs. 6,6'-dimycoloyl sucrose and methyl 6-mycoloyl α-D-glucoside. Eur. J. Biochem. *22*:364, 1971.

189. Kato, M., and Goren, M. B.: Synergistic action of cord factor and mycobacterial sulfatides on mitochondria. Infect. Immun. *10*:733, 1974.

190. Kato, M., and Maeda, J.: Isolation and biochemical activities of trehalose-6-monomycolate of *Mycobacterium tuberculosis.* Infect. Immun. *9*:8, 1974.

191. Keller, J. M., and Ballou, C. E.: The 6-O-methylglucose-containing lipopolysaccharide of *Mycobacterium phlei.* Identification of the lipid components. J. Biol. Chem. *243*:2905, 1968.

192. Kelly, M. T.: Plasma-dependent chemotaxis of macrophages toward BCG cell walls and the mycobacterial glycolipid P3. Infect. Immun. *15*:180, 1977.

193. Kelly, M. T., Granger, D. L., Ribi, E., Milner, K. C., Strain, S. M., and Stoenner, H. G.: Tumor regression with Q-fever rickettsia and a mycobacterial glycolipid. Cancer Immunol. Immunother. *1*:187, 1976.

194. Kervabon, A., Albert, B., and Etemadi, A. H.: Subunit composition and some properties of palmityl-Co A-ACP-transacylase of *Mycobacterium smegmatis.* Biochimie *59*:363, 1977.

195. Khuller, G. K., and Brennan, P. J.: Further studies on the lipids of corynebacteria: The mannolipids of *Corynebacterium aquaticum.* Biochem. J. *127*:369, 1972.

196. Khuller, G. K., and Subrahmanyam, D.: Antigenicity of phosphatidly inositomannoside of *Mycobacterium tuberculosis.* Immunochemistry *8*:251, 1971.

197. Kim, K.-S., Salton, M. R. J., and Barksdale, L.: Ultrastructure of superficial mycoside integuments of *Mycobacterium* sp. J. Bacteriol. *125*:739, 1976.

198. Knoche, H., Esders, T. W., Koths, K., and Bloch, K.: Palmityl coenzyme A inhibition of fatty acid synthesis. Relief by bovine serum albumin and mycobacterial polysaccharides. J. Biol. Chem. *248*:2317, 1973.

199. Knoche, H. W., and Koths, K. E.: Characterization of a fatty acid synthetase from *Corynebacterium diphtheriae.* J. Biol. Chem. *248*:3517, 1973.

200. Kochan, I.: The role of iron in bacterial infections, with special consideration of host-tubercle bacillus interaction. Curr. Top. Microbiol. Immunol. *54*:1, 1973.

201. Koga, T., Kato, K., Kotani, S, Tanaka, A., and Pearson, C. M.: Effect of degradation of arabinogalactan portion of a water soluble component from *M. tuberculosis* wax D on polyarthritis induction in the rat. Int.

Arch. Allergy Appl. Immunol. *51*:395, 1976.

202. Kondo, E., and Kanai, K.: Further demonstration of bacterial lipids in *Mycobacterium bovis* harvested from infected mouse lungs. Jpn. J. Med. Sci. Biol. *25*:105, 1972.

203. Kondo, E., and Kanai, K.: Some immunological and toxic properties of mycobacteria grown *in vivo.* Jpn. J. Med. Sci. Biol. *27*:53, 1974.

204. Kotani, S., Kitaura, T., Hirano, T., and Tanaka, A.: Isolation and chemical composition of the cell walls of BCG. Biken J. *2*:129, 1959.

205. Kotani, S., Kitaura, T., Higashigawa, M., Kato, K., Mori, Y., Matsubara, T., and Tsujimoto, T.: Studies on the immunological properties of the cell wall-, particle- and soluble-fractions of sonicated BCG cells. Biken J. *3*:159, 1960.

206. Kotani, S., Narita, T., Stewart-Tull, D. E. S., Shimono, T., Watanabe, Y., Kato, K., and Iwata, S.: Immunoadjuvant activities of cell walls and their water-soluble fractions prepared from various gram-positive bacteria. Biken J. *18*:77, 1975.

207. Kotani, S., Watanabe, Y., Narita, T., Shimono, T., Stewart-Tull, D. E. S., Iwata, S., et al.: Immunoadjuvant activities of fungal cell walls. Biken J. *18*:135, 1975.

208. Kotani, S., Watanabe, Y., Shimono, T., Kinoshita, F., Narita, T., et al.: Immunoadjuvant activities of peptidoglycan subunits from the cell walls of *Staphylococcus aureus* and *Lactobacillus plantarum.* Biken J. *18*:93, 1975.

209. Kotani, S., Watanabe, Y., Kinoshita, F., Shimono, T., Morisaki, I., et al.: Immunoadjuvant activities of synthetic N-acetyl muramyl-peptides or -amino acids. Biken J. *18*:105, 1975.

210. Kotani, S., Watanabe, T., Shimono, T., Harada, K., Shiba, T., et al.: Correlation between the immunoadjuvant activities and pyrogenicities of synthetic N-acetyl muramylpeptides of amino acids. Biken J. *19*:9, 1976.

211. Kusumoto, S., Okada, S., Shiba, T., Azuma, I., and Yamamura, Y.: Synthesis of 6-O-mycoloyl-N-acetylmuramyl-L-alanyl-D-isoglutamine with immunoadjuvant activity. Tetrahedron Lett. *47*:4287, 1976.

212. Lamonica, G., and Etemadi, A. H.: Sur la coupure specifique, en spectrometrie de masse, des aldehydes lineaires comportant des cycles propaniques. Bull. Soc. Chim. Fr. 1967:4275.

213. Lanéelle, G.: Étude de deux formes lipophiles d'acides aminés produites par des mycobactéries. Theses pour le Docteur Sciences Physiques. University of Toulouse, Toulouse France, 1967, p. 62.

214. Lanéelle, G., and Asselineau, J.: Structure

d'un glycoside de peptidolipide isolé d'une mycobactérie. Eur. J. Biochem. *5*:487, 1968.

215. Lanéelle, M. A., and Lanéelle, G.: Structure d'acides mycoliques et d'un intermediaire dans la biosynthèse d'acides mycoliques dicarboxyliques. Eur. J. Biochem. *12*:296, 1970.

216. Lanéelle, G., Asselineau, J., and Chamoiseau, G.: Presence de mycosides C' (formes simplifiées de mycoside C) dans les bactéries isolées de bovins atteints du farcin. FEBS Lett. *19*:109, 1971.

217. Leclerc, C., Lamensans, A., Chedid, L., Drapier, J. C., Petit, J.-F., Wietzerbin, J. and Lederer, E.: Non specific immunoprevention of L1210 leukemia cells by cord factor (6-6'-dimycolate of trehalose) administered in a metabolizable oil. Cancer Immunol. Immunother. *1*:227, 1976.

218. Lederer, E.: Glycolipids of mycobacteria and related microorganisms. Chem. Phys. Lipids *1*:294, 1967.

219. Lederer, E.: Mass spectrometry of natural and synthetic peptide derivatives. Pure Appl. Chem. *17*:489, 1968.

220. Lederer, E.: The mycobacterial cell wall. Pure Appl. Chem. *25*:135, 1971.

221. Lederer, E.: Cord factor and related trehalose esters. Chem. Phys. Lipids *16*:91, 1976.

222. Lederer, E.: Natural and synthetic immunostimulants relative to the mycobacterial cell wall. Med. Chem. *5*:257, 1977.

223. Lederer, E., Adam, A., Ciorbaru, R., Petit, J.-F., and Wietzerbin, J.: Cell walls of mycobacteria and related organisms: Chemistry and immunostimulant properties. Mol. Cell. Biochem. *7*:87, 1975.

224. Lee, Y. C.: Isolation and characterization of lipopolysaccharides containing 6-O-methyl-D-glucose from *Mycobacterium* species. J. Biol. Chem. *241*:1899, 1966.

225. Lee, Y. C., and Ballou, C. E.: 6-O-methyl-D-glucose from mycobacteria. J. Biol. Chem. *239*:PC 3602, 1964.

226. Lee, Y. C., and Ballou, C. E.: Structural studies on the myo-inositol mannosides from the glycolipids of *Mycobacterium tuberculosis* and *Mycobacterium phlei*. J. Biol. Chem. *239*:1316, 1964.

227. Lee, Y. C., and Ballou, C. E.: Complete structures of the glycophospholipids of mycobacteria. Biochemistry *4*:1395, 1965.

227a. Lehninger, A. L.: Biochemistry (2nd ed.). New York, Worth Publishers, 1975, p. 64.

228. Lenfant, M., Audier, H., and Lederer, E.: Sur une migration d'hydrogène au cours de la biosynthèse de l'acide tuberculostearique. Bull. Soc. Chim. France 1966:2775.

229. Lennarz, W. J.: The role of isoleucine in the biosynthesis of branched-chain fatty acids by *Micrococcus lysodeikticus*. Biochem. Biophys. Res. Commun. *6*:112, 1961.

230. Lennarz, W. J.: Lipid-linked sugars in glycoprotein synthesis. Science *188*:986, 1975.

231. Lennarz, W. J., Scheuerbrandt, G., and Bloch, K.: The biosynthesis of oleic acid and 10-methylstearic acids in *Mycobacterium phlei*. J. Biol. Chem. *237*:664, 1962.

232. Liaaen-Jensen, S., and Andrewes, G.: Microbial carotenoids. Ann. Rev. Microbiol. *26*:225, 1972.

233. Liu, T.-Y., Gotschlich, E. C.: Muramic acid phosphate as a component of the mucopeptide of gram-positive bacteria. J. Biol. Chem. *242*:471, 1967.

234. Lornitzo, F. A., and Goldman, D. S.: Intracellular location of a 6-O-methyl-D-glucose-containing soluble polysaccharide from *Mycobacterium tuberculosis*. Biochim. Biophys. Acta *158*:329, 1968.

235. Lowrie, D. B., Jackett, P. S., and Ratcliffe, N. A.: *Mycobacterium microti* may protect itself from intracellular destruction by releasing cyclic AMP into phagosomes. Nature *254*:600, 1975.

236. Macham, L. P., and Ratledge, C.: A new group of water-soluble iron-binding compounds from mycobacteria: the exochelins. J. Gen. Microbiol. *89*:379, 1975.

237. Macham, L. P., Ratledge, C., and Norton, J. C.: Extracellular iron acquisition by mycobacteria: Role of the exochelins and evidence against the participation of mycobactin. Infect. Immun. *12*:1242, 1975.

238. Machida, Y., and Bloch, K.: Complex formation between mycobacterial polysaccharides and fatty acyl CoA derivatives. Proc. Natl. Acad. Sci. U.S.A. *70*:1146, 1973.

239. MacLennan, A. P.: The monosaccharide units in specific glycolipids of *Mycobacterium avium*. Biochem. J. *82*:394, 1962.

240. MacLennan, A. P., Randall, H. M., and Smith, D. W.: The occurrence of methylesters of rhamnose and fucose in specific glycolipids of certain mycobacteria. Biochem. J. *80*:309, 1961.

240a. Maeda, J., Goren, M., and Macintyre, E.: Unpublished data.

241. Maitra, S. K., and Ballou, C. E.: Heterogeneity and refined structures of 3-O-methyl-D-mannose polysaccharides from *Mycobacterium smegmatis*. J. Biol. Chem. *252*:2459, 1977.

242. Markovits, J., Pinte, F., and Etemadi, A. H.: Sur la structure des acides mycoliques dicarboxyliques insaturés isolés de *Mycobacterium phlei*. C. R. Acad. Sci. (Paris) serie C *263*:960, 1966.

243. Marks, J., Jenkins, P. A., and Schaefer, W. B.: Thin layer chromatography of mycobacterial lipids as an aid to classification: Technical improvements; *Mycobacterium*

avium, M. intracellulare (Battey bacilli). Tubercle 52:219, 1971.

244. Marks, J., and Szulga, T.: Thin layer chromatography of mycobacterial lipids as an aid to classification: Technical procedures; *Mycobacterium fortuitum.* Tubercle 46:400, 1965.

245. Matsumura, S.: Conformation of acyl carrier protein from *Mycobacterium phlei.* Biochem. Biophys. Res. Commun. 38:238, 1970.

246. Matsumura, S., Brindley, D. N., and Bloch, K.: Acyl carrier protein from *Mycobacterium phlei.* Biochem. Biophys. Res. Commun. 38:369, 1970.

247. McCarthy, C.: Utilization of palmitic acid by *Mycobacterium avium.* Infect. Immun. 4:199, 1971.

248. McClatchy, J. K.: Mechanism of action of isoniazid on *Mycobacterium bovis* strain BCG. Infect. Immun. 3:530, 1971.

249. McLaughlin, C. A., Kelly, M. T., Milner, K. C., Parker, R., Ribi, E., Smith, R., and Toubiana, R.: Minimal structural requirements of defined microbial agents acting as immunopotentiators in protection against aerosol-induced tuberculosis and in tumor regression. *In* Proceedings, Eleventh Joint Meeting, Tuberculosis Panel, US-Japan Cooperative Medical Science Program, 1976, p. 167.

250. McLaughlin, C. A., Ribi, E., Goren, M. B., and Toubiana, R.: Tumor regression induced by defined microbial components in an oil-in-water emulsion is through their binding to oil droplets. Cancer Immunol. Immunother. 4:109, 1978.

251. McLaughlin, C. A., Strain, S. M., Bickel, W. D., Goren, M. B., Azuma, I., Milner, K., Cantrell, J. L., and Ribi, E.: Regression of line 10 hepatocellular carcinomas following treatment with aqueous soluble microbial extracts combined with trehalose or arabinose mycolates. Cancer Immunol. Immunother. 4:61, 1968.

252. Merser, C., Sinay, P., and Adam, A.: Total synthesis and adjuvant activity of bacterial peptidoglycan derivatives. Biochem. Biophys. Res. Commun. 66:1316, 1975.

253. Meyer, T. J., Ribi, E., Azuma, I., and Zbar, B.: Biologically active components from mycobacterial cell walls. II. Suppression and regression of strain-2 guinea pig hepatoma. J. Nat. Cancer Inst. 52:103, 1974.

253a. Middlebrook, G.: Unpublished data.

254. Middlebrook, G., Coleman, C. M., and Schaefer, W. B.: Sulfolipid from virulent tubercle bacilli. Proc. Natl. Acad. Sci., U. S. A. 45:1801, 1959.

255. Middlebrook, G., Dubos, R. J., and Pierce, C. H.: Virulence and morphological characteristics of mammalian tubercle bacilli. J. Exp. Med. 86:175, 1947.

256. Migliore-Samour, D., and Jollès, P.: Hydrosoluble adjuvant-active mycobacterial fractions of low molecular weight. FEBS Lett. 35:317, 1973.

257. Minnikin, D. E., and Polgar, N.: The methoxymycolic and ketomycolic acids from human tubercle bacilli. Chem. Commun. 22:1172, 1967.

258. Minnikin, D. E., and Polgar, N.: The mycolic acids from human and avian tubercle bacilli. Chem. Commun. 22:915, 1967.

259. Minnikin, D. E., and Polgar, N.: Structural studies on the mycolic acids. Chem. Commun. 1967:312.

260. Misaki, A., Seto, N., and Azuma, I.: Structure and immunological properties of D-arabino-D-galactans isolated from *Mycobacterium* species. J. Biochem. 76:15, 1974.

261. Mitchison, D. A.: The virulence of tubercle bacilli from patients with pulmonary tuberculosis in India and other countries. Bull. Int. Union Tuberc. 35:287, 1964.

262. Modolell, M., Luckenbach, G. A., Parant, M., and Munder, B. G.: The adjuvant activity of a mycobacterial water soluble adjuvant (WSA) *in vitro.* I. The requirements of macrophages. J. Immunol. 113:395, 1974.

263. Moore, V. L., Myrvik, Q. S., and Kato, M.: Role of cord factor (trehalose-6,6'-dimycolate) in allergic granuloma formation in rabbits. Infect. Immun. 6:5, 1972.

264. Motomiya, M., Mayama, A., Fujimoto, M., Sato, H., and Oka, S.: Chemistry and biology of phospholipids from an unclassified mycobacteria, P_6. Chem. Phys. Lipids 3:159, 1969.

265. Murohashi, T., Kondo, E., and Yoshida, K.: The role of lipids in acid-fastness of mycobacteria. Am. Rev. Respir. Dis. 99:794, 1969.

266. Nacash, C., and Vilkas, E.: Sur la présence simultanée de deux types de mycosides dans *Mycobacterium kansasii.* C. R. Acad. Sci. (Paris) serie C 265:413, 1967.

267. Narumi, K., Keller, J. M., and Ballou, C. E.: Biosynthesis of a mycobacterial lipopolysaccharide: Incorporation of [^{14}C]-acyl groups by whole cells *in vivo.* Biochem. J. 132:329, 1973.

268. Navalkar, R. G., Wiegeshaus, E., Kondo, E., Kim, H. K., and Smith, D. W.: Mycoside G, a specific glycolipid in *Mycobacterium marinum* (Balnei). J. Bacteriol. 90:262, 1965.

269. Nojima, S.: Studies on the chemistry of wax D of BCG. II. On the chemical structure of oligomannoinositides. J. Biochem. (Tokyo) 46:607, 1959.

270. Nojima, S., Kataoka, T., and Inoue, K.: Haptenic activity of phospholipids. Jpn. J. Med. Sci. Biol. 23:129, 1970.

271. Noll, H.: The chemistry of cord factor, a

toxic glycolipid of *M. tuberculosis*. Adv. Tuberc. Res. *7*:149, 1956.

272. Noll, H.: The chemistry of some native constituents of the purified wax of *Mycobacterium tuberculosis*. J. Biol. Chem. 224:149, 1957.

273. Noll, H., Bloch, H., Asselineau, J., and Lederer, E.: The chemical structure of the cord factor of *Mycobacterium tuberculosis*. Biochim. Biophys. Acta *20*:299, 1956.

274. Ohara, T., Shimmyo, Y., Sekikawa, I., Morikawa, K., and Sumikawa, E.: Studies on the cord factor, with special reference to its immunological properties. Jpn. J. Tuberc. *5*:128, 1957.

275. Oka, S., Fukushi, K., Fujimoto, M., Sato, H., and Motomiya, M.: La distribution subcellulaire des phospholipides de la mycobacterie. C. R. Soc. Biol. *162*:1648, 1968.

276. Okuda, S., Suzuki, N., and Suzuki, S.: Isolation and structure of cytidine diphosphate 6-deoxy-3-C-methyl-2-O-methyl-L-aldohexopyranoside (cytidine diphosphate vinelose) from *Azotobacter vinelandii*. J. Biol. Chem. *242*:958, 1967.

277. Okuda, S., Suzuki, N., and Suzuki, S.: Biosynthesis of branched chain deoxysugars. IV Isolation of cytidine diphosphate 6-deoxy-3-C-methyl-4-O-(O-methyl-glycolyl)-L-aldohexopyranoside from *Azotobacter vinelandii*. J. Biol. Chem. *243*:6353, 1968.

278. Okuyama, H., Kankura, T., and Nojima, S.: Positional distribution of fatty acids in phospholipids from *Mycobacteria*. J. Biochem. (Tokyo) *61*:732, 1967.

279. Pangborn, M. C., McKinney, J. A.: Purification of serologically active phosphoinositides of *Mycobacterium tuberculosis*. J. Lipid Res. *7*:627, 1966.

280. Parish, C. R.: Immune response to chemically modified flagellin IV. Further studies on the relationship between humoral and cell-mediated immunity. Cell. Immunol. *6*:66, 1973.

281. Petit, J.-F., Adam, A., Wietzerbin-Falszpan, J.: Isolation of UDP-N-glycolyl-muramyl-(ALA, GLU, DAP) from *Mycobacterium phlei*. FEBS Lett. *6*:55, 1970.

282. Pigretti, M., Vilkas, E., Lederer, E., and Bloch, H.: Proprietes chimiques et biologiques de fractions phosphatidiques isolées de ''l'antigène methylique'' de *Mycobacterium tuberculosis*. Bull. Soc. Chim. Biol. *47*:2039, 1965.

283. Polgar, N.: Constituents of the lipids of tubercle bacilli. Part III. Mycolipenic acid. J. Chem. Soc. 1954:1008.

284. Polgar, N.: Constituents of the lipids of tubercle bacilli. Part IV. Mycoceranic acid. J. Chem. Soc. 1954:1011.

285. Polgar, N., and Robinson, R.: The constitution of mycolipenic acid — I. Chem. Ind. 1951:685.

286. Promé, J.-C.: Localisation d'une cycle propanique dans une substance aliphatique par examen du spectre de masse des cetones obtenues par oxydation. Bull. Soc. Chim. Fr. 1968:655.

287. Promé, J.-C., Lacave, C., Ahibo-Coffy, A., and Savagnac, A.: Séparation et étude structurale des espèces moleculaires de monomycolates et de dimycolates des α-D-trehalose présents chez *Mycobacterium phlei*. Eur. J. Biochem. *63*:543, 1976.

288. Promé, J.-C., Walker, R. W., and Lacave, C.: Condensation de deux molecules d'acide palmitique chez *Corynebacterium diphtheriae*: formation d'un β-ceto-ester de trehalose. C. R. Acad. Sci. (Paris) serie C *218*:1065, 1974.

289. Rapp, H. J.: A guinea pig model for tumor immunology. A summary. Isr. J. Med. Sci. *9*:366, 1973.

290. Ratledge, C.: The physiology of the mycobacteria. Adv. Microb. Physiol. *13*:115, 1976.

290a. Reznikov, M., and Dawson, D. J.: Serological examination of some strains that are in the *Mycobacterium avium-intracellular-scrofulaceum* complex, but do not belong to Schaefer's complex. App. Microbiol. *26*:470, 1973.

291. Ribi, E., Anacker, R. L., Brehmer, W., Goode, G., Larson, C. L., List, R. H., Milner, K. C., and Wicht, W. C.: Factors influencing protection against experimental tuberculosis in mice by heat-stable cell wall vaccines. J. Bacteriol. *92*:869, 1966.

292. Ribi, E., Anacker, R. L., Barclay, W. R., Brehmer, W., Middlebrook, G., Milner, K. C., and Tarmina, D. F.: Structure and biological functions of mycobacteria. Ann. N. Y. Acad. Sci. *154*:41, 1968.

293. Ribi, E., Granger, D. L., Milner, K. C., Yamamoto, K., Strain, S. M., Parker, R., Smith, R. F., Brehmer, W., and Azuma, I.: Induction of resistance to tuberculosis in mice with defined components of mycobacteria and with some unrelated materials. J. Infect. Dis. (in press) 1977.

294. Ribi, E., Granger, D. L., Milner, K. C., and Strain, S. M.: Tumor regression caused by endotoxins and mycobacterial fractions. J. Nat. Cancer. Inst. *55*:1253, 1975.

295. Ribi, E., Milner, K. C., Granger, D. L., Kelly, M. T., Yamamoto, K.-I., Brehmer, W., Parker, R., Smith, R. F., and Strain, S. M.: Immunotherapy with nonviable components. International Conference on Immunotherapy Cancer. Ann. N. Y. Acad. Sci. *277*:228, 1976.

296. Ribi, E., Parker, R., and Milner, K.: Microparticulate gel chromatography accelerated by centrifugal force and pressure. Methods Biochem. Anal. *22*:355, 1974.

297. Rouser, G., Kritchevsky, G., Heller, D., and Lieber, E.: Lipid composition of beef brain, beef liver, and the sea anemone:

Two approaches to quantitative fractionation of complex lipid mixtures. J. Am. Oil Chem. Soc. 40:425, 1963.

298. Runyon, E. H.: Anonymous mycobacteria in pulmonary disease. Med. Clin. North Am. 43:273, 1959.

299. Runyon, E. H.: Pathogenic mycobacteria. Adv. Tuberc. Res. 14:235, 1965.

300. Sabin, F. R., and Smithburn, K. C.: Cellular reactions to fractions isolated from tubercle bacilli. Physiol. Rev. 12:141, 1932.

301. Saier, M. H., and Ballou, C. E.: The 6-O-methylglucose-containing lipopolysaccharide of *Mycobacterium phlei*. Identification of D-glyceric acid and 3-O-methyl-D-glucose in the polysaccharide. J. Biol. Chem. 243:992, 1968.

302. Saier, H. M., and Ballou, C. E.: The 6-O-methylglucose-containing lipopolysaccharide of *Mycobacterium phlei*. Structure of the reducing end of the polysaccharide. J. Biol. Chem. 243:4319, 1968.

303. Saier, M. H., and Ballou, C. E.: The 6-O-methylglucose-containing lipopolysaccharide of *Mycobacterium phlei*. Complete structure of the polysaccharide. J. Biol. Chem. 243:4332, 1968.

304. Saito, R., Tanaka, A., Sugiyama, K., Azuma, I., Yamamura, Y., Kato, M., and Goren, M. B.: Adjuvant effect of cord factor, a mycobacterial lipid. Infect. Immun. 13:776, 1976.

305. Sarda, P., and Gastambide-Odier, M.: Structure chimique de l'aglycone du Mycoside G de *Mycobacterium marinum*. Chem. Phys. Lipids 1:434, 1967.

306. Sarma, G. R., Chandramouli, V., and Venkitasubramanian, J. A.: Occurrence of phosphonolipids in mycobacteria. Biochim. Biophys. Acta 218:561, 1970.

307. Sasaki, A., and Takahashi, Y.: Activité serologique des phospholipides purifiés de *Mycobacterium tuberculosis*. C. R. Soc. Biol. 168:626, 1974.

308. Schaefer, W. B.: Serological classification of mycobacteria and extracts of their type-specific antigens. Bact. Proc. M80:58, 1964.

309. Schaefer, W. B.: Serologic identification and classification of atypical mycobacteria by their agglutination. Am. Rev. Respir. Dis. 92 (suppl.):85, 1965.

310. Schaefer, W. B.: Serologic identification of the atypical mycobacteria and its value in epidemiologic studies. Am. Rev. Respir. Dis. 96:115, 1967.

311. Schaefer, W. B.: Serological identification of atypical mycobacteria. Methods in Microbiology (in press), 1977.

312. Schaefer, W. B., and Lewis, C. W.: Effect of oleic acid on growth and cell structure of mycobacteria. J. Bacteriol. 90:1438, 1965.

313. Scheuerbrandt, G., Goldfine, H., Baronowsky, P., and Bloch, K.: A novel mechanism for the biosynthesis of unsaturated fatty acids. J. Biol. Chem. 236:PC70, 1961.

314. Schleifer, K. H., and Kandler, O.: Peptidoglycan types of bacterial cell walls and their taxonomic implications. Bacteriol. Rev. 36:407, 1972.

315. Schultz, J., and Elbein, A. D.: Biosynthesis of mannosyl- and glucosyl-phosphoryl polyprenols in *Mycobacterium smegmatis*: Evidence for oligosaccharide-phosphoryl-polyprenols. Arch. Biochem. Biophys. 160:311, 1974.

316. Segal, W.: Comparative study of *Mycobacterium* grown *in vivo* and *in vitro*. V. Differences in staining properties. Am. Rev. Respir. Dis. 91:285, 1965.

317. Segal, W., and Bloch, H.: Pathogenic and immunogenic differentiation of *Mycobacterium tuberculosis* grown *in vitro* and *in vivo*. Am. Rev. Tuberc. Pulm. Dis. 75:495, 1957.

318. Segal, W., and Miller, W. T.: Comparative study of *in vivo* and *in vitro* grown *Mycobacterium tuberculosis*. III. Lipid composition. Proc. Soc. Exp. Biol. Med. 118:613, 1965.

319. Sehrt, I., Kappler, W., and Lange, A.: Differentiation and identification of mycobacteria by means of thin layer chromatography of their lipids. II. Application for the classification of slowly growing mycobacteria: *M. avium* and *M. intracellulare*. Z. Erkr. Atm. 144:146, 1976.

320. Seibert, F. B.: The isolation of three different proteins and two polysaccharides from tuberculin by alcohol fractionation: their chemical and biological properties. Am. Rev. Tuberc. 59:86, 1949.

321. Shankaran, R., and Venkitasubramanian, T. A.: Effect of cord factor on carbohydrate metabolism in mice. Am. Rev. Respir. Dis. 101:401, 1970.

322. Shaw, N.: Bacterial glycolipids and glycophospholipids. Adv. Microb. Physiol. 12:141, 1975.

323. Smith, D. W., Harrell, W. K., and Randall, H. M.: Correlation of biologic properties of strains of mycobacterium with their infrared spectrums. III. Differentiation of bovine and human varieties of *M. tuberculosis* by means of their infrared spectrums. Am. Rev. Tuberc. 69:505, 1954.

324. Smith, D. W., Randall, H. M., Gastambide-Odier, M. M., and Koevoet, A. L.: The characterization of mycobacterial strains by the composition of their lipide extracts. Ann. N. Y. Acad. Sci. 69:145, 1957.

325. Smith, D. W., Randall, H. M., MacLennan, A. P., and Lederer, E.: Mycosides: a new class of type-specific glycolipids of mycobacteria. Nature 186:887, 1960.

326. Smith, D. W., Randall, H. M., MacLennan,

A. P., Putney, R. K., and Rao, S. V.: Detection of specific lipids in mycobacteria by infrared spectroscopy. J. Bacteriol. 79:217, 1960.

327. Smith, W. L., and Ballou, C. E.: The 6-O-methylglucose-containing lipopolysaccharides of *Mycobacterium phlei*. Locations of the neutral and acidic acyl groups. J. Biol. Chem. 248:7118, 1973.

328. Snow, G. A.: Mycobactins: Iron-chelating growth factors from mycobacteria. Bacteriol. Rev. 34:99, 1970.

329. Spikes, J. D., and Straight, R.: Sensitized photochemical processes in biological systems. Ann. Rev. Phys. Chem. 18:409, 1967.

330. Stewart-Tull, D. E. S., Shimono, T., Kotani, S., Kato, M., Ogawa, Y., Yamamura, Y., Koga, T., and Pearson, C. M.: The adjuvant activity of a non-toxic, water-soluble glycopeptide present in large quantities in the culture filtrate of *Mycobacterium tuberculosis* strain DT. Immunology 29:1, 1975.

331. Stewart-Tull, D. E. S., and White, R. G.: The occurrence of muramic acid in wax D preparations of mycobacteria. J. Gen. Microbiol. 34:43, 1964.

332. Stewart-Tull, D. E. S., and White, R. G.: The influence of age of culture on the production of adjuvant-active peptidoglycolipids by saprophytic mycobacteria. Immunology 12:349, 1967.

333. Strain, S. M., Toubiana, R., Ribi, E., and Parker, R.: Separation of the mixture of trehalose 6,6'-dimycolates comprising the mycobacterial glycolipid, fraction "P3." Biochem. Biophys. Res. Commun. 77:449, 1977.

334. Suzuki, T., Tanaka, H., and Itoh, S.: Sucrose lipids of Arthrobacter, Corynebacteria, and Nocardia grown on sucrose. Agr. Biol. Chem. (Tokyo) 38:557, 1974.

335. Szulga, T., Jenkins, P. A., and Marks, J.: Thin layer chromatography of mycobacterial lipids as an aid to classification; *Mycobacterium kansasii*; and *Mycobacterium marinum* (balnei). Tubercle 47:130, 1966.

335a. Takayama, K.: Personal communication, 1977.

336. Takayama, K., and Armstrong, E. L.: Mannolipid synthesis in a cell-free system of *M. smegmatis*. FEBS Letters 18:67, 1971.

337. Takayama, K., and Armstrong, E. L.: Isolation, characterization, and function of 6-mycolyl-6'-acetyltrehalose in the H37Ra strain of *Mycobacterium tuberculosis*. Biochemistry 15:441, 1976.

338. Takayama, K., Armstrong, E. L., and David, H. L.: Restoration of mycolate synthetase activity in *M. tuberculosis* exposed to INH. Am. Rev. Respir. Dis. 110:43, 1974.

339. Takayama, K., David, H. L., Wang, L., and Goldman, D. S.: Isolation and characterization of uridine diphosphate-N-glycolyl

muramyl-L-alanyl-α-D-glutamyl-meso-α,α' diaminopimelic acid from *Mycobacterium tuberculosis*. Biochem. Biophys. Res. Commun. 39:7, 1970.

340. Takayama, L., and Goldman, D. S.: Pathway for the synthesis of mannophospholipids in *Mycobacterium tuberculosis*. Biochim. Biophys. Acta 176:196, 1969.

341. Takayama, K., and Goldman, D. S.: Enzymatic synthesis of mannosyl-1-phosphoryl-decaprenol by a cell-free system of *Mycobacterium tuberculosis*. J. Biol. Chem. 245:6251, 1970.

342. Takayama, K., Qureshi, N., Schnoes, H. K., and Valicenti, A. J.: Pathway to the synthesis of mero-acid and site of inhibition of isoniazid in *Mycobacterium tuberculosis* H37Ra. *In* Proceedings, Twelfth U.S.-Japan Cooperative Medical Science Program, Tuberculosis Conference. 1977, p. 425.

343. Takayama, K., and Schnoes, H. K.: Inhibition in the synthesis of C_{28}-C_{40} fatty acids in *Mycobacterium tuberculosis* by isoniazid. Fed. Proc. 33:1425, 1974.

344. Takayama, K., Schnoes, H. K., and Semmler, E. J.: Characterization of the alkali-stable mannophospholipids of *Mycobacterium smegmatis*. Biochim. Biophys. Acta 316:212, 1973.

345. Takayama, K., Schnoes, H. K., Armstrong, E. L., and Boyle, R. W.: Site of inhibitory action of isoniazid in the synthesis of mycolic acids in *Mycobacterium tuberculosis*. J. Lipid Res. 16:308, 1975.

346. Takayama, K., Wang, L., and David, H. L.: Effects of isoniazid on the *in vivo* mycolic acid synthesis, cell growth, and viability of *Mycobacterium tuberculosis*. Antimicrob. Agents Chemother. 2:29, 1972.

347. Takeya, K., and Hisatsune, K.: Mycobacterial cell walls. I. Methods of preparation and treatment with various chemicals. J. Bacteriol. 85:16, 1963.

348. Takeya, K., Hisatsune, K., and Inoue, Y.: Mycobacterial cell walls. II. Chemical composition of the "basal" layer. J. Bacteriol. 85:24, 1963.

349. Takeya, K., Hisatsune, K., and Nakashima, K.: A cell-wall mucopeptide complex obtained from the culture filtrate of tubercle bacilli. Biochim. Biophys. Acta 54:595, 1961.

350. Tanaka, K., Tanaka, A., and Sugiyama, K.: Immunological adjuvants. I. Adjuvant activity and immunogenicity of acetylated wax D and its subfractions. Int. Arch. Allergy 34:495, 1968.

351. Tarnok, I., and Tarnok, Z.: Carotenes and xanthophylls in mycobacteria. I. Technical procedures; thin layer chromatographic patterns of mycobacterial pigments. Tubercle 51:305, 1970.

352. Thomas, D. W., Das, B. C., Gero, S. D., and Lederer, E.: Advantages and limitations

of the mass spectrometric determination of permethylated oligopeptide derivatives. Biochem. Biophys. Res. Commun. *32*:199, 1968.

353. Tocanne, J.-F.: Sur une nouvelle voie de synthèse du cord-factor, glycolipide toxique de *Mycobacterium tuberculosis* (Esters du tréhalose et d'acides gras α-ramifiés β-hydroxylés) Carbohydr. Res. *44*:301, 1975.

354. Toida, I.: Effects of cord factor on pyrazinamide deamidase. Am. Rev. Respir. Dis. *108*:694, 1973.

355. Toida, I.: Effects of cord factor on microsomal enzymes. Am. Rev. Respir. Dis. *110*:641, 1974.

356. Tokunaga, T., Kataoka, T., and Suga, K.: Phage inactivation by an ethanol-ether extract of *Mycobacterium smegmatis*. Am. Rev. Respir. Dis. *101*:309, 1970.

357. Tokunaga, T., Sellers, M. I., and Furuchi, A.: Phage receptor of *Mycobacterium smegmatis*. In Juhasz, J. E., and Plummer, G. (eds.): Host Virus Relationships in *Mycobacterium, Nocardia* and *Actinomycetes*. Springfield, Ill., Charles C Thomas, 1970, p. 119.

357a. Toubiana, R.: Personal communication, 1974.

358. Toubiana, R., Das, B. C., Defaye, J., Mompon, B., and Toubiana, M.-J.: Étude du cord-factor et de sa analogues. III. Synthèse du cord-factor (6,6'-di-O-mycoloyl trehalose) et du 6,6'-di-O-palmitoyl-α,α-trehalose. Carbohydr. Res. *44*:308, 1975.

359. Toubiana, R., Ribi, E., McLaughlin, C., and Strain, S. M.: The effect of synthetic and naturally occurring trehalose fatty acid esters in tumor regression. Cancer Immunol. Immunother. *2*:189, 1977.

360. Tsukamura, S.: Biological significance of pigments of bacteria. III. Resistance to ultra violet irradiation of various unclassified mycobacteria. Jpn. J. Tuberc. *12*:7, 1964.

361. Tung, K. K., and Ballou, C. E.: Biosynthesis of a mycobacterial lipopolysaccharide. Properties of the polysaccharide: acyl CoA acyltransferase reaction. J. Biol. Chem. *248*:7126, 1973.

362. Ungar, J.: Granuloma-producing properties of synthetic fatty acids. In Wolstenholme, G. E. W., Cameron, M. P., and O'Connor, C. M. (eds.): Experimental Tuberculosis. Ciba Foundation Symposia, 1955, p. 69.

363. Vance, D. E., Esders, T. W., and Bloch, K.: Purification and properties of the fatty acid synthetase from *Mycobacterium phlei*. J. Biol. Chem. *248*:2303, 1973.

364. Vilkas, E.: Sur divers types de phospholipides présents dans le Bacille Calmette-Guèrin. Bull. Soc. Chim. Biol. *42*:1005, 1960.

365. Vilkas, E.: Analogie des structures des my-cosides C_2 de *Mycobacterium avium* et C_b de *Mycobacterium butyricum*. C. R. Acad. Sci. (Paris) serie C *262*:786, 1966.

366. Vilkas, E., Amar, C., Markovits, J., Vliegenthart, J. F. G., and Kamerling, J. P.: Occurrence of a galactofuranose disaccharide in immunoadjuvant fractions of *Mycobacterium tuberculosis*. Biochim. Biophys. Acta *297*:423, 1973.

367. Vilkas, E., Adam, A., and Senn, M.: Isolément d'un nouveau type de diester de trehalose à partir de *Mycobacterium fortuitum*. Chem. Phys. Lipids *2*:11, 1968.

368. Vilkas, E., Gros, C., and Massot, J.-C.: Sur la structure chimique d'un mycoside C isolé de *Mycobacterium scrofulaceum*. C. R. Acad. Sci. (Paris) serie C, *266*:837, 1968.

369. Vilkas, E., and Lederer, E.: N-methylation de peptides par la methode de Hakomori. Structure du mycoside C_{b1}. Tetrahedron Lett. *26*:3089, 1968.

370. Vilkas, E., Rojas, A., Das, B. C., Wolstenholme, W. A., and Lederer, E.: Determination de séquences d'acides aminés dans des oligopeptides par la spectrometrie de masse. VI. Structure du mycoside C_b, peptidoglycolipide de *Mycobacterium butyricum*. Tetrahedron Lett. *22*:2809, 1966.

371. Vilkas, E., Rojas, A., and Lederer, E.: Sur un nouvel acide aminé naturel, la N-méthyl O-méthyl-L-serine des mycosides de *Mycobacterium butyricum* et *Mycobacterium avium*. C. R. Acad. Sci. (Paris) serie C, *261*:4258, 1965.

372. Ville, C., and Gastambide-Odier, M.: Le 3-O-methyl-L-rhamnose, sucre isolé du mycoside G de *Mycobacterium marinum*. Carbohydr. Res. *12*:97, 1970.

373. Voiland, A., Bruneteau, M., and Michel, G.: Étude du mycoside C_2 de *Mycobacterium avium*. Eur. J. Biochem. *21*:285, 1971.

374. Volpe, J. J., and Vagelos, P. R.: Saturated fatty acid biosynthesis and its regulation. Ann. Rev. Biochem. *42*:21, 1973.

375. Walczak, E., and Etemadi, A. H.: Sur la structure et la biogenèse des acids α-avimycoliques de *Mycobacterium avium*. C. R. Acad. Sci. *261*:2771, 1965.

376. Walker, R. W., Barakat, H., and Hung, J. G. C.: The positional distribution of fatty acids in the phospholipids and triglycerides of *Mycobacterium smegmatis* and *M. bovis* BCG. Lipids *5*:684, 1970.

377. Walker, R. W., Promé, J.-C., and Lacave, C. S.: Biosynthesis of mycolic acids. Formation of a C_{32} β-keto ester from palmitic acid in a cell-free system of *Corynebacterium diphtheriae*. Biochim. Biophys. Acta *326*:52, 1973.

378. Weir, M..P., Langridge, W. H. R., and Walker, R. W.: Relationships between oleic acid uptake and lipid metabolism in *Mycobacterium smegmatis*. Am. Rev. Respir. Dis. *106*:450, 1972.

379. Weiss, D. W., and Yashphe, D. J.: Nonspe-

cific stimulation of anti-microbial and anti-tumor resistance and of immunological responsiveness by the MER fraction of tubercle bacilli. *In* Weiss, D. W., and Zuckerman, A. (eds.): Dynamic Aspects of Host-Parastie Relationships. New York, Academic Press, 1973.

380. White, R. G.: Discussion (following Ungar, 1955). *In* Wolstenholme, G. E., Cameron, M. P., and O'Connor, C. M. (eds.): Experimental Tuberculosis. Ciba Foundation Symposia, 1955, p. 82.

381. White, R. G.: Role of adjuvants in the production of delayed hypersensitivity. Brit. Med. Bull. *23*:39, 1967.

382. White, R. G., Bernstock, L., Johns, R. G. S., and Lederer, E.: The influence of components of *M. tuberculosis* and other *Mycobacteria* upon antibody production to ovalbumin. Immunology *1*:54, 1958.

383. White, R. G., Jollès, P., Samour, O., and Lederer, E.: Correlation of adjuvant activity and chemical structure of wax D fractions of mycobacteria. Immunology *7*:158, 1964.

384. Wietzerbin-Falszpan, J., Das, B. C., Azuma, I., Adam, A., Petit, J.-F., and Lederer, E.: Isolation and mass spectrometric identification of the peptide subunits of mycobacterial cell walls. Biochem. Biophys. Res. Commun. *40*:57, 1970.

385. Wietzerbin, J., Das, B. C., Petit, J.-F., Lederer, E., Leyh-Bouille, M., and Ghuysen, J.-M.: Occurrence of D-alanyl-(D)-*meso*-diaminopimelic acid and *meso*-diaminopimelyl-*meso*-diaminopimelic acid interpeptide linkages in the peptidoglycan of Mycobacteria. Biochemistry *13*:3471, 1974.

386. Winder, F. G.: The antibacterial action of streptomycin, isoniazid and PAS. *In* Barry, V. C. (ed.): Chemotherapy of Tuberculosis. London, Butterworths, 1964, p. 111.

387. Winder, F. G., and Collins, P. B.: Inhibition by isoniazid of synthesis of mycolic acids in *Mycobacterium tuberculosis*. J. Gen. Microbiol. *63*:41, 1970.

388. Winder, F. G., Tighe, J. J., and Brennan, P. J.: Turnover of acylglucose, acyltrehalose and free trehalose during growth of *Mycobacterium smegmatis* on glucose. J. Gen. Microbiol. *73*:539, 1972.

389. Winder, F. G., and Rooney, S. A.: Effects of isoniazid on the triglycerides of BCG. Am. Rev. Respir. Dis. *97*:938, 1968.

390. Wolinsky, E., and Schaefer, W. B.: Proposed numbering scheme for mycobacterial serotypes by agglutination. Int. J. Syst. Bacteriol. *23*:182, 1976.

391. Woodward, R. B.: Neuere entwicklungen in der chemie der naturstoffe. Angew Chem. *68*:13, 1956.

391a. Yarkoni, E.: Personal communication, 1977.

392. Yarkoni, E., Meltzer, M. S., and Rapp, H. J.: Tumor regression after intralesional injection of emulsified trehalose-6,6'-dimycolate (cord factor): Efficacy increases with oil concentration. Int. J. Cancer *19*:818, 1977.

392a. Yarkoni, E., Goren, M. B., and Rapp, H. J.: Regression of a transplanted guinea pig hepatoma after intralesional injection of an emulsified mixture of endotoxin and mycobacterial sulfolipid. (Submitted).

393. Yarkoni, E., Wang, L., and Bekierkunst, A.: Suppression of growth of Ehrlich ascites tumor cells in mice by trehalose-6,6'-dimycolate (cord factor) and BCG. Infect. Immun. *9*:977, 1974.

394. Yarkoni, E., Wang, L., and Bekierkunst, A.: Stimulation of macrophages by cord factor (trehalose-6,6'-dimycolate) and by heat-killed and living BCG. Infect. Immun. *16*:1, 1977.

395. Yegian, D., and Vanderlinde, R. J.: The nature of acid-fastness. J. Bacteriol. *54*:777, 1947.

396. Youatt, S.: A review of the action of isoniazid. Amer. Rev. Respir. Dis. *99*:729, 1969.

397. Youmans, G. P., and Youmans, A. S.: An acute pulmonary granulomatous response in mice produced by mycobacterial cells and its relation to increased resistance and increased susceptibility to experimental tuberculous infection. J. Infect. Dis. *114*:135, 1964.

398. Zbar, B., Bernstein, I. D., Bartlett, G. L., Hanna, M. G., and Rapp, H. J.: Immunotherapy of cancer: regression of intradermal tumors and prevention of growth of lymph node metastases after intralesional injection of living *Mycobacterium bovis*. J. Natl. Cancer Inst. *49*:119, 1972.

399. Zbar, B., Ribi, E., Meyer, T. J., Azuma, I., and Rapp, H. J.: Immunotherapy of cancer: Regression of established intradermal tumors after intralesional injection of mycobacterial cell walls attached to oil droplets. J. Natl. Cancer Inst. *52*:1571, 1974.

5

Virulence of Mycobacteria

INTRODUCTION

One of the most puzzling features of the host-parasite interaction in tuberculosis has been the nature of the mechanism or mechanisms, that permits the tubercle bacillus to produce disease. With many bacteria, their capacity to produce an exotoxin, a capsule that prevents phagocytosis, or extracellular enzymes can be correlated with their capacity to produce disease. No similar situation exists in the case of *Mycobacterium tuberculosis.* Therefore, most workers have ascribed the capacity of the tubercle bacillus to produce disease merely to its capacity to multiply within host tissues and, at the same time, to be able to withstand host defense mechanisms. The fact that mycobacteria are appreciably more resistant to deleterious agents, such as acids, alkalis, and germicides, supports this concept. In addition, relatively enormous numbers[46] of living or

killed cells of *M. tuberculosis* can be injected into animals by any one of a variety of routes without causing obvious distress. Naturally, animals so injected with living virulent cells will eventually develop progressive disease and die.

The point we wish to emphasize here is that little or no sign of toxicity can be detected, even though, for example, as many as 10^7 or 10^8 living cells are injected intravenously into mice.[46] Such findings suggest that the tubercle bacillus elaborates no exotoxins, endotoxins, or extracellular enzymes that are deleterious, and since viable tubercle bacilli are rapidly phagocytosed even in the absence of antibody, no capsular material is produced that might interfere with phagocytosis. Actually, the microorganism not only is rapidly phagocytosed by reticuloendothelial cells but also multiplies within these cells, almost without hindrance, until the de-

194

velopment of acquired immunity (see Chapter 8).

However, the situation is not quite as simple or straightforward as outlined in the preceding paragraphs, because toxic factors have been isolated from mycobacterial cells and some of these factors may play a role in the pathogenesis of the disease. The substance that has received the greatest attention is cord factor, trehalose 6,6'-dimycolate. (Cord factor was referred to briefly in Chapter 3 and is fully described and discussed in Chapter 4.)

CORD FACTOR

The discovery of cord factor stemmed from the observation by Middlebrook and his colleagues in 1947[32] that there was a high correlation between the virulence of strains of mycobacteria and their capacity to grow in cords (Fig. 2–3). Middlebrook and his associates[32] noted that the highly virulent strains, such as *M. tuberculosis* and *M. bovis,* regularly grew in cords when cultivated on artificial media, whereas the attenuated and avirulent strains did not. These investigators inferred from their findings that virulent tubercle bacilli produce a cell surface substance that made them stick together after cell division, and Middlebrook and his coworkers felt that this substance might be a virulence factor.

Bloch in 1950[3] found that certain organic solvents and in particular, petroleum ether, when added to cultures of cord-forming mycobacteria, rapidly abolished cord formation because, after treatment with petroleum ether, the cells were dispersed in a rather heterogeneous manner. From petroleum ether extracts of large quantities of virulent mycobacterial cells, Bloch isolated a lipid fraction, which he termed "cord factor." Cord factor in single large doses of up to 50 milligrams, in-

jected intraperitoneally into mice, had no apparent deleterious effect on these animals. However, if given repeatedly, very small doses of cord factor—as little as 0.02 milligrams — had profound toxic effects; mice rapidly lost weight and died within a few days. Cord factor was also found to inhibit the migration of leukocytes.

In a series of subsequent studies, Bloch and his collaborators as well as other researchers[1, 2, 3, 5, 34-36] identified the active agent in their petroleum ether extracts as trehalose 6,6'-dimycolate. Thus, a toxic substance from virulent mycobacterial cells had been identified and isolated. Therefore, there was reason to think that a virulence factor had been identified. Unfortunately, it was soon found[33] that cord factor was present in completely avirulent mycobacteria, such as *M. phlei* and *M. smegmatis,* and in certain atypical mycobacteria. It follows, then, that while cord factor may play a role in disease production by virulent mycobacteria and may even be a necessary factor for pathogenicity, it certainly is not the only or necessarily the most important factor in disease production by mycobacteria.

Direct evidence of a role for cord factor in disease production by virulent mycobacteria was lacking until 1972, when Kato[20, 21] found that cord factor complexed with methylated bovine serum albumin became antigenic and that antibodies could be produced specific for cord factor. When mice were immunized against cord factor, up to the point at which antibodies were produced, and then challenged with virulent tubercle bacilli, the animals showed a much greater resistance to tuberculous infection than was demonstrated previously. Kato postulated that the extended survival of animals immunized against cord factor was a consequence of the neutralization of the toxicity of cord factor by antibody. That antibody to cord factor was the actual agent involved in the prolonged survival was shown by the fact that increased resistance to tuberculous infection could be induced by passively immunizing mice with antibody to cord factor. These results suggest that cord factor does play some role in disease production by mycobacteria. Of particular interest were the findings of Kato,[20, 21] which showed that no cord factor-specific antibodies were produced in animals immunized with viable BCG cells containing cord factor. However, these animals did develop appreciable increased resistance to infection. Therefore, immunity to tuberculosis induced by BCG vaccines or by other living mycobacterial cells cannot be ascribed to the production of antibody against cord factor. All in all, while cord factor contributes something to the virulence of mycobacterial cells, it is probably safe to assume that it is not a major factor in their capacity to produce disease. More information on cord factor — its toxicity, relation to virulence, mode of action on mammalian cells, and biologic effects — will be found in Chapter 4.

OTHER TOXIC LIPIDS

Spitznagel and Dubos[43] reported the isolation of another toxic lipid from mycobacterial cells. However, Bloch and colleagues[4] found that the toxicity of the Spitznagel and Dubos lipid fraction was due to the presence of small amounts of cord factor.

Other lipids have been implicated in the virulence of mycobacteria. In 1959 Middlebrook and coworkers reported the isolation of sulfolipids,[31] which are a group of several multiacylated trehalose sulfate derivatives[11-13] that do not contain mycolic acids or exhibit the type of toxicity characteristic of cord factor. However, according to Goren and his coworkers,[14] the sulfolipids will enhance the toxicity of cord factor. Furthermore, Gangadharam and colleagues examined a series of strains of *M. tuberculosis* isolated in Britain and India.[9, 10] Using aerogenic infection in guinea pigs, they found that these strains varied considerably in virulence. The researchers were able to rank the strains according to their virulence and found a high correlation between the sulfolipid content of the strains and the order of infectivity for guinea pigs. In 1974 Goren and his colleagues[15] confirmed that there was a high correlation between sulfolipid concentration and degree of virulence of the mycobacterial strains for guinea pigs.

The sulfolipids may not only promote virulence of mycobacteria by enhancing toxicity of cord factor, but they may also enhance infection by inhibiting lysosome-phagosome fusion. It has recently been shown that lysosome-phagosome fusion after ingestion of tubercle bacilli by macrophages is markedly less when virulent tubercle bacilli are involved than when avirulent mycobacteria are phagocytosed.[18] Thus, the capacity of virulent tubercle bacilli to grow within macrophages might conceivably be conditioned by the failure of lysosome-phagosome fusion. Such fusion may be required for the inhibition of multiplication of the ingested mycobacteria. It has been shown recently by Goren and coworkers[15] that the sulfolipids are potent inhibitors of lysosome-phagosome fusion and, therefore, might conceivably promote the virulence of tubercle bacilli in this manner (see Chapter 4 for further details).

The sulfolipids,[14] together with the phospholipids, probably account for the binding of neutral red dye in the "Neutral Red" virulence test of Middlebrook and colleagues.[32] Therefore, in view of the high correlation between the production of sulfolipids by mycobacterial strains and their virulence for man, the validity of the Neutral Red test as a measure for virulence of *M. tuberculosis* is greatly enhanced (see Chapter 4 for additional information).

As we have just seen, strains of *M. tuberculosis* can vary considerably in their capacity to produce disease in man. Whether or not this variation in disease-producing power is directly related to the capacity of different strains to produce certain lipids and other substances is not known for certain, in spite of the correlation between sulfolipid production and virulence. The situation is a complicated one because mycobacterial virulence can be defined just as easily in terms of host response, and perhaps more validly, than in terms of some property or characteristic of the bacillus. By this we mean that host immune responses may be more rapid and complete against some strains of *M. tuberculosis* than others. Thus, the more rapid and complete the immune response, the less virulent the infecting strain of *M. tuberculosis* will appear to be. (More will be said about this in Chapter 8, where it will be pointed out that the rapidity of the immune response appears to be responsible for the varying susceptibility of various species of animals to infection with mycobacteria.)

Goren and coworkers[15] also obtained findings that suggested phthiocerol dimycocerosate may play a role in the virulence of tubercle bacilli. Interestingly, the attenuated mycobacterial strains studied by Goren and his colleagues[15] contained another substance — phenolic phthioceroldiester. This lipid was not seen in any of the more virulent strains studied. Thus, the absence of a lipid might be of importance in the virulence of *M. tuberculosis*. A more detailed consideration of the relation to virulence and of the structure and biologic activities of these mycobacterial lipids can be found in Chapter 4.

ROLE OF IRON IN VIRULENCE

Other factors that might be concerned in the virulence of mycobacteria should be considered. For example, Kochan[24, 24a] and Kochan and coworkers[25] have pointed out the absolute dependence of mycobacteria on the presence of sufficient iron for growth. When growing in vivo, the tubercle bacillus depends upon the production of mycobactin (see Fig. 4–33), a substance that can retrieve iron from transferrin, thus allowing the virulent tubercle bacilli to grow. Since according to Kochan,[24] mycobactin is essential for this purpose, it might be referred to as a virulence factor, although it exerts no untoward effect directly on the host.

On the other hand, Macham and coworkers[27, 28] have shown that mycobactin serves only as a means of transporting iron across the mycobacterial cell wall. Macham and associates[27, 28] isolated two substances from cultures of mycobacteria. These substances, which they called "exochelins," would chelate with and solubilize iron. The exochelins could remove iron from ferritin and make it available to mycobacterial cells. These exochelins were soluble and dialyzable and were recovered from the culture medium in which mycobacteria, such as BCG or *M. smegmatis,* were grown. The exochelins were not precursors or breakdown products of mycobactin. Although they have no deleterious effect on animal hosts, the exochelins might also be thought of as virulence factors (see Chapter 4 for further discussion).

ROLE OF OXYGEN IN VIRULENCE

As we pointed out in Chapter 2, *M. tuberculosis* — like most, if not all, mycobacteria — is a strict aerobe. This can be recognized because of the following observation: although *M. tuberculosis* will grow at reduced oxygen tensions, all growth ceases when the supply of oxygen is exhausted, even though other nutritional conditions are favorable (see Chapter 2).

One might suspect that this dependence upon molecular oxygen for growth would play a role in the capacity of M. tuberculosis to multiply in vivo. A number of features of the growth of M. tuberculosis in vivo, both in natural disease and under experimental conditions, confirm this theory. For example, the lung is the favorite site of infection with M. tuberculosis. This predilection can probably be accounted for on the basis of the higher oxygen tension found in that organ. It has also been suggested that the apices of the lungs are the commonest site of reinfection tuberculosis because of their higher oxygen tension. The blood flow is less in the apices, and oxygen is less readily removed from the alveoli.[8, 29, 38]

The role of oxygen tension in the development of mycobacterial disease in the lungs was shown experimentally by Sever and Youmans.[42] These investigators infected mice intravenously with the H37Rv strain of M. tuberculosis and housed the mice in artificial atmospheres containing different amounts of oxygen. When these mice were maintained in an atmosphere containing 40 percent oxygen instead of the 20 percent found in air, the pulmonary disease progressed much more rapidly and became more extensive than when they were housed in a normal atmosphere. On the other hand, when the mice were housed in an artificial atmosphere containing only 10 percent oxygen, the pulmonary disease progressed more slowly.

Rich and Follis had previously obtained similar results, using 10 percent oxygen atmosphere.[40]

Of particular interest in these studies of Sever and Youmans[42] was the following fact: when mice were infected intravenously with either BCG cells or viable cells of the H37Ra strain and then housed in an atmosphere with a high oxygen content (40 percent), the attenuated mycobacterial cells grew more rapidly and reached a larger number in the lungs of the animals than when mice were housed in air containing the normal amount (20 percent) of oxygen. Thus, the capacity of attenuated strains to multiply in the lungs of mice is, in part, dependent upon the oxygen tension.

Similar observations have been made by a number of investigators when cultivating M. tuberculosis in vitro. It can readily be shown[16, 23, 26, 37] that the rate and amount of growth in vitro is directly proportional to the oxygen content of the atmosphere in which the cells are grown. This acceleration of growth continued in concentrations of oxygen ranging up to about 40 percent by volume (see Chapter 2). Above this level, however, increasing concentrations of oxygen actually inhibit growth. Growth is completely prevented when an atmosphere of 100 percent oxygen is provided.[16, 37]

Heplar and colleagues[19] and Guy and his coworkers[17] compared the effect of oxygen on the growth of the virulent H37Rv strain of M. tuberculosis and its attenuated variant, the H37Ra strain. They noted that the respiration of the virulent cells was not as readily inhibited at low oxygen concentrations as that of the avirulent H37Ra cells. They speculated that the capacity of the H37Rv strain to produce progressive disease might be due to the ability of this strain to respire, grow, and multiply at lower oxygen tensions. This attractive explanation for the virulence of some mycobacterial strains is not supported, however, by the work of Sever and Youmans, previously referred to. These investigators[42] found that while attenuated strains, such as BCG and H37Ra, would multiply to a slight degree in the lungs of mice maintained in an atmosphere containing 20 percent oxygen, they multiplied to a greater extent when the oxygen tension in the lungs was increased. Nevertheless, even under these conditions of maximal availability of oxygen, neither of these attenuated strains was able to produce progressive disease. Therefore, it is reasonable to conclude that although the oxygen requirement of mycobacteria may be very important in production of disease, it cannot be the sole factor involved in the capacity of virulent strains to multiply in tissue.

In earlier years, investigators thought that the dependence of tubercle bacilli on oxygen derived from the requirement for the direct oxidation of substrates such as glycerol and glucose. It has been shown by Ramakrishnan and colleagues[39] that tubercle bacilli and other mycobacteria do have a glycolytic system and, therefore, are able to dissimulate glucose anaerobically. These investigators measured the capacity of the glycolytic system to function in virulent and attenuated mycobacterial cells. They found that the glycolytic system functioned more effectively in the virulent H37Rv strain than in the attenuated H37Ra strain. They speculated that virulence might be dependent upon the ability of certain mycobacterial cells to utilize anaerobic methods for the dissimilation of glucose.

When considering any metabolic basis for virulence of mycobacteria, we must note that many isoniazid-resistant strains of *M. tuberculosis* have a markedly reduced virulence for guinea pigs; at the same time, these strains have a markedly reduced catalase activity.[22, 30] The basis for this low virulence is assumed to be the lack of capacity of these strains to break down hydrogen peroxide, since it is known that hydrogen peroxide production by phagocytic cells is a critical factor in their capacity to kill ingested bacteria.[7] Virulent mycobacteria, on the other hand, have high catalase activity, and this may contribute to their virulence. Once again, this cannot be regarded as the sole or even a major factor in virulence, since a variety of saprophytic mycobacteria and strains of low virulence also can have high catalase activity.[41]

In Chapter 2, we described the results of Wayne's experiments,[44] in which he obtained synchronous growth of virulent tubercle bacilli by allowing the mycobacterial cells to settle slowly to the bottom of a tube of culture medium that contained Tween 80. In the process of settling, the tubercle bacilli were exposed to decreasing concentrations of oxygen. In the oxygen-free sediment, the tubercle bacilli ceased multiplying but remained viable for prolonged periods. Apparently, the slow exposure to decreasing concentrations of oxygen allowed the microorganisms to adjust in such a manner that viability was retained, but ability to reproduce was lost. When restored to an environment that contained adequate oxygen, multiplication resumed, but the cells divided synchronously. In contrast, Wayne and Diaz[45] reported that if virulent tubercle bacilli were suddenly deprived of oxygen, rapid death and autolysis of the mycobacterial cells occurred. Wayne and Diaz[45] considered the possibility that the dormant state of tubercle bacilli in culture, produced as described here, might be equivalent to the dormant state known to occur in vivo. In this state, tubercle bacilli can remain viable, without multiplying, for prolonged periods of time (see Chapter 8). This may also have an important relationship to the nature of the acquired immune response in tuberculosis (see Chapter 12). The capacity of the tubercle bacillus to adjust its metabolism so as to remain viable but nonmultiplying in vivo for long periods of time might well be thought of as a virulence mechanism. In this connection, there is some evidence that tubercle bacilli may increase in virulence by residence in vivo. When tubercle bacilli harvested from the lungs of infected mice were reinjected into normal mice, Collins and Montalbine[6] reported that in the lungs of the recipient mice, a significantly greater number of the lung-grown tubercle bacilli had settled than had cells of the same strain of tubercle bacilli grown in vitro. The nature of this increased lung tropism produced by residence of bacilli in vivo is not known.

CONCLUSIONS

We can conclude that the capacity of *M. tuberculosis* to produce progressive disease may involve certain toxic factors, such as cord factor, perhaps other lipid constituents, oxygen requirement, catalase activity, and ability to solubilize iron. However, none of these, singly or together, can account completely for virulence; nor can any one or all of these account for the high virulence of certain strains, the low virulence of others, or the lack of virulence of mutants of virulent strains.

REFERENCES

1. Asselineau, J., Bloch, H., and Lederer, E.: A toxic lipid component of the tubercle bacillus ("cord factor"). III. Occurrence and distribution in various bacterial extracts. Am. Rev. Tuberc. 67:853, 1953.
2. Asselineau, J., and Lederer, E.: Sur la constitution du "cord factor" isolé d'une souche humaine de bacille tuberculeux. Biochim. Biophys. Acta 17:161, 1955.
3. Bloch, H.: Studies on the virulence of tubercle bacilli. Isolation and biological properties of a constituent of virulent organisms. J. Exp. Med. 91:197, 1950.
4. Bloch, H., Defaye, J., Lederer, E., and Noll, H.: Constituents of a "toxic-lipid" obtained from *Mycobacterium tuberculosis*. Biochim. Biophys. Acta 23:312, 1957.
5. Bloch, H., Sorkin, E., and Erlenmeyer, H.: A toxic lipid component of the tubercle bacillus ("cord factor"). I. Isolation from petroleum ether extracts of young bacterial cultures. Am. Rev. Tuberc. 67:629, 1953.
6 Collins, F. M., and Montalbine, V.: Distribution of mycobacteria grown *in vivo* in the organs of intravenously infected mice. Am. Rev. Respir. Dis. 113:281, 1976.

7. Davis, A. T., and Quie, P. G.: Phagocytes and phagocytosis. *In* Stiehm, E. R., and Fulginiti, V. A.: Immunologic Disorders in Infants and Children. Philadelphia, W. B. Saunders Co., 1973.
8. Dock, W.: Apical localization of phthisis. Its significance in treatment by prolonged rest in bed. Am. Rev. Tuberc. 53:297, 1946.
9. Gangadharam, P. R. J., Cohn, M. L., Davis, C. L., and Middlebrook, G.: Infectivity and pathogenicity of Indian and British strains of tubercle bacilli studied by aerogenic infection of guinea pigs. Am. Rev. Respir. Dis. 87:200, 1963.
10. Gangadharam, P. R. J., Cohn, M. L., and Middlebrook, G.: Infectivity, pathogenicity and sulpholipid fraction of some Indian and British strains of tubercle bacilli. Tubercle 44:452, 1963.
11. Goren, M. B.: Mycobacterial sulfolipids: Spontaneous desulfation. Lipids 6:40, 1971.
12. Goren, M. B.: Sulfolipid I of *Mycobacterium tuberculosis*, strain $H_{37}Rv$. I. Purification and properties. Biochim. Biophys. Acta 210:116, 1970.
13. Goren, M. B., Brokl, O., Das, B. C., and Lederer, E.: Sulfolipid I of *Mycobacterium tuberculosis*, strain H37Rv. Nature of the acyl substituents. Biochemistry 10:72, 1971.
14. Goren, M. B., Brokl, O., and Schaefer, W. B.: Lipids of putative relevance to virulence in *Mycobacterium tuberculosis*: correlation of virulence with elaboration of sulfatides and strongly acidic lipids. Infect. Immun. 9:142, 1974.
15. Goren, M. B., Brokl, O., and Schaefer, W. B.: Lipids of putative relevance to virulence in *Mycobacterium tuberculosis*: phthiocerol dimycocerosate and the attenuation indicator lipid. Infect. Immun. 9:150, 1974.
16. Gottlieb, S. F., Rose, N. R., Maurizi, J., and Lanphier, E. H.: Oxygen inhibition of growth of *Mycobacterium tuberculosis*. J. Bacteriol. 87:838, 1964.
17. Guy, L. R., Raffel, S., and Clifton, C. E.: Virulence of the tubercle bacillus. II. Effect of oxygen tension upon growth of virulent and avirulent bacilli. J. Infect. Dis. 94:99, 1954.
18. Hart, P. D., and Armstrong, J. A.: Strain virulence and the lysosomal response in macrophages infected with *Mycobacterium tuberculosis*. Infect. Immun. 10:742, 1974.
19. Heplar, J. Q., Clifton, C. E., Raffel, S., and Futrelle, C. M.: Virulence of the tubercle bacillus. I. Effect of oxygen tension upon respiration of virulent and avirulent bacilli. J. Infect. Dis. 94:90, 1954.
20. Kato, M.: Antibody formation to trehalose-6,6'-dimycolate (cord factor) of *Mycobac-*

terium tuberculosis. Infect. Immun. 5:203, 1972.

21. Kato, M.: Effect of anti-cord factor antibody on experimental tuberculosis in mice. Infect. Immun. 7:14, 1973.

22. Knox, R., Meadow, P. M., and Worssam, A. R. H.: The relationship between the catalase activity, hydrogen peroxide sensitivity, and isoniazid resistance of mycobacteria. Am. Rev. Tuberc. 73:726, 1956.

23. Knox, R., Thomas, C. G. A., Lister, A. J., and Saxby, C.: The effect of oxygen on the growth of *Mycobacterium tuberculosis* in semi-solid agar. Guy's Hospital Reports 110:174, 1961.

24. Kochan, I.: The role of iron in bacterial infections, with special consideration of host-tubercle bacillus interaction. Curr. Top. Microbiol. Immunol. 60:1, 1973.

24a. Kochan, I.: Nutritional regulation of antibacterial resistance. *In* Schlessinger, D. (ed.): Microbiology — 1974. Washington, D.C., American Society for Microbiology, 1974.

25. Kochan, I., Cahall, D. L., and Golden, C. A.: Employment of tuberculostasis in serum-agar medium for the study of production and activity of mycobactin. Infect. Immun. 4:130, 1971.

26. Lebek, G.: Die Abhängigkeit der Sauerstoffoptimums der beiden Säugetiertypen des Mycobacterium tuberculosis von den angebotenen Nährstoffen. Zbl. Bakt. (Orig) 176:530, 1959.

27. Macham, L. P., and Ratledge, C.: A new group of water-soluble iron-binding compounds from mycobacteria: the exochelins. J. Gen. Microbiol. 89:379, 1975.

28. Macham, L. P., Ratledge, C., and Nocton, J. C.: Extracellular iron acquisition by mycobacteria: Role of the exochelins and evidence against the participation of mycobactin. Infect. Immun. 12:1242, 1975.

29. Medlar, E. M., and Sasano, K. T.: A study of the pathology of experimental pulmonary tuberculosis in the rabbit. Am. Rev. Tuberc. 34:456, 1936.

30. Middlebrook, G., and Cohn, M. L.: Some observations on the pathogenicity of isoniazid-resistant variants of tubercle bacilli. Science 118:297, 1953.

31. Middlebrook, G., Coleman, C., and Schaefer, W. B.: Sulfolipid from virulent tubercle bacilli. Proc. Natl. Acad. Sci. U.S.A. 45:1801, 1959.

32. Middlebrook, G., Dubos, R. J., and Pierce, C.: Virulence and morphological characteristics of mammalian tubercle bacilli. J. Exp. Med. 86:175, 1947.

33. Nagasuga, T., Terai, T., and Yamamura, Y.: Studies on the toxic lipid of isoniazid-resistant human tubercle bacilli. Am. Rev. Respir. Dis. 83:248, 1961.

34. Noll, H., and Bloch, H.: Studies on the chemistry of the cord factor of *Mycobacterium tuberculosis*. J. Biol. Chem. 214:251, 1955.

35. Noll, H., and Bloch, H.: A toxic lipid component of the tubercle bacillus ("cord factor"). II. Occurrence in chloroform extracts of young and older bacterial cultures. Am. Rev. Tuberc. 67:828, 1953.

36. Noll, H., Bloch, H., Asselineau, J., and Lederer, E.: The chemical structure of the cord factor of *Mycobacterium tuberculosis*. Biochim. Biophys. Acta 20:299, 1956.

37. Novy, F. G., and Soule, M. H.: Microbic respiration. II. Respiration of the tubercle bacillus. J. Infect. Dis. 36:168, 1925.

38. Olson, B. J., Scott, H. W., Jr., Hanlon, C. R., and Mattern, C. F. T.: Experimental tuberculosis. III. Further observations on the effects of alteration of the pulmonary arterial circulation on tuberculosis in monkeys. Am. Rev. Tuberc. 65:48, 1952.

39. Ramakrishnan, T., Indira, M., and Maller, R. K.: Evaluation of the routes of glucose utilization in virulent and avirulent strains of *Mycobacterium tuberculosis*. Biochim. Biophys. Acta 59:529, 1962.

40. Rich, A. R., and Follis, R. H., Jr.: The effect of low oxygen tension upon the development of experimental tuberculosis. Bull. John Hopkins Hosp. 71:345, 1942.

41. Russell, W. F., and Middlebrook, G.: Chemotherapy of Tuberculosis. Springfield, Ill., Charles C Thomas, 1961.

42. Sever, J. L., and Youmans, G. P.: The relation of oxygen tension to virulence of tubercle bacilli and to acquired resistance in tuberculosis. J. Infect. Dis. 101:193, 1957.

43. Spitznagel, J. K., and Dubos, R. J.: A fraction of tubercle bacilli possessing primary toxicity. J. Exp. Med. 101:291, 1955.

44. Wayne, L. G.: Synchronized replication of *Mycobacterium tuberculosis*. Infect. Immun. 17:528, 1977.

45. Wayne, L. G., and Diaz, G. A.: Autolysis and secondary growth of *Mycobacterium tuberculosis* in submerged culture. J. Bacteriol. 93:1374, 1967.

46. Youmans, G. P., and Youmans, A. S.: The relation between the size of the infecting dose of tubercle bacilli and the survival time of mice. Am. Rev. Tuberc. 64:534, 1951.

6

Natural Resistance to Tuberculous Infection

INTRODUCTION

A great deal has been said and written about "natural resistance" to tuberculous infection. In fact, Rich,[21] in his book, *The Pathogenesis of Tuberculosis,* devotes 126 pages to this subject. However, much of what has been written about natural resistance to infection, and particularly tuberculous infection, is confusing because writers have not clearly differentiated between what is truly natural resistance to infection and what is acquired.

EXTERNAL DEFENSE MECHANISMS

The phrase "natural resistance to infection" should include only those normal anatomic structures and physiologic processes that play a part in preventing or eliminating infection. These can be conveniently divided into external and internal defense mechanisms. External defense mechanisms include the skin and the mucous membranes, which present external barriers to infection. Other examples of this type of mechanism are as follows: the ciliary action in the upper respiratory tract, which propels material to the oropharynx where it is swallowed; the mucociliary stream of the lower respiratory tract, which keeps it free of foreign bodies; the acidity of the stomach; the peristalsis of the small and large bowel; and the flushing action of urine, which keeps the urinary tract free of infection. Even such things as the washing action of tears and the pha-

202

gocytic action of leukocytes found on mucus membranes, as well as the presence of lysozyme in bodily secretions, can be regarded as natural resistance mechanisms. A more detailed discussion of such natural defense mechanisms can be found in the book by Youmans and associates.[25]

INTERNAL DEFENSE MECHANISMS

Internal natural defense mechanisms include the following: inflammation; the phagocytic activity of leukocytes; the opsonizing activity of natural antibodies (large globulin molecules that have the capacity to opsonize a wide variety of substances including bacteria); complement, which promotes phagocytosis and lysis of bacteria; germicidal substances such as lysozyme and beta lysin; and other bacteriocidal agents found in tissues and body fluids.[25]

There is little doubt that the external defense mechanisms play a significant role in the prevention of tuberculosis, especially those, such as the skin and mucous membrane, that impose a barrier between host and parasite. These are the true mechanisms of natural resistance to infection. Once the external barriers are breached, internal defense mechanisms must be brought into play. It can be stated categorically that in the person who has never had a previous experience with mycobacteria, none of the internal defense mechanisms will be very effective in preventing the growth and multiplication of virulent tubercle bacilli. Virulent tubercle bacilli are facultative intracellular parasites and will grow almost as well within phagocytic cells as they do in a tissue environment free of such cells. Therefore, for practical purposes, there really are few effective natural internal defense mechanisms against infection by *M. tuberculosis* or other virulent mycobacteria.

VARIATION IN RESISTANCE AMONG ANIMAL SPECIES

Assuming the correctness of the hypothesis that there are no really significant natural internal defense mechanisms against tuberculosis, we are left with the problem of explaining satisfactorily the well-documented differences in the susceptibility of different species and races of animals to tuberculous infection. Without question, species of animals vary widely in their susceptibility to infection with *M. tuberculosis*. For example, man, monkeys, and guinea pigs are far more susceptible to infection with *M. tuberculosis* than are mice and rats.[24] These differences in susceptibility can easily be demonstrated experimentally, except for man. Even within a given species of animal, different strains may show considerable variation in susceptibility. Among human beings, it is clear that blacks have less resistance than whites to tuberculous infection and that among whites, Jews are appreciably more resistant.[21] Among the lower animals, certain strains of rabbits, are more resistant than others.[14] Also, certain strains of inbred mice can be shown experimentally to be more susceptible than other strains.[5, 16, 26, 27]

EFFECT OF SEX, AGE, AND PREGNANCY UPON RESISTANCE TO TUBERCULOSIS

Within a given species or strain of animal, it has been shown that females are somewhat more susceptible than males to tuberculous infection.[9] Also less resistant are the very young and very old members of a strain.[21] Among human beings, it has long been recognized that the extremes in age, i.e., the very young and the old, are more susceptible to tuberculosis and that certain conditions, such as pregnancy, may appreciably lower resistance to tuberculous infection.[21] Also, among human beings there is relatively little difference in mortality from tuberculosis between males and females until the age of puberty; at which time, a higher mortality is noted in females. Following ages 35 to 45, the mortality is appreciably greater for males. A detailed discussion of the relation of sex to susceptibility to tuberculosis will be found in the work of Rich.[21]

The variations in susceptibility to tuberculosis have usually been ascribed to differences in natural resistance — in other words, to unique, innate (genetically determined) characteristics that decrease the capacity of virulent tubercle bacilli to grow and multiply.[14] For example, the highly resistant rat might be more resistant to tuberculous infection because the intracellular milieu of the animal may not provide appropriate or sufficient metabolites for optimal growth of tubercle bacilli. The rat also might be more resistant to tuberculosis because its phagocytic cells have some unique inherent capacity for inhibiting the multiplication of tubercle bacilli.

PHYSIOLOGIC RESISTANCE TO TUBERCULOUS INFECTION

That certain physiologic differences among species of animals can account for variation in susceptibility to infection has long been known. For example, the high body temperature of domestic fowl apparently makes them resistant to infection with *Bacillus anthracis*[24] and, in the same manner, probably accounts for the domestic fowl's great resistance to infection with *M. tuberculosis*. They are highly susceptible to *M. avium,* a microorganism with a higher optimal temperature requirement for growth. The variation in

susceptibility to tuberculosis of most mammalian species, however, cannot be accounted for by such physiologic differences.

NATURE OF NATURAL RESISTANCE TO TUBERCULOUS INFECTION

An explanation for the differences in susceptibility among species of animals and races of man, considering the fact that there are few natural internal defenses to *M. tuberculosis*, can be found in the experimental studies of Ratcliffe[18] and Ratcliffe and Palladino.[19] By the pulmonary route, Ratcliffe and Palladino infected mice, Syrian hamsters, rats, and guinea pigs with small numbers of either the Ravenel strain of *M. bovis* or the H37Rv strain of *M. tuberculosis*. The intrapulmonary infection was accomplished by making an aerosol of the virulent mycobacteria, then allowing the animals to inhale droplets containing single mycobacterial cells. In this manner, calculated numbers of mycobacterial cells were deposited, more or less uniformly within the pulmonary alveoli throughout the lung. The animals were infected in groups; then, three or more of each group were killed at different intervals after infection. The lungs were removed and, after fixation, were embedded in paraffin, sectioned at 5μ, and stained to demonstrate the bacilli and histologic changes associated with infection.

The results of these experiments showed that for approximately three weeks after the bacilli were deposited in the lungs, the progress of the infection and the reaction of all the animal species to it followed a highly uniform developmental pattern. During the fourth week of the infection, the rate and pattern of tubercle formation changed in each species of animal and, thereafter, became distinctive for each species of animal and each species of infecting parasite. The authors[18, 19] concluded that the highly uniform initial response was evidence that the various species of animals did not differ in their inherent (natural) resistance to tuberculous infection with either *M. tuberculosis* or *M. bovis*. Rather, the species differed widely only in their capacity to acquire resistance to the tubercle bacilli. This was shown by the variation in progression of tuberculous disease in the later stages.

In 1973, Lefford and colleagues[12] in-investigated the time of appearance of acquired immunity in rats infected either with the attenuated R1Rv strain of tuberculosis or with the H37Rv strain. Development of immunity in the infected rats was determined by collecting thoracic duct lymphocytes at various times after infection and transferring these to noninfected rats, which, in turn, were challenged with the R1Rv strain. The researchers found that as early as four days after infection, thoracic duct lymphocytes that would confer some immunity on normal animals could be obtained. Because of this very rapid development of immunity, these authors concluded that the apparent natural resistance of the rat to tuberculosis is actually due to the rapid induction of acquired immunity. Unfortunately, Lefford and his coworkers did not directly compare the rate of development of acquired immunity in the highly resistant rat to that in a highly susceptible species, such as the guinea pig. In view of the earlier findings of Ratcliffe and Palladino,[19] however, there is little reason to doubt the conclusions of Lefford and his coworkers.[12]

Thus, it is becoming increasingly clear that much, probably most, of what has been called natural resistance to tuberculosis actually is due to acquired immunity. This is in line with what we are beginning to learn about all infections — that it is the immune response of the host that de-

termines the outcome of an infectious process. Of course, if the ability to mount an immune response to an agent (such as *M. tuberculosis*) varies widely among species and races of animals, this variation must be genetically determined and in this sense, then, is "natural" to that species or race. The feature that is not natural is dependence upon the development of immunity. The immune response is, therefore, acquired, since it does not appear until after an antigenic stimulus is provided.

The variations noted in susceptibility to tuberculosis in persons of different ages and between males and females may also be due to variations in the capacity to mount a cellular immune response. The greater susceptibility of pregnant women clearly falls in the same category, since some workers have demonstrated that pregnancy depresses cellular immunity,[1, 3, 6-8, 10, 11, 13, 22, 23] although there are others who have not been able to demonstrate a depression of tuberculin hypersensitivity during pregnancy.[15, 17]

We must point out that the view that natural resistance in tuberculosis could be dependent, at least in part, upon the ability to develop acquired immunity to the infecting tubercle bacilli was suggested as early as 1917 by Cobbett.[2] Cummins in 1935[4] further stressed this possibility, and Rich[20] felt that some aspects of natural resistance might actually be due to acquired immunity.

The extensive investigations of Lurie and his colleagues[14] can also be interpreted in a manner supporting the thesis that much of what has been called natural resistance to tuberculosis actually depends upon the capacity of the infected host to mount an acquired immune response to *M. tuberculosis*. By selective brother-and-sister and parent-and-offspring breeding of rabbits of different derivation, rabbit families that exhibited degrees of resistance to infection with tubercle bacilli were developed.[14] The resistance of these rabbit families to tuberculous infection was determined in three ways: 1) by exposing the rabbits to natural airborne infection-derived rabbit roommates, which had been artificially infected with *M. bovis*; 2) by exposing the rabbits to the inhalation of known numbers of *M. bovis*, using an aerosol; and 3) by the parenteral injection of known numbers of *M. bovis*. Following infection, the more susceptible strains of rabbits died as the consequence of rapidly progressive and disseminated tuberculosis. There was little evidence of encapsulation of the pulmonary lesions or limitation of spread of the disease. In the more resistant strains of rabbits the pulmonary lesions progressed more slowly and became encapsulated, and the rabbits eventually died from a slowly progressive tuberculous disease. One of Lurie's observations is particularly pertinent to the present discussion.[14]

Contrary to expectation the transport of bacilli from the portal of entry in the lung to the draining lymph nodes was greater in the natively resistant animal than in the natively susceptible. The failure of the disease to disseminate to the rest of the body in the resistant strain was not due to fixation of the bacilli in the primary lesion but to the effective inhibition of multiplication of the bacilli in the metastatic foci.

Although Lurie[14] felt that natural genetically controlled factors were primarily responsible for the observed differences in susceptibility of his strains of rabbits to infection with *M. bovis*, he also recognized that acquired immunity must play a role. As a matter of fact, Lurie's observation on the differences between his susceptible and resistant species during the course of the disease can be much better explained by assuming that the more resistant rabbits were able to control the infection better because of a much greater capacity to develop acquired immunity to the infecting dose of bacilli. In view of what we now know about the acquired immune response in tuberculosis (see Chapters 8, 9, 10, 11, 12, and 13), it is clear that in Lurie's experiments, the lymphocytes and macrophages had acquired a much greater capacity to control the intracellular multiplication of *M. bovis* than had the same cells in the more susceptible animals. From Lurie's observations, we can see that dissemination of virulent tubercle bacilli was not prevented in the more resistant rabbits; rather, multiplication of the disseminated tubercle bacilli was inhibited within the cells of the tissues in which they lodged — a characteristic manifestation of acquired immunity to tuberculosis. Therefore, the major difference between the susceptible and resistant strains of rabbits was their capacity to mount an effective immune response; this capacity obviously must be genetically controlled. Thus, it should come as no surprise that different species or races of animals have been found to differ markedly in their capacity to develop immunity to tuberculosis and that this characteristic is responsible for what has been referred to as species or racial resistance to tuberculous disease.

Rich,[20, 21] though, expressed the belief that there were many instances of natural resistance that did not depend upon acquired immunity. This may well be the case, but we would like to express, just as strongly, the belief that most of the internal defense mechanisms in tuberculosis depend upon the acquisition by the host of specific cellular immunity. Unfortunately, the earlier writers who considered the question of natural resistance to tuberculosis did not have available the results of investigations such as those of Ratcliffe and Palladino[19] and of Lefford and his coworkers,[12] which we have just outlined; nor were the findings of Lurie[14] usually interpreted in the manner just discussed.

There is another aspect of the question of natural resistance to infection, and especially tuberculous infection, which we should consider. As we have already shown, it is quite possible to explain the variation in susceptibilities to tuberculosis on the basis of different capacities to develop acquired immunity to a parasite, such as *M. tuberculosis*. We then should ask the question: Can the variation among species or races in susceptibility to infection with different mycobacteria be explained in the same manner? We know of no evidence on this point, but we see no reason why this should not be the case. Here, of course, we are not referring to these situations where an obvious physiologic difference, such as body temperature or availability of oxygen or iron to the parasite, will determine the capacity of a mycobacterial species to multiply within the cells of a certain host. Rather, we are thinking of situations in which a potent pathogen such as *M. tuberculosis* readily produces progressive disease in human beings and guinea pigs but does so with difficulty in rabbits and cattle in which *M. bovis*, which readily produces progressive disease in cattle, human beings, and rabbits, has difficulty producing progressive disease in mice and rats. It would be of great interest to study the magnitude of the immune response to infection with a number of mycobacterial parasites in various species of animals.

The picture of natural resistance to tuberculous infection that we have just described will be considered greatly oversimplified by many people. Undoubtedly, this is correct because there are a multitude of factors that will influence the progression of tuberculous disease. However, it is highly probable that most of these factors, whether they operate locally (i.e., necrosis) or systemically (i.e., hormones)[14] to reduce resistance, are effective in this regard because they either impair the ability of the host to develop a specific immune response or inter-

fere with the operation of an already developed immune response.

REFERENCES

1. Bonnard, G. D., Glauser, A., Chappuis, M., Lemos, L., Gautier, E., Barrelet, V., and Jeannet, M.: *In vitro* induction of cytotoxic lymphocytes using lymphoid cells of parents and their newborn or adult children. *In* Centaro, A., and Carretti, N. (eds.): Immunology in Obstetrics and Gynecology: Proceedings of the First International Congress (June, 1973). New York, American Elsevier Publishing Co., Inc., 1974.
2. Cobbett, L.: The Causes of Tuberculosis; Together with Some Account of the Prevalence and Distribution of the Disease. Cambridge, Cambridge University Press, 1917.
3. Conn, R. W.: Effect of pregnancy upon tuberculin reaction. Am. Rev. Tuberc. *46*:350, 1942.
4. Cummins, S. L.: Acquired immunity as a clue to clinical differences in tuberculosis. Bull. Int. Union Tuberc. *12*:234, 1935.
5. Donovick, R., McKee, C. M., Jambor, W. P., and Rake, G.: The use of the mouse in a standardized test for antituberculous activity of compounds of natural or synthetic origin. II. Choice of mouse strain. Am. Rev. Tuberc. *60*:109, 1949.
6. Dossetor, J. B., Kovithavongs, T., Boyd, J. J., Lockwood, B., Lao, V., Schlaut, J., Liburd, E. M., Olson, L., and Russell, A. S.: Humoral and cell-mediated immunity in parous women. *In* Centaro, A., and Carretti, N. (eds.): Immunology in Obstetrics and Gynecology: Proceedings of the First International Congress (June, 1973). New York, American Elsevier Publishing Co., Inc., 1974.
7. Fabris, N., and Serri, F.: Immunological reactivity during pregnancy in the mouse. *In* Centaro, A., and Carretti, N. (eds.): Immunology in Obstetrics and Gynecology: Proceedings of the First International Congress (June, 1973). New York, American Elsevier Publishing Co., Inc., 1974.
8. Finn, R., St. Hill, C. A., Govan, A. J., Ralfs, I. G., Gurney, F. J., and Denye, V.: Immunological responses in pregnancy and survival of fetal homograft. Br. Med. J. *3*:150, 1972.
9. Hoyt, A., Moore, F. J., Knowles, R. G., and Smith, C. R.: Sex differences of normal and immunized mice in resistance to experimental tuberculosis. Am. Rev. Tuberc. *75*:618, 1957.
10. Jenkins, D. M., and Scott, J. S.: Immuno-

logical responses in pregnancy. Br. Med. J. *3*:528, 1972.

11. Kasakura, S.: Suppressive activities of pregnancy and fetal plasmas on the reactivity of lymphocytes to various stimulants. *In* Centaro, A., and Carretti, N. (eds.): Immunology in Obstetrics and Gynecology: Proceedings of the First International Congress (June, 1973). New York, American Elsevier Publishing Co., Inc., 1974.

12. Lefford, M. J., McGregor, D. D., and Mackaness, G. B.: Immune response to *Mycobacterium tuberculosis* in rats. Infect. Immun. *8*:182, 1973.

13. Lichtenstein, M. R.: Tuberculin reaction in tuberculosis during pregnancy. Am. Rev. Tuberc. *46*:89, 1942.

14. Lurie, M. B.: Resistance to Tuberculosis: Experimental Studies in Native and Acquired Defensive Mechanisms. Cambridge, Mass., Harvard University Press, 1964.

15. Montgomery, W. P., Young, R. C., Jr., Allen, M. P., and Harden, K. A.: The tuberculin test in pregnancy. Am. J. Obstet. Gynecol. *100*:829, 1968.

16. Pierce, C., Dubos, R. J., and Middlebrook, G.: Infection of mice in mammalian tubercle bacilli grown in Tween-albumin liquid medium. J. Exp. Med. *86*:159, 1947.

17. Present, P. A., and Comstock, G. W.: Tuberculin sensitivity in pregnancy. Am. Rev. Respir. Dis. *112*:413, 1975.

18. Ratcliffe, H. L.: Tuberculosis induced by droplet nuclei infection. Pulmonary tuberculosis of predetermined initial intensity in mammals. Am. J. Hyg. *55*:36, 1952.

19. Ratcliffe, H. L., and Palladino, V. S.: Tuberculosis induced by droplet nuclei infection. Initial homogeneous response of small mammals (rats, mice, guinea pigs, and hamsters) to human and to bovine bacilli, and the rate and pattern of tubercle development. J. Exp. Med. *97*:61, 1953.

20. Rich, A. R.: Immunity in tuberculosis. *In* New York Academy of Medicine: Diseases of the Respiratory Tract. Philadelphia, W. B. Saunders Co., 1936.

21. Rich, A. R.: The Pathogenesis of Tuberculosis. 2nd ed. Springfield, Ill., Charles C Thomas, 1951.

22. Smith, J. K., Caspary, E. A., and Field, E. J.: Immune responses in pregnancy. Lancet *1*:96, 1972.

23. Wade, L. J.: The effect of pregnancy upon experimental tuberculosis in rabbits. Am. Rev. Tuberc. *46*:93, 1942.

24. Wilson, G. S., and Miles, A.: Topley and Wilson's Principles of Bacteriology, Virology, and Immunity. 6th ed. Baltimore, The Williams & Wilkins Company, 1975.

25. Youmans, G. P., Paterson, P. Y., and Sommers, H. M.: The Biologic and Clinical Basis of Infectious Diseases. Philadelphia, W. B. Saunders Co., 1975.

26. Youmans, G. P., and Youmans, A. S.: Response of vaccinated and nonvaccinated syngeneic C57B1/6 mice to infection with *Mycobacterium tuberculosis*. Infect. Immun. *6*:748, 1972.

27. Youmans, G. P., Youmans, A. S., and Kanai, K.: The difference in response of four strains of mice to immunization against tuberculous infection. Am. Rev. Respir. Dis. *80*:753, 1959.

7

Development of Delayed (Tuberculin) Hypersensitivity in Tuberculosis

INTRODUCTION

One of the major manifestations of host response to tuberculous infection is the development of delayed hypersensitivity to protein antigens of the tubercle bacillus.[51] The presence of this altered state of host tissue reactivity can be demonstrated by the local delayed acute inflammatory reaction, which occurs when tuberculoprotein is injected intradermally, and by the systemic reactions of fever, malaise, and shock, if tuberculoprotein is introduced into the circulation and distributed widely to sensitive tissues.[51] It can also be shown that lymphocytes taken from a tuberculin-sensitive an-

imal or person will become activated and show blast transformation when exposed to tuberculoprotein.[18]

This altered state of tissue reactivity to tuberculin is of enormous importance to the tuberculous subject. In the first place, the acute inflammatory reaction that occurs in the hypersensitive person following exposure to tuberculoprotein can probably account for most of the tissue destruction, which is such a pronounced feature of tuberculous disease, whatever organ or tissue is involved.[51] For example, the necrosis occurring in tubercles in the lung and the resulting cavitation can be accounted for on the basis of the acute necrotizing inflammatory reaction that

209

occurs when tuberculoprotein from viable tubercle bacilli encounters hypersensitive tissue (see Chapter 14). Second, since tuberculin hypersensitivity is a specific immunologic reaction, the presence of the hypersensitivity, as elicited by skin tests or certain in vitro tests, will provide an indication of previous exposure to the tubercle bacillus or related mycobacteria. This then becomes, in turn, a very important and very useful diagnostic test (more will be said about this in Chapter 14). Third, there has been a school of thought that has equated immunity to tuberculous infection with tuberculin hypersensitivity.[70] That is, the hypersensitive state and the ensuing inflammatory reaction that occurs when tuberculoprotein encounters sensitive cells, are thought to account in full for the immunity that develops following infection with tubercle bacilli. This possible relationship of tuberculin hypersensitivity to immunity to tuberculosis is fully discussed in Chapter 13, where we provide evidence that we feel separates the two phenomena.

The initial observations on the altered reactivity that develops in animals infected with tubercle bacilli were made by Robert Koch in 1891.[31] His classical description, as given by Rich,[51] of what later became known as the "Koch Phenomenon" is as follows:

If a normal guinea pig is inoculated with a pure culture of tubercle bacilli, the wound, as a rule, closes and in the first few days seemingly heals. After ten to fourteen days, however, there appears a firm nodule which soon opens, forming an ulcer that persists until the animal dies. Quite different is the result if a tuberculous guinea pig is inoculated with tubercle bacilli. For this purpose it is best to use animals that have been infected four to six weeks previously. In such an animal, also, the little inoculation wound closes at first, but in this case no nodule is formed. On the next or second day, however, a peculiar change occurs at the inoculation site. The area becomes indurated and assumes a dark color, and these changes do not remain limited to the inoculation point, but

spread to involve an area 0.5 to 1.0 cm. in diameter. In the succeeding days it becomes evident that the altered skin is necrotic. It finally sloughs, leaving a shallow ulcer which usually heals quickly and permanently, and the regional lymph nodes do not become infected. The action of tubercle bacilli upon the skin of a normal guinea pig is thus entirely different from their action upon the skin of a tuberculous one. This striking effect is produced not only by living tubercle bacilli, but also by dead bacilli, whether killed by prolonged low temperature, by boiling, or by certain chemicals.

Following this description by Koch, interest was aroused in the nature of this altered reactivity. This interest has persisted, resulting in the recognition of what is known today as cellular immunity—one of the two major immune responses.

Actually, delayed hypersensitivity is a feature, or characteristic, of all bacterial, protozoan, fungal, and viral infections. In fact, the initial observation on increased reactivity to infectious agents was made by Jenner in 1798.[28] Jenner noted the increased reactivity to vaccinia virus occurring in persons who had previously been vaccinated or who had had smallpox.

NATURE OF TUBERCULIN

It is generally agreed that the active principle from the tubercle bacillus, which elicits the tuberculin reaction, is a protein, or polypeptide, but only recently has the exact nature of one of the highly reactive tuberculopolypeptides become known.[32, 33]

The original tuberculin preparation described by Koch in 1891 and named "Old Tuberculin" (OT) was merely a culture filtrate of *Mycobacterium tuberculosis*, which had been heated and concentrated by evaporation and then preserved with glycerol. This material was grossly impure since it contained all of the products of growth of tubercle bacilli, plus many materials that entered the medium because of autolysis of mycobacterial cells. Different preparations of Old Tuberculin varied markedly, and standardization was difficult. In the hope that a more purified product could be obtained for use in tuberculin testing of human beings and animals, considerable effort has been expended on the purification of Old Tuberculin. The initial studies of Seibert and her colleagues[39, 60] utilized ammonium sulfate to precipitate the proteins. The proteins after ammonium sulfate precipitation, were concentrated and dialyzed and thus could be standardized on the basis of protein content. This preparation was called *purified protein derivative* (PPD) and has proved much more useful for tuberculin testing than Old Tuberculin. It must be clearly recognized, however, that PPD itself is far from being a pure substance. It contains many proteins and polypeptides of different molecular weight. In addition, a number of polysaccharides may be present in some preparations.[34, 57] The molecular weights of the protein components of PPD can range from 10,000 or 20,000 to as high as 1,000,000. According to Landi and Held,[34] maximum biologic activity—that is, the capacity to elicit tuberculin reactions in sensitive subjects or animals—appears to reside in higher molecular weight components of from 60,000 to 125,000. However, considerable biologic activity is found even in some of the higher molecular weight polypeptides.[34, 57]

On the other hand, Kuwabara[32, 33] has purified an intracellular, tuberculin-active protein and has found it to be a thousand times more potent than PPD in eliciting dermal tuberculin reactions in guinea pigs and human beings. This product was purified by chromatography on DEAE cellulose and Sephadex G-200 and was obtained in crystalline form. Ultracentrifugation analysis showed only one major component with a calculated molecular weight of 9700. The specific activities of tuberculin-active protein were 6.33×10^9 tuberculin units per mg of protein-nitrogen for sensitized guinea pigs and 6.33×10^{11} tuberculin units per mg of protein-nitrogen for sensitized human beings. This crystalline tuberculoprotein might well be the long-needed, pure and specific agent for determining the tuberculin sensitivity of man and lower animals.

PPD originally was prepared from the heated culture filtrates of *M. tuberculosis*, which were used to prepare Old Tuberculin. It was recognized that the heating might result in hydrolysis of many of the proteins present and account in part for the heterogeneous molecular composition of PPD. In addition, the heating undoubtedly denatured many of the proteins, and this might result in loss of biologic activity. Therefore, a number of investigators[12, 13, 66, 69] have concentrated more recently on utilizing unheated culture filtrates of *M. tuberculosis* not only for the preparation of skin-testing antigens but also for the purpose of trying to characterize the many proteins produced by the tubercle bacillus. In all cases, however, these unheated culture filtrates or the precipitated proteins thereof also have been found to be very complex mixtures. Dozens of different types of proteins, as measured serologically or chemically, can be detected. These mixtures have biologic activity and are suitable for the production of tuberculin reactions in sensitive subjects; however, to date, no single protein (except for the crystalline material by Kuwabara)[32, 33] has been separated that can be utilized for routine tuberculin testing.[12, 13, 66, 69] The hope, of course, is that by chemical or physical means, it will be possible to isolate from culture filtrates of different species of mycobacteria a single protein, which, when utilized for detecting tuberculin hypersensitivity, may be specific for that particular species. Some degree of specificity has been achieved[12, 13, 66, 69] by utilizing proteins from culture filtrates of different mycobacteria; in addition, ribosomal proteins have been isolated from a number of mycobacterial species.[2, 44] Delayed hypersensitivity to these ribosomal proteins will develop in infected animals, and there is a possibility that utilization of ribosomal proteins may provide a more specific reagent for detection of delayed hypersensitivity in animals or human beings infected with tubercle bacilli. Some success has been claimed for this approach.[2, 44]

STANDARDIZATION OF TUBERCULIN

In view of the varying composition of different preparations of tuberculin, some kind of standardization based on biologic activity is necessary. The World Health Organization, for many years, has been aware of this need, and its various Expert Committees have considered the problem. As a consequence, the World Health Organization maintains stocks of standard preparations of OT and PPD. These are used as reference standards, and new preparations of either OT or PPD should be compared in their biologic activity to these standard prepara-

tions. Table 7–1 shows the World Health Organization standards in terms of amount of each preparation. A unit of OT is 10 micrograms of the standard preparation (0.1 milliliter of 1:100 dilution), and the standard PPD is regarded as having 50,000 units per milligram.

As pointed out by Outschoorn:[45]

[It was recognized by the World Health Organization] that the potency of tuberculin preparations cannot always be expressed in terms of international units by a biological assay that would be valid for all conditions of use. Each tuberculin product, therefore, should be assayed against a reference preparation of the same type and made in the same way as the test preparation. Each such reference preparation should be calibrated against the international standard for the tuberculin it more closely resembles in behaviour, i.e. PPD or OT. The calibration of the reference material should be done by a number of tests against the appropriate international standard, each test being made in the animal species in which the tuberculin is to be used in the case of tuberculins for veterinary testing or in man in the case of tuberculins for human use. The specific conditions under which such calibrations are made should be chosen in relation to each purpose for which the tuberculin preparation is to be used and at the dosage concerned. The comparison of activity of the proposed reference preparation with the relevant international standard, there-

TABLE 7–1.   **Comparable Doses of Old Tuberculin (OT) and Purified Protein Derivative (PPD)**

Dilution of OT	Tuberculin Injected (MG)*	PPD Injected (MG)**	Tuberculin Units (TU)	Strength
1:100,000	0.001		0.1	
1:10,000	0.01	.00002	1.0	First
1:2,000	0.05	.0001	5.0	Intermediate
1:1,000	0.1		10.0	
1:100	1.0	.005	250.0	Second

*Based on 1 ml of concentrated OT = 1000 mg.
**Based on milligrams of protein.
From Smith, D. T., et al. (eds.): Zinsser Microbiology. 14th ed. New York, Appleton-Century-Crofts, 1968, p. 541.

fore, would be at a particular dose level and under specific conditions for each of the types of use to which the preparation would be put in practice. In order to reduce the possible effect of a further variable, the Expert Committee also recommended that in such calibration procedures, if the International Standard for PPD (Mammalian) was used, it should be made up in phosphate-buffered saline, while the reference material which was being calibrated should be made up in the diluent in which the final product is to be used in tuberculin tests.

These recommendations were based upon observations showing that not only did the biologic activity of various tuberculin preparations differ quantitatively but also varied depending upon the species of animals used and the degree of hypersensitivity of the animal species employed.[45]

For example, standardization of tuberculin potency in animals given BCG vaccine, where a low degree of hypersensitivity is expected, would not be comparable to standardization conducted in animals infected with virulent tubercle bacilli. This same would be true in human beings. Also, biologic activity is not directly related to dose employed over a wide range; therefore, assumptions as to the biologic activity of the tuberculin preparation based upon tests using one dosage would not necessarily be valid for other dosages. The situation is also complicated by the knowledge that in low concentrations, PPD rapidly loses potency by absorption to glass.[45] For this reason, the most commonly employed PPD for tuberculin testing today is one in which the tuberculin concentrations have been made up in a medium containing small quantities of surface-active agent, Tween 80.[45]

From the preceding discussion, it follows that in any experimental work or in the testing of human populations for tuberculin sensitivity, only those PPD and OT preparations equivalent, in their capacity to elicit reactions, to the World Health Organization standard preparations should be used.

INDUCTION OF TUBERCULIN HYPERSENSITIVITY

In human beings and lower animals, hypersensitivity to tuberculin develops most readily after actual infection with virulent tubercle bacilli. The time of appearance of the hypersensitive state will depend upon the number of tubercle bacilli with which a person or animal becomes infected and, of course, upon the rate of multiplication of the virulent microorganisms. When large numbers of virulent tubercle bacilli are introduced into a suitable host, tuberculin hypersensitivity may appear as early as five to seven days later. When very small numbers are introduced, however, it may be a matter of two to three weeks before detectable tuberculin hypersensitivity is present. Even in persons in whom, after infection with virulent tubercle bacilli, no clinical signs of disease can be detected, a degree of tuberculin hypersensitivity will develop that is sufficient to give, for the most part, reactions to five TU of PPD that are in excess of 10 mm in diameter. The persistence of tuberculin hypersensitivity in an infected human being also will depend upon the persistence of viable tubercle bacilli in the body. If the infecting microorganisms are all killed and disposed of, after a period of months or several years, the tuberculin hypersensitivity will decrease and be undetectable by standard testing procedures. On the other hand, since tubercle bacilli do persist in the tissues of most persons infected, tuberculin hypersensitivity will be present in the majority of people even years after the initial infection. The clinical significance of a positive dermal tuberculin test and the significance of the size of the dermal tuberculin reaction will be given in detail in Chapter 14. It should be pointed out here, though, that caution must be exercised in assuming that active, progressive tuberculous disease is present merely because a person has a positive dermal reaction to tuberculin.

Although tubercle bacilli killed by heat or by chemicals will induce tuberculin hypersensitivity in certain experimental animals, their capacity to do so is much less than that of viable cells. This has been ascribed to the fact that killed tubercle bacilli cannot multiply in vivo; therefore, the required mass of tuberculoprotein for the development of tuberculin hypersensitivity is not achieved. However, the injection into experimental animals of enormous numbers of dead tubercle bacilli does not entirely compensate for the lack of capacity of smaller numbers of killed cells to induce tuberculin hypersensitivity. Between living and dead tubercle bacilli, therefore, there must be a qualitative difference that is responsible for the lack of capacity of the latter to induce tuberculin hypersensitivity. The ability of dead tubercle bacilli or of products of tubercle bacilli (such as cell walls) to induce tuberculin hypersensitivity can be increased greatly by incorporation of the dead bacilli or cell walls in Freund's incomplete adjuvant or in mineral oil alone. The exact role of mineral oil in this regard is not known, but possibly it may compensate in some manner for the loss of some adjuvant activity when tubercle bacilli are killed. One likely candidate is the mycobacterial RNA, which we have found to be a potent adjuvant for the induction of delayed hypersensitivity. This material would be denatured or degraded when mycobacteria are killed, and its loss might easily account for the failure of dead cells to be effective inducers of tuberculin hypersensitivity, particularly since it is known that the tuberculoprotein to which the hypersensitivity develops is relatively stable.

As we will see in the next chapter, the markedly reduced capacity of killed mycobacterial cells to induce tuberculin hypersensitivity is paralleled by their reduced capacity to produce immunity to infection. In extensive studies (see Chapter 8), we have reported that the inability of killed mycobacterial cells to induce immunity to tuberculous infection may be due to the destruction of some labile immunizing substance by the process that kills the mycobacterial cells. We have, we feel, identified this labile substance as mycobacterial, and presumably ribosomal, RNA (see Chapter 9).

In this connection, it is of great interest to examine the capacity of viable attenuated or avirulent strains of mycobacteria to induce immunity to tuberculous infection as well as tuberculin hypersensitivity. It is well documented (see Chapter 8) that viable attenuated or avirulent mycobacterial cells are extremely potent inducers of immunity to tuberculous infection. These same viable cells are also very able inducers of tuberculin hypersensitivity in both experimental animals and in human beings. The attenuated strain that has received the most attention in this regard is the BCG strain of _Mycobacterium bovis_. The vaccination of literally hundreds of millions of human beings since its introduction as a vaccine in 1922 thoroughly attests to the capacity of this strain to induce tuberculin hypersensitivity in human beings. The tuberculin hypersensitivity induced in human beings following vaccination with BCG tends to be of lower degree than that following natural infection with _M. tuberculosis_, and it usually does not persist quite as long.[56] BCG strains used as vaccines in human beings only have a limited capacity to multiply in vivo. It might be that the lower degree of tuberculin hypersensitivity that is engendered is a consequence of this reduced ability to multiply. On the other hand, it well may be that it is the viability of the mycobacterial cells, and the consequent integrity of the mycobacterial RNA, which is of greater importance. This latter hypothesis is supported by the fact that certain mycobacterial strains, such as the H37Ra mutant of the H37Rv strain of *M. tuberculosis,* have practically no capacity to multiply in vivo, and yet they are potent inducers of both tuberculin hypersensitivity and immunity. It is of importance in this connection that for adjuvant activity, the mycobacterial RNA does not require the presence of mineral oil, as is the case with the lipids of mycobacterial cells.[10, 26, 71] Thus, the mycobacterial RNA may well play a dual role, serving as an adjuvant for the induction of tuberculin hypersensitivity and functioning in some as yet unknown manner as the inducer of specific immunity to tuberculous infection. More detailed discussion of the role of RNA in the induction of immunity will be found in Chapter 9.

THE HISTOLOGY OF THE LOCAL TUBERCULIN REACTION

The characteristic feature of the local reaction, which occurs when tuberculoprotein is introduced into the tissue of an animal hypersensitive to this protein, is an acute inflammatory reaction. This will follow the injection of an amount of tuberculoprotein which when injected into a nonsensitized subject will produce little or no reaction. A second feature of the tuberculin reaction is that the appearance of the acute inflammatory reaction is delayed as compared to those inflammatory reactions seen with the immediate allergic reactions. In the tuberculin reaction, gross evidence of inflammation can be seen within a few hours. This inflammatory reaction continues and reaches its maximum in from 24 to 72 hours. When the degree of hypersensitivity is high or the amount of antigen injected is large, necrosis may eventually occur.

Histologically, the inflammatory response differs in no way from that produced by nonspecific irritants. The succession of events described by investigators who have studied the tuberculin reaction has been that of typical dilatation of capillaries and the exudation of fluids and cells, with an initial predominance of segmented neutrophils. This is followed by an increase in the number of mononuclear cells, until the lesion consists predominantly of macrophages and lymphocytes. It is this accumulation of mononuclear cells that provides the typical histologic picture of a developed tuberculin reaction and also accounts for the indurated nature of the lesion. Rich[51] and textbooks of pathology should be consulted for more details on the histologic appearance of typical tuberculin reactions.

Reactions of tuberculin hypersensitivity can be obtained in any tissue in a sensitive subject into which tuberculoprotein is introduced. For example, tuberculin reactions have been elicited in the testes,[37] the lung,[54] the meninges,[9a] the kidney,[38] and even the cornea.[52]

Systemic tuberculin shock can be produced by injecting sensitive animals intravenously with tuberculin. This shock also is characteristically delayed since it comes on several hours after the administration of the tuberculin. The exact mechanism of the shock-like picture in such animals is not known.[51]

Focal reactions around areas of infection also can occur in tuberculous animals or human beings when tuberculin is administered and reaches the site of infection. This is characterized by an increase in the inflammatory reaction around the site of the infection. Presumably, the increased amount of tuberculoprotein at the sites of infection causes a flare-up of the smoldering allergic reaction. For more details on both systemic shock and focal reactions, refer to Rich.[51]

MECHANISM OF THE TUBERCULIN REACTION

Delayed hypersensitivity will develop to a wide variety of protein antigens, both bacterial and nonbacterial. In addition, delayed hypersensitivity can be induced to a wide variety of simple chemicals and low molecular weight polypeptides. Much of the work on the mechanism of delayed hypersensitivity has been done using antigens such as these. It is not our intention here to dwell at length on the basic mechanisms of delayed hypersensitivity in general. For this purpose a variety of other books or review articles should be consulted.[4, 6, 9, 16, 35, 36, 43, 63, 65, 68]

What is important for us here is to delineate as carefully as possible the events that take place in the body during the induction of tuberculin hypersensitivity and the events that occur when reactions of tuberculin hypersensitivity are elicited either by the injection of tuberculoprotein or during the course of the disease. This is important because a major portion of the pathology of tuberculosis and the various features of the disease can be readily ascribed to this state of hypersensitivity to tuberculoprotein. The inflammatory reactions that take place in an infected and, therefore, sensitized person may markedly accelerate the progress of the disease (see Chapter 14). It is also important, as we shall see, because acquired immunity to tuberculous infection, which brings about the control of the infectious process, has been ascribed to tuberculin hypersensitivity.[40] This view is probably incorrect (see Chapter 13), but there is such a close relationship between tuberculin hypersensitivity and acquired immunity in tuberculosis that only by understanding to the fullest degree the nature of both processes can we provide a rational basis for the role of each in the pathogenesis of tuberculosis. The relationship between these two and the pathogenesis of the disease will be taken up in Chapters 13 and 14. Here we will only briefly review what is known about the nature of tuberculin hypersensitivity and the nature of the inflammatory reaction that occurs when tuberculoprotein encounters the tissue of a sensitized subject.

It is clear that the effector limb of the response to tuberculin in the sensitized person is mediated by thymus-derived lymphocytes and, in particular, by small circulating lymphocytes.[64, 67] Macrophages do not appear to be greatly involved except insofar as they may contribute to the inflammatory reaction by the release of lysosomal contents following their destruction by the inflammatory process. That these active lymphocytes are T-cells has also been demonstrated. The role of lymphocytes has been demonstrated by the passive transfer of tuberculin hypersensitivity to nonsensitive guinea pigs using spleen cells and lymph node cells.[21] Furthermore, tuberculin hypersensitivity can be markedly reduced by the administration of antilymphocyte serum to sensitive animals.[27] As we will note in another chapter (see Chapter 8), this is also true of immunity to tuberculosis.

Careful studies by Feldman and Najarian[21] have also defined the dynamics of the induction of tuberculin hypersensitivity by the transfer of lymphocytes. The investigators took spleen cells from guinea pigs sensitized to tuberculin and injected them intravenously into nonsensitized guinea pigs. Prior to injection, these cells were labeled with tritiated thymidine. At the time that the passive transfer of cells was made, the animals were also given an intracutaneous injection of tuberculin. When tuberculin reactions developed at the site of injection of the tuberculoprotein in these passively sensitized animals, the lesions were excised, and the number of passively transferred lymphocytes in the lesions was calculated from the radioactivity found. The researchers found, in parallel with what happens with the inflammatory reaction, that the radioactivity increased to a peak in the tuberculin injected sites at 18 to 24 hours and then declined over the next two days. In control skin sites and in untreated skin, radioactivity was low or negligible throughout the period of observation. The absolute numbers of cells contributed by donor and host were also calculated. Less than 1 percent of the transferred sensitized cells arrived at the site of antigen deposition and, therefore, contributed only a minor proportion of all the infiltrating mononuclear elements in the test lesion.

Feldman and Najarian concluded that the skin lesions of tuberculin sensitivity were composed of two concurrent processes: 1) an accumulation of sensitized cells, apparently in response to specific antigen; and 2) an infiltration of mononuclear cells contributed by the host, probably as a response to the injury. From studies such as these, we can reasonably conclude that in the actively sensitized animal or human being as well as in the passively sensitized animal, when antigen such as tuberculoprotein is introduced into the tissue, time is required for the accumulation at the site of antigen injection of a sufficient number of circulating sensitized lymphocytes to trigger the inflammatory reaction. Also, since only a small proportion of the lymphocytes that accumulate at the site of the antigen injection are sensitized, it must be that other nonsensitized lymphocytes also participate in the reaction. Presumably, the sensitized lymphocytes following exposure to antigen can produce a substance, or substances, that, in turn, will activate nonsensitized lymphocytes. Therefore, the delay in the occurrence of the inflammatory reaction can be accounted for on the basis of the time required for the ac-

cumulation at the site of antigen deposition of a sufficient number of sensitized circulating T-lymphocyte cells.

It is assumed that the inflammatory reaction occurs when lymphocytes are exposed to the antigens to which they are sensitized; they then are stimulated to undergo blast transformation and begin the elaboration of a wide variety of soluble substances having a number of biologic actions, including the attraction and immobilization of macrophages.[18] Some of the substances produced have been shown to have direct toxic action on cells.[18] Presumably, a small number of sensitized lymphocytes in the lesion would activate nonsensitized lymphocytes to produce these substances; thus, the inflammatory reaction would be potentiated. The chemotactic factors would bring about further accumulation of lymphocytes and macrophages with the production of toxic factors which, in turn, would result in the destruction of these cells. In this manner, the cellular contents, including the lysosomes of ruptured macrophages, would magnify the inflammatory reaction and perhaps account in large part for the necrosis so frequently observed.

These soluble lymphocyte factors have been termed by some, "mediators," and by others, "lymphokines," and a large number have been described.[18] Most of our information about them has come from studies in which lymphocytes maintained in tissue culture have been exposed to antigen to which the cells are sensitive, or to certain mitogens. The cells can be centrifuged out at appropriate times after exposure to the antigen or mitogen, and the supernatant tissue culture fluid can then be tested for lymphokine activities. Any role that these lymphokines might play in producing the inflammatory reactions of delayed hypersensitivity has been inferred rather than directly demonstrated. Since lymphokines are produced when sensitized lymphocytes are exposed to specific antigen in vivo, it is reasonable to assume that they do play a significant role in the reactions of delayed hypersensitivity. The exact role of each will only be defined after further extensive investigation. It is worth pointing out here — as will be seen in Chapters 9, 10, and 12 — that a lymphokine is most probably also involved in acquired immunity to tuberculosis.

A number of the lymphocyte mediators that appear following exposure of sensitized cells to antigens are of greater significance in relation to the reactions of delayed hypersensitivity, and in particular tuberculin hypersensitivity, than others. Since they are always produced following stimulation of lymphocytes with specific antigen, these lymphocyte mediators can serve as in vitro correlates of delayed hypersensitivity. This means that much information can be obtained on mechanisms involved in delayed hypersensitivity without resorting to complex in vivo situations. The best studied and most important of these lymphocyte mediators is *macrophage migration inhibitory factor* (MIF).[18] Detection of MIF, or observation of inhibition of migration of macrophages when exposed to sensitized lymphocytes exposed to antigen, is today regarded as a valid in vitro correlate of delayed hypersensitivity.[18] Therefore, the features of and the basis for tests for macrophage migration inhibitory activity are given here.

One of the earliest in vitro models for studying delayed hypersensitivity was the inhibition of cell migration from tissue explants occurring when antigen was added, as described by Rich and Lewis.[53] These investigators prepared spleen fragments and buffy coat cells from guinea pigs that had been sensitized to avirulent human tubercle bacilli. Old Tuberculin (OT) would consistently inhibit the migration of cells from these explants, while

OT had no effect on spleen explants from normal animals. Migration of macrophages and segmented neutrophils was inhibited, but lymphocytes migrated normally.

The findings of Rich and Lewis were confirmed by Aronson.[1] Aronson sensitized guinea pigs to virulent tubercle bacilli and horse serum. Cell migration from explants of spleen and bone marrow cells were inhibited by OT, whereas cells migrated normally in the presence of horse serum. Their studies emphasized the difference between the tuberculin and Arthus reactions, since cells from animals sensitized so that they exhibited an Arthus reaction to horse serum were not inhibited from migrating when cultured in the presence of guinea pig anti-horse serum and horse serum.

In 1962, George and Vaughan[24] introduced a modification of this system in which the inhibition of migration by antigen of peritoneal exudate cells from capillary tubes was measured. In the presence of PPD, peritoneal exudate cells from animals sensitized to PPD failed to migrate normally. Inhibition of migration of peritoneal exudate cells in the presence of egg albumin occurred if sensitization had been performed so that delayed skin reactions to egg albumin occurred.

The capillary tube system of migration inhibition was expanded and popularized by the work of David and colleagues.[17] These investigators demonstrated that the migration of peritoneal exudate cells from guinea pigs with delayed hypersensitivity to PPD, ovalbumin, and diphtheria toxoid was inhibited by the respective antigen, with the inhibition being specific. Migration of cells from guinea pigs that produced precipitating antibodies was not inhibited by antigen. Only a small percentage of cells (2.5 percent of the total cell population) from a sensitized animal was required to inhibit the migration of normal peritoneal exudate cells.[19] It was demonstrated that two cell types were important in this system: 1) a sensitive lymphocyte population; and 2) macrophages, which served as indicator cells and did not need to be obtained from a sensitive animal.[14]

Bloom and Bennett[7] confirmed these findings with experiments using separated populations of lymphocytes and macrophages obtained from peritoneal exudates. Normal peritoneal exudate cells were inhibited by PPD when only a few sensitive peritoneal lymphocytes were present in the mixture. Furthermore, macrophages from exudates (obtained from sensitized animals) rendered free of lymphocytes were no longer inhibited from migrating by specific antigen.

Studies by Heise and Weiser in 1970,[27] using antilymphocyte and antimacrophage sera, showed that lymphocytes were essential for the migration inhibition response, but a decrease in the number of macrophages had no effect on the overall reaction. The lymphocyte is, therefore, the reactive cell in migration inhibition, while the macrophage is the secondary reactor cell.[20]

The fact that few sensitive lymphocytes, upon exposure to antigen, can attract and involve large numbers of nonsensitive cells suggested that lymphocytes may produce various biologic effects through soluble mediators. The isolation of a soluble cell-free substance that was elaborated by sensitive lymphocytes in response to antigen and that was capable of inhibiting normal macrophage migration was reported independently by Bennett and Bloom[5] and by David.[14]

Bloom and Bennett[7] incubated purified peritoneal lymphocytes from PPD-sensitive guinea pigs in the presence of PPD. After 24 hours, the cells were removed by centrifugation, and the resulting supernatant fluids were found to inhibit the migration of normal peritoneal exudate cells. No inhibitory supernatant fluids were produced by lymphocytes obtained from guinea pigs that did not exhibit delayed hypersensitivity but did produce high titers of antibody to ovalbumin, bovine serum albumin, and PPD.

Similar results were obtained by others,[14, 18] using lymph node lymphocytes from guinea pigs sensitized to o-chlorobenzyl-bovine globulin, or ovalbumin. Cell-free supernatant fluids inhibited migration of normal peritoneal cells only if they were obtained from cultures of sensitive lymphocytes and specific antigen. Supernatant fluids from cultures of sensitive lymphocytes not incubated with antigen or incubated with unrelated antigen did not produce migration inhibition.

Therefore, the soluble substance that is produced when sensitized lymphocytes are cultured in the presence of specific antigen and that will inhibit the migration of normal peritoneal exudate cells has been appropriately designated as *migration inhibitory factor* (MIF).

The chemical and physical characteristics, as well as kinetics of MIF production, have been extensively examined. MIF is nondialyzable, stable for 30 minutes at 56° C, and resistant to RNase and DNase, but its activity is abolished by trypsin treatment.[15] The elaboration of MIF is inhibited by puromycin[7, 14] and mitomycin,[7] indicating that active protein synthesis is required for its production. MIF activity is first detected in supernatant culture fluids, at six[55] or eight hours[5] following antigenic stimulation of sensitive lymphocytes. More recently, Rocklin[55] demonstrated that treatment of human lymphocytes with 5-bromo-2-deoxyuridine eliminated lymphocyte proliferation in response to antigen while MIF production remained unaffected, indicating that MIF was elaborated by nondividing lymphocytes.

David[15] filtered MIF-rich supernatant fluids on Sephadex G-200 or G-100 columns and demonstrated that MIF activity was recovered in fractions that eluted with molecules approximately the size of albumin, therefore having a molecular weight between 35,000 and 55,000. No activity was recovered from fractions containing high molecular weight proteins, such as immunoglobulins.

When MIF-rich fractions from Sephadex gels were chromatographed on DEAE cellulose, activity was eluted in fractions containing albumin.[8] Remold and coworkers,[50] using acrylamide gel discontinuous electrophoresis, demonstrated that MIF activity was consistently recovered from fractions containing proteins migrating anodally to albumin. When MIF was centrifuged in cesium chloride gradients, it had a buoyant density slightly greater than that of rabbit serum albumin.[50] This, together with the fact that neuraminidase abolished MIF activity, indicates that MIF is a glycoprotein and that sialic acid is necessary for its biologic activity.[48]

Although initial investigations by David[14] and by Bloom and Bennett[7] indicated MIF was elaborated by sensitized lymphoid cells in response to stimulation with specific antigen, it has now been demonstrated that MIF can be produced nonspecifically under a variety of conditions. MIF production by nonsensitized cells has been demonstrated following stimulation with nonspecific mitogens.[16, 22, 29, 47, 49, 58, 61] It has been detected in supernatant fluids from several established cell lines.[25, 46, 62] MIF has also been produced by mixed cultures of allogeneic peripheral lymphocytes from guinea pigs[3] and from mixed human lymphocyte cultures.[11]

In a review by David and David,[18] many of the clinical and immunologic applications of the migration inhibition system are discussed. Migration inhibition has been adapted to study diseases such as experimental allergic encephalomyelitis in guinea pigs, rats, and monkeys; thyroiditis in guinea pigs; and nephrosis in rats. It has been employed in studies on homograft sensitivity in mice, guinea pigs, and rats. It also has been applied to studies of cellular hypersensitivity to influenza and mumps in mice, and to vaccinia in guinea pigs. Sensitivity to many bacterial and tumor antigens in man and animals has been demonstrated using this technique.

Following the identification of MIF as a soluble product released by sensitive lymphocytes into culture supernatant fluids, many other lymphocyte products have been identified. David and David[18] have reviewed these products, which include chemotactic factor, macrophage activating factor, cytotoxic factors, human and mouse lymphotoxin, cloning inhibitory factor, proliferation inhibitory factor, skin reactive factors, blastogenic factors, interferon, and lymph node permeability factor. A question of major concern is whether or not these soluble mediators are chemically and biologically distinct molecules, or if one lymphocyte product may indeed be responsible for several in vitro phenomena.

We have already pointed out that a lymphokine is most probably also involved in acquired immunity to tuberculosis (see Chapters 9, 10, and 12).

SPECIFICITY OF IN VITRO AND IN VIVO TESTS FOR TUBERCULIN HYPERSENSITIVITY

Since both in vivo (skin tests) and in vitro tests for tuberculin hypersensitivity may now be used, it is worth exploring the relative sensitivity of the two procedures. In highly sensitive guinea pigs, it has been reported that based upon the amount of PPD needed to elicit a reaction, skin tests are more sensitive; i.e., appreciably less tuberculin is necessary to produce a skin reaction than is required to stimulate sensitive lymphocytes so that enough MIF is produced to bring about inhibition of macrophage migration. Usually, this is also the case when lymphocytes from tuberculin-sensitive human beings are employed. Results such as these indicate that tests for dermal hypersensitivity are far more sensitive than in vitro tests, such as inhibition of macrophage migration.

On the other hand, Galindo and Myrvik[23] have shown that rabbits sensitized by the subcutaneous injection of BCG in mineral oil routinely developed dermal hypersensitivity to PPD but failed to develop pulmonary granulomas. In contrast, the majority of the rabbits sensitized by the injection of BCG in oil, using the intravenous route, developed a marked pulmonary granulomatous response but did not develop dermal hypersensitivity to PPD. However, alveolar cells were obtained from the granulomas of rabbits sensitized by the intravenous route. These cells were consistently inhibited in their migration when exposed to PPD. Also, supernatant fluids, obtained from cultures of these pulmonary cells stimulated with PPD, inhibited the migration of macrophages obtained from nonsensitized rabbits. These observations show that an animal may be PPD-negative by skin test but may still possess focal collections of cells that are sensitive to PPD, as measured by the migration-inhibition test. Under these conditions, the migration-inhibition test for tuberculin hypersensitivity is more sensitive than dermal tests for hypersensitivity.

In guinea pigs sensitized to dinitrophenyl lysine attached to a carrier protein and desensitized with haptene alone, Schlossman and colleagues[59] observed that dermal sensitivity was lost but that lymphocytes obtained from lymph nodes were still able to respond when stimulated with antigen. These authors suggest that under certain conditions, sensitized lymphocytes may be compartmentalized in the body and not available in the circulation in sufficient numbers to initiate a positive dermal test.

In our work,[30, 41, 42] we have found that the intravenous injection of PPD into mice sensitive to tuberculin reduced the dermal reaction to tuberculin but, at the same time, increased the capacity of splenic lymphocytes to produce MIF.

Therefore, under certain conditions, dermal tests may be more sensitive than in vitro tests for delayed hypersensitivity, since they can be elicited with smaller amounts of antigen, but in vitro tests may be more sensitive than intradermal tests in circumstances where there is such a degree of internal compartmentalization of lymphocytes that dermal tests will be reduced in intensity or will be negative.

This is of some importance from the clinical standpoint because it is not too unusual to encounter patients with active tuberculosis who do not react to the intradermal administration of PPD. These same patients, though, will frequently regain intradermal reactivity to PPD when given adequate chemotherapy. Presumably, with the decrease in internal load of antigen brought about with therapy, the internal compartmentalization of lymphocytes will decrease, and the number of circulating lymphocytes will increase to the point where sufficient numbers can accumulate at the intradermal site of antigen deposition and will produce a positive skin test.

REFERENCES

1. Aronson, J. D.: Tissue culture studies on the relation of the tuberculin reaction to anaphylaxis and the Arthus phenomenon. J. Immunol. 25:1, 1933.
2. Baker, R. E., Hill, W. E., and Larson, C. L.: Delayed hypersensitivity reactions provoked by ribosomes from acid-fast bacilli. I. Ribosomal isolation, characterization,

delayed hypersensitivity, and specificity. Infect. Immun. *6*:258, 1972.

3. Bartfeld, H., and Atoynatan, T.: Activity and properties of macrophage migration inhibitory factor produced by mixed lymphocyte cultures. Nature *230*:246, 1971.

4. Bellanti, J. A.: Immunology. Philadelphia, W. B. Saunders Co., 1971.

5. Bennett, B., and Bloom, B. R.: Studies on the migration inhibitory factor associated with delayed-type hypersensitivity: Cytodynamics and specificity. Transplantation *5*:996, 1967.

6. Bloom, B. R.: *In vitro* approaches to the mechanisms of cell-mediated immune reactions. Adv. Immunol. *13*:101, 1971.

7. Bloom, B. R., and Bennett, B.: Mechanism of a reaction *in vitro* associated with delayed-type hypersensitivity. Science *153*:80, 1966.

8. Bloom, B. R., and Bennett, B.: Relation of the migration inhibitory factor (MIF) to delayed-type hypersensitivity reactions. Ann. N. Y. Acad. Sci. *169*:258, 1970.

9. Bloom, B. R., and Glade, P. (eds.): *In Vitro* Methods in Cell-Mediated Immunity. New York, Academic Press, 1971.

9a. Burn, C. G., and Finley, K. H.: The role of hypersensitivity in the production of experimental meningitis. J. Exp. Med. *56*:203, 1932.

10. Casavant, C. H., and Youmans, G. P.: The induction of delayed hypersensitivity in guinea pigs to poly U and poly A:U. J. Immunol. *114*:1506, 1975.

11. Clausen, J. E.: Migration inhibitory effect of cell-free supernatants from mixed human lymphocyte cultures. J. Immunol. *108*:453, 1972.

12. Daniel, T. M., and Ferguson, L. E.: Purification and characterization of two proteins from culture filtrates of *Mycobacterium tuberculosis* H$_{37}$Ra strain. Infect. Immun. *1*:164, 1970.

13. Daniel, T. M., and Hinz, C. F., Jr.: Reactivity of purified proteins and polysaccharides from *Mycobacterium tuberculosis* in delayed skin test and cultured lymphocyte mitogenesis assays. Infect. Immun. *9*:44, 1974.

14. David, J. R.: Delayed hypersensitivity *in vitro:* Its mediation by cell-free substances formed by lymphoid cell-antigen interaction. Proc. Natl. Acad. Sci. U.S.A. *56*:72, 1966.

15. David, J. R.: Macrophage migration. Fed. Proc. *27*:6, 1968.

16. David, J. R.: Mediators produced by sensitized lymphocytes. Fed. Proc. *30*:1730, 1971.

17. David, J. R., Al-Askari, S., Lawrence, H. S., and Thomas, L.: Delayed hypersensitivity *in vitro*. I. The specificity of inhibition of cell migration by antigens. J. Immunol. *93*:264, 1964.

18. David, J. R., and David, R. R.: Cellular hypersensitivity and immunity. Inhibition of macrophage migration and the lymphocyte mediators. Prog. Allergy *16*:300, 1972.

19. David, J. R., Lawrence, H. S., and Thomas, L.: Delayed hypersensitivity *in vitro*. II. Effect of sensitive cells on normal cells in the presence of antigen. J. Immunol. *93*:274, 1964.

20. Dumonde, D. C.: The role of the macrophage in delayed hypersensitivity. Br. Med. Bull. *23*:9, 1967.

21. Feldman, J. D., and Najarian, J. S.: Dynamics and quantitative analysis of passively transferred tuberculin hypersensitivity. J. Immunol. *91*:306, 1963.

22. Gadol, N., and Waldman, R. H.: Migration inhibitory factor induction by nonspecific mitogenic stimulation of mouse lymphocytes. J. Reticuloendothel. Soc. *14*:398, 1973.

23. Galindo, B., and Myrvik, Q. N.: Migratory response of granulomatous alveolar cells from BCG-sensitized rabbits. J. Immunol. *105*:227, 1970.

24. George, M., and Vaughan, J. H.: *In vitro* cell migration as a model for delayed hypersensitivity. Proc. Soc. Exp. Biol. Med. *111*:514, 1962.

25. Granger, G. A., Moore, G. E., White, J. G., Matzinger, P., Sundsmo, J. S., Shupe, S., Kolb, W. P., Kramer, J., and Glade, P. R.: Production of lymphotoxin and migration inhibitory factor by established human lymphocytic cell lines. J. Immunol. *104*:1476, 1970.

26. Gumbiner, C., Paterson, P. Y., Youmans, G. P., and Youmans, A. S.: Adjuvanticity of mycobacterial RNA and poly A:U for induction of experimental allergic encephalomyelitis in guinea pigs. J. Immunol. *110*:309, 1973.

27. Heise, E. R., and Weiser, R. S.: Tuberculin sensitivity: The effect of antilymphocyte and antimacrophage serum on cutaneous, systemic and *in vitro* reactions. J. Immunol. *104*:704, 1970.

28. Jenner, E.: An inquiry into the causes and effects of the variolae vaccinae. London, Low, 1801.

29. Kaplin, J.: Staphylococcal enterotoxin B induced release of macrophage migration inhibition factor from normal lymphocytes. Cell. Immunol. *3*:245, 1972.

30. Klun, C. L., Neiburger, R. G., and Youmans, G. P.: Relationship between mouse mycobacterial growth-inhibitory factor and mouse migration inhibitory factor in supernatant fluids from mouse lymphocyte cultures. J. Reticuloendothel. Soc. *13*:310, 1973.

31. Koch, R.: Fortsetzung der Mittheilungen uber ein Heilmittel gegen Tuberkulose. Deutsche Med. Wochenschr. *17*:101, 1891.

32. Kuwabara, S.: Amino acid sequence of tuberculin-active protein from *Mycobacterium tuberculosis*. J. Biol. Chem. *250*:2563, 1975.

33. Kuwabara, S.: Purification and properties of tuberculin-active protein from *Mycobacterium tuberculosis*. J. Biol. Chem. *250*:2556, 1975.

34. Landi, S., and Held, H. R.: Present status of tuberculin. Ann. Sclavo *13*:862, 1971.

35. Lawrence, H. S.: Introductory remarks. Intersociety symposium: *In vitro* correlates of delayed hypersensitivity. Fed. Proc. *27*:3, 1968.

36. Lawrence, H. S.: Transfer factor. Adv. Immunol. *11*:195, 1969.

37. Long, E. R.: Tuberculous reinfection and the tuberculin reaction in the testicle of the tuberculous guinea pig. Am. Rev. Tuberc. *9*:215, 1924.

38. Long, E. R., and Finner, L. L.: Experimental glomerulonephritis produced by intrarenal tuberculin reactions. Am. J. Pathol. *4*:571, 1928.

39. Long, E. R., Seibert, F. B., and Aronson, J. D.: A standardized tuberculin (purified protein derivative) for uniformity in diagnosis and epidemiology. Tubercle *16*:304, 1935.

40. Mackaness, G. B.: The immunology of antituberculous immunity. Am. Rev. Respir. Dis. *97*:337, 1968.

41. Neiburger, R. G., and Youmans, G. P.: Inhibition of migration of mouse macrophages by tuberculin-sensitive mouse lymphocytes and by mouse migration inhibitory factor. Infect. Immun. *7*:190, 1973.

42. Neiburger, R. G., Youmans, G. P., and Youmans, A. S.: Relationship between tuberculin hypersensitivity and cellular immunity to infection in mice vaccinated with viable attenuated mycobacterial cells or with mycobacterial ribonucleic acid preparations. Infect. Immun. *8*:42, 1973.

43. Opie, E. L.: The significance of allergy in disease. Medicine *15*:489, 1936.

44. Ortiz-Ortiz, L., Solarolo, E. B., and Bojalil, L. F.: Delayed hypersensitivity to ribosomal protein from BCG. J. Immunol. *107*:1022, 1971.

45. Outschoorn, A. S.: Standardization of tuberculins. Ann. Sclavo *13*:884, 1971.

46. Papageorgiou, P. S., Henley, W. L., and Glade, P. R.: Production and characterization of migration inhibitory factor(s) (MIF) of established lymphoid and non-lymphoid cell lines. J. Immunol. *108*:494, 1972.

47. Pick, E., Brostoff, J., Krejci, K., and Turk, J. L.: Interaction between "sensitized lymphocytes" and antigen *in vitro*. II. Mitogen-induced release of skin reactive and macrophage migration inhibitory factors. Cell. Immunol. *1*:92, 1970.

48. Remold, H. G., and David, J. R.: Further studies on migration inhibitory factor (MIF): Evidence for its glycoprotein nature. J. Immunol. *107*:1090, 1971.

49. Remold, H. G., David, R. A., and David, J. R.: Characterization of migration inhibitory factor (MIF) from guinea pig lymphocytes stimulated with concanavalin A. J. Immunol. *109*:578, 1972.

50. Remold, H. G., Katz, A. B., Haber, E., and David, J. R.: Studies on migration inhibitory factor (MIF): Recovery of MIF activity after purification by gel filtration and disc electrophoresis. Cell. Immunol. *1*:133, 1970.

51. Rich, A. R.: The Pathogenesis of Tuberculosis. 2nd ed. Springfield, Ill., Charles C Thomas, 1951.

52. Rich, A. R., and Follis, R. H., Jr.: Studies on the site of sensitivity in the Arthus phenomenon. Bull. Johns Hopkins Hosp. *66*:106, 1940.

53. Rich, A. R., and Lewis, M. R.: The nature of allergy in tuberculosis as revealed by tissue culture studies. Bull. Johns Hopkins Hosp. *50*:115, 1932.

54. Rich, A. R., and McCordock, H. A.: An enquiry concerning the role of allergy, immunity and other factors of importance in the pathogenesis of human tuberculosis. Bull. Johns Hopkins Hosp. *44*:273, 1929.

55. Rocklin, R. E.: Production of migration inhibitory factor by non-dividing lymphocytes. J. Immunol. *110*:674, 1973.

56. Rosenthal, S. R.: BCG Vaccination Against Tuberculosis. Boston, Little, Brown and Company, 1957.

57. Saletti, M., Barnabe, R., Lenzini, L., and Ricci, A.: Preparazione, proprietá fisico-chimiche ed attivitá biologica delle tubercoline purificate. Ann. Sclavo *13*:838, 1971.

58. Salvin, S. B.: Occurrence of delayed hypersensitivity during the development of Arthus type hypersensitivity. J. Exp. Med. *107*:109, 1958.

59. Schlossman, S. F., Levin, H. A., Rocklin, R. E., and David, J. R.: The compartmentalization of antigen-reactive lymphocytes in desensitized guinea pigs. J. Exp. Med. *134*:741, 1971.

60. Seibert, F. B., Aronson, J. D., Reichel, J., Clark, L. T., and Long, E. R.: Purified protein derivative. A standardized tuberculin for uniformity in diagnosis and epidemiology. Am. Rev. Tuberc. *30*:Supplement, 1934.

61. Svejcar, J., Johanovsky, J., and Pekarek, J.: Studies on the mechanism of delayed type hypersensitivity in tissue cultures. X. The ability of substances released during cultivation of hypersensitive spleen cells with antigen to influence migration activity of normal cells. Z. Immunitaetsforsch. *133*:187, 1967.

62. Tubergen, D. G., Feldman, J. D., Pollock, E.

M., and Lerner, R. A.: Production of macrophage migration inhibition factor by continuous cell lines. J. Exp. Med. *135*:255, 1972.

63. Turk, J. L.: Delayed Hypersensitivity. Amsterdam, North-Holland Publishing Company, 1967.

64. Turk, J. L., and Polak, L.: Studies on the origin and reactive ability *in vivo* of peritoneal exudate cells in delayed hypersensitivity. Int. Arch. Allergy Appl. Immunol. *31*:403, 1967.

65. Uhr, J. W.: Delayed hypersensitivity. Physiol. Rev. *46*:359, 1966.

66. Wayne, L. G.: Phenol-soluble antigens from *Mycobacterium kansasii, Mycobacterium gastri,* and *Mycobacterium marinum.* Infect. Immun. *3*:36, 1971.

67. Wesslen, T.: Passive transfer of tuberculin hypersensitivity by viable lymphocytes

from thoracic duct. Acta Tuberc. Scandinav. *26*:38, 1952.

68. Wilson, G. S., and Miles, A.: Topley and Wilson's Principles of Bacteriology, Virology and Immunity. 6th ed. Baltimore, The Williams & Wilkins Company, 1975.

69. Wright, G. L., Jr., Affronti, L. F., and Reich, M.: Characterization and comparison of mycobacterial antigens by two-dimensional polyacrylamide gel electrophoresis. Infect. Immun. *5*:482, 1972.

70. Youmans, G. P.: Relation between delayed hypersensitivity and immunity in tuberculosis. Am. Rev. Respir. Dis. *111*:109, 1975.

71. Youmans, G. P., and Youmans, A. S.: The effect of mycobacterial RNA on the primary antibody response of mice to bovine γ globulin. J. Immunol. *109*:217, 1972.

8

Acquired Immunity in Tuberculosis

INTRODUCTION

In addition to the appearance of delayed hypersensitivity to tuberculoprotein, persons infected with either virulent or attenuated tubercle bacilli will develop a markedly increased resistance to reinfection. This state of tuberculoimmunity is specific (although it may be accompanied by an element of nonspecificity), and it persists for an extended period. The nature of this immune response will be considered at length in Chapter 12; here, we wish only to stress the major features of tuberculoimmunity, since it is so different from that which is used by the immune host to deal with extracellular parasites. Specific tuberculoimmunity is characterized by intracellular (intramacrophagic) bacteriostasis, rather than by intracellular killing, which characterizes the manner in which the immune host copes with extracellular parasites. This process has been ascribed to a cytophilic antibody,[22] to delayed hypersensitivity,[16] or merely to hyperactive macrophages.[9]

Pertinent to the determination of the acquired immune response is the definition of the substance, or substances, in the tubercle bacillus responsible for the stimulation of immunity. A large amount of effort by a number of investigators over the years has revealed that a variety of poorly defined substances, extracted by chemical or physical means from mycobacterial cells, will induce some increase in resistance to infection in some species of animal, under appropriate conditions of testing. This large literature has been reviewed by Crowle,[8] more recently by Kanai,[14] by Smith and his coworkers,[24] and by Youmans and Youmans.[39] None of these substances has been completely

225

characterized and identified as the inducer of the specific immune response. In fact, there is no agreement that acquired immunity in tuberculosis is specific, since some believe that it operates equally well against other facultative intracellular parasites.[16] This point of view, however, is not supported by the work of Coppel and Youmans[4-6] and by other researchers.[12]

Relevant to the question of the specificity of the immune response is the solution of the still-unsettled problem of whether living attenuated mycobacterial cells and killed attenuated cells are equally immunogenic. The very large literature on this subject, reviewed by Weiss,[26] Youmans and Youmans,[39] Smith and colleagues,[24] and Kanai,[14] generally supports the view that living cells are far more active in this respect than are killed cells. However, Weiss[26] points out that this may be an invalid conclusion because it does not take into account the fact that when comparable numbers of living and killed attenuated mycobacterial cells are injected into experimental animals, the living cells multiply and metabolize for a long enough period to produce far more immunizing substance than could be present in the dead cells. The validity of this position, in turn, rests upon establishing that 1) attenuated viable mycobacterial cells actually multiply to a significant extent in vivo; and 2) the substance, or substances, in killed and viable cells is the same — in other words, that there is no labile immunogen in viable cells.

This is of particular importance because if killed mycobacterial cells, regardless of the method of killing, are far less effective as immunizing agents than are viable mycobacterial cells, the possibility of extracting a potent immunogen from killed mycobacterial cells is remote. The starting material for the preparation of mycobacterial immunogens should logically be the most immunogenic material available; that is, living mycobacterial cells.

Some studies have purported to show that cobalt-60 irradiated tubercle bacilli[19] and ethylene oxide-killed tubercle bacilli[7] are as effective immunizing agents as are living cells, but the evidence is far from convincing.

It generally has been assumed that attenuated strains, such as BCG, multiply in vivo and that the immunizing capacity is directly proportional to the extent to which multiplication takes place.[2, 3, 7, 10, 11, 20, 21] On the other hand, it is clear that certain attenuated or avirulent mycobacterial strains, such as the H37Ra mutant, do not multiply significantly in vivo (in fact, they are rapidly destroyed); yet these strains produce nearly as great an immune response in experimental animals as do the viable and supposedly multiplying BCG strains.[15, 17, 25, 37] As for the second point, evidence has now accumulated that clearly shows the presence of at least two immunizing moieties in the mycobacterial cells. One of these is heat-stable and located predominantly in the cell wall, inducing a low-grade immune response to tuberculous infection; it is responsible for the nonspecific immunity noted to other intracellular parasites.[5, 38] The second immunogen is quite labile and is found in the ribosomal fraction when viable broken mycobacterial cells are fractionated by differential centrifugation under the proper conditions.[30-35, 38]

However, in spite of the evidence, the opinion is still widely held that the only difference in the immunizing capacity of dead and living attenuated mycobacterial cells is quantitative. Therefore, much meaningless effort has been expended in the chemical fractionation of cells killed by harsh extraction methods or cells killed with a germicide before the analytic procedure is begun. Part of the reason for the persistance of this concept is that a number of workers have compared the immunizing potency of dead and living cells, such as BCG,[13, 27] and have noted that large immunizing doses of dead cells will produce a degree of immunity to tuberculous infection in experimental animals comparable to that produced by a small number of living cells. The unfortunate feature of these studies is that although graded immunizing doses of killed cells may be used, they are usually compared with only a single, much smaller dose of living cells, apparently on the assumption that the living cells will multiply and produce the maximum immune response possible. The pitfall in this type of experimentation lies in the real possibility that the living cells do not multiply or metabolize appreciably *in vivo*, thus making the conclusion from the comparison invalid because larger immunizing doses of living cells should then be even more effective than the larger doses of killed cells. Collins and Miller[2] have stated that mycobacterial cells do not contain a heat-labile immunizing substance because the immunogenicity of heat-killed cells is restored by incorporation into Freund's incomplete adjuvant. As we will soon see, this is incorrect.

COMPARATIVE IMMUNIZING POTENCY OF KILLED AND LIVING MYCOBACTERIAL CELLS

The proper resolution of this problem should involve the determination of the immunizing dose-immune response relationship, using both living and killed cells and using an in vivo model in which it is known that the viable cells used for vaccination do not multiply significantly but, on the contrary, are rapidly destroyed.[23] In such a system, other factors, such as the age of cells used to immunize, the time of challenge, the route of challenge, the method of killing cells, and the effect of adjuvants, also can be measured more validly.

Over a number of years, we have collected such data in a mouse infection system. These data show that at least in this one system, attenuated mycobacterial cells killed by a variety of methods are never as immunogenic as living cells. The evidence will therefore support the thesis that living cells are more immunogenic because of the possession of a labile immunizing antigen (see Chapter 9).[30-33]

In our studies,[36] the H37Ra attenuated strain of *M. tuberculosis* was used for the preparation of all vaccines. The virulent H37Rv strain of *M. tuberculosis* was used in all cases for challenge of control and vaccinated mice. Both of these cultures were maintained by weekly subculture on a modified Proskauer and Beck medium.[34, 35] The preparation and standardization of suspensions of mycobacterial cells for vaccination or challenge has been described in detail (see also Chapter 9).[34] A 1.0 mg amount, moist weight (0.2 mg dry weight), of both mycobacterial strains contained approximately 10^7 viable particles, as determined by plating.[23]

The vaccines consisted of either viable cells of the H37Ra strain or cells of the same strain killed by heat or chemicals. Most of the experiments were conducted with cells killed by autoclaving for 15 minutes at 121° C, although in certain instances lower temperatures were used. Treated suspensions of mycobacterial cells were tested for viability by subculture of several 0.1 ml portions on egg yolk agar, with incubation at 37° C for 8 to 12 weeks. The H37Ra cells were killed by phenol by exposing large numbers of H37Ra cells to a large volume of 2 percent phenol solution for 24 hours, after which they were washed three times with large volumes of distilled water. Acetone-dried cells were prepared by washing, on a sintered glass filter, large numbers of H37Ra cells with three 500 ml volumes of cold acetone. Viability tests were carried out as before. Viability tests were done on all chemically treated cells, and all were sterile, except for the vaccine prepared by treating with acetone alone from which a few viable cells were cultivated. Accurate counts were not done, but estimation from gross observations indicated that the vast majority of the cells were killed by the acetone treatment. All mice were vaccinated intraperitoneally with the appropriate vaccine contained in 0.2 ml of 0.01 M phosphate buffer solution (pH 7.0). Freund's incomplete adjuvant was prepared by the use of aquaphor and heavy mineral oil,[32] and 0.4 ml of adjuvant vaccine mixture was injected intraperitoneally.

Male mice, CF-1, weighing between 18 and 22 g, were used exclusively. Both vaccinated and control mice were infected by the intravenous injection of 1.0 mg of a fine suspension of the virulent H37Rv strain of *M. tuberculosis*. The mice were observed daily, and a record was kept of the time of death of each experimental animal. The surviving animals were sacrificed 31 days after infection, and the number of 30-day survivors (S-30 mice) in each experimental group was compared with the number of S-30 mice in the other experimental groups and in the nonvaccinated animals. The rationale for and the validity of this evaluation procedure have been covered thoroughly elsewhere (see Chapter 15).[37]

Figure 8–1 presents the immune response of CF-1 mice to immunization intraperitoneally with different numbers of living and heat-killed (autoclaved), four-week-old cells of the attenuated H37Ra strain of *M. tuberculosis*. In this graph, the data obtained from different experiments were pooled. The number of animals represented by each point on the graph varies from 58 to 394 with the living cells, and from 59 to 90 with the heat-killed cells. All animals were challenged with the virulent strain four weeks after vaccination. The data clearly show that the response to immunization with both living and heat-killed cells is dose dependent and that living cells are several hun-

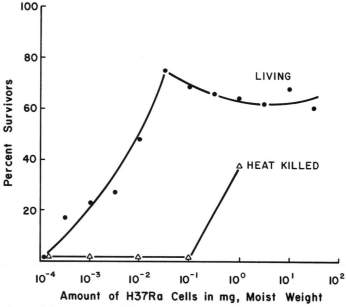

FIGURE 8–1. Immunizing capacity of living and heat-killed 4-week-old H37Ra cells. (From Youmans, G. P., and Youmans, A. S.: Immunizing capacity of viable and killed attenuated mycobacterial cells against experimental tuberculous infection. J. Bacteriol. 97:107, 1969.)

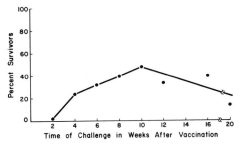

FIGURE 8–2. Effect of time upon immune response of CF-1 mice vaccinated with 0.001 mg viable H37Ra cells. (From Youmans, G. P., and Youmans, A. S.: Relative effectiveness of living and non-living vaccines. *In* Status of Immunization in Tuberculosis in 1971. National Institutes of Health, Bethesda, Md., October, 1971. DHEW Publication No. (NIH) 72-68.)

To further explore the relationship of time of challenge to immune response, the small 10^{-3} mg immunizing dose of viable cells was selected because the immune response produced at four weeks was poor; therefore, mice were vaccinated intraperitoneally and challenged at regular intervals over a period of 20 weeks. The results are shown in Table 8–1 and Figure 8–2. Also shown in Table 8–1 is the response of mice given a thousandfold higher immunizing dose of H37Ra. It is evident that the response following intraperitoneal immunization with the small dose did not reach a maximum until 10 weeks after vaccination. In contrast, companion experiments showed that when the same numbers of viable H37Ra were injected intravenously, a higher immune response was obtained in a shorter time, since 90 percent of the vaccinated animals survived challenge at 4 weeks. This emphasizes the importance of the route of vaccination. The findings did not result from multiplication in vivo of the few viable cells initially injected. This was covered by exhaustive experiments in which mice injected intraperitoneally or intravenously with the same small number of viable cells were sacrificed at weekly intervals;

dred times more effective than heat-killed cells. Also, the larger dose of living cells appeared to suppress the immune response. To test this hypothesis, some of the mice of the groups vaccinated with 1.0, 10.0, and 50.0 mg were challenged 8 weeks after vaccination. At this time, the percentages of S-30 mice were found to be 92, 95, and 90 respectively, establishing the point that the response to immunization of mice with living mycobacterial cells is not only dose but also time dependent.

TABLE 8–1. **Immune Response of Mice Vaccinated Intraperitoneally with Viable H37Ra Cells***

Time of challenge After Vaccination (Weeks)	Mice Injected With 0.001 mg of Vaccine			Mice Injected With 1.0 mg of Vaccine		
	No. of Mice	No. of S-30 Mice	Per-cent of S-30 Mice	No. of Mice	No. of S-30 Mice	Per-cent of S-30 Mice
2	94	2	2	100	70	70
4	139	17	24	137	115	84
6	97	31	32	47	41	87
8	135	53	39	130	104	80
10	134	64	48	135	94	70
12	134	45	34	133	92	69
16	38	15	40	39	27	69
20	29	4	14	24	18	75

*The percent of nonvaccinated S-30 mice ranged from 4 to 11, except at 20 weeks when it increased to 24 percent. (From Youmans, G. P., and Youmans, A. S.: Immunizing capacity of viable and killed attenuated mycobacterial cells against experimental tuberculous infection. J. Bacteriol. 97:107, 1969.)

then the spleens, livers, lungs, and kidneys were homogenized, and samples of appropriate dilutions were plated on suitable media. In all cases, the number of viable cells that could be detected this way rapidly decreased and had disappeared by four weeks.

All of these experiments were conducted using mice that had been vaccinated with H37Ra cells harvested four weeks after the medium had been inoculated. We have found that cells harvested two weeks after inoculation not only immunize mice more effectively but have a much higher content of ribonucleic acid and protein and serve as a much better source of immunizing ribosomal fraction.[34] Therefore, the immunizing dose-immune response relationship in mice to tuberculous infection was reinvestigated using two-week-old cells (Fig. 8–3). These data confirm the greater immunizing activity of viable two-week-old cells not only in respect to the minimal number of viable cells that will provoke an immune response but also in

respect to the rate at which the immune response develops and the magnitude of the response with the larger doses. Since a maximal response occurred with the three highest doses of viable cells, the enormous numbers employed with four-week-old cells were not used. Heat-killed two-week-old cells, on the other hand, did not differ significantly in immunizing power from heat-killed four-week-old cells when comparable doses were used. In these experiments, mice vaccinated with even larger doses (10.0 and 50.0 mg) of heat-killed cells were challenged at two, four, and eight weeks (Table 8–2). The results at four weeks were used to plot the curve in Figure 8–3. The data and the graph show that even these enormous immunizing doses did not greatly increase the immune response. Furthermore, the immune response engendered by these massive doses was approximately the same at two, four, and eight weeks (Table 8–2). This is in contrast to the observations made when the same

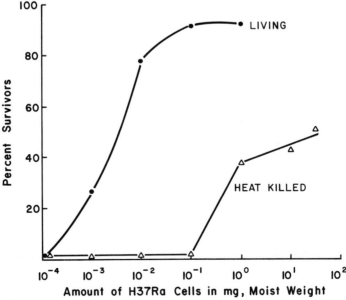

FIGURE 8–3. Immunizing capacity of living and heat-killed two-week-old H37Ra cells. (From Youmans, G. P., and Youmans, A. S.: Immunizing capacity of viable and killed attenuated mycobacterial cells against experimental tuberculous infection. J. Bacteriol. *97*:107, 1969.)

TABLE 8–2. Immune Response of Mice Vaccinated Intraperitoneally with Heat-killed 2-week-old H37Ra Cells and Challenged at Different Times After Vaccination

Moist Weight of Vaccine	Challenged at 2 Weeks		Challenged at 4 Weeks		Challenged at 8 Weeks	
	No. of Mice	Per-cent of S-30 Mice	No. of Mice	Per-cent of S-30 Mice	No. of Mice	Per-cent of S-30 Mice
mg						
50	19	53	54	56	19	64
10	28	57	59	42	25	43
1	18	44	88	38	25	32
0.1	29	3	90	8	53	23
0.01	30	0	89	10	55	22
0.001	30	13	59	5	55	13
None	30	13	90	1	55	22

From Youmans, G. P., and Youmans, A. S.: Immunizing capacity of viable and killed attenuated mycobacterial cells against experimental tuberculous infection. J. Bacteriol. 97:107, 1969.

large vaccinating dose of viable cells was employed (Fig. 8–1).

An objection might be raised to the use of such a high temperature for the killing of the cells, since a lower temperature might destroy viability but leave a moderately labile immunogen untouched. Therefore, experiments were conducted in which cells were killed by boiling (98° C) for 30 minutes or by being held at 65° C for 30 minutes. These cells were then injected intraperitoneally into mice as before. The cells heated at 98° C were no more immunogenic than those that had been autoclaved (Table 8–3). Those cells held at 65° C produced an immune response with the 1.0 mg dose but were inactive when the dose was lowered to 0.1 mg. The viable H37Ra cells, from which the heated cells were prepared, produced a substantial immune response when 0.01 mg was given (52 percent S-30 mice).

Also included in Table 8–3 is the immune response obtained at four weeks when four-week-old H37Ra cells killed by phenol or dried with acetone were used as vaccines. These two organic reagents were chosen because it has been claimed that phenol-killed cells are not only as effective

immunizing agents as living cells but also because they have been used to prepare immunogenic fractions of tubercle bacilli.[27] Acetone is frequently used to dry mycobacterial cells used as vaccines or as sources of immunogenic fractions. The results show that both reagents destroyed the immunizing activity more effectively than did autoclaving, even though minute numbers of viable cells were detected in the cell suspensions exposed to acetone.

EFFECT OF FREUND'S INCOMPLETE ADJUVANT ON THE IMMUNOGENIC ACTIVITY OF LIVING AND KILLED H37Ra CELLS

Finally, the effect of Freund's incomplete adjuvant on the immunogenic activity of heat-killed and viable H37Ra cells was tested. This adjuvant is frequently used as a vehicle to increase the immunizing activity of mycobacterial cell fractions.[13] In addition, Bloch and Ferreira[1] and Hoyt and colleagues[13] have reported that Freund-type adjuvants significantly decrease

TABLE 8-3. Immune Response of Mice Vaccinated with H37Ra Cells Killed by Heat and Chemicals

Method of Treatment of H37Ra Cells	Amount of Vaccine Injected									
	1.0 MG		0.1 MG		0.01 MG		0.001 MG		NONE	
	No. of Mice	Percent of S-30 Mice	No. of Mice	Percent of S-30 Mice	No. of Mice	Percent of S-30 Mice	No. of Mice	Percent of S-30 Mice	No. of Mice	Percent of S-30 Mice
Boiling at 98° C for 30 min	39	31	38	11	39	8	35	11	40	3
Holding at 65° C for 30 min	29	79	29	14	19	5	18	0	30	17
Phenol (2.0 Percent)	40	13	37	0	19	16	15	20	37	11
Acetone-dried	36	17	34	1					37	11

From Youmans, G. P., and Youmans, A. S.: Immunizing capacity of viable and killed attenuated mycobacterial cells against experimental tuberculous infection. J. Bacteriol. 97:107, 1969.

TABLE 8-4. Effect of Freund's Incomplete Adjuvant on the Immunizing Capacity of Viable and Heat-killed H37Ra Cells

Amount of Vaccine mg	Viable H37Ra Cells				Heat-killed H37Ra Cells			
	Without Adjuvant		With Adjuvant		Without Adjuvant		With Adjuvant	
	No. of Mice	Percent of S-30 Mice	No. of Mice	Percent of S-30 Mice	No. of Mice	Percent of S-30 Mice	No. of Mice	Percent of S-30 Mice
1.0	148	90	119	93	120	68	120	58
0.1	117	89	117	91	119	28	117	32
0.01	120	79	117	85	120	26	118	19
0.001	149	26	148	36	114	11	117	17
0.0001	117	12	117	23				
None	139	14						

From Youmans, G. P., and Youmans, A. S.: Immunizing capacity of viable and killed attenuated mycobacterial cells against experimental tuberculous infection. J. Bacteriol. 97:107, 1969.

the immunizing capacity of mycobacterial whole cells for mice. We have shown that both the composition and method of preparation of Freund's incomplete adjuvant significantly affect the adjuvant activity.[32] Table 8–4 shows the effect of Freund's incomplete adjuvant on the immunizing activity of both heat-killed and viable H37Ra cells when tested by challenge four weeks after vaccination. There is little indication from the data that immunizing activity of whole cells, whether viable or killed, was affected appreciably by being administered in Freund's incomplete adjuvant. Statistically, living cells given in adjuvant in doses of 0.01 or 0.001 mg were slightly more effective ($P = 0.05$). These results are in conflict with those reported by Collins and Miller.[2] However, the procedures used by Collins and Miller could not be expected to reveal the lack of effect of Freund's incomplete adjuvant because graded doses of the immunizing agents were not used (see also Chapter 15).

Results such as these help to clarify the situation regarding the relative immunizing activity of living, attenuated mycobacterial cells and the same cells killed by heat or certain chemicals. It is clear that the immune response produced by both types of cells is dose and time dependent. Also when the respective dose-response curves are compared, living cells prove to be several hundred times more effective. It is possible to obtain an immune response with dead cells equivalent to that produced by living cells, but only when the immunizing dose of dead cells is several hundred times larger. Expressed in another way, no matter how large the immunizing doses of killed cells, there will be a smaller number of living cells that will be far more immunogenic. Therefore, the statement that killed mycobacterial cells are as effective immunizing agents as living cells is incorrect unless these quantitative factors are taken into consideration.

It is important to emphasize that the present studies were done employing an in vivo system in which the viable immunizing mycobacterial cells did not increase significantly in number; instead, viability was rapidly lost and, depending upon the number of cells used for vaccination, could no longer be detected in the tissues after a four- to six-week period. Our own studies[23] completely confirm the original findings of Middlebrook and colleagues[18] that the H37Ra strain does not multiply in certain strains of mice, regardless of the number of cells injected. Yamamura and coworkers[28, 29] have also shown that the H37Ra mycobacterial strain does not increase in number in CF-1 mice. The only contrary findings are those of Larson and Wicht,[15] who reported that H37Ra cells multiply extensively in the organs of the RML mouse strain.

The greater efficacy, therefore, in these experiments of viable cells for vaccination cannot be ascribed to in vivo multiplication. The production of an immunizing metabolic product in vivo by the viable cells cannot be ruled out. However, the rapidity with which viability is lost in vivo and the fact that very small doses of viable cells (0.001 mg) will immunize as well as enormous doses (1.0 to 50 mg) of killed cells makes this seem very unlikely, especially in view of the fact that a labile substance equal in immunizing capacity to that of viable mycobacterial cells can be isolated from living cells of the H37Ra strain.[30-33]

SPECIFICITY OF THE IMMUNE RESPONSE TO VIABLE AND KILLED MYCOBACTERIAL CELLS

From the results of this study and from the experience of many others over the years,[26] the method of killing appears inconsequential; once mycobacterial cells are dead, they are poor immunizing agents. However, a factor that usually is not taken into consideration is the time of exposure to the lethal agent; to be certain that all cells are dead, maximal exposure time is usually used rather than the minimal time required to kill all cells. It might be that with certain germicides, a brief exposure, although killing all the cells, might leave the labile immunizing component unaffected.

The marked superiority of living mycobacterial cells over killed cells for immunization is not noted when vaccinated mice are challenged with *Listeria monocytogenes* and *Klebsiella pneumoniae*[4-6] instead of *M. tuberculosis*. In fact, living and heat-killed mycobacterial cells perform equally well in inducing protection against these heterologous microorganisms and the magnitude of the immune response is equivalent only to that noted with the killed cells when challenge is with *M. tuberculosis*. This emphasizes again the necessity of recognizing that there are at least two immunizing moieties in attenuated mycobacterial cells. One is a relatively stable cell wall component, which immunizes equally well against homologous and heterologous infection and is possibly similar in its action to *Escherichia coli* endotoxin; the other is a labile material that has a much greater capacity to immunize, but only against mycobacterial infection. Therefore, living and killed mycobacterial cells differ not only quantitatively in their capacity to immunize against tuberculous infection but also qualitatively. In addition, the techniques used for measurement of the immune response may seriously affect measurement of immunity to tuberculosis in experimental animals (see Chapter 15 for a detailed discussion of these procedures).

REFERENCES

1. Bloch, H., and Ferreira, I.: The effect of adjuvants on antituberculosis vaccination with live mycobacteria. J. Immunol. *83*:372, 1959.
2. Collins, F. M., and Miller, T. E.: Growth of a drug-resistant strain of *Mycobacterium bovis* (BCG) in normal and immunized mice. J. Infect. Dis. *120*:517, 1969.
3. Collins, F. M., and Montalbine, V.: Relative immunogenicity of streptomycin-sensitive and -resistant strains of BCG. Infect. Immun. *8*:381, 1973.
4. Coppel, S., and Youmans, G. P.: Specificity of acquired resistance produced by immunization with *Listeria monocytogenes* and listeria fractions. J. Bacteriol. *97*:121, 1968.
5. Coppel, S., and Youmans, G. P.: Specificity of acquired resistance produced by immunization with mycobacterial cells and mycobacterial fractions. J. Bacteriol. *97*:114, 1968.
6. Coppel, S. and Youmans, G. P.: Specificity of the anamnestic response produced by *Listeria monocytogenes* or *Mycobacterium tuberculosis* to challenge with *Listeria monocytogenes*. J. Bacteriol. *97*:127, 1968.
7. Costello, R. and Dubos, R. J.: Comparative vaccination studies in mice with BCG and mycobacteria killed by ethylene oxide. Japan-United States Cooperative Medical Science Program Abstracts. Leprosy and Tuberculosis Conference, May 18–20, Tokyo, 1965.
8. Crowle, A. J.: Immunizing constituents of the tubercle bacillus. Bacteriol. Rev. *22*:183, 1958.
9. Dannenberg, A. M., Jr., Meyer, O. T., Esterly, J. R., and Kambara, T.: The local nature of immunity in tuberculosis, illustrated histochemically in dermal BCG lesions. J. Immunol. *100*:931, 1968.
10. Dubos, R. J., and Pierce, C. H.: Differential characteristics *in vitro* and *in vivo* of several substrains of BCG. I. Multiplication and survival *in vitro*. Am. Rev. Tuberc. *74*:655, 1956.
11. Dubos, R. J., and Pierce, C. H.: Differential characteristics *in vitro* and *in vivo* of several substrains of BCG. IV. Immunizing effectiveness. Am. Rev. Tuberc. *74*:699, 1956.
12. Frenkel, J. K., and Caldwell, S. A.: Specific immunity and nonspecific resistance to infection: *Listeria*, protozoa, and viruses in mice and hamsters. J. Infect. Dis. *131*:201, 1975.
13. Hoyt, A., Thompson, M. A., Moore, F. J., and Smith, C. R.: The effect of adjuvants on a nonviable antituberculosis vaccine and on live BCG. Am. Rev. Respir. Dis. *91*:565, 1965.
14. Kanai, K.: Review. Acquired resistance to tuberculous infection in experimental model. Jpn. J. Med. Sci. Biol. *20*:21, 1967.
15. Larson, C. L., and Wicht, W. C.: Infection

of mice with *Mycobacterium tuberculosis,* strain H37Ra. Am Rev. Respir. Dis. *90:*742, 1964.

16. Mackaness, G. B.: The immunology of antituberculous immunity. Am. Rev. Respir. Dis. *97:*337, 1968.

17. Meyer, S. N.: Animal studies on effects of BCG, H37Ra and *Mycobacterium phlei* in tuberculosis immunization. Tubercle *37:*11, 1956.

18. Middlebrook, G., Dubos, R. J., and Pierce, C.: Virulence and morphological characteristics of mammalian tubercle bacilli. J. Exp. Med. *86:*175, 1947.

19. Nishihara, H., Lawrence, C. A., Taplin, G. V., and Carpenter, C. M.: Immunogenicity of gamma-irradiated *Mycobacterium tuberculosis* H37Rv (GIV) in mice. Am. Rev. Respir. Dis. *88:*827, 1963.

20. Pierce, C. H., and Dubos, R. J.: Differential characteristics *in vitro* and *in vivo* of several substrains of BCG. II. Morphologic characteristics *in vitro* and *in vivo*. Am. Rev. Tuberc. *74:*667, 1956.

21. Pierce, C. H., Dubos, R. J., and Schaefer, W. B.: Differential characteristics *in vitro* and *in vivo* of several substrains of BCG. III. Multiplication and survival *in vivo*. Am. Rev. Tuberc. *74:*683, 1956.

22. Rowley, D.: Phagocytosis and immunity. Experientia 22:1, 1966.

23. Sever, J. L., and Youmans, G. P.: The enumeration of nonpathogenic viable tubercle bacilli from the organs of mice. Am. Rev. Tuberc. *75:*280, 1957.

24. Smith, D. W., Grover, A. A., and Wiegeshaus, E.: Nonliving immunogenic substances of mycobacteria. Adv. Tuberc. Res. *16:*191, 1968.

25. Steiner, M., and Zuger, B.: Allergy and immunity in tuberculosis. I. Immunization and reinfection of guinea pigs with homologous variants of the human tubercle bacillus H37. J. Immunol. *46:*83, 1943.

26. Weiss, D. W.: Vaccination against tuberculosis with nonliving vaccines. I. The problem and its historical background. Am. Rev. Respir. Dis. *80:*340–358, 495–509, 676–688, 1959.

27. Weiss, D. W., and Wells, A. Q.: Vaccination against tuberculosis with nonliving vaccines. II. Vaccination of guinea pigs with phenol-killed tubercle bacilli. Am. Rev. Respir. Dis. *81:*518, 1960.

28. Yamamura, Y., Kato, M., Ikuta, S., Okuyama, T., and Watanabe, S.: A homogenate technique of whole body of mice. Med. J. Osaka Univ. *6:*501, 1955.

29. Yamamura, Y., Walter, A., and Bloch, H.: Bacterial populations in experimental murine tuberculosis. I. Studies in normal mice. J. Infect. Dis. *106:*211, 1960.

30. Youmans, A. S., and Youmans, G. P.: Effect of trypsin and ribonuclease on the immunogenic activity of ribosomes and ribonucleic acid isolated from *Mycobacterium tuberculosis.* J. Bacteriol. *91:*2146, 1966.

31. Youmans, A. S., and Youmans, G. P.: Immunogenic activity of a ribosomal fraction obtained from *Mycobacterium tuberculosis.* J. Bacteriol. *89:*1291, 1965.

32. Youmans, A. S., and Youmans, G. P.: Preparation and effect of different adjuvants on the immunogenic activity of mycobacterial ribosomal fraction. J. Bacteriol. *94:*836, 1967.

33. Youmans, A. S., and Youmans, G. P.: Preparation of highly immunogenic ribosomal fractions of *Mycobacterium tuberculosis* by use of sodium dodecyl sulfate. J. Bacteriol. *91:*2139, 1966.

34. Youmans, A. S., and Youmans, G. P.: Ribonucleic acid, deoxyribonucleic acid, and protein content of cells of different ages of *Mycobacterium tuberculosis* and the relationship to immunogenicity. J. Bacteriol. *95:*272, 1968.

35. Youmans, G. P., and Karlson, A. G.: Streptomycin sensitivity of tubercle bacilli. Studies on recently isolated tubercle bacilli and the development of resistance to streptomycin *in vivo*. Am. Rev. Tuberc. *55:*529, 1947.

36. Youmans, G. P., and Youmans, A. S.: Immunizing capacity of viable and killed attenuated mycobacterial cells against experimental tuberculous infection. J. Bacteriol. *97:*107, 1969.

37. Youmans, G. P., and Youmans, A. S.: The measurement of the response of immunized mice to infection with *Mycobacterium tuberculosis* var. *hominis*. J. Immunol. *78:*318, 1957.

38. Youmans, G. P., and Youmans, A. S.: Nonspecific factors in resistance of mice to experimental tuberculosis. J. Bacteriol. *90:*1675, 1965.

39. Youmans, G. P., and Youmans, A. S.: Recent studies on acquired immunity in tuberculosis. Curr. Top. Microbiol. Immunol. *48:*129, 1969.

9

Biologic Activities of Mycobacterial Ribosomal and RNA Vaccines

ANNE S. YOUMANS, Ph.D.

INTRODUCTION

Since 1965, when Youmans and Youmans[99] first reported that ribosomal preparations obtained from ruptured cells of the H37Ra strain of *M. tuberculosis* were immunogenic in mice against infection with virulent tubercle bacilli, there has been a great deal of interest in the immunizing capacity of ribosomal and RNA prepara-

236

tions obtained from other bacterial species. It has been shown by a number of investigators that ribosomal and RNA vaccines prepared from a variety of bacteria, fungi, and protozoa will immunize well against infection with virulent microorganisms of the same species.[1, 23, 30, 39, 44, 57, 59, 60, 67-70, 76-85, 89, 90, 99]

In this chapter we will give the hypothesis that led to the initiation of the work that resulted in the first preparation of ribosomal and RNA vaccines from the attenuated H37Ra strain of *M. tuberculosis*. Considerable emphasis will be placed on the methods required for the production of highly active vaccines and on the chemical and the physical characteristics of the ribosomes and RNA in the vaccine. The immunizing moiety contained in the ribosomal and RNA vaccines has been found to be very labile. Therefore, special care must be taken with the manipulative procedures required for isolation and preparation in order for potent vaccines to be obtained. In the following chapter (Chapter 10), a discussion will be given of the possible modes of action of RNA and ribosomal vaccines obtained from a number of microbial species. Apparently, the type of immunity stimulated by injection of these vaccines will depend, in large part, on the nature of the immune response required to control disease production by the parasite from which the vaccine is prepared.

PREPARATION OF THE PARTICULATE FRACTION

When this research project was started approximately 25 years ago, it was generally recognized that living cells of *M. tuberculosis* were far more potent immunogens than killed cells. We have already discussed this in detail in Chapter 8. As outlined in that chapter, it seemed reasonable to hypothesize that the living cells might be more effective immunizing agents because of the presence of a substance that could easily be destroyed by heat or chemicals. An opportunity arose to test this hypothesis when Dr. Irving Millman was a graduate student in our laboratory. At that time, Dr. Millman was mechanically breaking cells of the attenuated H37Ra strain of *M. tuberculosis* to determine the enzymatic activities of various cellular components. We de-

cided to test some of these cellular components to determine if any of them might be immunogenic in mice against a standardized infection by the virulent H37Rv strain of *M. tuberculosis*. Three fractions were tested: a pellet, which was sedimented after high-speed centrifugation and which contained particles of various sizes (particulate fraction); the supernatant fluid from this centrifugation; and a fluid fatty layer, which appeared on top of the supernatant fluid. An immunogenic substance was detected only in the particulate fraction.[106] This immunogen turned out to be very labile, and we found it difficult to consistently obtain active preparations. In addition, with active material as much as 20 mg per mouse was needed to give good protection. Obviously, methods had to be devised not only to stabilize the immunizing activity but also to increase the immunogenic potency.

Dr. Koomi Kanai joined our group in the late 1950s, and he compared the protection produced in mice when vaccinated with mycobacterial cell walls with that produced with the particulate fraction. Based on weight, the particulate fraction was more immunogenic than the cell walls, as shown in Table 9–1.[32] While Dr. Kanai was with us, we also explored the capacities of particulate fraction, cell walls, and viable H37Ra cells to produce delayed hypersensitivity to tuberculoprotein in guinea pigs. Little or no skin reaction occurred in guinea pigs vaccinated with the particulate fraction, but large areas of erythema and induration as well as some necrosis occurred in guinea pigs vaccinated with the cells or the cell walls. This comparison is shown in Table 9–2.[33]

After Dr. Kanai left in 1960, we spent several years trying to determine the conditions required to obtain more stable preparations. At the time, little was known about intracellular bacterial components. Since the particulate fraction showed consider-

TABLE 9–1. Response of CF-1 Mice to Immunization with Mycobacterial Intracellular Particles and Cell Walls

	Cell Walls				Particulate Fraction		
AMOUNT INJECTED (MG)	NUMBER OF MICE	NUMBER OF S-30[a] MICE	S-30[a] MICE (PERCENT)	AMOUNT INJECTED (MG)	NUMBER OF MICE	NUMBER OF S-30[a] MICE	S-30[a] MICE (PERCENT)
40	32	3	9.3	40	16	7	43.8
30	10	0	0.0	30	84	49	58.3
20	30	1	3.3	20	20	8	40.0
10	30	5	16.6	10	97	59	60.8
4	18	2	11.1	5	40	16	40.0
2	39	3	7.7	2.5	20	1	5.0
				0	139	7	5.0
H37Ra, 1.0	193	131	67.8				

[a]S-30 = Survived 30 days.

From Kanai, K., and Youmans, G. P.: Immunogenicity of intracellular particles and cell walls from *Mycobacterium tuberculosis*. J. Bacteriol. *80:*607, 1960.

TABLE 9–2. Tuberculin Hypersensitivity Induced in Guinea Pigs by H37Ra Living Cells, Cell Walls, and Particulate Fraction

		Size of Induration Induced by 1:50 Dilution of Old Tuberculin[a]		
Sensitizing Agent	Animal Number	3 WEEKS (MM)	6 WEEKS (MM)	9 WEEKS (MM)
None (control)	1	0	0	0
	2	0	0	0
	3	0	5 × 5	0
Particulate fraction	4	0	0	0
	5	0	0	5 × 5
	6	0	0	0
	7	0	0	0
	8	0	15 × 15	0
Cell walls	9	30 × 25	20 × 20	15 × 10
	10	30 × 28	25 × 25	10 × 10
	11	21 × 22	25 × 25	10 × 10
	12	23 × 23	25 × 25	15 × 10
	13	20 × 20	20 × 20	10 × 10
H37Ra cells	14	25 × 25	35 × 30[b]	25 × 25
	15	25 × 25	30 × 30	20 × 20
	16	35 × 35	40 × 40[b]	20 × 20
	17	30 × 30	25 × 25[b]	20 × 20
	18	25 × 25	30 × 35[b]	25 × 25

[a]The tuberculin reactions were read 43 hr after tuberculin injection.
[b]Induration accompanied by central necrosis.

From Kanai, K., Youmans, G. P., and Youmans, A. S.: Allergenicity of intracellular particles, cell walls, and cytoplasmic fluid from *Mycobacterium tuberculosis*. J. Bacteriol. *80:*615, 1960.

able enzymatic activity,[45] we took much of our research direction from the work that was being done with mammalian mitochondria, thinking that the active moiety of the particulate fraction might be the bacterial equivalent of mammalian mitochondria.

Therefore, the effect on the particulate fraction of a number of substances and conditions known to affect mitochondrial activity was tested.

The immunogenicity of the particulate fraction, which had been exposed to different temperatures and hydrogen-ion concentrations, was first determined. We found that the immunogenic activity was greater if the particulate fraction was kept at 4° C and at a pH of 7.0.[98] The effect of various mitochondrial stabilizers on the immunogenic activity was measured.[93] It was noted that increasing the level of sucrose from 0.25 M to 0.44 M in the buffer in which the cells were broken improved immunogenicity to the point where protection in mice could be induced with as little as 5 mg. The effect of magnesium ions on immunogenicity was next defined. Magnesium ions improved immunogenicity, and the amounts used were critical. Magnesium ions in a concentration of 3×10^{-2} M in the 0.44 M sucrose buffer increased the potency of the particulate fraction to the point where 1.0 mg vaccinating dose immunized the mice. Other mitochondrial stabilizers were tried, but they either had no effect on immunogenicity or decreased the potency of the vaccine.

Next, the nature of the particulate fraction was explored[101] by exposing it to deoxyribonuclease and ribonuclease. The immunizing activity was susceptible to ribonuclease but was not affected by deoxyribonuclease. The particulate fraction then was differentially centrifuged to separate particles of different sizes, and the larger and most immunogenic particles were tested by different procedures in order to solubilize or rupture the membranes, since the results indicated that some structure had to be intact for immunogenic activity.

Preparations were subjected to sonic oscillation (10 kc, with a Raytheon sonic oscillator; 1.0 amp) for 15 minutes at 2 to 4° C. Sonic oscillation markedly reduced the immunogenic activity.[101]

These larger particles were treated with a number of agents in order to solubilize or rupture the membranes. The effect of freezing and thawing on the immunogenic activity of the 144,000 × g particles also was determined. It was found that this treatment also significantly reduced the immunogenic activity, as did distilled water when it was used to prepare the particulate fraction.[101]

Particulate fraction was treated with the two surface-active agents, sodium deoxycholate and sodium dodecyl sulfate (SDS), and the immunogenic activity was significantly reduced compared with the non-detergent-treated particulate fraction.[101]

Therefore, at that time (1964), we felt the enzymatically active, mitochondria-like particles were the labile immunogen and that an intact membrane was necessary for immunogenicity. No immunizing activity at this time was found in the ribosomal fraction.[101]

PREPARATION OF IMMUNOGENIC RIBOSOMAL FRACTION

In the course of some of these experiments, we had found during preparation of the particulate fraction a small amount of white, waxy substance, which was insoluble in organic

TABLE 9–3. **Immunogenic Activity of the Particulate Fraction and a Ribosomal Fraction, With and Without Freund's Incomplete Adjuvant**

Immunizing Preparation	Freund's Adjuvant Added	Amount Injected[a] (mg)	Number of Mice	Number of S-30 Mice[b]	Percent of S-30 Mice
Particulate fraction	−	20	126	90	71
	+	20	94	65	69
	−	1	112	40	36
	+	1	84	33	39
Ribosomal fraction	−	20	117	45	39
	+	20	120	81	68
	−	1	29	3	10
	+	1	52	18	35
H37Ra cells		1	115	93	81
None		0	118	4	3

[a] Moist weight.
[b] S-30 mice = number of mice that survived >30 days.
From Youmans, A. S., and Youmans, G. P.: Immunogenic activity of a ribosomal fraction obtained from *Mycobacterium tuberculosis*. J. Bacteriol. *89*:1291, 1965.

solvents, in NaOH, or in HCl but was soluble in physiologic saline and sodium bicarbonate solution — solutions in which RNA is soluble. It also was hydrolyzed by ribonuclease; this suggested that the material might be RNA. We found that this material, when incorporated into Freund's incomplete adjuvant (FIA), was very immunogenic but when injected alone, was inactive.[101]

In view of this finding, we repeated the experiments in which fractions were obtained by differential centrifugation. Half of each fraction was incorporated into FIA and injected into mice. Other mice were injected with the fraction alone. The results were quite different from those obtained previously. This time, the ribosomal fraction (the pellet collected after three hours of centrifugation at 144,000 × g) was highly

TABLE 9–4. **Effect of Sodium Deoxycholate on the Immunogenic Activity of the Particulate Fraction, With and Without Freund's Incomplete Adjuvant**

Immunizing Preparation	Freund's Adjuvant Added	Amount Injected[a] (mg)	Number of Mice	Number of S-30 Mice[b]	Percent of S-30 Mice
Particulate fraction	−	20	107	54	51
	+	20	70	47	67
Particulate fraction treated with sodium deoxycholate (recentrifuged sediment)	−	20	96	30	31
	+	20	67	35	52
H37Ra cells		1	112	70	63
Controls		0	118	12	10

[a] Moist weight.
[b] S-30 mice = number of mice that survived >30 days.
From Youmans, A. S., and Youmans, G. P.: Immunogenic activity of a ribosomal fraction obtained from *Mycobacterium tuberculosis*. J. Bacteriol. *89*:1291, 1965.

TABLE 9–5. **Immunogenic Activity of the Particulate Fraction,
With and Without Freund's Incomplete Adjuvant, After Being Mixed
With 0.25 Percent Sodium Dodecyl Sulfate**

Immunizing Preparation	Freund's Adjuvant Added	Amount Injected[a] (mg)	Number of Mice	Number of S-30 Mice[b]	Percent of S-30 Mice
Particulate fraction + sodium lauryl sulfate (recentrifuged sediment)	−	20	59	13	22
	+	20	76	53	70
H37Ra	−	1	83	55	66
Controls		0	90	1	1

[a] Moist weight.
[b] S-30 mice = number of mice that survived > 30 days.
From Youmans, A. S., and Youmans, G. P.: Immunogenic activity of a ribosomal fraction obtained from *Mycobacterium tuberculosis.* J. Bacteriol. 89:1291, 1965.

immunogenic, but only when it was emulsified in FIA; it was not immunogenic when injected alone (Table 9–3).[99] We could only speculate that apparently the membranes of the larger particles had been acting as a protective adjuvant for the ribosomes. This provided the first direct evidence that the ribosomes constituted the active immunizing ingredient of the particulate fraction.

A ribosomal fraction then was prepared more directly by treating the particulate fraction with agents that would dissolve membranes. Ribosomal fractions of *M. tuberculosis*, strain H37Ra, were prepared by treatment of the particulate fraction with sodium deoxycholate (Table 9–4). Table 9–5 shows the effect of 0.25 percent sodium dodecyl sulfate followed by centrifugation at 144,000 × g for three hours on the particulate fraction. Freezing and thawing also had no effect on the immunogenicity of the particulate fraction (Table 9–6).

The addition of small concentrations (10^{-4} M) of $MgCl_2$ to the final diluent

TABLE 9–6. **Effect of Freezing and Thawing on the Immunogenicity
of the Particulate Fraction, With and Without Freund's Incomplete Adjuvant**

Immunizing Preparation	Freund's Adjuvant Added	Amount Injected[a] (mg)	Number of Mice	Number of S-30 Mice[b]	Percent of S-30 Mice
Particulate fraction	−	20	30	26	87
	+	20	29	19	66
Particulate fraction frozen and thawed six times (recentrifuged sediment)	−	20	22	10	46
	+	20	17	15	88
H37Ra cells		1	27	18	67
Controls		0	28	1	4

[a] Moist weight.
[b] S-30 mice = number of mice that survived > 30 days.
From Youmans, A. S., and Youmans, G. P.: Immunogenic activity of a ribosomal fraction obtained from *Mycobacterium tuberculosis.* J. Bacteriol. 89:1291, 1965.

increased immunogenic activity, whereas larger concentrations (10^{-3} M) of the substance reduced immunogenic activity.[103] Preparation of the ribosomal fraction from the ruptured cells performed in one continuous process during the course of a single day, also increased the activity of the ribosomal fraction,[103] since degradation of the RNA appeared to occur if the solution was left overnight at 4° C.

It also appeared that the membrane-bound ribosomes were more immunogenic than those present in the cytoplasmic material, since these preparations were as much as 100 times more immunogenic than ribosomal fractions prepared by differential centrifugation; 1 μg per mouse induced some immunity. Using ribosomal fractions treated with SDS, the effect of trypsin and ribonuclease on immunogenic activities was again determined to see if the immunogen was the protein or the RNA moiety of the ribosome (Table 9–7).[95] The portions treated with trypsin were as immunogenic as the untreated ribosomal fractions. No protein was detected chemically in the trypsin-treated groups. In contrast, ribonuclease decreased the immunogenic activity by approximately 50 percent (Table 9–8). These results suggested that the RNA might be the immunogen.

We also found that SDS was the best detergent of the several we tested to solubilize the mycobacterial membrane. The concentration of the SDS was important, since for optimal immunizing activity the final concentration in the suspending fluid could be no more than 0.25 percent.

PREPARATION OF MYCOBACTERIAL RNA

To isolate the ribosomal RNA, and thereby determine its immunogenicity, posed somewhat of a problem, since we did not want to use a phenol extraction method. We knew from previous experience[109] that whole cells of the H37Ra strain killed by exposure to phenol lost their immunogenicity, and we reasoned that the caustic phenol might well have degraded the

TABLE 9–7. **Effect of Trypsin on the Immunogenic Activity of the Ribosomal Fraction**

Immunizing Preparation	Amount Injected (mg)[a]	Number of Mice	Number of S-30 Mice[b]	Percent of S-30 Mice	Amount (μg) of Protein/ mg[a] of Immunizing Preparation
Ribosomal fraction	20.0	67	56	84	35
	1.0	142	97	69	
	0.1	130	78	60	
Ribosomal fraction treated with trypsin	20.0	66	51	77	0
	1.0	114	89	78	
	0.1	140	59	42	
H37Ra	1.0	140	132	94	
Controls		144	24	17	

[a]Moist weight.

[b]S-30 mice = number of mice that survived > 30 days.

From Youmans, A. S., and Youmans, G. P.: Effect of trypsin and ribonuclease on the immunogenic activity of ribosomes and ribonucleic acid isolated from *Mycobacterium tuberculosis*. J. Bacteriol. 91:2146, 1966.

TABLE 9–8. Effect of Ribonuclease on the Immunogenic Activity of
Mycobacterial RNA

Immunizing Preparation	Amount Injected (mg)[a]	Number of Mice	Number of S-30 Mice[b]	Percent of S-30 Mice
RNA	1.0	30	21	70
	0.1	30	13	43
	0.01	30	8	27
RNA (24 C°, 30 min)	1.0	30	22	73
	0.1	30	11	37
	0.01	30	7	23
RNA (24 C°, 30 min + ribonuclease)	1.0	30	12	40
	0.1	21	4	19
	0.01	30	4	13
H37Ra	1.0	30	28	93
Controls		30	0	0

[a] Moist weight.
[b] S-30 mice = number of mice that survived > 30 days.
From Youmans, A. S., and Youmans, G. P.: Effect of trypsin and ribonuclease on the immunogenic activity of ribosomes and ribonucleic acid isolated from *Mycobacterium tuberculosis*. J. Bacteriol. *91*:2146, 1966.

labile RNA. Therefore, we decided to use the mild ethanol extraction method of Crestfield and colleagues.[18] We modified their method so that fewer steps were involved and obtained RNA that was as immunogenic as the original ribosomal fraction and the H37Ra cells from which it had been extracted (Table 9–9).[95, 96] This material consisted of approximately two-thirds RNA and one-third protein. If treated with trypsin to remove the protein, the remaining RNA was just as immunogenic as the nontreated RNA.

TABLE 9–9. Immunogenic Activity of Mycobacterial Ribosomal and
RNA Preparations and Viable H37Ra Cells

Immunizing Preparation	RNA Injected (µg)	Number of Mice	Number of S-30 Mice[a]	Percent of S-30 Mice	Range Between Experiments
Ribosomal fraction	50.0[b]	334	191	87	76 to 100
	5.0	303	194	64	47 to 86
	0.5	252	123	49	21 to 86
RNA preparation	50.0	239	193	81	73 to 89
	5.0	234	171	73	64 to 90
	0.5	157	87	55[c]	47 to 78
H37Ra cells	50.0[b]	272	229	84	77 to 100
	5.0	236	201	85	72 to 97
	0.5	239	156	65[c]	60 to 87
Controls		270	42	16	

[a] S-30 mice = number of mice that survived > 30 days.
[b] 1.0 mg (moist weight).
[c] $P = <0.005, >0.001$.
From Youmans, A. S., and Youmans, G. P.: Factors affecting immunogenic activity of mycobacterial ribosomal and ribonucleic acid preparations. J. Bacteriol. *99*:42, 1969.

This procedure for the extraction of RNA turned out to be a fortunate choice, since the RNA usually was not appreciably degraded during preparation and there was a close correlation between the quality of the RNA and immunogenic activity. We have since prepared RNA using phenol,[96] but the immunogenic activity has never been as high as that obtained using the ethanol RNA preparations; at least in our hands, the RNA prepared by phenol extraction was always considerably degraded.

ROLE OF ADJUVANTS AND GROWTH PATTERN IN THE IMMUNIZING ACTIVITY OF MYCOBACTERIAL RNA

Since the mycobacterial RNA needs an adjuvant to protect it from being destroyed by the host's ribonucleases, a study was made of a number of adjuvants to determine the most effective. Several emulsified and two non-emulsified incomplete adjuvants were examined for their adjuvant activity using mycobacterial ribosome fractions as a substrate. It was found that FIA (heavy mineral oil and aquaphor) and arlacel A plus hexadecane were the best adjuvants tested.[102] Therefore, we have continued to use FIA. Also, five polybasic amines were later used to test the possibility of their adjuvant activity since they bind with nucleic acids.[94] The results were negative. A histone called spermidine was tried, since histones also combine with nucleic acid; the results were again negative. Cellulose gum alone and cellulose gum mixed with poly-L-lysine were tried. The cellulose gum alone was not effective but, when mixed with poly-L-lysine, gave some protection.[111]

During this time, we also determined the optimal growth conditions for the pellicle growth of H37Ra in order to obtain maximal yield of undegraded RNA. It is well known that during the logarithmic growth phase, the content of RNA in living bacterial cells is at its peak and the RNA is less degraded than in the stationary phase of growth. We measured, at different times, the RNA, DNA, and protein content of H37Ra cells grown as surface pellicles and found that after two weeks of incubation, the RNA content of these cells rapidly decreased.[105] Therefore, we decided to use 12-day-old H37Ra cells for the preparation of RNA to be sure that they were in the logarithmic growth phase; this led to a greater yield and a much greater consistency in immunizing power of our RNA preparations.

ROLE OF PROTEIN AND/OR A POSSIBLE CONTAMINANT IN THE IMMUNIZING ACTIVITY OF MYCOBACTERIAL RNA

We have extracted ribosomal protein with 2-chlorethanol and tested it for immunogenicity. The ribosomal protein was not immunogenic, whether or not it was incorporated into FIA. The double-stranded synthetic polyribonucleotide, poly A:U, was mixed with the protein to see if the protein needed a double-stranded ribonucleotide adjuvant in order to be immunogenic — a role possibly played by the mycobacterial RNA. However, this mixture, whether or not incorporated in FIA, also was not immunogenic.[97] In contrast, the ribosomal fraction from which it was extracted was immunogenic, as was the RNA left after the extraction of the protein.[97]

To test for the presence of a possible contaminant in the RNA preparations, that could not be detected chemically, the RNA was completely hydrolyzed by using dilute alkali, as recommended by Gottlieb.[26] Although the original RNA preparation was very immunogenic, the hydrolyzed material was not. The "contaminant," in order to be immunogenic, might have needed double-stranded RNA as an adjuvant; therefore, we mixed the hydrolyzed material with synthetic poly A:U, and this mixture was injected with and without FIA. These preparations also were not immunogenic.[97] In addition, no relationship could be found between the amount of protein and immunogenic activity; however, there was a direct relationship between the amount and the quality of the RNA and immunogenicity.[96] These results then strongly suggested that the RNA was the labile immunogen present in the living H37Ra cells. At that time (1969), based on the amount of RNA present, the immunogenic activity of RNA preparations and the viable H37Ra cells from which they were extracted were not significantly different (Table 9–9). A high degree of immunity could be obtained regularly with as little as 0.5 μg RNA per mouse, and at times with 0.0005 μg.

In summary, by following careful procedures, it was possible to obtain mycobacterial ribosomal fractions and ribonucleic acid, prepared by ethyl alcohol precipitation, that had immunogenic activity similar to that of the viable attenuated H37Ra cells of *M. tuberculosis* from which they came (Table 9–9). This comparison was based on the amount of RNA present. These preparations consisted of approximately 63 percent RNA and 37 percent protein; no deoxyribonucleic acid or polysaccharide was detected by chemical tests. A high correlation was found between the immunogenic activity of a preparation and the percent increase in hyperchromicity at 260 nm of a ribonuclease-hydrolyzed portion. Final concentrations of sodium dodecyl sulfate higher than 0.25 percent, when used for the preparation of the ribosomal fractions and RNA, resulted in significantly lower immune responses and greater variation between experiments. This was not related to the amount of protein present. The stability of the ribosomal and RNA preparations was tested under a variety of conditions. The need for a good protective adjuvant again was shown, since mouse serum readily hydrolyzed the RNA. Equal immunity was obtained after immunization by the intraperitoneal and subcutaneous routes; however, no immune response was obtained when the intravenous route was used. RNA prepared with phenol was much more easily degraded during preparation. This apparently accounts for the lower immune response to this material than was obtained with the RNA prepared with ethyl alcohol.

PHYSICAL AND CHEMICAL CHARACTERISTICS AND SEDIMENTATION PATTERNS OBTAINED WITH MYCOBACTERIAL RNA AND RIBOSOMES

Five to twenty percent linear sucrose gradients were used to obtain sedimentation patterns of mycobacterial ribosomes, ribosomal subfractions, and RNA preparations.[100] Classical 70S ribosomes were obtained when 10^{-1} M magnesium chloride was used (Fig. 9–1). These, when dialyzed against 10^{-4} M MgCl$_2$, yielded typical 50S, 30S, and smaller ribosomal subunits.

Physical and chemical evidence suggested that mycobacterial RNA preparations extracted with 65 percent ethyl alcohol from the ribosomes and diluted in distilled water were either double-stranded or had a highly organized secondary or tertiary structure.[100] This was based on the following observations:

1. Native RNA was resistant to trace amounts of ribonuclease (Fig. 9–2).
2. The approximate T_m value in SSC buffer (0.15 M NaCl plus 0.015 M sodium citrate) was greater than 85° C and was 55° C in 0.1 SSC buffer; the RNA diluted in SSC buffer produced a

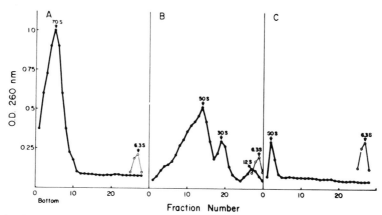

FIGURE 9–1. Sedimentation patterns of *A,* 70S mycobacterial ribosomes, sedimented in a 5 to 20 percent sucrose gradient containing 10^{-1} M MgCl$_2$; *B,* 70S ribosomes, dialyzed against 10^{-4} M MgCl$_2$ overnight and sedimented in a 5 to 20 percent sucrose gradient containing 10^{-4} M MgCl$_2$, and *C,* 80S mammalian brain ribosomes, sedimented in a 5 to 20 percent sucrose gradient containing 10^{-2} M MgCl$_2$. Alkaline phosphatase marker = ○. (From Youmans, A. S., and Youmans, G. P.: Immunogenic mycobacterial ribosomal and ribonucleic acid preparations: Chemicals and physical characteristics. Infect. Immun. 2:659, 1970.)

hypochromic effect on cooling at room temperature (Fig. 9–3).

3. Formaldehyde in the presence of SSC buffer decreased the T_m of the RNA to approximately 55° C, and there was no hypochromic effect on cooling (Fig. 9–3).

4. Formaldehyde did not increase the wave length of maximal adsorption of the RNA (Fig. 9–4).

5. The value of the purine/pyrimidine ratio was close to one.

6. The major peak of the RNA was 16S or 23S (Fig. 9–5).

There was a relationship between the sedimentation pattern obtained with mycobacterial RNA preparations on sucrose gradients and immunogenicity (Table 9–10).[104] When the mycobacterial preparations were treated with trace amounts of ribonuclease, the major peak changed from 16S to 23S. In addition, the 23S-peaking preparations appeared to produce the highest immune response. Smaller RNA-protein complexes, such as 6S, obtained when the RNA preparation was diluted in certain buffers, were

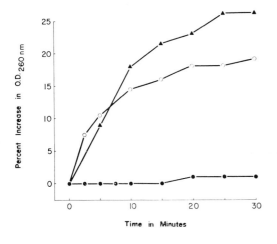

Figure 9–2. Effect of 0.2 μg of ribonuclease on 20 μg of RNA at 25° C. Undenatured mycobacterial RNA is shown by ●, heat-denatured mycobacterial RNA by ○, and yeast RNA by ▲. (From Youmans, A. S., and Youmans, G. P.: Immunogenic mycobacterial ribosomal and ribonucleic acid preparations: Chemical and physical characteristics. Infect. Immun. 2:659, 1970.)

FIGURE 9–3. Thermal transition curves of mycobacterial RNA in SSC buffer symbolized by ●; in 0.1 SSC buffer, by ○; and in SSC buffer containing 2.76 percent formaldehyde, by ▲. (From Youmans, A. S., and Youmans, G. P.: Immunogenic mycobacterial ribosomal and ribonucleic acid preparations: Chemical and physical characteristics. Infect. Immun. 2:659, 1970.)

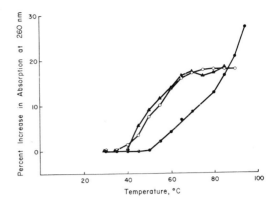

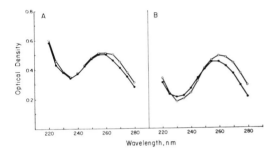

FIGURE 9–4. Effect of 1.5 percent formaldehyde on the ultraviolet absorption spectra of *A*, mycobacterial RNA in water (●) and in formaldehyde (○); and *B*, yeast RNA in water (●) and in formaldehyde (○). (From Youmans, A. S., and Youmans, G. P.: Immunogenic mycobacterial ribosomal and ribonucleic acid preparations: Chemical and physical characteristics. Infect. Immun. 2:659, 1970.)

FIGURE 9–5. Sedimentation patterns of mycobacterial RNA preparation (●—●); treated with ribonuclease (○—○); alkaline phosphatase marker (○--○). (From Youmans, A. S., and Youmans, G. P.: The relationship between sedimentation value and immunogenic activity of mycobacterial ribonucleic acid. J. Immunol. 110:581, 1973.)

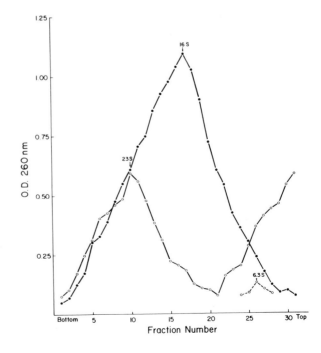

TABLE 9-10. The Relationship Between Sedimentation Value and
Immunogenic Activity of Mycobacterial RNA Preparations

Immunizing Preparation	S Values after Treatment with Ribonuclease	RNA Injected	Number of Mice	Number of S-30 Mice[a]	Percent of S-30 Mice	Range Between Experiments
Sucrose gradient sedimentation values						
16S (Group I)	23	50.0	147	126	86[b, c]	80 to 90
		5.0	145	115	79[c]	75 to 85
		0.5	48	34	71[b, d]	64 to 80
15 to 16S (Group II)	20 to 23	50.0	200	166	83[e]	70 to 97
		5.0	148	102	69[e, f]	50 to 85
		0.5	166	90	54[d, f]	50 to 60
14 to 15S (Group III)	19	50.0	129	71	55[h]	37 to 70
		5.0	137	59	43[c, g]	32 to 60
		0.5	138	57	41[c, h]	20 to 55
Controls			338	55	16[h]	

[a] S-30 = number of mice that survived > 30 days.
[b] Probability = < 0.02.
[c] Nonsignificant.
[d] Probability = < 0.05.
[e] Probability = < 0.005.
[f] Probability = < 0.01.
[g] Probability = < 0.05.
[h] Probability = < 0.001.

From Youmans, A. S., and Youmans, G. P.: The relationship between sedimentation value and immunogenic activity of mycobacterial ribonucleic acid. J. Immunol. *110*:581, 1973.

much less immunogenic. Immunogenic activity was apparently related to the structure of the RNA, since it was maximal when the RNA appeared either to be double-stranded or to have a highly organized secondary structure.

ALLERGENICITY OF MYCOBACTERIAL RIBOSOMES AND RNA

In view of the great theoretical as well as practical importance of the development of a vaccine against tuberculosis—one that is not only highly immunogenic but also incapable of inducing tuberculin hypersensitivity in man or lower animals—we continued our studies of the allergenicity of the ribosomal and RNA myco-

bacterial vaccine. In 1960,[33] we reported that the particulate fraction from which the ribosomal and RNA vaccines are prepared did not induce tuberculin hypersensitivity in guinea pigs. However, in view of the development of far more active immunizing preparations and the definition of the role of mycobacterial RNA in this activity, we felt that the allergenicity of such preparations should be carefully re-examined.[107]

Guinea pigs were injected subcutaneously with mycobacterial ribosomal fraction incorporated in FIA and tested 6 to 12 weeks later by the intradermal injection of 0.5 μg (25 TU) of purified protein derivative (PPD). No evidence of delayed-type hypersensitivity could be detected in these animals, although large necrotic reactions were obtained in the skins of guinea pigs sensitized with living, attenuated mycobacterial cells. Mice also were vaccinated by the intraperitoneal injection of mycobacterial ribosomal fraction or RNA and tested for sensitivity to tuberculin at subsequent times by injecting 2 μg (100 TU) into the footpad of the right hind foot. The thickness of the footpad was measured at 4, 24, and 48 hours after the injection of the PPD. No evidence of true tuberculin hypersensitivity could be detected at any time, although what appeared to be small Arthus-type reactions (increase in footpad thickness only at 4 hours) were seen in mice given the largest vaccinating doses. Mice vaccinated at the same time with viable H37Ra cells showed typical increase in footpad thickness 24 hours after PPD administration. Four weeks after vaccination with living cells, attempts to recall tuberculin sensitivity in vaccinated mice by the intravenous injection of viable cells of either the virulent or attenuated mycobacterial strains were unsuccessful. Instead, when the virulent cells were injected, a suppression of footpad reactivity was noted in animals made sensitive to tuberculin by the previous intraperitoneal injection of viable attenuated mycobacterial cells. Both guinea pigs and mice, vaccinated in the manner just described, also were skin-tested or footpad-tested, respectively, with 2 μg of the ribosomal fraction or RNA used for vaccination. No evidence of true tuberculin hypersensitivity could be obtained; instead, in both vaccinated and nonvaccinated guinea pigs, very small dermonecrotic areas were noted in the skin at the site of injection. Swelling and redness of the footpad occurred to an equal extent at 4 and 24 hours in both vaccinated and nonvaccinated mice.[107]

In addition, extensive experiments were carried out in which spleen cells were collected from both guinea pigs and mice following immunization with mycobacterial RNA preparations. These spleen cells were stimulated with PPD, and the supernatant fluids of the stimulated spleen cell cultures were tested for the presence of macrophage migration inhibitory activity by the capillary tube migration technique of David.[20] No migration inhibitory activity could ever be demonstrated in such supernatant fluids,[52] although good migration inhibitory activity could be found in the supernatant fluids of PPD-stimulated spleen cell cultures when the spleen cells were removed from animals that had been vaccinated with viable H37Ra cells.[52]

Thus, it would appear that neither ribosomal nor RNA mycobacterial vaccines will induce tuberculin hypersensitivity in guinea pigs or mice. Others[4, 53] have reported that ribosomal protein will induce delayed hypersensitivity to ribosomal protein, but we saw no evidence of this in these experiments. We were unable to elicit positive skin tests in immunized animals with either ribosomal or RNA preparations. Neither were we able to detect migration inhibitory activity after using ribosomal or RNA preparations to stimulate spleen cells taken from animals immunized with these materials.

Thus, not only is mycobacterial RNA an effective immunizing agent against tuberculous infection, but also it apparently does not induce significant degrees of tuberculin hypersensitivity in either mice or guinea pigs. Mycobacterial RNA, therefore, should be an appropriate agent for the immunization of human beings against tuberculosis, since the induction of tuberculin hypersensitivity by vaccines such as BCG has been one of the major drawbacks to their use in human beings. Unfortunately, in order to be effective, the RNA vaccine must be incorporated in a water-in-oil adjuvant such as FIA in order to prevent early degradation of the RNA within the body. Since such adjuvants are unsuitable for administration to human beings, the trial of this vaccine for the immunization of human beings must await the development of a nontoxic, biodegradable adjuvant. Conceivably, the immunizing activity of the vaccine might be maintained by some chemical manipulation that would prevent degradation but retain the immunizing activity. To date, however, all of our efforts in this direction have been unsuccessful.

VACCINATION OF GUINEA PIGS WITH MYCOBACTERIAL RNA

In collaboration with Dr. Robert Good,[25] we have recently completed studies which show that mycobacterial RNA preparations are also highly effective immunizing agents in guinea pigs. For these studies, we prepared mycobacterial RNA vaccine in Chicago and incorporated it there into FIA. We then transported this by hand to Washington, D. C., where, in cooperation with Dr. Good, guinea pigs were vaccinated subcutaneously. The vaccinating doses for different groups of guinea pigs were: 250 μg, 50 μg and 10 μg of RNA vaccine. Nine weeks later, half of these vaccinated guinea pigs were infected with the virulent Erdman strain of *M. tuberculosis* by the pulmonary route, using aerosolized suspensions of *M. tuberculosis*. The other half of the vaccinated animals were challenged by injecting them intraperitoneally with an appropriate dose of the Erdman strain of *M. tuberculosis*. Guinea pigs that had not been vaccinated and those that had been vaccinated subcutaneously with the viable H37Ra cells from which the RNA vaccine had been prepared were challenged with virulent tubercle bacilli in the same manner. These latter two groups served as the necessary controls for the evaluation of the immunizing activity of the RNA vaccine. Also in these experiments, prior to transporting the RNA vaccine to Washington, mice were vaccinated

with it in Chicago. In order to test for any loss of immunizing potency during the process of transportation, extra vaccine in FIA was carried back to Chicago, where mice were again vaccinated. Table 9–11 shows that no loss of potency occurred.

The results clearly showed that the RNA vaccine exerted a good protective effect against challenge with tubercle bacilli, although the protective effect did not quite equal that shown by the viable H37Ra cells. Table 9–12 provides further data on these experiments. It should be pointed out that in such protection experiments, all that can be expected of any vaccine used against tuberculosis is a prolongation of survival time. Experience has shown that no matter what the vaccine or the potency, vaccinated guinea pigs will eventually die of tuberculosis. The increase in survival time actually reflects a retardation in the rate of multiplication of the challenge dose of virulent tubercle bacilli.

In these guinea pig experiments, slight dermal reactions to PPD were seen in those animals vaccinated with the 250 μg dose of mycobacterial RNA. These results, in contrast to those which we reported on earlier and which we have just discussed, suggest that large doses of RNA vaccine may at times induce low degrees of tuberculin hypersensitivity to the protein present. The guinea pigs given the viable H37Ra cells, on the other hand, showed strong tuberculin hypersensitivity as measured by skin tests with PPD.

Experiments such as these with guinea pigs are of great importance. They clearly show that the mycobacterial RNA vaccine is an effective immunizing agent not only in mice — animals that are fairly resistant to tuberculous infection — but also in guinea pigs — animals that are extremely susceptible to infection with virulent tubercle bacilli. It is quite possible that the utilization of larger doses of vaccine or the administration

TABLE 9–11.   **The Immunogenic Activity of Mycobacterial RNA Obtained from Viable H37Ra Cells**[a]

Immunizing Preparation	Amount RNA Given (μg)	Number of Mice	Number of S-30 Mice[b]	Percent of S-30 Mice[b]	Nativeness
VACCINATED AT NORTHWESTERN NOVEMBER 15, 1974, PRIOR TO WASHINGTON, D.C., TRIP					
Mycobacterial RNA[c]	50.0	30	25	83	34
	5.0	30	18	60	
	0.5	29	18	62	
Freund's incomplete adjuvant	———	30	6	20	
H37Ra cells	5.0	30	30	100	
Controls	———	30	1	3	
VACCINATED AT NORTHWESTERN NOVEMBER 15, 1974, PRIOR TO WASHINGTON, D.C., TRIP					
Mycobacterial RNA[d, e] (Same as above but traveled to and from Washington, D.C.)	50.0	20	17	85	30
	5.0	20	16	80	
	0.5	20	11	55	
H37Ra cells	5.0	20	19	95	
Controls	———	20	1	5	

[a] In both parts of this experiment, challenge was January 7, 1975, I.V., with 0.4 mg/mouse H37Rv cells in 0.2 ml buffer. C57Bl/6 mice were used. These mice are more susceptible to infection with tubercle bacilli.

[b] S-30 Mice = number of mice that survived > 30 days.

[c] Sedimentation value on 5 to 20 percent sucrose gradients equals 16S. After treatment with trace amounts of ribonuclease, which hydrolyzes single-stranded RNA, the S value was 23 to 24. These figures indicate high-quality RNA.

[d] This material was also used to vaccinate guinea pigs at Dr. Good's laboratory in Washington (see Table 9–12 for his results).

[e] Sedimentation values were the same for this RNA as the RNA in the November 15, 1974, part of this experiment.

of multiple injections of vaccine might raise the level of immunity to that observed when guinea pigs are vaccinated with viable cells of BCG or the H37Ra strain.

SPECIFICITY OF IMMUNITY PRODUCED BY MYCOBACTERIAL RNA

We have been particularly interested in the specificity of the immune response to the mycobacterial RNA vaccine. This we felt was especially important because of the widely held view[40-42] that immunity to infection with facultative intracellular parasites is entirely nonspecific. If this view is correct, immunity to tuberculosis should be nonspecific, and animals vaccinated with the RNA vaccine would be expected to be equally resistant to infection with other bacteria. We have done extensive experiments[15-17] which show that administering RNA vaccine to mice does not induce any significant increased resistance to infection with bacteria

TABLE 9–12. **Response of Guinea Pigs to Vaccination With Viable H37Ra Cells, RNA Vaccine and Cholera Toxoid**

Vaccine	Amount of Vaccine	Route of Challenge	ST$_{50}$ In Days (95 Percent Confidence Limits)	Significantly Different from Controls
None	None	IP	125 (109 to 144)	0
H37Ra cells	1000.0 μg[a]	IP	210 (197 to 224)	+
RNA	10.0 μg	IP	155 (142 to 169)	+
RNA	50.0 μg	IP	185 (155 to 210)	+
RNA	250.0 μg	IP	195 (171 to 222)	+
Cholera toxoid		IP	150 (113 to 200)	−
None	None	Aerosol	85 (71 to 102)	0
H37Ra cells	1000.0 μg[a]	Aerosol	210 (178 to 245)	+
RNA	10.0 μg	Aerosol	106 (90 to 125)	+
RNA	50.0 μg	Aerosol	120 (103 to 140)	+
RNA	250.0 μg	Aerosol	128 (111 to 147)	+
Cholera toxoid		Aerosol	105 (93 to 119)	−

[a] 1000 μg moist weight of H37Ra cells = 50.0 μg mycobacterial RNA.

Published with the permission of Dr. Robert C. Good, Center for Disease Control, Atlanta, Georgia.

such as *Listeria monocytogenes* or *Klebsiella pneumoniae*. Also, through the courtesy of Dr. Nancy Bigley, we obtained ribosomal vaccine prepared from *Salmonella typhimurium* and have found that this vaccine did not induce immunity to tuberculous infection in mice.[110] Also, through the courtesy of Dr. Ram Tewari, we obtained ribosomal vaccine, which he prepared from *Histoplasma capsulatum*, and have found that the injection of this vaccine in mice did not induce any significant increase in resistance to infection with virulent tubercle bacilli.[110] We supplied mycobacterial RNA vaccine to Dr. Stuart Mudd; he and his coworkers have found that this vaccine did not induce increased resistance in mice to infection with *Staphylococcus aureus*.[70]

IMMUNIZING ACTIVITY OF MYCOBACTERIAL RNA AGAINST EXPERIMENTAL INFECTION WITH *MYCOBACTERIUM LEPRAE*

More recently we have had the opportunity to conduct an extensive collaborative study with Dr. Charles Shepard, who tested the immunizing power of mycobacterial RNA vaccine against footpad infection of mice with *Mycobacterium leprae*.[65] In this study, as in the one on guinea pigs previously mentioned, we prepared the mycobacterial RNA vaccine and incorporated it into FIA. In contrast to the guinea pig study, we shipped the vaccine in this form to Dr. Charles Shepard in Atlanta, Georgia. In this air express shipment, we included double the amount of vaccine needed by Dr. Shepard to vaccinate his mice. The remainder was returned to us so that we could vaccinate mice in our laboratory. This, again, was a test of the effect of transportation on the immunizing potency. The vaccine, of course, was also tested for its potency by means of injecting mice in our laboratory at the time that it was shipped to Dr. Shepard. In view of the lability of this material, we felt it wise to be sure that Dr. Shepard was vaccinating his animals with a potent preparation. Table 9–13 shows that there was no significant loss in vaccinating potency from the time that it was tested in our laboratory to when it was returned to us by

TABLE 9–13.   **Results of Challenge of Vaccinated Mice With**
Virulent *M. tuberculosis*

Vaccine	Dose (μg)	Number of Mice	S-30 Mice[a]	
			NUMBER	PERCENT
Before shipment to Atlanta				
myc RNA	50	20	15	75
myc RNA	5	30	14	47
myc RNA	0.5	30	7	23
FIA[b] + H$_2$O		30	2	7
H37Ra	100[c]	30	20	67
Nil		30	8	27
After return from Atlanta				
myc RNA	50	20	16	80
myc RNA	5	20	14	70
myc RNA	0.5	20	8	40
H37Ra	100	20	18	90
Nil		20	5	25

[a] S-30 mice were mice that survived 30 days.
[b] FIA, Freund incomplete adjuvant.
[c] A 100-μg portion of H37Ra is equivalent to 5 μg of myc RNA.
From Shepard, C. C., Youmans, A. S., and Youmans, G. P.: Lack of protection afforded by ribonucleic acid preparations from *Mycobacterium tuberculosis* against *Mycobacterium leprae* infections in mice. Infect. Immun. *15*:733, 1977.

Dr. Shepard. Dr. Shepard vaccinated his mice subcutaneously with this material. At the same time, he also included several groups of mice as controls. One of these groups received no vaccine; one was vaccinated with viable BCG cells, which he previously had found would favorably affect the course of the footpad infection in mice; and the third was vaccinated with an equivalent dose of the viable H37Ra cells, which had been used to prepare the vaccine.

Twenty-eight days after vaccination, mice were infected in one hind footpad with an appropriate dose of *M. leprae*. Dr. Shepard then followed the course of the infection in these mice by sacrificing animals in each group at appropriate intervals after infection (see Fig. 9–6). The number of *M. leprae* cells in the footpads was counted. The enumeration procedure was the standard one, devised by Dr. Shepard, in which footpad specimens were prepared, stained, and the number of leprae bacilli counted by microscopic observation. Figure 9–6 shows the re-sults at the end of 165 days and, again, after 90 more days. It is clear that the leprae bacilli grew very readily and that prior vaccination with BCG vaccine significantly retarded the development of *M. leprae*. However, the animals that received the mycobacterial RNA vaccine and the H37Ra cells showed no such protective effects from the vaccinating procedure. This negative effect occurred in spite of the fact that the material (the RNA vaccine and the H37Ra cells) used was highly effective for the protection of mice against infection with *M. tuberculosis* (Table 9–13).

It is not at all clear why viable BCG cells could induce some protection against infection with *M. leprae* while viable H37Ra cells failed to do so, especially when the viable cells of these two strains of mycobacteria are equally effective for the protection of mice against tuberculosis (see Chapter 8). It is, however,[55] well recognized that BCG cells have a greater capacity to multiply to a certain extent in the tissues of mice; whereas H37Ra

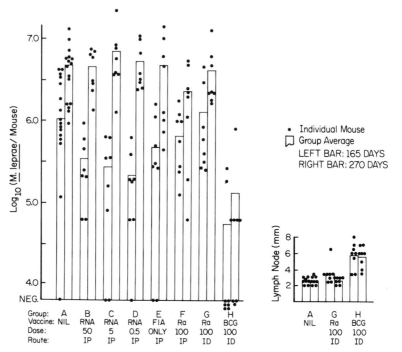

FIGURE 9–6. Results of challenge of vaccinated mice with *M. leprae*. The numbers of *M. leprae* harvested from individual mice near the end of the logarithmic phase in the controls (165 days) and again, 90 days later, are given on the left. In certain groups, the lymph nodes regional to the intradermal (flank) vaccination were measured at harvest, and these measurements are shown on the right. Abbreviations: RNA, mycobacterial RNA; FIA, Freund's incomplete adjuvant; Ra, H37Ra; IP, intraperitoneal; and ID, intradermal. The dose of vaccine is given in micrograms. (From Shepard, C. C., Youmans, A. S., and Youmans, G. P.: Lack of protection afforded by ribonucleic acid preparations from *Mycobacterium tuberculosis* against *Mycobacterium leprae* infections in mice. Infect. Immun. *15*:733, 1977.)

cells[63, 91, 92] have little or no capacity to do so. We have commented on this in Chapter 8. It might well be that the more intense inflammatory reaction engendered by multiplying BCG cells would impart a greater resistance to infection with *M. leprae* than would the nonmultiplying and dying H37Ra cells. This, however, is purely speculative at the moment.

In any event, it is clear that the RNA vaccine, which is highly effective for the protection of mice against *M. tuberculosis,* has no capacity to favorably influence the course of infection with *M. leprae*. This indicates a high order of specificity in the immune response to tuberculosis, on the one hand, and to leprosy, on the other.

Such results also do not lend support to the theory that immunity to infection with facultative intracellular parasites is entirely nonspecific.

The experiments mentioned previously, including those obtained with *M. leprae,* indicate conclusively that immunity produced to tuberculous infection by RNA vaccine is specific. This, in turn, means that immunity to tuberculosis is specific except for the cross-protection that is observed between closely related mycobacterial species, such as the immunity to infection with virulent tubercle bacilli induced by BCG cells, *M. kansasii,* and *M. intracellulare*. The results that we obtained, showing no cross-protection between the mycobacterial RNA vaccine and *M. leprae* infection, suggest that these two species of mycobacteria are not very closely related.

THE ADJUVANT ACTIVITY OF MYCOBACTERIAL RNA

Our interest in the possibility that mycobacterial RNA vaccine might function as an immunologic adjuvant was aroused by the work of Braun and his coworkers,[11, 12] who have shown that oligo- and polynucleotides will markedly stimulate antibody production in animals to a number of antigens. In particular, the work of Johnson and colleagues[31] and of Schmidtke and Johnson[61] showed that synthetic polynucleotides will stimulate antibody formation to bovine gamma globulin (BGG). These polynucleotides, however, only exhibited adjuvant activity if they were injected in the double-stranded form. For example, poly-adenylic acid (poly A) would not stimulate antibody production to BGG, nor would poly-uridylic acid (poly U). However, if these two were mixed to form the double-stranded complex, poly A:U, and were then injected into animals receiving BGG, a marked increase in the amount of antibody formed was noted over the amount formed after the injection of the equivalent amount of BGG alone.

In our study of the chemical and physical characteristics of the immunizing mycobacterial RNA outlined in the earlier part of this chapter, we found that this material reacted in a manner that suggested it might be double-stranded, or at least have some highly organized secondary or tertiary structure. In view of these findings and the fact that the synthetic polynucleotides will stimulate antibody formation *in vivo* only when injected in the double-stranded form, we felt that it would be of interest to determine whether mycobacterial RNA preparation would increase antibody production to a protein antigen in the same manner as double-stranded synthetic polynucleotides. The well-known potent adjuvant activity of intact mycobacterial cells made such studies of special interest.

In these experiments, CF-1 mice were injected intraperitoneally with BGG, either alone or together with mycobacterial RNA.[108] At appropriate times after immunization, the mice were bled after pentabarbital anesthesia from the inferior vena cava. The serum was collected, and the antibody response to BGG measured by a modification of the micro-titer passive hemagglutination test described by Weir.[86] BGG was adsorbed to tanned red blood cells. Table 9–14 gives some of our initial results. It is clear that

TABLE 9–14. Mean[a] Antibody Titers Obtained With the Sera of CF-1 Mice Injected Intraperitoneally With 3 mg BGG and Mycobacterial RNA, or Poly A:U, or Freund's Incomplete Adjuvant

Materials Injected	Time in Days		
	7	14	21
1. BGG	20	256	51
2. BGG + myc RNA (0.05 mg)	406	1290	1024
3. BGG + poly A:U (0.3 mg)	161	812	322
4. BGG + FIA (0.4 ml)	512	256	161
5. BGG + FIA (0.4 ml) + myc RNA (0.05 mg)	406	1613	645

[a] Reciprocal of the geometric mean of the highest dilution of serum which agglutinated SRBC coated with BGG.

From Youmans, G. P., and Youmans, A. S.: The effect of mycobacterial RNA on the primary antibody response of mice to bovine γ globulin. J. Immunol. *109*:217, 1972.

mycobacterial RNA exerted an adjuvant activity on antibody formation in CF-1 mice that was equivalent, if not superior, to that produced by poly A:U. In other experiments, the adjuvant activity of the mycobacterial RNA was compared with a number of other substances, such as poly I:C, *E. coli* endotoxin, and viable H37Ra cells. Table 9–15 shows the results of these experiments. Again, mycobacterial RNA showed adjuvant activity, which, interestingly, was considerably inferior to the adjuvant activity exhibited by endotoxin. It is noteworthy that in these experiments, treatment of the mycobacterial RNA with trypsin or with ribonuclease did not affect the adjuvant activity. In addition, we tested the adjuvant activity of mycobacterial RNA extracted with phenol; this material proved to have no adjuvant activity whatsoever. This is of particular importance because it is known that phenol treatment of RNA will reduce or eliminate secondary or tertiary structures. We therefore assumed that the double-stranded areas in the mycobacterial RNA molecule are responsible for the adjuvant activity. It is also noteworthy in these experiments that the mycobacterial RNA exhibited adjuvant activity without being incorporated into FIA. This is in marked contrast to the requirement for such a protective adjuvant in order for this RNA to be an effective immunizing agent against tuberculosis. We can only assume that the adjuvant effect of the RNA is exerted very rapidly in the body before any significant degradation of the RNA by the host nucleases can occur. Johnson and colleagues[31] and Schmidtke and Johnson[61] came to the same conclusion in their study of the adjuvant activity of poly A:U.

In view of the potent adjuvant activity of mycobacterial RNA preparations for the enhancement of antibody formation, we, together with Dr. Carl Gumbiner and Dr. Philip Paterson of Northwestern University Medical School, explored the possibility that mycobacterial RNA might serve as an adjuvant for the induction of experimental allergic encephalomyelitis (EAE) in guinea pigs. Mycobacteria[38, 54, 64, 87, 88] or certain mycobacterial cell wall fractions have been recognized as essential for the induction of EAE in guinea pigs. Intact mycobacterial cells, however, have been found to be far superior in this respect to any mycobacterial fraction.

Rather extensive studies were con-

TABLE 9–15.   **Mean[a] Antibody Titers Obtained With the Sera of CF-1 Mice Injected Intravenously With 3 mg BGG and Polynucleotides or Other Substances**

Materials Injected	Time in Days		
	7	14	21
1. BGG	40	181	40
2. BGG + myc RNA (0.05 mg)	106	407	81
3. BGG + poly A:U (0.05 mg)	161	256	102
4. BGG + poly I:C (0.05 mg)	203	362	323
5. BGG + endotoxin (0.05 mg)	3251	8190	2048
6. BGG + viable H37Ra cells (0.05 mg)[b]	81	256	81
7. BGG + heat-killed H37Ra cells (0.05 mg)	40	214	161
8. BGG + Mu-9 ds-RNA (0.05 mg)	102	3445	512
9. BGG + H37Ra cell walls (0.05 mg)	40	609	161

[a] Reciprocal of the geometric mean of the highest dilution of serum which partially agglutinated SRBC coated with BGG.

[b] This value represents the amount of myc RNA present in 1.0 mg H37Ra cells, moist weight.

From Youmans, G. P., and Youmans, A. S.: The effect of mycobacterial RNA on the primary antibody response of mice to bovine γ globulin. J. Immunol. *109*:217, 1972.

TABLE 9–16. Adjuvanticity of Mycobacterial RNA and Synthetic
Polynucleotide for Production of Experimental Allergic
Encephalomyelitis (EAE) in Guinea Pigs

Type and Amount of Adjuvant Component Injected[a] (μg)		Nervous Tissue Antigen Injected[b]	Clinical Signs of EAE	Lesions of EAE
Mycobacteria	200	Cord	16/16[c]	16/16
	200	MBP	9/9	9/9
Mycobacteria cell walls	200	Cord	3/3	3/3
Mycobacteria RNA	200	Cord	8/10	10/10
	200	MBP	3/6	4/6
	20	Cord	0/3	2/3
	20	MBP	0/3	3/3
	2	Cord	0/3	0/3
	2	MBP	0/3	1/3
KOH-treated myco- bacteria RNA	200	MBP	0/3	0/3
Poly A:U	200	Cord	0/3	2/3
	200	MBP	0/3	1/3

[a] Incorporated into Freund's incomplete adjuvant.

[b] Guinea pig whole spinal cord homogenate 13 mg (wet weight) or myelin basic protein (MBP) 10 μg (dry weight) combined with adjuvant.

[c] Numerator, number of animals exhibiting clinical signs of EAE or shown to have histologic evidence of EAE; denominator, number of animals injected.

From Gumbiner, C., Paterson, P. Y., Youmans, G. P., and Youmans, A. S.: Adjuvanticity of mycobacterial RNA and poly A:U for induction of experimental allergic encephalomyelitis in guinea pigs. J. Immunol. *110*:309, 1973.

ducted in which the adjuvant activity of mycobacterial RNA and poly A:U for the induction of experimental allergic encephalomyelitis was examined.[27] Table 9–16 shows that mycobacterial RNA at the maximum dosage was just as effective for this purpose as intact mycobacterial cells. Poly A:U also was effective but did not seem as active in this regard as the mycobacterial RNA. It is of considerable interest that as little as 2 μg of mycobacterial RNA together with nervous tissue antigen would induce signs of EAE in guinea pigs.

Finally, the capacity of mycobacterial RNA preparations to induce delayed hypersensitivity to protein antigens was explored. This work, done in our laboratory by Dr. Conrad Casavant, clearly shows that small amounts of mycobacterial RNA together with tuberculoprotein would induce delayed hypersensitivity to the tuberculoprotein.[13] Similar results were obtained with ovalbumin. An outstanding feature of this study was that evidence of the presence of delayed hypersensitivity was not limited to the elicitation of dermal reactions. The delayed hypersensitive state in these animals also was revealed by passive transfer of this delayed hypersensitivity with spleen cells from sensitized guinea pigs and by the presence, as detected in tissue sections of the dermal lesions, of the typical histologic picture of delayed hypersensitivity reactions.

THE ANTITUMOR ACTIVITY OF MYCOBACTERIAL RNA

One of the most interesting developments in recent years has been the realization that viable mycobacterial cells in the form of BCG vaccine are capable, under appropriate conditions, of exerting a considerable suppressive effect on the growth of tumors in both experimental animals and man. Early work has shown that BCG vaccine will inhibit the development of certain tumors in mice, rats, hamsters, and guinea pigs and will occasionally inhibit the development of spontaneous tumors in animals. (See the reviews of Bast et al.[5-7] for the early literature.) These studies originated from the demonstration by Bradner and coworkers[10] that stimulation of the reticuloendothelial system has a beneficial effect on the development of tumors in experimental animals and from the findings of Biozzi and colleagues[8] that BCG was a potent stimulator of the reticuloendothelial system. Capacity to stimulate the reticuloendothelial system is a property of all mycobacterial cells, so mycobacteria other than BCG will also favorably influence the course of experimental tumors.[46-48] Actually, the stimulating effect of mycobacterial cells on the reticuloendothelial system has long been known,[58] but the usefulness of this action for the suppression of tumor growth was not recognized until recently.

BCG vaccine also has been found to effectively suppress growth of tumors in human beings.[6, 7] It is most effective under conditions where the tumor has been accessible to the injection of the BCG vaccine right into the tumor mass. Thus, the most striking results have been obtained in the treatment of melanoma.[3, 9, 29, 37, 49, 56, 62, 66, 75] Other cutaneous neoplastic conditions, however, such as basal and squamous cell carcinoma, lymphangiosarcoma, reticulum cell sarcoma, and Kaposi's sarcoma, have been favorably influenced by BCG administration.[34-36] Certain systemic neoplastic conditions, such as acute lymphocytic leukemia,[21, 22, 24] acute myelogenous leukemia,[19] and chronic myelogenous leukemia,[71-74] have been found to respond at least partially to BCG treatment.

The effectiveness of BCG vaccine in producing a favorable effect on tumor progression apparently lies in the vaccine's capacity to stimulate the cells of the reticuloendothelial system. We have noted in Chapters 3 and 4 that mycobacterial cells are stimulators of the reticuloendothelial system. Mycobacterial cells are potent producers of macrophage activation; they stimulate the accumulation of large numbers of lymphocytes and macrophages (the granulomatous response), and when tuberculin hypersensitivity exists, an acute inflammatory response is mounted to the injection of mycobacterial cells. In addition, mycobacterial cells have been found to be potent stimulators of immune responses; in other words, they are excellent adjuvants (see Chapters 3 and 4). All of these reactions to mycobacterial cells undoubtedly play some part in the favorable effect of BCG vaccine on tumor progression. Depending upon the nature of the tumor, the site of tumor growth, and the route of injection of BCG cells, one or more may predominate in the antitumor action. Certainly, under conditions where tumor-specific antigens are present, the adjuvant activity by mycobacterial cells will stimulate the host immune response. Chapter 4 discusses the antitumor activity of a variety of mycobacterial lipids and cell fractions and elaborates on the manner whereby mycobacterial cells and cell components exert antitumor activity.

We should recall at this point that the stimulation of the reticuloendothelial system, in the manner just described, by mycobacterial cells will bring about a marked increase in the nonspecific resistance of a host to bacterial infection (see Chapter 8). In fact, with mycobacterial cells such as those present in BCG vaccine, there is a parallel between the capacity to nonspecifically increase resistance to heterologous infection and the capacity to modify or suppress tumor formation. Therefore, in view of the capacity of these cells to nonspecifically increase resistance to invasion by all foreign living cells, the favorable effect noted on progression of tumor growth following the injection of BCG vaccine or other mycobacterial cells is only what would be expected.

It must be emphasized that the administration of large numbers of mycobacterial cells in the form, for example, of BCG vaccine may be accompanied by marked untoward local and systemic reactions in the host so injected. Serious reactions are noted particularly in persons who already are sensitive to tuberculin or who become sensitive in response to the injection of the massive doses of mycobacterial cells usually employed.[2, 9, 14, 28, 43, 50, 51, 56, 75]

It is not our intention here to dwell at length on the many results that have been reported on the use of BCG vaccine either experimentally or clinically for the suppression of cancer. The literature has been extensively reviewed by Bast and colleagues,[5-7] and these reviews should be consulted for details.

Because of the adverse reactions just noted to the use of BCG vaccine and because it is eminently desirable to avoid the induction of tuberculin hypersensitivity in cancerous patients treated with BCG vaccine, considerable attention has been given to the capacity of certain mycobacterial products to favorably influence the growth of tumors in experimental animals. Many of these are of lipid nature, and their anticancer effects will be found in Chapter 4.

Our major purpose in this section is to briefly describe the effect of mycobacterial RNA vaccine on the growth of tumors in experimental animals. The RNA vaccines described in this chapter and in Chapter 10 are also potent stimulators of the reticuloendothelial system; if it should be found that these materials have antitumor effects, their use in human beings would be particularly advantageous because they do not induce tuberculin hypersensitivity nor do they elicit delayed hypersensitivity reactions in subjects sensitive to tuberculin (see Chapters 7 and 8). Thus, many of the untoward reactions noted in patients treated with BCG vaccine could be avoided. This favorable aspect of the use of RNA vaccines for the treatment of cancer has been commented upon at greater length by Millman and his coworkers.[46-48]

Initially, in our own laboratory we studied the effect of mycobacterial RNA vaccine on the development of spontaneous leukemia in AKR mice. In one out of three experiments, the results indicated that the administration of RNA vaccine to adult AKR mice did delay significantly the appearance of spontaneous leukemia. In two other experiments, no such favorable effect was noted.

The effect of RNA vaccine on experimentally induced leukemia in AKR mice has been studied rather extensively. In these experiments, regardless of the route of injection or the number of tumor cells injected, the administration of RNA vaccine only served to enhance somewhat the rate of growth of the leukemia cells. Many other factors, including the amount of RNA vaccine administered and the time of administration in relation to the challenge dose of tumor, were studied and under all circumstances, only an enhancing effect or no effect on tumor growth was noted. Furthermore, administration of RNA vaccine to AKR mice prior to challenge with tumor cells did not inhibit in any way the development of the neoplastic disease.[111]

In other studies, conducted by Dr. Irving Millman and his associates at the Institute for Cancer Research in Philadelphia, using other experimental systems, more promising results were obtained.[46-48] Initial studies were conducted to determine the effect of viable cells of the H37Ra strain and that of our mycobacterial RNA fraction on tumor growth.[46, 47] The tumors used were three chemically induced transplantable fibrosarcomas. Before use, tumors were routinely passaged by subcutaneous

TABLE 9–17. **Experimental Protocol**[a]

| | | **Prechallenge** | | | |
Group	Mice	Treatment	Amount Injected per Mouse	Volume Injected	Route
1	18	Living H37Ra	8×10^6	0.4 ml	IP
2	18	RNA fraction	$50 \mu g$	0.1 ml	IP
3	18	Medium 199	Control	0.4 ml	IP
4	18	BCG (Tice)	5×10^6	0.05 ml	IC

| **Challenge Group** | | | |
1	2	3	4
H37Ra (4×10^6 viable particles/0.1 ml)	RNA Fraction ($50 \mu g/0.1$ ml)	Medium 199 (Control)	BCG (5×10^6 viable particles/0.1 ml)

[a]Five weeks after the prechallenge procedure, the four groups of normal syngeneic mice were challenged with tumor cell suspension ($10^6/0.1$ ml) mixed with equal volumes of the respective materials listed above. The challenge dose was 0.2 ml given subcutaneously (dorsally). All injections were randomly spaced by cage and the entire procedure lasted no longer than 1 hour.

From Millman, I., Maguire, H. C., Youmans, G. P., and Youmans, A. S.: Effect of the H37Ra strain of *M. tuberculosis* and of a mycobacterial RNA fraction on tumor growth. Proc. Soc. Exp. Biol. Med. *147*:765, 1974.

transplantation in syngeneic female mice. Tumor cells were dispersed enzymatically by using pronase, washed three times, and made up to a concentration of 10^6 tumor cells per 0.1 milliliter. In these experiments the mice were pretreated with tubercle bacilli or the RNA fraction and then challenged with the tumor cells five weeks later. Included with the challenge injection was another dose of the pretreatment agent. In these experiments the effectiveness of the H37Ra cells and the RNA were compared to that of viable BCG cells.

Table 9–17 shows the type of experimental protocol that was used, and

Table 9–18 compares the effects of the various agents on tumor growth. It is clear from these experiments that both the viable H37Ra microorganisms and the RNA fraction derived from this strain of *Mycobacterium* inhibited the growth of tumor cells. They were, in fact, more effective than BCG cells.

In the continuation of these studies, by Millman and colleagues, a further comparison was made of the effectiveness of mycobacterial RNA and intact mycobacteria for the suppression of murine tumor growth.[46] The effect of these agents, including BCG cells, on the chemically induced fibrosarcomas is

TABLE 9–18. **Comparison of Various Treatments for Effect on Tumor Growth**

| | **7 Days** | | | **14 Days** | | | **21 Days** | | |
	Tumor Free	<5mm	≥5mm	Tumor Free	<5mm	≥5mm	Tumor Free	<5mm	≥5mm
RNA	17	0	0	11	4	2	5	5	7
H37Ra	18	0	0	17	1	0	17	0	1
BCG	0	2	16	0	2	16	1	0	17
Media	13	3	1	0	2	15	0	3	14

From Millman, I., Maguire, H. C., Youmans, G. P., and Youmans, A. S.: Effect of the H37Ra strain of *M. tuberculosis* and of a mycobacterial RNA fraction on tumor growth. Proc. Soc. Exp. Biol. Med. *147*:765, 1974.

shown in Figure 9–7. In these experiments the mice also were preimmunized, and the challenge dose of fibrosarcoma cells was again mixed with the appropriate immunizing preparation. Table 9–19 shows the results of similar experiments in which mice were immunodepressed by thymectomy and irradiation.

To summarize the results, the data show that the RNA fraction isolated from H37Ra cells, as well as the intact H37Ra cells, is an effective agent for suppression of tumor growth. However, for the suppression of the chemically induced tumors, direct contact with the tumor is necessary. There is no way of knowing, however, whether this would be the case with other tumors and with other strains of syngeneic mice. Furthermore, the immunologic system of the host is a necessary component for inhibition of tumor growth by these agents since there is no tumor suppression in immunologically impaired mice.

In other experiments, the immunosuppressive activity of the mycobacterial RNA fraction was compared with mycobacterial cell wall fractions.[48] In these studies, a mastocytoma (P-815) was used. The RNA preparation and the cell wall skeleton were able to produce regression of the mastocytoma in Dba-2 mice, provided that the animals were presensitized with freshly harvested, living H37Ra cells. In the absence of presensitization, only the RNA fraction was inhibitory. Cell wall skeleton, under these conditions, stimulated tumor growth. A few experiments were done with lipid material taken from the cell walls. When these were added to the H37Ra cell wall skeleton fraction, no increase in the inhibitory activities of the cell wall skeleton fraction could be detected. Also, mycobacterial RNA appeared to be an effective inhibitor of mastocytoma metastases because the inhibition of a second foot pad lesion distant from the one treated could be observed and because an increase in the survival time of the mice was noted (Table 9–20).

Thus, although a great deal more work needs to be done, it appears that the mycobacterial RNA fraction, under certain conditions, does have an adverse effect on the progression of certain

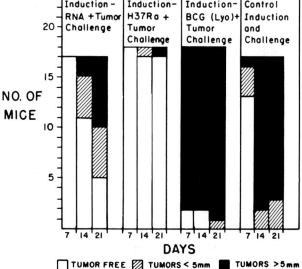

FIGURE 9–7. The effect of mycobacteria and mycobacterial RNA on tumor growth. The mice used were BALB/c × C3H syngeneic males, 18 per group, presensitized with RNA (IFA), H37Ra, BCG (lyophilized, Tice) and HBSS. The tumor involved was T-1967 MCA fibrosarcoma. Measurements were made twice weekly under ether anesthesia using microcaliper. Differences in numbers of mice in each bar graph were due to ether deaths. (From Millman, I., Maguire, H. C., Pass, M. (Kavanaugh), Youmans, A. S., and Youmans, G. P.: Mycobacterial RNA. A comparison with intact mycobacteria for suppression of murine tumor growth. J. Med. 7:249, 1976.)

TABLE 9–19. The Effect of Mycobacteria and Mycobacterial
RNA on Tumor[a] Growth

	Tumor Size (Mean $L + W)^2$			
	O-trace	<25	<100	>100
Hanks' BSS (depressed)[b]	0/5	0/5	1/5	4/5
Hanks' BSS (normal)	0/6	1/6	0/6	5/6
RNA fraction (depressed)[b]	0/6	0/6	0/6	6/6
RNA fraction (normal)	7/12	3/12	1/12	1/12
H37Ra (depressed)[b]	1/5	0/5	0/5	4/5
H37Ra (normal)	11/12	0/12	0/12	1/12
BCG (fresh harvest) (depressed)[b]	0/5	0/5	1/5	4/5
BCG (fresh harvest) (normal)	12/12	0/12	0/12	0/12

[a] Tumor cells (10^5) were mixed with RNA (50 μg) or mycobacterial cells (0.2 mg wet wt) in HBSS in a total volume of 0.2 ml. The mixture was injected in the dorsal flank subcutaneously into C3H syngeneic male mice. Groups of mice were randomized for injection. Tumor = T-2060 MCA fibrosarcoma.
[b] Mice were thymectomized and irradiated (400 r).
From Millman, I., Maguire, H. C., Pass, M. (Kavanaugh) Youmans, A. S., and Youmans, G. P.: Mycobacterial RNA. A comparison with intact mycobacteria for suppression of murine tumor growth. J. Med. 7:249, 1976.

tumors in mice. Not only are such results extremely encouraging from the standpoint of therapy but also because the RNA mycobacterial fraction neither elicits reactions of tuberculin hypersensitivity in tuberculous animals nor does it induce tuberculin hypersensitivity; however, further quantitative studies are needed. The use of such preparations in human beings would not be attended by many of the complications noted when intact BCG cells are used.

REFERENCES

1. Andron, L. A., II, and Eigelsbach, H. T.: Biochemical and immunological properties of ribonucleic acid-rich extracts from *Francisella tularensis*. Infect. Immun. 12:137, 1975.
2. Aungst, C. W., Sokal, J. E., and Jager, B. V.: Complications of BCG vaccination. Proceedings of the American Association for Cancer Research 14:108, 1973.
3. Baker, M. A., and Taub, R. N.: B.C.G. in malignant melanoma. Lancet 1:1117, 1973.
4. Baker, R. E., Hill, W. E., and Larson, C. L.: Ribosomes of acid-fast bacilli: Immunogenicity, serology, and *in vitro* correlates of delayed hypersensitivity. Infect. Immun. 8:236, 1973.
5. Bast, R. C., Jr., Bast, B. S., and Rapp, H. J.: Critical review of previously reported animal studies of tumor immunotherapy with nonspecific immunostimulants. International Conference on Immunotherapy of Cancer. Ann. N.Y. Acad. Sci. 277:60, 1976.
6. Bast, R. C., Jr., Zbar, B., Borsos, T., and Rapp, H. J.: BCG and cancer (first of two parts). N. Engl. J. Med. 290:1413, 1974.
7. Bast, C. R., Jr., Zbar, B., Borsos, T., and Rapp, H. J.: BCG and cancer (second of two parts). N. Engl. J. Med. 290:1458, 1974.
8. Biozzi, G., Benacerraf, B., Grumbach, F., Halpern, B. N., Levaditi, J., and Rist, N.: Étude de l'activité granulopexique du système réticulo-endothélial au cours de l'infection tuberculeuse expérimentale de la souris. Ann. Inst. Pasteur (Paris) 87:291, 1954.
9. Bornstein, R. S., Mastrangelo, M. J., Sulit, H., Chee, D., Yarbro, J. W., Prehn, L. (Melartin), and Prehn, R. T.: Immunotherapy of melanoma with intralesional BCG. Conference on the Use of BCG in Therapy of Cancer. Natl. Cancer Inst. Monogr. 39:213, 1973.
10. Bradner, W. T., Clarke, D. A., and Stock, C. C.: Stimulation of host defense against experimental cancer. I. Zymosan and sarcoma 180 in mice. Cancer Res. 18:347, 1958.
11. Braun, W., and Nakano, M.: Antibody formation: stimulation by polyadenylic and polycytidylic acids. Science 157:819, 1967.

TABLE 9–20. Results of Treatment With RNA and Cell Wall Skeleton Fractions[a]

Treatment	Tumor Growth (mm)									
	14[b]		21		25		28		32	
	RIGHT	LEFT	RIGHT	LEFT	RIGHT	LEFT	RIGHT	LEFT	RIGHT	LEFT
RNA	2.88 ± 0.45[c]	2.72 ± 0.67	4.78 ± 0.72	4.6 ± 1.1	5.17 ± 0.93	4.57 ± 1.1	6.68 ± 1.1	5.72 ± 1.2	7.76 ± 1.1	6.03 ± 1.3
Cell wall skeleton	3.44 ± 0.41	3.66 ± 0.40	6.47 ± 0.54	7.14 ± 0.75	7.17 ± 0.53	7.46 ± 0.78	8.65 ± 0.48[d]	9.28 ± 0.89[d]	9.53 ± 0.41	8.82 ± 0.89
Control	3.23 ± 0.36	3.35 ± 0.32	5.47 ± 0.70	6.24 ± 0.63	5.99 ± 0.79	6.23 ± 0.71	7.65 ± 0.85	7.98 ± 0.67	8.29 ± 0.91	8.95 ± 0.57

Determination	Mann-Whitney (2-Tailed Probability) Significance of Difference (Groups)									
	14		21		25		28		32	
	RIGHT	LEFT	RIGHT	LEFT	RIGHT	LEFT	RIGHT	LEFT	RIGHT	LEFT
RNA vs. control	0.012		0.014		0.058		0.011	0.007 (E)[e]	0.057	
Cell wall skeleton vs. control	0.133		0.034 (E)[e]		0.015 (E)[e]		0.44		0.279	

[a] Syngeneic DBA/2 female mice, 19 to 22 g were used. RNA (lyophilized) was wetted with heavy mineral oil (Squibb) and diluted with 0.2 percent Tween 80 dissolved in HBSS. Cell wall skeleton was prepared from crude walls of H37Ra by the procedure described for BCG by Ribi and colleagues (Natl. Cancer Inst. Monogr. 39:115, 1973.) Dose per mouse was 50 μg/0.05 ml. Control is mineral oil-HBSS-Tween 80 mixture used as diluent for above. Twelve mice per group were injected with 10^5 P-815 mastocytoma cells into each rear footpad. In 7 days, when tumor growth was visible, the left rear footpad was injected (intralesionally) with the preparation. A week after the first treatment, a second dose was administered intraperitoneally. A week after the second dose, a third was administered subcutaneously. Footpads were measured twice weekly, using a Schnelltaster caliper.
[b] Day after injection of tumor cells.
[c] Mean ± standard error of the mean.
[d] Difference between footpads significant ($P = 0.034$).
[e] E = Enhancement.

From Millman, I., Scott, A. W., Halbherr, T., Youmans, A. S., and Youmans, G. P.: Mycobacterial ribonucleic acid: comparison with mycobacterial cell wall fractions for regression of murine tumor growth. Infect. Immun. 14:929, 1976.

12. Braun, W., Nakano, M., Jaraskova, L., Yajima, Y., and Jimenez, L.: Stimulation of antibody-forming cells by oligonucleotides of known composition. *In* Plescia, O. J., and Braun, W. (eds.): Nucleic Acids in Immunology. New York, Springer-Verlag, Inc., 1968.

13. Casavant, C. H., and Youmans, G. P.: The induction of delayed hypersensitivity in guinea pigs to poly U and poly A:U. J. Immunol. *114*:1506, 1975.

14. Chess, L., Bock, G. N., Ungaro, P. C., Buchholz, D. H., and Mardiney, M. R.: Immunologic effects of BCG in patients with malignant melanoma: Specific evidence for stimulation of the "secondary" immune response. J. Natl. Cancer Inst. *51*:57, 1973.

15. Coppel, S., and Youmans, G. P.: Specificity of acquired resistance produced by immunization with *Listeria monocytogenes* and listeria fractions. J. Bacteriol. *97*:121, 1969.

16. Coppel, S., and Youmans, G. P.: Specificity of acquired resistance produced by immunization with mycobacterial cells and mycobacterial fractions. J. Bacteriol. *97*:114, 1969.

17. Coppel, S., and Youmans, G. P.: Specificity of the anamnestic response produced by *Listeria monocytogenes* or *Mycobacterium tuberculosis* to challenge with *Listeria monocytogenes*. J. Bacteriol. *97*:127, 1969.

18. Crestfield, A. M., Smith, K. C., and Allen, F. W.: The preparation and characterization of ribonucleic acids from yeast. J. Biol. Chem. *216*:185, 1955.

19. Crowther, D., Powles, R. L., Bateman, C. J. T., Beard, M. E. J., Gauci, C. L., Wrigley, P. F. M., Malpas, J. S., Fairley, G. H., and Scott, R. B.: Management of adult acute myelogenous leukaemia. Br. Med. J. i:131, 1973.

20. David, J. R.: Delayed hypersensitivity *in vitro*: Its mediation by cell-free substances formed by lymphoid cell-antigen interaction. Proc. Natl. Acad. Sci. U.S.A. *56*:72, 1966.

21. Davignon, L., Lemonde, P., St.-Pierre, J., and Frappier, A.: B.C.G. vaccination and leukaemia mortality. Lancet *1*:80, 1971.

22. Davignon, L., Lemonde, P., St.-Pierre, J., and Frappier, A.: B.C.G. vaccination and leukaemia mortality. Lancet *1*:799, 1971.

23. Feit, C., and Tewari, R. P.: Immunogenicity of ribosomal preparations from yeast cells of *Histoplasma capsulatum*. Infect. Immun. *10*:1091, 1974.

24. Frei, E., III, and Freireich, E. J.: Progress and perspectives in the chemotherapy of acute leukemias. Adv. Chemotherapy *2*:269, 1965.

25. Good, R. C., Youmans, G. P., Youmans, A. S., and McCarroll, N. E.: Immunogenic activity of mycobacterial RNA in guinea pigs. Abstracts of the Annual Meeting of the American Society for Microbiology, 1977. p. 86.

26. Gottlieb, A. A.: Macrophage ribonucleoprotein: nature of the antigenic fragment. Science *165*:592, 1969.

27. Gumbiner, C., Paterson, P. Y., Youmans, G. P., and Youmans, A. S.: Adjuvanticity of mycobacterial RNA and poly A:U for induction of experimental allergic encephalomyelitis in guinea pigs. J. Immunol. *110*:309, 1973.

28. Gutterman, J. U., Mavligit, G., McBride, C., Frei, E., III, Freireich, E. J., and Hersh, E. M.: Active immunotherapy with B.C.G. for recurrent malignant melanoma. Lancet *1*:1208, 1973.

29. Hersh, E. M.: Modification of host defense mechanisms. *In* Holland, J. F., and Frei, E., III, (eds.): Cancer Medicine. Philadelphia, Lea and Febiger, 1973.

30. Jensen, R., Gregory, B., Naylor, J., and Actor, P.: Isolation of protective somatic antigen from *Vibrio cholerae* (Ogawa) ribosomal preparations. Infect. Immun. *6*:156, 1972.

31. Johnson, A. G., Schmidtke, J., Merritt, K., and Han, I.: Enhancement of antibody formation by nucleic acids and their derivatives. *In* Plescia, O. J., and Braun, W. (eds.): Nucleic Acids in Immunology. New York, Springer-Verlag, Inc., 1968.

32. Kanai, K., and Youmans, G. P.: Immunogenicity of intracellular particles and cell walls from *Mycobacterium tuberculosis*. J. Bacteriol. *80*:607, 1960.

33. Kanai, K., Youmans, G. P., and Youmans, A. S.: Allergenicity of intracellular particles, cell walls, and cytoplasmic fluid from *Mycobacterium tuberculosis*. J. Bacteriol. *80*:615, 1960.

34. Klein, E.: Immunotherapy of cancer in man, a reality. Conference on the Use of BCG in Therapy of Cancer. Natl. Cancer Inst. Monogr. *39*:139, 1973.

35. Klein, E., and Holtermann, O. A.: Immunotherapeutic approaches to the management of neoplasms. Natl. Cancer Inst. Monogr. *35*:379, 1972.

36. Klein, E., Holtermann, O. A., Papermaster, B., Milgrom, H., Rosner, D., Klein, L., Walker, M. J., and Zbar, B.: Immunologic approaches to various types of cancer with the use of BCG and purified protein derivatives. Conference on the Use of BCG in Therapy of Cancer. Natl. Cancer Inst. Monogr. *39*:229, 1973.

37. Levy, N. L., Mahaley, M. S., Jr., and Day, E. D.: Serum-mediated blocking of cell-mediated anti-tumor immunity in a melanoma patient: Association with BCG immunotherapy and clinical deterioration. Int. J. Cancer *10*:244, 1972.

38. Lipton, M. M., and Steigman, A. J.: *Pseudomonas pseudomallei* and *Pseudomonas aeru-*

ginosa as adjuvants in the production of experimental allergic encephalomyelitis. J. Immunol. *90*:512, 1963.

39. Lynn, M., Tewari, R. P., and Solotorovsky, M.: Immunoprotective activity of ribosomes from *Haemophilus influenzae*. Infect. Immun. *15*:453, 1977.

40. Mackaness, G. B.: Cellular resistance to infection. J. Exp. Med. *116*:381, 1962.

41. Mackaness, G. B.: The immunological basis of acquired cellular resistance. J. Exp. Med. *120*:105, 1964.

42. Mackaness, G. B.: The immunology of antituberculous immunity. Am. Rev. Respir. Dis. *97*:337, 1968.

43. Mansell, P. W. A., and Krementz, E. T.: Reactions to BCG. J.A.M.A. *226*:1570, 1973.

44. Margolis, J. M., and Bigley, N. J.: Cytophilic macroglobulin reactive with bacterial protein in mice immunized with ribonucleic acid-protein fractions of virulent *Salmonella typhimurium*. Infect. Immun. *6*:390, 1972.

45. Millman, I., and Darter, R. W.: Intracellular localization of enzymes in *Mycobacterium tuberculosis* var. *hominis*. Proc. Soc. Exp. Biol. Med. *91*:271, 1956.

46. Millman, I., Maguire, H. C., Pass, M. (Kavanaugh), Youmans, A. S., and Youmans, G. P.: Mycobacterial RNA. A comparison with intact mycobacteria for suppression of murine tumor growth. J. Med. *7*:249, 1976.

47. Millman, I., Maguire, H. C., Jr., Youmans, G. P., and Youmans, A. S.: Effect of the H37Ra strain of *M. tuberculosis* and of a mycobacterial RNA fraction on tumor growth. Proc. Soc. Exp. Biol. Med. *147*:765, 1974.

48. Millman, I., Scott, A. W., Halberr, T., Youmans, A. S., and Youmans, G. P.: Mycobacterial ribonucleic acid: Comparison with mycobacterial cell wall fractions for regression of murine tumor growth. Infect. Immun. *14*:929, 1976.

49. Minton, J. P.: Mumps virus and BCG vaccine in metastatic melanoma. Arch. Surg. *106*:503, 1973.

50. Morton, D. L., Holmes, E. C., Eilber, F. R., and Wood, W. C.: Immunological aspects of neoplasia: A rational basis for immunotherapy. Ann. Intern. Med. *74*:587, 1971.

51. Nathanson, L.: Regression of intradermal malignant melanoma after intralesional injection of *Mycobacterium bovis* strain BCG. Cancer Chemother. Rep. *56*:659, 1972.

52. Neiburger, R. G., Youmans, G. P., and Youmans, A. S.: Relationship between tuberculin hypersensitivity and cellular immunity to infection in mice vaccinated with viable attenuated mycobacterial cells or with mycobacterial ribonucleic acid preparations. Infect. Immun. *8*:42, 1973.

53. Ortiz-Ortiz, L., Solarolo, E. B., and Bojalil, L.

F.: Delayed hypersensitivity to ribosomal protein from BCG. J. Immunol. *107*:1022, 1971.

54. Paterson, P. Y.: Experimental allergic encephalomyelitis and autoimmune disease. Adv. Immunol. *5*:131, 1966.

55. Pierce, C. H., Dubos, R. J., and Schaefer, W. B.: Multiplication and survival of tubercle bacilli in the organs of mice. J. Exp. Med. *97*:189, 1953.

56. Pinsky, C. M., Hirshaut, Y., and Oettgen, H. F.: Treatment of malignant melanoma by intratumoral injection of BCG. Conference on the Use of BCG in Therapy of Cancer. Natl. Cancer Inst. Monogr. *39*:225, 1973.

57. Preston, P. M., and Dumonde, D. C.: Immunogenicity of a ribosomal antigen of *Leishmania enriettii*. Trans. R. Soc. Trop. Med. Hyg. *65*:18, 1971.

58. Rich, A. R.: The Pathogenesis of Tuberculosis. 2nd ed. Springfield, Ill., Charles C Thomas, 1951.

59. Saunders, E. S., Solotorovsky, M., and Tewari, R. P.: Immunization against experimental candidosis with ribosomal preparations from *Candida albicans*. Abstracts of the Annual Meeting of the American Society for Microbiology, 1975. p. 89.

60. Schalla, W. O., and Johnson, W.: Immunogenicity of ribosomal vaccines isolated from group A, type 14, *Streptococcus pyogenes*. Infect. Immun. *11*:1195, 1975.

61. Schmidtke, J. R., and Johnson, A. G.: Regulation of the immune system by synthetic polynucleotides. I. Characteristics of adjuvant action on antibody synthesis. J. Immunol. *106*:1191, 1971.

62. Seigler, H. F., Shingleton, W. W., Metzgar, R. S., Buckley, C. E., Bergoc, P. M., Miller, D. S., Fetter, B. F., and Phaup, M. B.: Non-specific and specific immunotherapy in patients with melanoma. Surgery *72*:162, 1972.

63. Sever, J. L., and Youmans, G. P.: The enumeration of nonpathogenic viable tubercle bacilli from the organs of mice. Am. Rev. Tuberc. *75*:280, 1957.

64. Shaw, C. M., Alvord, E. C., Jr., Fahlberg, W. J., and Kies, M. W.: Substitutes for the mycobacteria in Freund's adjuvants in the production of experimental "allergic" encephalomyelitis in the guinea pig. J. Immunol. *92*:28, 1964.

65. Shepard, C. C., Youmans, A. S., and Youmans, G. P.: Lack of protection afforded by ribonucleic acid preparations from *Mycobacterium tuberculosis* against *Mycobacterium leprae* infections in mice. Infect. Immun. *15*:733, 1977.

66. Smith, G. V., Morse, P. A., Jr., Deraps, G. D., Raju, S., and Hardy, J. D.: Immunotherapy of patients with cancer. Surgery *74*:59, 1973.

67. Smith, R. A., and Bigley, N. J.: Detection of

delayed hypersensitivity in mice injected with ribonucleic acid-protein fractions of *Salmonella typhimurium*. Infect. Immun. 6:384, 1972.

68. Smith, R. A., and Bigley, N. J.: Inability of RNA-protein fractions of *Salmonella typhimurium* to induce immune deviation. Abstracts of the Annual Meeting of the American Society for Microbiology, 1973. p. 114.

69. Smith, R. A., and Bigley, N. J.: Ribonucleic acid-protein fractions of virulent *Salmonella typhimurium* as protective immunogens. Infect. Immun. 6:377, 1972.

70. Smith, R. L., Wysocki, J. A., Brunn, J. N., DeCourcy, S. J., Jr., Blakemore, W. S., and Mudd, S.: Efficacy of ribosomal preparations from *Pseudomonas aeruginosa* to protect against intravenous pseudomonas challenge in mice. J. Reticuloendothel. Soc. 15:22, 1974.

71. Sokal, J. E., Aungst, C. W., and Grace, J. T., Jr.: Immunotherapy of chronic myelocytic leukemia. Conference on the Use of BCG in Therapy of Cancer. Natl. Cancer Inst. Monogr. 39:195, 1973.

72. Sokal, J. E., Aungst, C. W., and Grace, J. T., Jr.: Immunotherapy of myeloid leukemia. Ann. Intern. Med. 76:878, 1972.

73. Sokal, J. E., Aungst, C. W., and Han, T.: Use of *Bacillus Calmette-Guérin* as adjuvant in human cell vaccines. Cancer Res. 32:1584, 1972.

74. Sokal, J. E., and Grace, J. T.: An attempt to protect patients with chronic myelocytic leukemia (CML) against blastic transformation. Proc. Am. Assoc. Cancer Research 10:85, 1969.

75. Sparks, F. C., Silverstein, M. J., Hunt, J. S., Haskell, C. M., Pilch, Y. H., and Morton, D. L.: Complications of BCG immunotherapy in patients with cancer. N. Engl. J. Med. 289:827, 1973.

76. Sundararaj, T., and Agarwal, S. C.: Cell-mediated immunity to *Nocardia asteroides* induced by its ribonucleic acid protein fraction. Infect. Immun. 18:253, 1977.

77. Suzuki, K.: Cellular fractions of *Listeria monocytogenes* in relation to the localization of a protective antigen and monocytosis producing factor. Yonago Acta Med. 14:52, 1970.

78. Tewari, R. P.: Immunization against histoplasmosis. *In* Neter, E., and Milgrom, F. (eds.): The Immune System and Infectious Diseases. 4th International Convocation on Immunology, Buffalo, N. Y., 1974. Basel, S. Karger, 1975.

79. Thomas, D. W., and Weiss, E.: Response of mice to injection of ribosomal fraction from group B *Neisseria meningitidis*. Infect. Immun. 6:355, 1972.

80. Thompson, H. C. W., and Eisenstein, T. K.: Biological properties of an immunogenic

pneumococcal subcellular preparation. Infect. Immun. 13:750, 1976.

81. Thompson, H. C. W., and Snyder, I. S.: Protection against pneumococcal infection by a ribosomal preparation. Infect. Immun. 3:16, 1971.

82. Venneman, M. R.: Purification of immunogenically active ribonucleic acid preparations of *Salmonella typhimurium:* Molecular-sieve and anion-exchange chromatography. Infect. Immun. 5:269, 1972.

83. Venneman, M. R., and Berry, L. J.: Cell-mediated resistance induced with immunogenic preparations of *Salmonella typhimurium*. Infect. Immun. 4:381, 1971.

84. Venneman, M. R., and Berry, L. J.: Experimental salmonellosis: Differential passive transfer of immunity with serum and cells obtained from ribosomal and ribonucleic acid-immunized mice. J. Reticuloendothel. Soc. 9:491, 1971.

85. Venneman, M. R., Bigley, N. J., and Berry, L. J.: Immunogenicity of ribonucleic acid preparations obtained from *Salmonella typhimurium*. Infect. Immun. 1:574, 1970.

86. Weir, D. M. (ed.): Handbook of Experimental Immunology. Philadelphia, F. A. Davis Company, 1967.

87. White, R. G., and Marshall, A. H. E.: The role of various chemical fractions of *M. tuberculosis* and other mycobacteria in production of allergic encephalomyelitis. Immunology 1:111, 1958.

88. Wiener, S. L., Tinker, M., and Bradford, W. L.: Experimental meningoencephalomyelitis produced by *Hemophilus pertussis*. Arch. Pathol. 67:694, 1959.

89. Winston, S. H., and Berry, L. J.: Antibacterial immunity induced by ribosomal vaccines. J. Reticuloendothel. Soc. 8:13, 1970.

90. Winston, S. H., and Berry, L. J.: Immunity induced by ribosomal extracts from *Staphylococcus aureus*. J. Reticuloendothel. Soc. 8:66, 1970.

91. Yamamura, Y., Kato, M., Ikuta, S., Okuyama, T., and Watanabe, S.: A homogenate technique of whole body of mice. Med. J. Osaka Univ. 6:501, 1955.

92. Yamamura, Y., Walter, A., and Bloch, H.: Bacterial populations in experimental murine tuberculosis. I. Studies in normal mice. J. Infect. Dis. 106:211, 1960.

93. Youmans, A. S., and Youmans, G. P.: Effect of mitochondrial stabilizers on the immunogenicity of the particulate fraction isolated from *Mycobacterium tuberculosis*. J. Bacteriol. 87:1346, 1964.

94. Youmans, A. S., and Youmans, G. P.: Effect of polybasic amines on the immunogenicity of mycobacterial ribonucleic acid. Infect. Immun. 6:798, 1972.

95. Youmans, A. S., and Youmans, G. P.: Effect of trypsin and ribonuclease on the immunogenic activity or ribosomes and ribonucleic acid isolated from *Mycobacterium tuberculosis*. J. Bacteriol. *91*:2146, 1966.

96. Youmans, A. S., and Youmans, G. P.: Factors affecting immunogenic activity of mycobacterial ribosomal and ribonucleic acid preparations. J. Bacteriol. *99*:42, 1969.

97. Youmans, A. S., and Youmans, G. P.: Failure of synthetic polynucleotides to affect the immunogenicity or mycobacterial ribonucleic acid and ribosomal protein preparations. Infect. Immun. *3*:149, 1971.

98. Youmans, A. S., and Youmans, G. P.: Further studies on a labile immunogenic particulate substance isolated from *Mycobacterium tuberculosis*. J. Bacteriol. *87*:278, 1964.

99. Youmans, A. S., and Youmans, G. P.: Immunogenic activity of a ribosomal fraction obtained from *Mycobacterium tuberculosis*. J. Bacteriol. *89*:1291, 1965.

100. Youmans, A. S., and Youmans, G. P.: Immunogenic mycobacterial ribosomal and ribonucleic acid preparations: Chemical and physical characteristics. Infect. Immun. *2*:659, 1970.

101. Youmans, A. S., and Youmans, G. P.: Nature of the labile immunogenic substance in the particulate fraction isolated from *Mycobacterium tuberculosis*. J. Bacteriol. *88*:1030, 1964.

102. Youmans, A. S., and Youmans, G. P.: Preparation and effect of different adjuvants on the immunogenic activity of mycobacterial ribosomal fraction. J. Bacteriol. *94*:836, 1967.

103. Youmans, A. S., and Youmans, G. P.: Preparation of highly immunogenic ribosomal fractions of *Mycobacterium tuberculosis* by use of sodium dodecyl sulfate. J. Bacteriol. *91*:2139, 1966.

104. Youmans, A. S., and Youmans, G. P.: The relationship between sedimentation value and immunogenic activity of mycobacterial ribonucleic acid. J. Immunol. *110*:581, 1973.

105. Youmans, A. S., and Youmans, G. P.: Ribonucleic acid, deoxyribonucleic acid, and protein content of cells of different ages of *Mycobacterium tuberculosis* and the relationship to immunogenicity. J. Bacteriol. *95*:272, 1968.

106. Youmans, G. P., Millman, I., and Youmans, A. S.: The immunizing activity against tuberculous infection in mice of enzymatically active particles isolated from extracts of *Mycobacterium tuberculosis*. J. Bacteriol. *70*:557, 1955.

107. Youmans, G. P., and Youmans, A. S.: Allergenicity of mycobacterial ribosomal and ribonucleic acid preparations in mice and guinea pigs. J. Bacteriol. *97*:134, 1969.

108. Youmans, G. P., and Youmans, A. S.: The effect of mycobacterial RNA on the primary antibody response of mice to bovine γ globulin. J. Immunol. *109*:217, 1972.

109. Youmans, G. P., and Youmans, A. S.: Immunizing capacity of viable and killed attenuated mycobacterial cells against experimental tuberculous infection. J. Bacteriol. *97*:107, 1969.

110. Youmans, G. P., and Youmans, A. S.: Implications of immunization against infectious diseases with ribosomal and RNA vaccines. *In* Neter, E., and Milgrom, F. (eds.): The Immune System and Infectious Diseases. 4th International Convocation on Immunology, Buffalo, N. Y., 1974. Basel, S. Karger, 1975.

111. Youmans, G. P., and Youmans, A. S.: Unpublished data.

10

The Nature of the Immunizing Activity of Mycobacterial and Other Ribosomal and RNA Vaccines

INTRODUCTION

Since we first published on mycobacterial ribosomal and RNA vaccines, the question has been asked repeatedly, "How do they immunize?" Although no final answer to this question is yet available, we do have an hypothesis that if correct, might account for the immunizing activity of mycobacterial RNA. The experimental procedures and results that led to the development of this hypothesis will be described in this chapter.[41]

In view of our considerable experi-

ence in the experimental chemotherapy of tuberculosis,[54] we decided to treat vaccinated mice with doses of metabolic inhibitors that had been shown to be active, in one way or another, in vivo to see whether they would affect the induction of the immune response. From the results of these experiments, we hoped to gain some insight into the mechanism by which mycobacterial RNA immunized against tuberculosis in mice, since the metabolic processes inhibited by many of these compounds are well known.

EFFECT OF METABOLIC INHIBITORS ON IMMUNITY TO TUBERCULOSIS PRODUCED BY RNA VACCINES

Streptomycin sulfate, an inhibitor of protein synthesis (primarily in bacterial cells), was the first compound used. It is also an effective chemotherapeutic agent against tuberculosis.[54] Although the dose used was effective for the treatment of tuberculosis, this drug had no effect on the immune response in mice vaccinated with RNA (see Table 10–1). Another protein inhibitor, chloramphenicol (inhibitor of protein synthesis in both bacterial and mammalian cells), was tried; it also had no effect on the immune response. Cycloheximide (inhibitor of protein synthesis in mammalian cells) was mixed with RNA, and mice were vaccinated with this mixture. Cycloheximide alone was injected at various times around the time of vaccination and daily for four days after vaccination. None of these treatments affected the immune response in the vaccinated mice, although all three compounds in the same dosages markedly inhibited antibody formation in mice to sheep red blood cells (SRBC) (see Table 10–1). These results suggested that protein synthesis was not involved in the immune mechanism. Therefore, neither antibody nor adaptive enzymes should be involved in the immune process.

Rifampin, which inhibits DNA-dependent RNA polymerase, was used in concentrations that inhibit the enzyme in both mammalian and bacterial cells. However, this compound also had no effect on the high immune response obtained in the vaccinated mice, even though the concentration of rifampin used inhibited antibody formation to SRBC and inhibited the growth of virulent tubercle bacilli in vivo (see Table 10–1). These results tend to rule out this enzyme as being involved in the immune response.

TABLE 10–1. **Effect of Metabolic Inhibitors on Replication of RNA Oncogenic Viruses, Immune Response to Mycobacterial RNA, and Antibody Formation**

Metabolic Inhibitor	Virus Replication	Immune Response to RNA	Antibody Formation
Streptomycin sulfate	−	−	+
Chloramphenicol	−	−	+
Cycloheximide	−	−	+
Rifampin	−	−	+
5-fluoro-deoxyuridine			
1 h before vaccination	+	+	−
18 h after vaccination	−	−	+
Ethidium bromide	+	+	−
Proflavin	+	+	−
Chloroquine			
1 h before vaccination	−	−	−
1 h after vaccination	+	+	−
18 h after vaccination	+	+	−
Actinomycin D			
1 h before vaccination	−	−	+
1 h after vaccination	−	−	+
18 h after vaccination	+	+	+

From Youmans, A. S., and Youmans, G. P.: Mycobacterial extracts and immunity to tuberculosis. *In* Neter, E., and Milgrom, F. (eds.): The Immune System and Infectious Diseases—Fourth International Convocation on Immunology (Buffalo, N.Y., 1974). Basel, S. Karger, 1975.

Merritt and Johnson[17] measured the effect of 5-fluoro-deoxyuridine (FUDR) on antibody formation. FUDR inhibits thymidine synthetase and, thereby, inhibits DNA synthesis. They found that antibody formation was stimulated if FUDR was injected into the mice up to 14 hours after vaccination but was markedly reduced if FUDR was injected 18 hours after vaccination.

Our experiments were based on those of Merritt and Johnson. We used the same concentration of FUDR and, by the same route, injected it just before vaccination and 1 and 18 hours after vaccination. The results (see Table 10–1) were just the opposite of those found by Merritt and Johnson.[17] We obtained a significant reduction in the immune response of vaccinated mice if the FUDR was injected near the time of vaccination but found no effect on the immune response if FUDR was injected 18 hours after vaccination. These unexpected results implied that DNA formation was important at the beginning of the immune response. Therefore, we tried three other compounds — ethidium bromide, proflavin, and chloroquine — that inhibit DNA synthesis primarily by binding with the DNA. All of these compounds significantly reduced the immune response (see Table 10–1). These results strongly suggested that DNA played an important role in the manner by which mycobacterial RNA immunized mice.

Actinomycin D, which inhibits DNA-primed RNA synthesis, was injected at various times into vaccinated and nonvaccinated mice. It had no effect on the immune response obtained in the vaccinated mice if injected at the time of vaccination or 1 hour after vaccination, but it significantly inhibited the immune response if given 18 hours after vaccination. These results indicated that the transcription of RNA from a DNA template might be involved in the immune response.

The results we have just described assume much greater significance when they are compared with the effect of the same metabolic inhibitors on the replication of the RNA oncogenic viruses (see Table 10–1).[8] Since the RNA tumor viruses replicate in a unique manner, the analogy is even more interesting. Table 10–1 shows a summary of the effect of these compounds on the immune response to mycobacterial RNA and on the replication of the RNA oncogenic viruses. The table also includes the manner in which these compounds affect antibody formation. From this table it can be seen that:

1. The replication of the RNA tumor viruses is not inhibited by inhibitors of protein synthesis; neither was the immune response produced in mice vaccinated with mycobacterial RNA.

2. Rifampin had no effect on either system, indicating that DNA-dependent RNA polymerase was not involved.

3. Inhibitors of DNA synthesis inhibited both systems.

4. The need for DNA synthesis is transient for both systems, but there is a need for functioning DNA at all times after infection or vaccination, as is shown by the results with FUDR and the other DNA inhibitors.

5. A unique characteristic of RNA tumor viruses is the inhibition of their replication by actinomycin D after some viral replication has occurred. The same time sequence of inhibition was noted following immunization with mycobacterial RNA. Actinomycin D inhibits DNA-dependent RNA transcription by combining with the DNA template.

6. These results suggested the presence of RNA-dependent DNA polymerase in mycobacterial RNA. It is of interest that in support of this possibility, Müller and coworkers[20] found that *several* of these metabolic inhibitors inhibited RNA-dependent DNA polymerase of an oncogenic RNA virus.

7. In addition, there is a close correlation between the pathogenicity of *M.*

tuberculosis and RNA tumor viruses.[38, 41] Both reproduce intracellularly; both can transform normal cells, form tumors, and remain latent for various periods of time; and the immunity againt both diseases is cellular.

In contrast, as is seen in Table 10–1, there is no correlation between these disease entities and the formation of antibody. Those compounds that inhibit antibody formation have no effect on either viral replication or induction of the immune response. The compounds affecting the latter had no effect on antibody formation with the exception of FUDR and actinomycin D, and in those cases, the time at which inhibition occurred was different.

In view of the close parallels just noted between the replication of RNA tumor viruses and the induction of the immune response to tuberculous infection by mycobacterial RNA, it is tempting to hypothesize that the development of the immune response in mice may involve replication of RNA by a process analogous to the replication of the RNA tumor viruses. If true, the RNA would form a DNA template that might then transcribe RNA in the mammalian cell, which would transform from a normal cell into an immune cell.

Difficult as it may be to accept the possibility that a bacterial RNA may replicate in mammalian cells, it is supported by the work of Anker and Stroun,[2] who have shown that both plant and animal cells will synthesize bacterial RNA by using bacterial DNA as a template. It is only a small step to make the starting material RNA instead of DNA, especially with the example of the oncogenic viruses in front of us. In other words, if viral RNA can replicate in mammalian cells, why not bacterial RNA?

While mycobacterial RNA may immunize by some other fashion than replication, such as acting as a potent adjuvant[9, 53] for some other mycobac-

terial component, it would seem unlikely that this type of immunity would be as specific as the type that we find induced by mycobacterial RNA.

How, given the hypothesis that mycobacterial RNA may replicate in mammalian cells, this could lead to increased resistance to infection with virulent tubercle bacilli is far from clear. Conceivably, cells might be transformed to a more resistant state in which they no longer served as a suitable culture medium for virulent tubercle bacilli. Or, the increase in amount of RNA might maintain a specific state of activation of macrophages or lymphocytes or both for prolonged periods. Finally, if we carry the analogy with viral infection to the extreme, specific resistance due to the presence of mycobacterial RNA and the DNA derived from it in the genomes of reticuloendothelial cells might result in preventing the RNA or DNA from virulent mycobacteria from functioning in host cells, much in the same manner as viral genomes do, and thus interrupt some essential step in the replication of virulent mycobacteria in vivo. In this connection, these data may provide a new concept that could serve as a basis for an explanation of the nature of the specific phase of cellular immunity to mycobacterial infection.

MODE OF ACTION OF OTHER RIBOSOMAL AND RNA VACCINES

There has been an increasing interest in bacterial ribosomal and RNA vaccines since the reports of Youmans and Youmans[41-53, 55-57] on the immunizing activity against tuberculous infection of ribosomal and RNA preparations obtained from the attenuated H37Ra strain of *M. tuberculosis*. Since then, ribosomal or RNA vaccines prepared from a number of other pathogenic microorganisms have been found to be effective immunizing agents in experimental animals.[1, 3-7, 10, 12-16, 18, 19, 21-37, 39, 40] (See Chapter 9.)

The effectiveness of these materials for the prevention of infection in experimental animals immediately raises the question of whether they would be equally effective immunizing agents in human beings. Because of the importance of the answer to this question, we should examine the characteristics of these immunizing agents and make some kind of preliminary assessment of their suitability for injection into human beings. For example, we first must be concerned with their capacity to elicit local or systemic toxic reactions. Secondly, we should have some information on the antigenicity of the substances present in these vaccines. Will they induce either immediate or delayed-type hypersensitivity, with the consequent risk of serious allergic reactions? Also, what effect, if any, may they have on other biologic situations, such as tumor progression and autoimmune disease? Finally, what is the nature of the immune response to those vaccines? Is it mediated by either a circulating or cell-bound antibody, or is it purely cellular immunity, or both? Is it specific? What is the nature of the active ingredient in each vaccine?

Answers to these questions should help greatly in assessing possible usefulness for the prevention of infectious disease in human beings.

It is our opinion that at least two immune responses may be involved in the immunity engendered by ribosomal or RNA vaccines. The nature of the response will depend upon the bacterial species from which the vaccine is prepared. Our feeling arises from the following considerations. *M. tuberculosis* is the classical example of a facultative intracellular parasite that, when producing infection, stimulates the production of a purely cellular type of immunity. Ability to be passively transferred by cells (i.e., lymphocytes) but failure to be passively trans-

ferred by serum characterizes this type of immunity (see Chapter 8). Another important characteristic of cellular immunity is that killed bacterial cells do not readily stimulate its development; whereas living cells — either virulent or attenuated — induce a high degree of immunity. Initially, we were testing the hypothesis that cellular immunity in tuberculosis might require some very labile substance for its induction (see Chapter 8), thereby accounting for the much greater immunizing activity of living microorganisms. The discovery that the major immunogen in *M. tuberculosis* was located in ribosomal and RNA preparations led us to believe that there was some relationship between the nature of the immunizing material and the type of immune response found in tuberculosis; that is, cellular immunity to infection. Also, the demonstration by Venneman and colleagues[37] that ribosomal fractions from *Salmonella typhimurium* were immunogenic supported the notion that there was some relationship between cellular immunity to infection and the effectiveness of ribosomal vaccines. In rapid succession, immunizing ribosomal preparations were obtained from staphylococci,[40] *Pseudomonas*,[27, 39] *Vibrio cholerae*,[12] pneumococci,[32, 33] group A streptococci,[23] and *Neisseria meningitidis*.[31] All of these bacteria are extracellular parasites because they are killed once they have been phagocytosed. It follows that the only requirement for a high degree of immunity to extracellular parasites is opsonizing antibody to a surface antigen. Furthermore, in a number of these preparations, notably those of *Vibrio cholerae*[12] and staphylococci,[40] the active ingredient has tentatively been identified as a protein. In the mycobacterial system, on the other hand, the protein constituents are completely inactive; instead, there is a high correlation between degree of immunizing activity and nativeness of the RNA (see Chapter 9). It is possible that the immunogenicity of ribosomal vaccines of those bacteria that are true extracellular parasites is merely a consequence of the method of preparation. The mechanical breakage of the bacterial cell may release and help solubilize cell wall antigens, which then could complex with the ribosomal RNA or ribosomal protein and be carried down with the ribosomes during the subsequent necessary centrifugations. These cell wall materials —most likely polysaccharides or proteins, possibly in the form of polysaccharide-protein complexes —might easily stimulate the formation of enough antibody to act as an opsonin that would promote phagocytosis and, therefore, the killing of the virulent challenge inoculum. This is supported by the recent studies of Thompson and Eisenstein,[32] who found that the immunity produced in mice by pneumococcal ribosomal vaccine could be transferred to nonimmunized mice with the serum of immunized animals. This suggests that an opsonizing antibody is responsible for the immunity.

Superficially, such an explanation would not appear to be adequate for the activity of the *S. typhimurium* vaccine, although Smith and Bigley[26] have reported that the immunogenicity of *S. typhimurium* ribosomal vaccine also resides in the protein portion. The salmonellae have long been regarded as true facultative intracellular parasites. Therefore, one would expect the response to salmonella ribosomal vaccines to resemble that to mycobacterial ribosomal and RNA vaccines, but it is not so. This apparent contradiction can be resolved if we recognize that the salmonellae, at least *S. typhimurium*, are not really facultative intracellular parasites after all. Several lines of evidence support this conclusion. The most convincing evidence will be found in a paper by Hsu and Mayo.[11] These workers found that in guinea pigs, immunity to *S. typhimurium* was mediated by an antibody cytophilic for macrophages. The major function of this cytophilic antibody

appeared to be to act as an opsonin, since once ingested by macrophages, the bacterial cells were readily killed. Thus, since *S. typhimurium* apparently is truly an extracellular parasite, the findings using ribosomal vaccines should parallel those obtained with ribosomal vaccines prepared from other extracellular parasites, and they do. Of great importance in this respect is the finding by Douglas and Berry[5] that the ribosomal vaccines which they prepared from *S. typhimurium* do contain small amounts of sugars known to be present in O antigen. However, Misfeldt and Johnson have shown that O antigen cannot account for the immunogenicity of ribosomal vaccines prepared from *S. typhimurium*.[18]

Margolis and Bigley[16] found a macroglobulin that reacted specifically with the ribosomal vaccine in mice immunized with ribosomal vaccines prepared from *S. typhimurium*. Since this macroglobulin promoted phagocytosis of *S. typhimurium*, it is possible that this is the opsonin that would be required for protection of these vaccinated mice against challenge with *S. typhimurium*.

We conclude, therefore, that ribosomal vaccines may induce either antibody-mediated immune responses or cellular immunity, depending upon the parasitic nature of the bacterial species from which they are prepared. It also follows that there is no special relationship between ribosomal and RNA vaccines and cellular immunity to infection. The type of immunity that will develop in response to RNA vaccines will be that required to cope with the particular pathogen involved.

Although the above explanation is the most attractive to us at this time, there are three alternatives that should be considered. First, it is conceivable that the RNA vaccines could be such potent activators of the reticuloendothelial system that these cells would more actively phagocytose virulent cells at the time of challenge. It is possible that activated macrophages will phagocytose extracellular parasites more readily, even in the absence of specific opsonin. Such increased resistance would, of course, be nonspecific and of a much lower grade than that mediated by opsonin.

Second, it is possible that the RNA vaccines direct the immune response toward cell-mediated immunity and that cell-mediated immunity is more effective for the control of infection due to extracellular parasites than is generally realized.

Third, perhaps these ribosomal materials are biologically so active that they prime the immune systems in such a way that they will respond much more rapidly to stimulation by an antigen at some later date. In this case, the immune response, because of the priming, would be so rapid to the challenge infection itself that adequate amounts of antibody would be formed before the disease became fatal, and the animals would appear to have been effectively immunized.

It would be most helpful, and might be revealing, if experimenters who are working with ribosomal vaccines obtained from extracellular parasites would enlarge their studies to include detection of opsonizing antibody, either circulating in the serum or cell-bound.

ARE RIBOSOMAL AND RNA VACCINES TOXIC?

There is very little information available on possible toxic reactions following the injection of ribosomal vaccines. Most investigators have used mice, and deleterious effects have not been reported. In the mycobacterial system, we have had occasion to use both mice and guinea pigs. In guinea pigs, the ribosomal or RNA preparations have been used both for the induction of immunity and as skin test agents for the detection of hypersensitivity (see Chapter 9 for further de-

tails). Large doses of ribosomal material or RNA from mycobacteria produced no detectable adverse effects when incorporated in Freund's incomplete adjuvant and injected subcutaneously into guinea pigs. On the other hand, small doses (1.0 μg) injected intradermally produced small inflammatory reactions, 5 to 6 mm in diameter, and central necrosis within 24 hours. The necrotic areas seldom exceeded 2 or 3 mm. No evidence of allergy was noted, as these reactions were of the same size in normal and vaccinated animals.[52]

Mice injected subcutaneously or intraperitoneally with these preparations in Freund's incomplete adjuvant usually showed no adverse effects. Sometimes with the largest doses employed (50.0 μg), mice appeared somewhat listless for the first few days after vaccination. They rapidly recovered and, four weeks after vaccination, appeared as healthy as the nonvaccinated control mice.

REFERENCES

1. Andron, L. A., II, and Eigelsbach, H. T.: Biochemical and immunological properties of ribonucleic acid-rich extracts from *Francisella tularensis.* Infect. Immun. 12:137, 1975.
2. Anker, P., and Stroun, M.: Bacterial ribonucleic acid in the frog brain after a bacterial peritoneal infection. Science *178*:621, 1972.
3. Baba, T.: Immunogenic activity of a ribosomal fraction obtained from *Pasteurella multocida.* Infect. Immun. 15:1, 1977.
4. Berry, L. J., Douglas, G. N., Hoops, P., and Prather, N. E.: Immunization against salmonellosis. *In* Neter, E., and Milgrom, F. (eds.): The Immune System and Infectious Diseases — Fourth International Convocation on Immunology (Buffalo, N.Y., 1974). Basel, S. Karger, 1975.
5. Douglas, G. N., and Berry, L. J.: Partial characterization of highly immunogenic RNA fractions from *Salmonella typhimurium* SR-11 using gas-liquid chromatography. Abstract No. 36 of the Annual Meeting of the Reticuloendothelial Society (December 5–8, 1973, Williamsburg, Virginia). J. Reticuloendothel. Soc. *15*:21a, 1974.

6. Eisenstein, T. K.: Evidence for O antigens as the antigenic determinants in "ribosomal" vaccines prepared from *Salmonella*. Infect. Immun. *12*:364, 1975.

7. Feit, C., and Tewari, R. P.: Immunogenicity of ribosomes from *Histoplasma capsulatum*. Infect. Immun. *10*:1091, 1974.

8. Green, M.: Oncogenic viruses. Annu. Rev. Biochem. *39*:701, 1970.

9. Gumbiner, C., Paterson, P. Y., Youmans, G. P., and Youmans, A. S.: Adjuvanticity of mycobacterial RNA and poly A:U for induction of experimental allergic encephalomyelitis in guinea pigs. J. Immunol. *110*:309, 1973.

10. Hoops, P., Prather, N. E., Berry, L. J., and Ravel, J. M.: Evidence for an extrinsic immunogen in effective ribosomal vaccines from *Salmonella typhimurium*. Infect. Immun. *13*:1184, 1976.

11. Hsu, H. S., and Mayo, D. R.: Interactions between macrophages of guinea pigs and samonellae. III. Bactericidal action and cytophilic antibodies of macrophages of infected guinea pigs. Infect. Immun. *8*:165, 1973.

12. Jensen, R., Gregory, B., Naylor, J., and Actor, P.: Isolation of protective somatic antigen from *Vibrio cholerae* (Ogawa) ribosomal preparations. Infect. Immun. *6*:156, 1972.

13. Johnson, W.: Ribosomal vaccines. I. Immunogenicity of ribosomal fractions isolated from *Salmonella typhimurium* and *Yersinia pestis*. Infect. Immun. *5*:947, 1972.

14. Johnson, W.: Ribosomal vaccines. II. Specificity of the immune response to ribosomal ribonucleic acid and protein isolated from *Salmonella typhimurium*. Infect. Immun. *8*:395, 1973.

15. Lynn, M., Tewari, R. P., and Solotorovsky, M.: Immunoprotective activity of ribosomes from *Haemophilus influenzae*. Infect. Immun. *15*:453, 1977.

16. Margolis, J. M., and Bigley, N. J.: Cytophilic macroglobulin reactive with bacterial protein in mice immunized with ribonucleic acid-protein fractions of virulent *Salmonella typhimurium*. Infect. Immun. *6*:390, 1972.

17. Merritt, K., and Johnson, A. G.: Studies on the adjuvant action of bacterial endotoxins on antibody formation. VI. Enhancement of antibody formation by nucleic acids. J. Immunol. *94*:416, 1965.

18. Misfeldt, M. L., and Johnson, W.: Role of endotoxin contamination in ribosomal vaccines prepared from *Salmonella typhimurium*. Infect. Immun. *17*:98, 1977.

19. Misfeldt, M. L., and Johnson, W.: Variability of protection in inbred mice induced by a ribosomal vaccine prepared from *Salmonella typhimurium*. Infect. Immun. *14*:652, 1976.

20. Müller, W. E. G., Zahn, R. K., and Seidel, H. J.: Inhibitors acting on nucleic acid synthesis in an oncogenic RNA virus. Nature *232*:143, 1971.

21. Preston, P. M., and Dumonde, D. C.: Immunogenicity of a ribosomal antigen of *Leishmania enriettii*. Trans. R. Soc. Trop. Med. Hyg. *65*:18, 1971.

22. Saunders, E. S., Solotorovsky, M., and Tewari, R. P.: Immunization against experimental candidosis with ribosomal preparations from *Candida albicans*. Abstracts of the Annual Meeting of the American Society for Microbiology, 1975. p. 89.

23. Schalla, W. O., and Johnson, W.: Immunogenicity of ribosomal preparations isolated from group A, type 14, *Streptococcus pyogenes*. Infect. Immun. *11*:1195, 1975.

24. Smith, R. A., and Bigley, N. J.: Detection of delayed hypersensitivity in mice injected with ribonucleic acid-protein fractions of *Salmonella typhimurium*. Infect. Immun. *6*:384, 1972.

25. Smith, R. A., and Bigley, N. J.: Inability of RNA-protein fractions of *Salmonella typhimurium* to induce immune deviation. Abstracts of the Annual Meeting of the American Society for Microbiology, 1973. p. 114.

26. Smith, R. A., and Bigley, N. J.: Ribonucleic acid-protein fractions of virulent *Salmonella typhimurium* as protective immunogens. Infect. Immun. *6*:377, 1972.

27. Smith, R. L., Wysocki, J. A., Bruun, J. N., De Courcy, S. J., Jr., Blakemore, W. S., and Mudd, S.: Efficacy of ribosomal preparations from *Pseudomonas aeruginosa* to protect against intravenous pseudomonas challenge in mice. J. Reticuloendothel. Soc. *15*:22, 1974.

28. Suzuki, K.: Cellular fractions of *Listeria monocytogenes* in relation to the localization of a protective antigen and monocytosis producing factor. Yonago Acta Med. *14*:52, 1970.

29. Tewari, R. P.: Immunization against histoplasmosis. *In* Neter, E., and Milgrom, F. (eds.): The Immune System and Infectious Diseases. Fourth International Convocation on Immunology (Buffalo, N.Y., 1974). Basel, S. Karger, 1975.

30. Tewari, R. P., Sharma, D., Solotorovsky, M., Lafemina, R., and Balint, J.: Adoptive transfer of immunity from mice immunized with ribosomes of live yeast cells of *Histoplasma capsulatum*. Infect. Immun. *15*:789, 1977.

31. Thomas, D. W., and Weiss, E.: Response of mice to injection of ribosomal fraction from group B *Neisseria meningitidis*. Infect. Immun. *6*:355, 1972.

32. Thompson, H. C. W., and Eisenstein, T. K.:

Biological properties of an immunogenic pneumococcal subcellular preparation. Infect. Immun. *13*:750, 1976.

33. Thompson, H. C. W., and Snyder, I. S.: Protection against pneumococcal infection by a ribosomal preparation. Infect. Immun. *3*:16, 1971.

34. Venneman, M. R.: Purification of immunogenically active ribonucleic acid preparations of *Salmonella typhimurium*: Molecular-sieve and anion-exchange chromatography. Infect. Immun. *5*:269, 1972.

35. Venneman, M. R., and Berry, L. J.: Cell-mediated resistance induced with immunogenic preparations of *Salmonella typhimurium*. Infect. Immun. *4*:381, 1971.

36. Venneman, M. R., and Berry, L. J.: Experimental salmonellosis: Differential passive transfer of immunity with serum and cells obtained from ribosomal and ribonucleic acid-immunized mice. J. Reticuloendothel. Soc. *9*:491, 1974.

37. Venneman, M. R., Bigley, N. J., and Berry, L. J.: Immunogenicity of ribonucleic acid preparations obtained from *Salmonella typhimurium*. Infect. Immun. *1*:574, 1970.

38. Vigier, P.: RNA oncogenic viruses. Structure, replication, and oncogenicity. Prog. Med. Virol. *12*:240, 1970.

39. Winston, S. H., and Berry, L. J.: Antibacterial immunity induced by ribosomal vaccines. J. Reticuloendothel. Soc. *8*:13, 1970.

40. Winston, S. H., and Berry, L. J.: Immunity induced by ribosomal extracts from *Staphylococcus aureus*. J. Reticuloendothel. Soc. *8*:66, 1970.

41. Youmans, A. S., and Youmans, G. P.: The effect of metabolic inhibitors and hydroxylamine on the immune response in mice to mycobacterial ribonucleic acid vaccines. J. Immunol. *112*:271, 1974.

42. Youmans, A. S., and Youmans, G. P.: Effect of polybasic amines on the immunogenicity of mycobacterial ribonucleic acid. Infect. Immun. *6*:798, 1972.

43. Youmans, A. S., and Youmans, G. P.: Effect of trypsin and ribonuclease on the immunogenic activity of ribosomes and ribonucleic acid isolated from *Mycobacterium tuberculosis*. J. Bacteriol. *91*:2146, 1966.

44. Youmans, A. S., and Youmans, G. P.: Factors affecting immunogenic activity of mycobacterial ribosomal and ribonucleic acid preparations. J. Bacteriol. *99*:42, 1969.

45. Youmans, A. S., and Youmans, G. P.: Failure of synthetic polynucleotides to affect the immunogenicity of mycobacterial ribonucleic acid and ribosomal protein preparations. Infect. Immun. *3*:149, 1971.

46. Youmans, A. S., and Youmans, G. P.: Immunogenic activity of a ribosomal fraction obtained from *Mycobacterium tuberculosis*. J. Bacteriol. *89*:1291, 1965.

47. Youmans, A. S., and Youmans, G. P.: Immunogenic mycobacterial ribosomal and ribonucleic acid preparations: Chemical and physical characteristics. Infect. Immun. *2*:659, 1970.

48. Youmans, A. S., and Youmans, G. P.: Preparation and effect of different adjuvants on the immunogenic activity of mycobacterial ribosomal fraction. J. Bacteriol. *94*:836, 1967.

49. Youmans, A. S., and Youmans, G. P.: Preparation of highly immunogenic ribosomal fractions of *Mycobacterium tuberculosis* by use of sodium dodecyl sulfate. J. Bacteriol. *91*:2139, 1966.

50. Youmans, A. S., and Youmans, G. P.: The relationship between sedimentation value and immunogenic activity of mycobacterial ribonucleic acid. J. Immunol. *110*:581, 1973.

51. Youmans, A. S., and Youmans, G. P.: Ribonucleic acid, deoxyribonucleic acid, and protein content of cells of different ages of *Mycobacterium tuberculosis* and the relationship to immunogenicity. J. Bacteriol. *95*:272, 1968.

52. Youmans, G. P., and Youmans, A. S.: Allergenicity of mycobacterial ribosomal and ribonucleic acid preparations in mice and guinea pigs. J. Bacteriol. *97*:134, 1969.

53. Youmans, G. P., and Youmans, A. S.: The effect of mycobacterial RNA on the primary antibody response of mice to bovine gamma globulin. J. Immunol. *109*:217, 1972.

54. Youmans, G. P., and Youmans, A. S.: Experimental chemotherapy of tuberculosis and other mycobacterial infections. *In* Schnitzer, R. J., and Hawking, F. (eds.): Experimental Chemotherapy, Vol. II. New York, Academic Press, 1964.

55. Youmans, G. P., and Youmans, A. S.: Immunizing antigens of mycobacteria. *In* Nowotny, A. (ed.): Cellular Antigens. New York, Springer-Verlag, 1972.

56. Youmans, G. P., and Youmans, A. S.: *Mycobacterium tuberculosis* immunogens. Ann. Sclavo *13*:707, 1971.

57. Youmans, G. P., and Youmans, A. S.: Recent studies on acquired immunity in tuberculosis. Curr. Top. Microbiol. Immunol. *48*:129, 1969.

11

Other Immunizing Substances Found in Mycobacteria

INTRODUCTION

The search for immunizing components from mycobacterial cells was spurred in the early 1950s by Salton and Horne's demonstration[45] that ruptured bacterial cells could be separated into major structural components by differential centrifugation. Millman and Youmans[35, 36] ruptured living H37Ra mycobacterial cells, either by grinding in a ball mill or by sonic oscillation, and separated the broken cells by high-speed differential centrifugation into a "red fraction," consisting of intracellular particulate matter, and a "supernatant fraction," from which all particulate matter had been removed. These fractions were then tested for enzymatic activity (see Chapter 2).

In a companion study, Youmans and coworkers[49] in 1955 reported upon the capacity of these same fractions to induce immunity in mice to challenge with virulent tubercle bacilli. Only the "red fraction" was an effective immunizing agent. It was from this "red fraction" that the highly immunogenic RNA vaccine was eventually produced. The production and activity of the RNA vaccine is described in detail in Chapter 9.

MYCOBACTERIAL CELL WALLS

In 1960 Kanai and Youmans[29] reported that mycobacterial cell walls isolated by differential centrifugation from disrupted H37Ra cells had little or no capacity to immunize mice against intravenous challenge with the H37Rv strain. The cell walls were purified by the method described by Ribi and coworkers.[40] Larson and colleagues[30] also found that neither mycobacterial cell walls nor a mixture of cell walls and cytoplasm were able to immunize mice to aerosol challenge with virulent tubercle bacilli.

OIL-DISRUPTION PRODUCT

Interest in mycobacterial cell walls as possible immunogens was reawakened when Larson and colleagues,[30] using a technique developed by Smith,[30] reported that when BCG cells were suspended in light mineral oil and passed through a Sorvall-Ribi disruption press, the "oil-disruption product" of mycobacterial cells was highly immunogenic against aerosol challenge with virulent mycobacteria, provided the vaccine was administered intravenously. The same disruption product of similar cells suspended in water was without immunizing activity.

Further investigations by this group[37-42] revealed that not only was the "oil-disruption product" immunogenic when given to mice by the intravenous route but also cell walls prepared by disruption of the mycobacterial cells in water, then dried and resuspended in mineral oil, were immunogenic when given intravenously. Neither "oil-disruption product" nor oil-coated cell walls gave protection against aerosol infection when the vaccinating doses were given subcutaneously or intraperitoneally. On the other hand, following intravenous, subcutaneous, or intraperitoneal vaccination, protection was noted when the challenge dose of virulent tubercle bacilli was administered intravenously.

PULMONARY GRANULOMAS PRODUCED BY OIL-COATED MYCOBACTERIAL CELL WALLS

Thus, we have the peculiar situation of an immunizing moiety that is active against aerosol infection with virulent tubercle bacilli only when administered intravenously. Kanai in 1967 suggested that "granulomatous lesions caused by oil-coated cell walls in the lungs may be the site of a strong local immunity, where virulent tubercle bacilli inhaled would be most effectively destroyed."[28] This explanation was later found to be correct by Barclay and colleagues[1] in 1967. These investigators reported that the intravenous injection of mycobacterial cell wall-oil vaccine induced an intense granulomatous response in the lungs of mice. It is well known that the intravenous injection of viable or killed mycobacterial cells into mice or rabbits will induce a pulmonary granulomatous response (see Chapter 3). Broken mycobacterial cells or cell components isolated by centrifugation from broken cells, such as intracellular membranes, intracellular fluid, ribosomes, and other cellular particulates, have no capacity to do so.[52] With the initiation of the granulomatous response, there is an increase in resistance to tuberculous infection, which, in turn, is directly proportional to the magnitude of the granulomatous response.[50] It has been shown that mineral oil increases the pulmonary granulomatous response produced by whole cells and that the macrophages that accumulate are metabolically more active and have a greater capacity to destroy mycobacterial cells.[24, 31] Therefore, the pulmonary granulomatous response can account for the increased resistance noted following intravenous vaccination of mice with oil-cell wall preparations, whether challenge is by the pulmonary or intravenous route.

What remains unexplained is why, in mice, no evidence of immunity can be demonstrated following vaccination with viable attenuated mycobacterial cells by the subcutaneous or intraperitoneal route if challenge is by the pulmonary route, when it can be demonstrated by intravenous challenge. This is of interest especially since guinea pigs,[46] rabbits,[33] monkeys,[27] and man[44] can show an appreciable degree of increased resistance under similar conditions of vaccination and challenge. Technical factors may be partly responsible, but the explanation may be that whole cells do not induce a significant pulmonary granulomatous response in mice when administered by any route other than intravenous. Under these other conditions, however, these whole cells will prime the animal in such a fashion that it will respond more rapidly and with a greater granulomatous response when mycobacterial cells subsequently are given intravenously (the accelerated granulomatous response). This could account for the increased resistance noted following subcutaneous or intraperitoneal vaccination with oil-cell wall preparations or with whole cells when a large intravenous challenge is employed. The minute numbers of virulent cells usually used for aerosol challenge, deposited on what is essentially an external body surface, might not initially constitute an adequate secondary stimulus of the reticuloendothelial system. Only when sufficient multiplication and tissue destruction has taken place would these microorganisms be distributed to the reticuloendothelial system in sufficient numbers to restimulate the defensive forces of the vaccinated animal. This, for unknown reasons, may occur appreciably later after aerosol infection in mice than in the other animal species just mentioned. A further discussion of the granulomatous response is given in Chapters 3 and 4.

On the other hand, the recent work of Lefford[32] would indicate that following vaccination of mice subcutaneously or intraperitoneally, sufficient committed lymphocytes do not accumulate in the lung to give an immune response to intrapulmonary challenge.

TRYPSIN-EXTRACTED IMMUNOGEN

An immunizing substance from mycobacterial cells that in recent years has received considerable attention is the trypsin-extracted antigen of Crowle. Crowle has described this antigen in a number of papers and in a summarizing review article.[10-21] These publications should be consulted for complete details.

Trypsin-extracted immunizing antigen was prepared by Crowle by treating acetone-killed mycobacterial cells (H37Ra, BCG and virulent cells) with trypsin. This treatment apparently releases water-soluble cell wall components into the medium. Figure 11–1, taken from Crowle,[12] shows the steps involved in the production of the trypsin-extracted antigen.

According to Crowle,[12] his results indicate that the digestion of killed, acetone-washed tubercle bacilli with trypsin releases a water-soluble, low molecular weight complex of peptides and a polysaccharide that can immunize experimental animals specifically against tuberculosis without, at the same time, sensitizing them against tuberculin. Although a polysaccharide appears to be the major immunizing moiety, peptides also appear to be important. Involvement of polysaccharide is indicated by the resistance of the trypsin extract to all digestive pro-

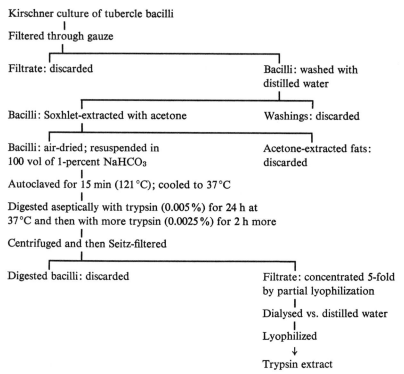

FIGURE 11–1.   Current procedure for preparing trypsin extract. Generally, the starting bacilli are H37Ra strain, but virulent and bovine strains can be used. The yield from bovine strains is low. (From Crowle, A. J.: Trypsin-extracted immunizing antigen of the tubercle bacillus: A practical vaccine? Adv. Tuberc. Res. *18*:31, 1972.)

cedures except hydrolysis with pancreatic amylase and oxidation with periodic acid and by the presence of three sugars in the chromatographically purified immunogen. The importance of peptides is suggested by the diminution of immunogenicity that occurs with pronase but not with other proteolytic enzymes, by the purified immunogen's strong negative charge, and by the presence in chromatographically purified immunogen of four amino acids. Of particular importance is the fact that trypsin-extracted immunogen does not sensitize either guinea pigs or mice to tuberculin, although it can induce a delayed-type hypersensitivity specific for some component in itself.

We should take particular note of the fact that trypsin-extracted immunogen is prepared from killed mycobacterial cells. Therefore, it should be a far less effective immunizing agent than viable cells of the mycobacterial strain from which it is prepared. At least, it should not be more effective in equal doses than the killed mycobacterial cells from which it is extracted. As a matter of fact, this generally appears to be the case.[12] The important question then becomes: Are the killed cells from which trypsin-extracted antigen is prepared equal to or inferior to the viable cells of the same strain in capacity to immunize? From the data we have presented in Chapter 8, we would expect the killed cells to be much poorer in immunizing power, and therefore, no extracts of these cells could be expected to be very potent immunizing agents. Crowle[12] addressed himself to this problem and published data that he felt showed that killed BCG cells and fractions were almost as effective immunizing agents in guinea pigs as viable BCG cells. Examination, however, of the data provided by Crowle raises some question about the correctness of this conclusion. In Figure 11–2, taken from Crowle,[18] it is clear that the viable BCG cells are far more effective immunizing agents than killed BCG cells. Unfortunately, in these experiments apparently only single arbitrarily selected doses of the different immunizing preparations were compared. As we have seen from the data provided in Chapter 8, valid comparisons of immunizing potency can only be made by employing graded doses of each immunizing agent and then constructing a dose-response curve of immunizing potency for each. Only comparison of these dose-response curves will provide a valid basis for judging relative immunzing potency. The data found in the publications of other investigators, cited in support of the contention that killed bacilli immunize as well as living cells, are similarly too inadequate to justify such a conclusion (see also Chapter 8).[9,47]

In spite of the questions raised in the preceding paragraph, it is clear that trypsin-extracted immunogen in suitable doses will produce a significant increase in resistance to tuberculous infection when given to mice or guinea pigs. In addition, the immuni-

ty so engendered is specific, since no immunity develops to infection with *Klebsiella pneumoniae* or *Streptococcus pneumoniae*.[12] Furthermore, trypsin extracts prepared using saprophytic mycobacteria have no immunizing action against infection with *Mycobacterium tuberculosis*. Also, trypsin-extracted antigen does not induce hypersensitivity to tuberculin in mice or guinea pigs.[12] These characteristics make this material well worth further investigation because of its potential for use in human beings. Detailed comparisons of the immunizing activity of trypsin extract with viable BCG, with viable H37Ra cells, and with mycobacterial RNA should be made so that there can be an assessment of its immunizing capacity as compared with the best agents now available. Although RNA vaccine is apparently far more effective at lower doses than is the trypsin-extracted material (see Chapter 9), these two vaccines compare favorably in respect to their specificity and their failure to produce tuberculin hypersensitivity.

It would be interesting indeed if the polysaccharide in the trypsin extract should be a haptene that, in the RNA preparation, is complexed with the RNA and, because of the potent adjuvant activity of mycobacterial RNA, has had its specific immunizing activity markedly increased; at least, this possibility should be explored.

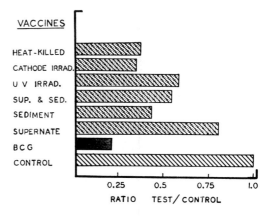

FIGURE 11–2. Results against tuberculosis where protection in guinea pigs is expressed as the ratio of mean gross tuberculosis in a test group to the same measure in the control group vaccinated with water-in-oil emulsion alone. (From Crowle, A. J.: Tuberculoimmunity induced by killed tubercle bacilli and their constituents. Acta Tuberc. Scand. Suppl. 58:27, 1964.)

MISCELLANEOUS IMMUNIZING SUBSTANCES

A great deal of effort by investigators over the years has revealed that a variety of poorly defined substances obtained from mycobacterial cells will induce some increase in resistance to infection with tubercle bacilli in some species of animal, under appropriate conditions of testing. This large literature has been well reviewed by Crowle[9] and, more recently, by Kanai[28] and by Smith and co-workers.[47] None of these substances have been defined chemically, except for perhaps cord factor, and none of the preparations have been pure. For the most part, they consist of material extracted from killed mycobacterial cells by fat solvents of one kind or another; i.e., acetone, ethanol-ether, chloroform, methanol, and mineral oil. Even the residues from such extractions have been shown to be somewhat protective under certain conditions.[46] This indicates that the basic cell wall mucopeptide has some capacity to induce increased resistance to tuberculous infection.

Because of lack of purity of the material extracted, it is difficult to specify the chemical nature of the active substance or substances. However, it appears that wax D, a peptidoglycolipid, is slightly immunogenic in the hands of some workers,[25, 26] and there are a number of other preparations in which the predominant component appears to be a lipopolysaccharide or polysaccharide.[8, 43] A number of investigators have suggested that an immunizing moiety of killed and living mycobacterial cells is a lipopolysaccharide.[23, 34, 48, 51] The immunizing capacity of such preparations, however, is not great, since it does not exceed that of killed cells.[51]

It is well recognized that endotoxin, or lipopolysaccharide, from gram-negative bacteria will also induce some increased resistance in mice to infection with tubercle bacilli.[22, 51] We have found[51] that the magnitude and duration of the immune response to this agent is comparable to that produced with lipopolysaccharide preparations from mycobacteria. We have suggested, therefore, that mycobacterial cells contain a lipopolysaccharide as a cell wall component, which has the same capacity to stimulate the reticuloendothelial system as do lipopolysaccharides from gram-negative bacteria. This lipopolysaccharide, without possessing the toxic characteristics of endotoxin, induces increased resistance to infection.[22, 51]

Cord factor (trehalose 6,6'-dimycolate), when dissolved in mineral oil and injected intravenously as an oil-in-water emulsion, also will increase the resistance of mice to tuberculous infection.[2-7] When injected in this manner, cord factor will induce a profound pulmonary granulomatous response (see Chapter 2). The increased resistance to infection produced by cord factor is probably due to this pulmonary granulomatosis. (For more information on cord factor and its biologic activities, see Chapter 4.)

REFERENCES

1. Barclay, W. R., Anacker, R., Brehmer, W., and Ribi, E.: Effects of oil-treated mycobacterial cell walls on the organs of mice. J. Bacteriol. *94*:1736, 1967.
2. Bekierkunst, A., Levij, I. S., Yarkoni, E., Vilkas, E., Adam, A., and Lederer, E.: Granuloma formation induced in mice by chemically defined mycobacterial fractions. J. Bacteriol. *100*:95, 1969.
3. Bekierkunst, A., Levij, I. S., Yarkoni, E., Vilkas, E., and Lederer, E.: Cellular reaction in the footpad and draining lymph nodes of mice induced by mycobacterial fractions and BCG bacilli. Infect. Immun. *4*:245, 1971.
4. Bekierkunst, A., Levij, I. S., Yarkoni, E., Vilkas, E., and Lederer, E.: Suppression of urethan-induced lung adenomas in mice treated with trehalose 6,6'-dimycolate (cord factor) and living bacillus Calmette-Guérin. Science *174*:1240, 1971.

5. Bekierkunst, A., Wang, L., Toubiana, R., and Lederer, E.: Immunotherapy of cancer with nonliving BCG and fractions derived from mycobacteria: Role of cord factor (trehalose-6,6'-dimycolate) in tumor regression. Infect. Immun. *10*:1044, 1974.

6. Bekierkunst, A., and Yarkoni, E.: Granulomatous hypersensitivity to trehalose-6,6'-dimycolate (cord factor) in mice infected with BCG. Infect. Immun. *7*:631, 1973.

7. Bekierkunst, A., Yarkoni, E., Flechner, I., Morecki, S., Vilkas, E., and Lederer, E.: Immune response to sheep red blood cells in mice pretreated with mycobacterial fractions. Infect. Immun. *4*:256, 1971.

8. Choucroun, N.: Tubercle bacillus antigens. Biological properties of two substances isolated from paraffin oil extract of dead tubercle bacilli. Am. Rev. Tuberc. *56*:203, 1947.

9. Crowle, A. J.: Immunizing constituents of the tubercle bacillus. Bacteriol. Rev. *22*:183, 1958.

10. Crowle, A. J.: Immunogen extracted from tubercle bacilli with trypsin. Z. Immunitaetsforsch. *137*:71, 1969.

11. Crowle, A. J.: A study of the immunizing factors of the tubercle bacillus. Dissertation, Stanford University, 1954.

12. Crowle, A. J.: Trypsin extracted immunizing antigen of the tubercle bacillus: A practical vaccine? Adv. Tuberc. Res. *18*:31, 1972.

13. Crowle, A. J.: Tubercle bacillary extracts immunogenic for mice. 1. Factors affecting demonstration of their activity. Tubercle *42*:470, 1961.

14. Crowle, A. J.: Tubercle bacillary extracts immunogenic for mice. 2. Water-soluble proteinaceous extracts. Tubercle *42*:479, 1961.

15. Crowle, A. J.: Tubercle bacillary extracts immunogenic for mice. 3. Chemical degradation studies on the immunogen extracted from tubercle bacilli by trypsin digestion. Tubercle *43*:178, 1962.

16. Crowle, A. J.: Tubercle bacillary extracts immunogenic for mice. 4. Lipids. Proc. Soc. Exp. Biol. Med. *109*:969, 1962.

17. Crowle, A. J.: Tubercle bacillary extracts immunogenic for mice. 5. Specificity of tuberculo-immunity induced by trypsin extracts of tubercle bacilli. Tubercle *44*:241, 1963.

18. Crowle, A. J.: Tuberculoimmunity induced by killed tubercle bacilli and their constituents. Acta Tuberc. Scandinav. Suppl. *58*:27, 1964.

19. Crowle, A. J., and Hu, C. C: Tubercle bacillary extracts immunogenic for mice. 7. Electrophoretic analyses. Tubercle *46*:214, 1965.

20. Crowle, A. J., and Letcher, D. B.: Tubercle bacillary extracts immunogenic for mice.

8. Storage stability of trypsin-extracted immunogen. Tubercle *49*:304, 1968.

21. Crowle, A. J., and Teramura, F.: Tubercle bacillary extracts immunogenic for mice. 6. Comparative immunogenicity of trypsin extract of tubercle bacilli in mice and guinea pigs. Tubercle *45*:40, 1964.

22. Dubos, R. J., Schaedler, R. W., and Böhme, D.: Effects of bacterial endotoxins on susceptibility to infection with gram-positive and acid-fast bacteria. Fed. Proc. *16*:856, 1957.

23. Hedgecock, L. W.: Protective and serologically active fractions from phenol extract of *Mycobacterium tuberculosis*. Am. Rev. Respir. Dis. *92*:973, 1965.

24. Heise, E. R., Myrvik, Q. N., and Leake, E. S.: Effect of bacillus Calmette-Guérin on the levels of acid phosphatase, lysozyme and cathepsin in rabbit alveolar macrophages. J. Immunol. *95*:125, 1965.

25. Hoyt, A., Dennerline, R. L., Moore, F. J., and Smith, C. R.: Tubercle bacillus wax as an experimental vaccine against mouse tuberculosis. Am. Rev. Tuberc. *76*:752, 1957.

26. Hoyt, A., Moore, F. J., and Thompson, M. A.: Analysis of mixed distributions in antituberculosis vaccine assays. Am. Rev. Respir. Dis. *86*:733, 1962.

27. Janicki, B. W., Good, R. C., Minden, P., Affronti, L. F., and Hymes, W. F.: Immune responses in rhesus monkeys after bacillus Calmette-Guérin vaccination and aerosol challenge with *Mycobacterium tuberculosis*. Am. Rev. Respir. Dis. *107*:359, 1973.

28. Kanai, K.: Review. Acquired resistance to tuberculous infection in experimental model. Jpn. J. Med. Sci. Biol. *20*:21, 1967.

29. Kanai, K., and Youmans, G. P.: Immunogenicity of intracellular particles and cell walls from *Mycobacterium tuberculosis*. J. Bacteriol. *80*:607, 1960.

30. Larson, C. L., Ribi, E., Wicht, W. C., List, R. H., and Goode, G.: Resistance to tuberculosis in mice immunized with BCG disrupted in oil. Nature *198*:1214, 1963.

31. Leake, E. S., Gonzalez-Ojeda, D., and Myrvik, Q. N.: Enzymatic differences between normal alveolar macrophages and oil-induced peritoneal macrophages obtained from rabbits. Exp. Cell Res. *33*:553, 1964.

32. Lefford, M. J.: The induction and expression of immunity after BCG immunization. Infect. Immun. *18*:646, 1977.

33. Lurie, M. B.: Resistance to Tuberculosis: Experimental Studies in Native and Acquired Defensive Mechanisms. Cambridge, Mass., Harvard University Press, 1964.

34. Millman, I.: Nonspecific resistance to tuberculosis. Am. Rev. Respir. Dis. *83*:668, 1961.

35. Millman, I., and Youmans, G. P.: The characterization of the terminal respiratory enzymes of the H37Ra strain of *Mycobacterium tuberculosis* var. *hominis*. J. Bacteriol. *69*:320, 1955.

36. Millman, I., and Youmans, G. P.: Studies on the metabolism of *Mycobacterium tuberculosis*. VII. Terminal respiratory activity of an avirulent strain of *Mycobacterium tuberculosis*. J. Bacteriol. *68*:411, 1954.

37. Ribi, E., Anacker, R. L., Brehmer, W., Goode, G., Larson, C. L., List, R. H., Milner, K. C., and Wicht, W. C.: Factors influencing protection against experimental tuberculosis in mice by heat-stable cell wall vaccines. J. Bacteriol. *92*:869, 1966.

38. Ribi, E., Brehmer, W., and Milner, K.: Specificity of resistance to tuberculosis and to salmonellosis stimulated in mice by oil-treated cell walls. Proc. Soc. Exp. Biol. Med. *124*:408, 1967.

39. Ribi, E., and Larson, C.: Immunological properties of cell wall versus protoplasm from mycobacteria. Zentralbl. Bakteriol. Abt. I Referate *194*:673, 1964.

40. Ribi, E., Larson, C. L., List, R., and Wicht, W.: Immunologic significance of cell wall of mycobacteria. Proc. Soc. Exp. Biol. Med. *98*:263, 1958.

41. Ribi, E., Larson, C., Wicht, W., List, R., and Goode, G.: Effective nonliving vaccine against experimental tuberculosis in mice. J. Bacteriol. *91*:975, 1966.

42. Ribi, E., Larson, C. L., Wicht, W., List, R., and Goode, G.: Resistance to experimental tuberculosis stimulated by fractions from attenuated tubercle bacilli. Proc. Soc. Exp. Biol. Med. *118*:926, 1965.

43. Robson, J. M., and Smith, J. T.: Immunizing effects of a lipopolysaccharide in mice. Am. Rev. Respir. Dis. *84*:100, 1961.

44. Rosenthal, S. R.: BCG Vaccination against Tuberculosis. Boston, Little, Brown and Company, 1957.

45. Salton, M. R. J., and Horne, R. W.: Studies on the bacterial cell wall. II. Methods of preparation and some properties of cell walls. Biochim. Biophys. Acta *7*:177, 1951.

46. Smith, D. W., Fregnan, G. B., DeLaquerrière-Richardson, L., and Valdivia, E.: Induction of acquired resistance in guinea pigs with defatted *Mycobacterium tuberculosis* vaccines. J. Bacteriol. *88*:87, 1964.

47. Smith, D. W., Grover, A. A., and Wiegeshaus, E.: Nonliving immunogenic substances of mycobacteria. Adv. Tuberc. Res. *16*:191, 1968.

48. Suter, E., and White, R. G.: The response of the reticulo-endothelial system to the injection of the "purified wax" and the lipopolysaccharide of tubercle bacilli. Am. Rev. Tuberc. *70*:793, 1954.

49. Youmans, G. P., Millman, I., and Youmans, A. S.: The immunizing activity against tuberculous infection in mice of enzymatically active particles isolated from extracts of *Mycobacterium tuberculosis*. J. Bacteriol. *70*:557, 1955.

50. Youmans, G. P., and Youmans, A. S.: An acute pulmonary granulomatous response in mice produced by mycobacterial cells and its relation to increased resistance and increased susceptibility to experimental tuberculous infection. J. Infect. Dis. *114*:135, 1964.

51. Youmans, G. P., and Youmans, A. S.: Nonspecific factors in resistance of mice to experimental tuberculosis. J. Bacteriol. *90*:1675, 1965.

52. Youmans, G. P., and Youmans, A. S.: Unpublished data.

12

Nature of the *Specific* Acquired Immune Response in Tuberculosis

INTRODUCTION

In Chapters 8, 9, and 10, we have described how a variety of constituents of the tubercle bacillus will induce increased resistance to tuberculous infection when injected into experimental animals. First, there are those substances, derived from mycobacterial cell walls, that are relatively stable. They owe their capacity to induce increased resistance to tuber-

culous infection to the activation of macrophages and/or to the induction of a significant granulomatous response. We have seen that the immunity produced by the injection of these substances is of relatively low grade, only comparable to that produced by heat-killed mycobacterial cells. The immunity is relatively nonspecific because the macrophages of animals in which macrophage activation or a granulomatous response has been induced will

285

also cope with heterologous micro-organisms.

On the other hand, we have seen that viable mycobacterial cells will induce a much greater degree of specific immunity to tuberculous infection. Also, the immunity-inducing capacity of viable cells apparently is due to the presence in these cells of a very labile constituent. This labile constituent we have identified as being present in mycobacterial ribosomal or RNA preparations (see Chapter 9).

These facts — that a number of substances in the tubercle bacillus will induce increased resistance to tuberculosis and that the immune response varies both in nature and degree, depending upon the nature of the immunity-inducing substance of the tubercle bacillus — have led us to formulate a multiple response theory of immunity to tuberculosis.[66]

Although the nature of the immune response to mycobacterial cell wall constituents has been shown to be due to macrophage activation and the granulomatous response, the nature of the immune response to viable mycobacterial cells, and in particular to the labile immunizing RNA preparations, has not been fully elucidated. We have pointed out in Chapter 10 that the immune response to myco-bacterial RNA may possibly depend upon the replication of the mycobacterial RNA in vivo. This, of course, leaves unclear the cellular or molecular basis of the immune response to either viable cells or mycobacterial RNA preparations.

IMMUNITY TO FACULTATIVE INTRACELLULAR PARASITES

It has been recognized for some time that immunity to infection by facultative intracellular parasites is not mediated by an antibody. In the case of tuberculosis, the lack of any role for antibody is supported by the fact that in either the natural or experimental disease, there is no relationship between amount of antibody formed and immunity to tuberculosis.[53, 55] Also, experimentally, investigators have been unable to transfer immunity from immunized animals to nonimmunized animals by injecting serum that contains antibodies to constituents of the tubercle bacillus.[53, 67] Furthermore, it has now been shown that immunity to tuberculous infection can be transferred to nonimmune animals by using either peritoneal exudate cells or thoracic duct lymphoid cells.[35, 45, 56, 62, 63]

At this point, we should emphasize that the phenomenon of cellular immunity to infection is not limited to the control of tuberculous infection. There are many intracellular parasites, including not only bacteria but also protozoa, fungi, and viruses. While the basic mechanism involved in cellular immunity to infection may be the same against many facultative intracellular parasites, differences must exist, if for no other reason than to account for the specificity of the immunity produced. Also, some facultative intracellular parasites, such as pasteurella, brucella, and even *Listeria monocytogenes,* apparently require antibody (opsonin) in order to gain their intracellular position. Also, certain obligate intracellular parasites, such as rickettsiae, may require an antibody that neutralizes certain toxic substances before the parasites can be killed and digested by macrophages.[18, 65] A great deal of our information on host response to facultative intracellular parasites has been gained using bacteria other than *Mycobacterium tuberculosis.* For example, *Listeria monocytogenes* has been used to derive much of our current knowledge about the ability of an animal to mount an immune response to facultative intracellular parasites.[3, 4, 12, 26, 27, 33, 40-44] The validity of transferring such information to the tuberculosis system, however, has not been clearly documented.

THE INHIBITION OF MICROBIAL MULTIPLICATION WITHIN MACROPHAGES

In any event, it is essential that we now review the evidence, in more or less chronologic order, that has led to the recognition of the T-lymphocyte as the affector and the macrophage as the effector cell in immunity to tuberculosis.

Probably the first direct demonstration that cells were involved in immunity to tuberculosis was provided by Lurie in 1942.[36, 37] Using irritating substances, Lurie induced inflammatory peritoneal exudates in both normal and immunized rabbits. The peritoneal cells (approximately 75 percent mononuclear in type) were removed from the peritoneal cavities of the rabbits and then washed and mixed with virulent human-type tubercle bacilli. Phagocytosis of the tubercle bacilli was allowed to take place for one hour, after which the extracellular bacilli were removed. Normal or immune serum was then added to alliquots of the infected cell suspensions. These infected cell-serum mixtures were then injected into the anterior chamber of one eye of separate rabbits and allowed to incubate there for 10 to 14 days. At the end of this period, the number of tubercle bacilli in the eye of each rabbit was determined by removing the fluid and the iris and making direct counts microscopically. The number of mycobacteria found in the fluid and iris of those animals implanted with immune cells was *usually* lower than the number of tubercle bacilli found in the fluid and iris of rabbits that had been implanted with infected-normal cells (not from immunized animals). The ability of the bacilli to inhibit intracellular proliferation also seemed to be uniquely a property of the phagocytic cell present, since immune serum plus immune cells yielded results similar to those obtained with immune

cells mixed with normal serum. However, due to the use of too few animals and the variability of the data, the validity of Lurie's conclusions is questionable.

In 1952 and 1953,[59-61] Suter published data obtained by using tissue culture techniques, that enabled him to quantitate the in vitro multiplication of tubercle bacilli within peritoneal macrophages obtained from normal guinea pigs. Peritoneal exudate cells were suspended with tubercle bacilli and then allowed to adhere to coverslips. At the time of infection and after one, three, five, and seven days of incubation, coverslips were removed. The cells were fixed and stained, and the number of tubercle bacilli present within each of 100 infected cells was determined microscopically. Suter[59] utilized this technique to compare the multiplication of tubercle bacilli within macrophages obtained from BCG-immunized guinea pigs and rabbits with the multiplication of tubercle bacilli within cells obtained from normal rabbits and guinea pigs. The results of these experiments supported the previous observations (1942) of Lurie. Intracellular multiplication of tubercle bacilli was retarded or completely inhibited within the macrophages from animals immunized with BCG, as compared to the proliferation of tubercle bacilli within normal macrophages. The presence of immune or normal serum had no effect on the multiplication of tubercle bacilli within normal or immune macrophages. Suter also observed inhibition of growth of mycobacterial strains R1Rv, BCG-Phipps, BCG Tice, and Valle within macrophages from immunized animals.

In 1955, Raffel[53] reported on the multiplication of BCG within murine macrophages in vitro. Raffel employed Suter's tissue culture technique and concluded from the results that peritoneal macrophages from BCG-immunized mice inhibited the intracellular multiplication of BCG, when compared to the intracellular growth of BCG in normal mouse macrophages. Raffel[53] also reported results on infected-normal and BCG-immune macrophages placed in semipermeable chambers and implanted in the peritoneal cavities of normal and BCG-immune guinea pigs. Under these conditions, he observed no difference in the rate of intracellular bacillary multiplication between normal and BCG-immune macrophages.

Further support of Suter's observations was published by Berthrong and Hamilton in 1958 and 1959.[1, 2] Multiplication of virulent tubercle bacilli was inhibited within macrophages obtained from BCG-immunized guinea pigs and maintained in vitro. In contrast to these results, Mackaness[39] in 1954 observed no significant difference in the rate of multiplication of virulent tubercle bacilli within peritoneal macrophages from normal and immune rabbits in vitro.

Berthrong and Hamilton[1, 2] noted that BCG cells did not multiply within normal guinea pig exudate cells when 5 μg/ml of streptomycin was present in the medium. In the absence of the antibiotic, there was a slight suggestion of growth, which they attributed to phagocytosis of extracellular organisms. The human strain, H37Rv, did multiply in normal cells in the presence of streptomycin. Upon comparison of the growth of H37Rv cells in normal and BCG-immunized macrophages with streptomycin in the medium, they observed that the bacilli multiplied to approximately the same extent within both cell types but that cord formation was absent in "immune" cells; therefore, they concluded that "immune" macrophages had a greater ability to resist the intracellular proliferation of H37Rv cells than did normal cells.

BCG vaccination of natively susceptible rabbits by Hsu in 1965[24, 25] conferred upon the peritoneal macrophages of these animals the ability to restrain intracellular multiplication of the H37Rv strain. Hsu used strepto-

mycin to inhibit extracellular growth of the tubercle bacilli. Hsu also found that immune serum conferred on the natively susceptible macrophages the ability to resist degeneration caused by infection but did not alter the multiplication of the intracellular virulent bacilli.

Kochan and Smith in 1965[31] found that BCG cells multiplied in monocytes from normal and BCG-immunized guinea pigs, in the absence of streptomycin. When human serum possessing a tuberculostatic factor was added to BCG-infected "immune" cells, the intracellular BCG multiplication was inhibited; however, this human serum did not affect the growth of BCG cells in normal monocytes. It is interesting to note that human serum (transferrin?) alone inhibited the growth of BCG cells, even in the absence of the "immune" macrophages.

Fong and colleagues in 1956[14] and 1957[15] demonstrated that immune serum protected H37Rv-infected, normal rabbit peritoneal macrophages from degeneration for 48 hours in vitro, but by 72 hours, the amount of cellular degeneration was the same as that observed with normal cells in the presence of normal serum. In contrast, when peritoneal cells from immunized animals were cultured in the presence of immune serum, infection with H37Rv cells caused little or no cellular degeneration during 72 hours. Unfortunately, the number of intracellular mycobacteria was not counted.

THE ROLE OF STREPTOMYCIN IN THE INTRACELLULAR INHIBITION OF MICROBIAL GROWTH

In all the cases just mentioned in which it was found that inhibition of intracellular tubercle bacilli by cells from immunized animals occurred, streptomycin was incorporated in the medium to suppress extracellular bacillary multiplication. It is imperative to notice that in the two instances in which intracellular growth was reported within "immune" cells, streptomycin was not used in the culture medium.[31, 39]

Mackaness[38] and Suter[61] have stated that to completely inhibit intracellular proliferation of virulent tubercle bacilli within normal macrophages, 80 to 100 μg/ml of streptomycin was necessary. Suter[59] also stated that 5 μg/ml of the antibiotic had no effect on the intracellular multiplication of BCG cells within normal macrophages. However, the effect of streptomycin on the growth of virulent mycobacteria within "immune" macrophages was not investigated.

Shepard[57] found that HeLa cells infected with H37Rv cells could be used to assess the action of antimycobacterial agents. He employed two protocols of drug exposure — an early schedule, in which the test material was present during phagocytosis and throughout the experiment, and a delayed schedule, in which the test material was not added until sometime after phagocytosis. He observed that 4 to 16 μg/ml of streptomycin was the minimal inhibitory concentration for the early schedule and more than 2000 μg/ml was necessary for complete bacterial growth inhibition when the delayed schedule was followed. Thus, Shepard concluded that the intracellular location of the bacilli protected them from the deleterious effects of streptomycin. Kornegay and co-workers[32] explained the limited value of streptomycin in the therapy of infections caused by brucella by the apparent failure of the antibiotic to penetrate tissue in therapeutic quantities. In contrast, it must be noted that streptomycin is extremely effective as a chemotherapeutic agent for the treatment of tuberculosis in man and animals. If it is unable to penetrate the cells in which the bacilli are residing, how, then, can it be so effective?

Recently, investigations by Chang[9] and by Bonventre and Imhoff[5] have unequivocally established that streptomycin enters macrophages maintained in cell culture. Chang[9] infected peritoneal macrophages with *Mycobacterium lepraemurium* and followed the mycobacterial multiplication with various concentrations of streptomycin in the medium. As little as 0.05 μg/ml of the antibiotic caused a reduction in the number of intracellular bacilli compared to cultures not treated with streptomycin. Since *M. lepraemurium* is an obligate intracellular parasite and cannot grow in the culture medium, the influence of extracellular proliferation and rephagocytosis was ruled out. The effect of the antibiotic on the bacteria was dose-dependent. Bonventre and Imhoff[5] followed the uptake of tritiated dihydrostreptomycin into mouse peritoneal macrophages. They observed that the uptake of the antibiotic was delayed 2 to 4 hours, but a linear increase followed for several days until a plateau was reached. No uptake was observed at 4° C. Other investigators, Morello and Baker (1965),[46] Freeman and Vana (1958),[16] and Gerber and Watkins (1961),[20] have reported that macrophages are permeable to streptomycin; this indicates that the streptomycin can restrict intracellular microbial multiplication.

The literature reveals certain contradictions in regard to the multiplication of virulent tubercle bacilli within macrophages from immunized and nonimmunized animals. Two groups of investigators who did not use streptomycin in the medium found no difference between the ability of macrophages from immunized animals and macrophages from nonimmunized animals to inhibit the multiplication of tubercle bacilli. Therefore, in the late 1960s, Patterson and Youmans reinvestigated the effect of streptomycin on the multiplication of tubercle bacilli within macrophages. In 1970, Patterson and Youmans[51, 52] published data that clearly showed that in the absence of streptomycin in the medium, macrophages from immunized animals were no more effective than macrophages obtained from nonimmunized animals for the intracellular inhibition of multiplication of virulent tubercle bacilli (see Fig. 12–1).

These studies of Patterson and Youmans were conducted using peritoneal macrophages from both normal and immunized mice. The mice were immunized with 1.0 mg of viable cells of the attenuated H37Ra strain of *M. tuberculosis*. Approximately four weeks after immunization, the mice were sacrificed and peritoneal macrophages were obtained. These macrophages, after washing, were established in tissue culture on coverslips. The monolayers of macrophages were then infected by adding suspensions of cells of the virulent H37Rv strain of *M. tuberculosis* and sufficient time for phagocytosis of the mycobacterial cells was allowed. Macrophages were obtained from the peritoneal cavities of companion, nonimmunized mice at the same time. These were also established in tissue culture as monolayers and infected with tubercle bacilli. A number of such infected tissue cultures were established, and to one set

of immunized macrophages and one set of normal macrophages, streptomycin in a concentration of 5.0 μg/ml was added.

The rate of multiplication of the tubercle bacilli within macrophages was determined by withdrawing coverslips at suitable times (usually 3, 6, and 9 days after infection), staining these by modification of the Ziehl-Neelson technique, and counting the actual number of tubercle bacilli at each time within a hundred infected macrophages. With such data, graphs could be made showing the actual rate of multiplication intracellularly of virulent tubercle bacilli within macrophages kept under a variety of conditions. Figure 12–1 shows the results of one such early experiment. From Figure 12–1 it is clear that without streptomycin in the medium, the tubercle bacilli grew as rapidly within the macrophages obtained from immunized animals as they did within the macrophages obtained from nonimmunized animals. However, when streptomycin was included in the medium, there was appreciable inhibition of multiplication, particularly after five days of incubation. Noteworthy is the fact that in the presence of streptomycin,

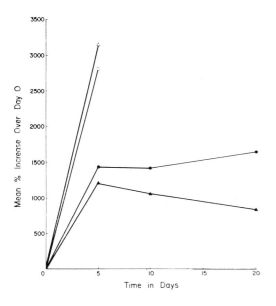

FIGURE 12–1. Mean percentage increase of virulent H37Rv cells within normal and "immune" macrophages cultured with and without streptomycin. Normal macrophages with streptomycin (●), without streptomycin (○). "Immune" macrophages with streptomycin (▲), without streptomycin (△). (From Patterson, R. J., and Youmans, G. P.: Multiplication of *Mycobacterium tuberculosis* within normal and "immune" mouse macrophages cultivated with and without streptomycin. Infect. Immun. *1*:30, 1970).

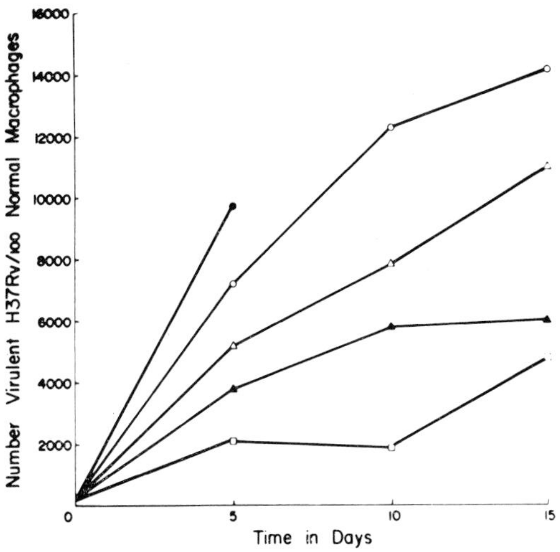

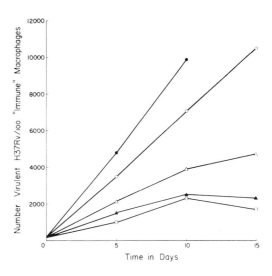

FIGURE 12–2. Effect of various concentrations of streptomycin on the intracellular proliferation of virulent H37Rv cells within normal macrophages. Units of streptomycin per ml: 0 (●), 1.25 (O), 2.5 (△), 5.0 (▲), 10.0 (□). (From Patterson, R. J., and Youmans, G. P.: Multiplication of *Mycobacterium tuberculosis* within normal and "immune" mouse macrophages cultivated with and without streptomycin. Infect. Immun. *1*:30, 1970.)

there was greater inhibition of multiplication of the tubercle bacilli within the macrophages from immunized animals than within the macrophages from normal animals.

These experiments were repeated with both normal macrophages and macrophages from immunized animals, but using several different concentrations of streptomycin. These results are shown in Figures 12–2 and 12–3. Once again, there was marked inhibition of growth in the macrophages that were kept in the medium with streptomycin, and particularly important, the inhibition of growth was directly proportional to the concentration of streptomycin in the medium. This showed beyond all doubt that it was the streptomycin that was inhibiting the growth of the tubercle bacilli within the macrophages. Once again, there was somewhat greater inhibition of growth by the streptomycin within the cells from immunized animals.

In all of the experiments in which macrophages from immunized animals have been placed in tissue culture and maintained in the presence of strepto-

FIGURE 12–3. Effect of various concentrations of streptomycin on the intracellular proliferation of virulent H37Rv cells within "immune" macrophages. Units of streptomycin per ml: 0 (●), 1.25 (O), 2.5 (△), 5.0 (▲), 10.0 (□). (From Patterson, R. J., and Youmans, G. P.: Multiplication of *Mycobacterium tuberculosis* within normal and "immune" mouse macrophages cultivated with and without streptomycin. Infect. Immun. *1*:30, 1970.)

mycin after being infected with tubercle bacilli, we have noted that the inhibition of intracellular growth of tubercle bacilli by the streptomycin in the medium was greater and occurred more rapidly in the macrophages from immunized animals. The explanation of this increased bacteriostasis within macrophages from immunized animals probably lies in the fact that macrophages obtained from animals immunized with viable mycobacterial cells are somewhat more activated than macrophages obtained from nonimmunized animals. By virtue of this activation, they are somewhat more phagocytic; they are more motile and metabolically more active; and they undoubtedly turn over membrane faster than do macrophages from nonimmunized animals. If the pinocytosis rate is greater in macrophages from immunized animals, we would expect these cells to take up the streptomycin in the medium more rapidly than would macrophages from nonimmunized animals. This, in turn, would result in a more rapid increase in the internal concentration of streptomycin and, therefore, an earlier and greater inhibition of growth of the susceptible tubercle bacilli.

Particular care was taken in these experiments to eliminate the possibility that the increase in numbers of tubercle bacilli noted within macrophages was a consequence of intracellular multiplication and not of extracellular multiplication with continued phagocytosis by the macrophages of the extracellular mycobacterial cells. This would be a particular risk in those experiments in which streptomycin was omitted from the medium because the growth inhibition effect of streptomycin on extracellular growth would not be noted. To circumvent this possibility, the cultures were washed frequently to remove extracellular bacteria and, at the time of removal of the supernatant fluids, actual counts were made of the number of tubercle bacilli in the extracellular fluid. This voluminous data will not be given here, but it showed that the increase in numbers of tubercle bacilli within macrophages in tissue culture without streptomycin could not be ascribed to extracellular growth and phagocytosis. In subsequent studies by Klun and colleagues[28] and by Klun and Youmans,[29, 30] the possibility that extracellular multiplication of tubercle bacilli might play an important role in these results was completely eliminated by using tissue culture medium in which tubercle bacilli would not multiply. This was accomplished by using batches of horse serum (40 percent horse serum was used in the tissue culture medium) that were inhibitory to the growth of tubercle bacilli probably because of inactivation of iron by transferrin (see Chapter 2). Identical results to those published by Patterson and Youmans were obtained under these conditions. In addition, other investigators have shown that streptomycin in the tissue culture medium will inhibit the growth of intracellular mycobacteria. Also, as we have already pointed out, a number of workers have found that streptomycin does penetrate within cells in concentrations sufficient to inhibit the growth of susceptible bacteria.[5, 16, 20, 46]

FATE OF TUBERCLE BACILLI WITHIN MACROPHAGES

In the experiments of Patterson and Youmans, the number of macrophages on the coverslips in the tissue cultures also were counted each time they were removed after infection. Infected macrophage tissue culture cells will die eventually from the infection with virulent tubercle bacilli; it is of particular interest that the rate of death is exponential. Actual counts of macrophages on the coverslips of both infected and noninfected tissue cultures are shown in Figure 12–4. It will be noted that

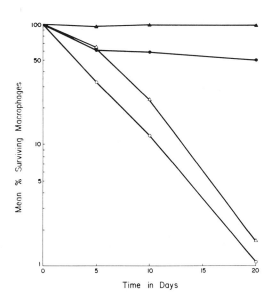

FIGURE 12–4. Mean percentage of surviving normal and "immune" macrophages cultured with and without streptomycin after in vitro infection with virulent H37Rv cells. Normal macrophages with streptomycin (●), without streptomycin (○). "Immune" macrophages with streptomycin (▲), without streptomycin (△). (From Patterson, R. J., and Youmans, G. P.: Multiplication of *Mycobacterium tuberculosis* within normal and "immune" mouse macrophages cultivated with and without streptomycin. Infect. Immun. 1:30, 1970.)

the decrease in number of viable macrophages due to the infection is exponential in character. This would be expected since the growth of the intracellular bacteria is itself exponential. However, of more than passing interest is the fact that the rate of increase in the number of tubercle bacilli within macrophages in such cultures can therefore be measured by determining the rate of decrease in number of surviving macrophages, provided that one wished to use this less direct enumeration procedure for determining the effect of agents on the intracellular growth of tubercle bacilli within macrophages.

Another finding of interest was that although the tubercle bacilli grew just as rapidly within macrophages from immunized animals as within macrophages from nonimmunized animals, they reached greater total numbers in the macrophages from immunized animals. In other words, although the macrophages from immunized animals had no more capacity to inhibit the multiplication of the tubercle bacilli, these macrophages did resist destruction by the tubercle bacilli to a greater extent than macrophages from nonim-

munized animals. This phenomenon of greater resistance of macrophages from immunized animals to physical agents has been noted before. Patnode and Hudgins,[50] for example, showed that macrophages from guinea pigs immunized with BCG were more resistant to destruction by sonic vibration than macrophages from nonimmunized guinea pigs.

These experiments and subsequent ones by Klun and colleagues,[28] by Klun and Youmans,[29, 30] and by Cahall and Youmans[6-8] have clearly shown that the prevailing concept of approximately the past 30 years — that immunity in tuberculosis is due to the "immune macrophage" — is incorrect. Furthermore, the accumulated evidence that pointed to the "immune macrophage" as the cell responsible for immunity to tuberculosis was derived under conditions where the intracellular inhibition of mycobacterial growth was due to the streptomycin in the medium. Thus, the whole concept of the "immune macrophage" arose because of an artifact introduced into the experimental conditions by the use of streptomycin in the tissue culture medium.

THE ROLE OF LYMPHOCYTES IN CELLULAR IMMUNITY TO INFECTION

Having ruled out the "immune macrophage" as the primary cell involved in immunity to tuberculosis, Patterson and Youmans were left with the problem of how to account for the fact that the multiplication of virulent tubercle bacilli is inhibited in the tissues of immunized animals. In tissues, the majority of the tubercle bacilli reside within macrophages, so the inhibition of multiplication that does occur—and that has been documented repeatedly—obviously had to involve some other type of cell or factor. In view of the considerable evidence indicating that lymphocytes might play some role in cellular immunity in general, and perhaps cellular immunity to infection in particular, Patterson and Youmans[51] investigated the effect of adding lymphocytes from normal and vaccinated mice to macrophage tissue cultures that had been infected with tubercle bacilli. For most of these studies, macrophages were taken from nonimmunized mice, placed in tissue culture, and infected with virulent

tubercle bacilli. Initially, whole spleen cells, predominantly lymphocytes, were added to the infected tissue culture system. When this was done, marked intracellular inhibition of the growth of the tubercle bacilli was noted. This is shown graphically in Figure 12–5. It is noteworthy that immune macrophages were not needed to show this effect; the only cells needed were lymphocytes from immunized animals and macrophages from nonimmunized animals infected with tubercle bacilli.

Next, after it had been shown that lymphocytes from immunized animals apparently were the affector cells, Patterson and Youmans[51] set up spleen cell tissue cultures and stimulated them with whole viable cells of tubercle bacilli. After stimulation, the spleen cells were centrifuged out and the tubercle bacilli removed by filtration. These supernatant fluids then were added to cultures of normal macrophages infected with tubercle bacilli. Once again, the intracellular growth of the tubercle bacilli was markedly inhibited. Needless to say, these experiments were all conducted under conditions in which streptomycin was not added to the macrophage tissue culture system. Thus, it appeared that

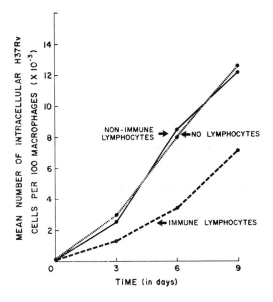

FIGURE 12–5. Growth of *M. tuberculosis* (H37Rv) within normal macrophages exposed to splenic lymphocytes from immunized and nonimmunized mice. (From Patterson, R. J., and Youmans, G. P.: Demonstration in tissue culture of lymphocyte-mediated immunity to tuberculosis. Infect. Immun. *1*:600, 1970.)

not only were lymphocytes the affector cells in this intracellular inhibition of multiplication of tubercle bacilli but also they produced an extracellular substance that when added to the infected macrophage tissue culture system would bring about, in one way or another, the intracellular inhibition of mycobacterial multiplication. In other words, immunity to tuberculosis, as demonstrated by this tissue culture system, apparently was lymphokine-mediated.

In the course of their studies, Patterson and Youmans made another very important observation.[51, 52] Mice were immunized with heat-killed, attenuated H37Ra cells and with the mycobacterial RNA preparations previously discussed in Chapter 9. Four weeks after immunization, spleens were removed from these animals and the lymphocytes collected, as before. These lymphocytes were added to tissue cultures of macrophages that had been infected with virulent tubercle bacilli. As a control for this experiment, lymphocytes that had come from mice immunized with viable, whole H37Ra cells were also used. The rate of multiplication of the tubercle bacilli within these macrophages was then measured by counting the number of tubercle bacilli within the cells. The infected macrophage tissue culture cells to which the lymphocytes from the viable H37Ra immunized mice had been added showed the marked inhibition of growth of the intracellular tubercle bacilli previously noted. However, the infected tissue cultures to which lymphocytes from the mice immunized with heat-killed cells had been added showed no inhibition of multiplication of the intracellular tubercle bacilli. On the other hand, when lymphocytes were taken from the animals immunized with the mycobacterial RNA preparations and were added to infected macrophage tissue cultures, there was a marked inhibition of the intracellular growth of the virulent tubercle bacilli. These findings strongly support the point

previously made in Chapter 8 that the nature of the immune response to killed and to living attenuated mycobacterial cells is very different. Furthermore, these findings support the hypothesis that the mycobacterial RNA contains the specific immunizing material of the tubercle bacilli. Similar findings subsequently were obtained by Klun and colleagues[28] and by Klun and Youmans.[29, 30] Furthermore, Klun and Youmans showed that exposure of lymphocytes from animals immunized with whole, viable H37Ra cells to tuberculin would induce formation of mycobacterial intracellular growth-inhibiting substance; whereas stimulation with PPD of lymphocytes from animals immunized with mycobacterial RNA did not result in the production of the mycobacterial growth-inhibiting substance. These results further emphasize the dichotomy between tuberculin hypersensitivity and immunity to tuberculosis (see Chapter 13).

THE RELATIONSHIP BETWEEN THE MYCOBACTERIAL GROWTH INHIBITORY FACTOR AND MIGRATION INHIBITORY FACTOR

Klun and coworkers[28] examined the relationship between mycobacterial growth inhibitory factor and mouse migration inhibitory factor in the supernatant fluids obtained from mouse lymphocyte cultures. These workers found that when lymphocyte supernatant fluids from immunized animals were simultaneously examined for the presence of migration inhibitory factor and mycobacterial growth inhibitory factor, both activities could not always be demonstrated. In some cases both activities were present, but the presence of migration inhibitory factor activity was not necessary for the demonstration of the inhibition of growth of intracellular tubercle bacilli. Therefore, since migration inhibitory factor could be found in certain of the lymphocyte supernatant fluids that did not inhibit the intracellular growth of tubercle bacilli and mycobacterial growth inhibitory factor was found in some lymphocyte supernatant fluids that did not inhibit the migration of macrophages, the results indicated that these two lymphokines were different. This further strengthens the dichotomy between delayed hypersensitivity and immunity to tuberculosis, since tuberculin hypersensitivity is thought to be mediated by migration inhibitory factor.[13]

THE EFFECT OF MYCOBACTERIAL GROWTH INHIBITORY FACTOR ON TUBERCLE BACILLI IN VITRO

Klun and coworkers[28] and Klun and Youmans[29, 30] also conducted experiments to determine whether mycobacterial growth inhibitory factor obtained from immunized lymphocytes would inhibit growth of virulent tubercle bacilli in vitro; that is, inhibit the growth of tubercle bacilli in a culture medium in the absence of macrophages. Although extensive experiments were conducted, no evidence that mycobacterial growth inhibitory factor would affect tubercle bacilli directly could be obtained. This, of course, suggested that the lymphokine that brought about the intracellular multiplication of tubercle bacilli acted by affecting some function of the macrophage.

NATURE OF THE MYCOBACTERIAL GROWTH INHIBITORY FACTOR

In 1975, Cahall and Youmans[6-8] reported on some of the conditions necessary for the production of mycobacterial growth inhibitory factor obtained from the spleen cells of immunized animals and on some of the physical and chemical properties of the agent.

When spleen cells from animals immunized with H37Ra viable cells were stimulated with H37Ra cells, 72 hours of incubation were required to produce spleen cell supernatant fluids that would cause intracellular inhibition of mycobacterial growth when added to infected macrophage cultures. Not even supernatant fluids from 48-hour mouse spleen cell cultures were able to induce intracellular inhibition of mycobacterial growth. Investigation of some of the culture conditions for production of mycobacterial growth inhibitory substance showed that at least 1.0 percent of human serum was required in the tissue culture medium for its production by spleen cells from immunized mice. The mycobacterial growth inhibitory factor was nondialyzable and was unaffected by freezing, lyophilization, or incubation at 60° C for 30 minutes. However, the factor was inactivated after incubation at 80° C for 30 minutes. The growth inhibitory activity was not affected by low hydrogen ion concentrations (pH of 7 to 12), but exposure to higher hydrogen ion concentrations (pH of 6 or 5) significantly decreased activity, and exposure to pH of 4 to 2 abolished all growth inhibitory activity. Some dilution of the factor, though was possible, since supernatant fluids diluted 1:32 were still able to produce significant intracellular inhibition of growth of virulent tubercle bacilli.

Exposure of mycobacterial growth inhibitory factor to trypsin, chymotrypsin, or neuraminidase appreciably decreased the ability to produce intracellular inhibition of mycobacterial growth within macrophages. This last finding suggested that mycobacterial growth inhibitory factor might be a glycoprotein. Mycobacterial growth inhibitory factor activity was unaffected by deoxyribonuclease or ribonuclease. Of particular interest was the finding that supernatant fluids from antigenically stimulated H37Ra mouse spleen cells exposed to puromycin were unable to produce significant intracellular inhibition. These results showed that for the production of the mycobacterial growth inhibitory substance, protein synthesis by lymphocytes is required.

The filtration of mycobacterial growth inhibitory factor containing supernatant fluids on Sephadex G-150 demonstrated that significant activity appeared only in those fractions that eluted on the downward side of the serum albumin peak. Based upon protein standards filtered through Sephadex gel, the molecular weight of mycobacterial growth inhibitory factor appeared to be between 20,000 and 35,000 daltons.

Further interesting and important findings by Cahall and Youmans[7] showed that partially purified eluates (from Sephadex G-150 columns) had no capacity to inhibit the migration of normal peritoneal exudate cells.

The experiments by Cahall and Youmans also showed that for inhibition of intracellular growth of virulent tubercle bacilli by the lymphocyte product, the infected macrophages had to be exposed to this material for at least three days. Less time than this did not result in intracellular inhibition of mycobacterial growth. Treatment of infected macrophages with trypsin before being exposed to the mycobacterial growth inhibitory factor abolished the ability of the lymphokine to inhibit intracellular multiplication of tubercle bacilli. Apparently, a protein receptor on the surface of the macrophages was removed by the trypsin treatment. Incubation of infected macrophages with goat antimouse globulin, before exposure to mycobacterial growth inhibitory factor, blocked the action of the lymphokine. Therefore, it appears that the surface receptor on the macrophage is some kind of an immunoglobulin.

The possibility that the mycobacterial growth inhibitory factor might be the mediator of the immune response against tuberculosis should be examined. There is little direct evidence on this point, but it is known that immunity in tuberculosis and immunity to other facultative intracellular parasites is mediated by T-lymphocytes. Therefore, it is not unreasonable to speculate that a lymphokine may be produced by T-lymphocytes, when stimulated with the proper antigen, that would either directly inhibit the growth of tubercle bacilli in macrophages or would indirectly bring about their growth inhibition by some action on the macrophages. If enough lymphokine could be produced from lymphocytes of immunized animals to use for testing its protective effect against tuberculous infection in nonimmunized animals, the direct evidence would be forthcoming. In this connection, Turcotte and coworkers[64] obtained a growth inhibitory factor from lymphocytes of immunized mice that also brought about the intracellular inhibition of growth of virulent tubercle bacilli within macrophages in tissue culture. These investigators, though, produced their inhibitory substance by disrupting the harvested spleen cells by repeated freezing and thawing. This frozen and thawed material was centrifuged to remove cellular debris, and the supernatant fluid, which they refer to as lymphocyte extract, was used for treatment of infected macrophages in tissue culture. They also found that this active agent was nondialyzable, that it was not affected by lyophilization, and that it was not inactivated by exposure to ribonuclease or deoxyribonuclease. However, heating at temperatures over 100° C completely eliminated all growth inhibitory activity. They reported that this lymphocyte extract did not inhibit the growth of BCG cells in culture. Mice infected with virulent tubercle bacilli were treated with rather small doses of their lymphocyte extract and a slightly statistically significant retardation of the disease process was noted. These findings, of course, support the possibility that products of immunized lymphocytes may mediate the intracellular inhibition of growth of virulent tubercle bacilli in immunized animals. Much more extensive experiments, however, need to be done in order to thoroughly establish this point.

From the previous paragraphs, it is clear that the prevailing concept that "immune macrophages" are the cells responsible for immunity to tuberculous infection is not tenable. The experiments conducted over a number of years that purportedly showed this were really describing the effect of streptomycin on the intracellular growth of the tubercle bacilli. We can assume, though, that T-lymphocytes from immunized animals probably are the cells that are primarily responsible for the mounting of the immune response to tuberculosis. The direct evidence for this comes from those experiments in which immunity to tuberculosis in experimental animals has been passively transferred using lymphocytes. This role of lymphocytes from immune animals, specifically T-lymphocytes, is further strengthened by the demonstration of their importance in immunity to disease due to other facultative intracellular parasites, such as leprosy,[21] histoplasmosis,[22, 23] disease due to *Listeria monocytogenes*,[26, 27, 58] toxoplasmosis,[17, 34] and infections with *M. microti* and *M. lepraemurium*.[21] It is supported also by the findings that the thymectomy,[10, 11, 47-49] or whole-body irradiation, or both, will markedly reduce resistance to tuberculous infection as well as to leprosy.[19, 54]

Whether the T-lymphocytes act through the agency of a lymphokine, such as the one we have just de-scribed, awaits confirmation from experiments involving treatment of tuberculous nonimmunized animals with lymphokine prepared from the lymphocytes of immunized animals. The experiments, though, of Turcotte and colleagues[64] are very suggestive in this regard. The role of mycobacterial RNA in the induction of a population of the immune T-cells also awaits further exploration.

REFERENCES

1. Berthrong, M., and Hamilton, M. A.: Tissue culture studies on resistance in tuberculosis. I. Normal guinea pig monocytes with tubercle bacilli of different virulence. Am. Rev. Tuberc. *77*:436, 1958.
2. Berthrong, M., and Hamilton, M. A.: Tissue culture studies on resistance in tuberculosis. II. Monocytes from normal and immunized guinea pigs infected with virulent human tubercle bacilli. Am. Rev. Tuberc. *79*:221, 1959.
3. Blanden, R. V.: T cell response to viral and bacterial infection. Transplant. Rev. *19*:56, 1974.
4. Blanden, R. V., and Langman, R. E.: Cell-mediated immunity to bacterial infection in the mouse. Thymus-derived cells as effectors of acquired resistance to *Listeria monocytogenes*. Scand. J. Immunol. *1*:379, 1972.
5. Bonventre, P. F., and Imhoff, J. G.: Uptake of ^{3}H-dihydrostreptomycin by macrophages in culture. Infect. Immun. *2*:89, 1970.
6. Cahall, D. L., and Youmans, G. P.: Conditions for production, and some characteristics, of mycobacterial growth inhibitory factor produced by spleen cells from mice immunized with viable cells of the attenuated H37Ra strain of *Mycobacterium tuberculosis*. Infect. Immun. *12*:833, 1975.
7. Cahall, D. L., and Youmans, G. P.: Macrophage migration inhibitory activity of mycobacterial growth inhibitory factor and the effect of a number of factors on mycobacterial growth inhibitory factor activity. Infect. Immun. *12*:851, 1975.
8. Cahall, D. L., and Youmans, G. P.: Molecular weight and other characteristics of mycobacterial growth inhibitory factor produced by spleen cells obtained from mice immunized with viable attenuated mycobacterial cells. Infect. Immun. *12*:841, 1975.
9. Chang, Y. T.: Suppressive activity of streptomycin on the growth of *Mycobacterium*

lepraemurium in macrophage cultures. Appl. Microbiol. *17*:750, 1969.

10. Collins, F. M., Congdon, C. C., and Morrison, N. E.: Growth of *Mycobacterium bovis* (BCG) in T lymphocyte-depleted mice. Infect. Immun. *11*:57, 1975.

11. Collins, F. M., and Mackaness, G. B.: The relationship of delayed hypersensitivity to acquired antituberculous immunity. 1. Tuberculin sensitivity and resistance to reinfection in BCG-vaccinated mice. Cell. Immunol. *1*:253, 1970.

12. Crum, E. D., and McGregor, D. D.: Functional properties of T and B cells isolated by affinity chromatography from rat thoracic duct lymph. Cell. Immunol. *23*:211, 1976.

13. David, J. R., and David, R. R.: Cellular hypersensitivity and immunity. Inhibition of macrophage migration and the lymphocyte mediators. Prog. Allergy *16*:300, 1972.

14. Fong, J., Schneider, P., and Elberg, S. S.: Studies on tubercle bacillus-monocyte relationship. I. Quantitative analysis of effect of serum of animals vaccinated with BCG upon bacterium-monocyte system. J. Exp. Med. *104*:455, 1956.

15. Fong, J., Schneider, P., and Elberg, S.: Studies on tubercle bacillus-monocyte relationship. II. Induction of monocyte degeneration by bacteria and culture filtrate: Specificity of serum and monocyte effects on resistance to degeneration. J. Exp. Med. *105*:25, 1957.

16. Freeman, B. A., and Vana, L. R.: Host-parasite relationships in Brucellosis. I. Infection of normal guinea pig macrophages in tissue culture. J. Infect. Dis. *102*:258, 1958.

17. Frenkel, J. K.: Adoptive immunity to intracellular infection. J. Immunol. *98*:1309, 1967.

18. Gambrill, M. R., and Wisseman, C. L., Jr.: Mechanisms of immunity in typhus infections. II. Multiplication of typhus rickettsiae in human macrophage cell cultures in the nonimmune system: Influence of virulence of rickettsial strains and of chloramphenicol. Infect. Immun. *8*:519, 1973.

19. Gaugas, J. M.: Enhancing effect of antilymphocytic globulin on human leprosy infection in thymectomized mice. Nature *220*:1246, 1968.

20. Gerber, D. F., and Watkins, H. M. S.: Growth of shigellae in monolayer tissue cultures. J. Bacteriol. *82*:815, 1961.

21. Godal, T., Rees, R. J. W., and Lamvik, J. O.: Lymphocyte-mediated modification of blood-derived macrophage function *in vitro*; inhibition of growth of intracellular mycobacteria with lymphokines. Clin. Exp. Immunol. *8*:625, 1971.

22. Howard, D. H., and Otto, V.: Experiments on lymphocyte-mediated cellular immunity in murine histoplasmosis. Infect. Immun. *16*:226, 1977.

23. Howard, D. H., Otto, V., and Gupta, R. K.: Lymphocyte-mediated cellular immunity in histoplasmosis. Infect. Immun. *4*:605, 1971.

24. Hsu, H. S.: *In vitro* studies on the interactions between macrophages of rabbits and tubercle bacilli. I. Cellular basis of native resistance. Am. Rev. Respir. Dis. *91*:488, 1965.

25. Hsu, H. S.: *In vitro* studies on the interactions between macrophages of rabbits and tubercle bacilli. II. Cellular and humoral aspects of acquired resistance. Am. Rev. Respir. Dis. *91*:499, 1965.

26. Jones, T., and Youmans, G. P.: The *in vitro* inhibition of growth of intracellular *Listeria monocytogenes* by lymphocyte products. Cell. Immunol. *9*:353, 1973.

27. Jones, T., and Youmans, G. P.: Nonspecific inhibition of growth of intracellular *Listeria monocytogenes* by lymphocyte culture products. Infect. Immun. *9*:472, 1974.

28. Klun, C. L., Neiburger, R. G., and Youmans, G. P.: Relationship between mouse mycobacterial growth-inhibitory factor and mouse migration-inhibitory factor in supernatant fluids from mouse lymphocyte cultures. J. Reticuloendothel. Soc. *13*:310, 1973.

29. Klun, C. L., and Youmans, G. P.: The effect of lymphocyte supernatant fluids on the intracellular growth of virulent tubercle bacilli. J. Reticuloendothel. Soc. *13*:263, 1973.

30. Klun, C. L., and Youmans, G. P.: The induction by *Listeria monocytogenes* and plant mitogens of lymphocyte supernatant fluids which inhibit the growth of *Mycobacterium tuberculosis* within macrophages *in vitro*. J. Reticuloendothel. Soc. *13*:275, 1973.

31. Kochan, I., and Smith, L.: Antimycobacterial activity of tuberculostatic factor on intracellular bacilli. J. Immunol. *94*:220, 1965.

32. Kornegay, G. B., Forgacs, J., and Henley, T. F.: Studies on streptomycin. II. Blood levels and urinary excretion in man and animals. J. Lab. Clin. Med. *31*:523, 1946.

33. Koster, F. T., and McGregor, D. D.: The mediator of cellular immunity. III. Lymphocyte traffic from the blood into the inflamed peritoneal cavity. J. Exp. Med. *133*:864, 1971.

34. Krahenbuhl, J. L., and Remington, J. S.: *In vitro* induction of nonspecific resistance in macrophages by specifically sensitized lymphocytes. Infect. Immun. *4*:337, 1971.

35. Lefford, M. J., McGregor, D. D., and Mack-

aness, G. B.: Immune response to *Myco-bacterium tuberculosis* in rats. Infect. Immun. *8*:182, 1973.

36. Lurie, M. B.: Resistance to Tuberculosis: Experimental Studies in Native and Acquired Defensive Mechanisms. Cambridge, Mass., Harvard University Press, 1964.

37. Lurie, M. B.: Studies on the mechanism of immunity in tuberculosis. The fate of tubercle bacilli ingested by mononuclear phagocytes derived from normal and immunized animals. J. Exp. Med. *75*:247, 1942.

38. Mackaness, G. B.: The action of drugs on intracellular tubercle bacilli. J. Pathol. Bacteriol. *64*:429, 1952.

39. Mackaness, G. B.: The growth of tubercle bacilli in monocytes from normal and vaccinated rabbits. Am. Rev. Tuberc. *69*:495, 1954.

40. McGregor, D. D., Koster, F. T., and Mackaness, G. B.: The mediator of cellular immunity. I. The life-span and circulation dynamics of the immunologically committed lymphocyte. J. Exp. Med. *133*:389, 1971.

41. McGregor, D. D., and Kostiala, A. A. I.: Role of lymphocytes in cellular resistance to infection. Contemp. Top. Immunobiol. *5*:237, 1976.

42. McGregor, D. D., and Logie, P. S.: The mediator of cellular immunity. VI. Effect of the antimitotic drug vinblastine on the mediator of cellular resistance to infection. J. Exp. Med. *137*:660, 1973.

43. McGregor, D. D., and Logie, P. S.: The mediator of cellular immunity. VII. Localization of sensitized lymphocytes in inflammatory exudates. J. Exp. Med. *139*:1415, 1974.

44. McGregor, D. D., and Logie, P. S.: The mediator of cellular immunity. VIII. Effect of mitomycin C on specifically sensitized lymphocytes. Cell. Immunol. *15*:69, 1975.

45. Millman, I.: Nonspecific resistance to tuberculosis. Am. Rev. Respir. Dis. *83*:668, 1961.

46. Morello, J. A., and Baker, E. E.: Interaction of salmonella with phagocytes *in vitro*. J. Infect. Dis. *115*:131, 1965.

47. Morrison, N. E., and Collins, F. M.: Restoration of T-cell responsiveness by thymosin: Development of antituberculous resistance in BCG-infected animals. Infect. Immun. *13*:554, 1976.

48. North, R. J.: Cell mediated immunity and the response to infection. *In* McCluskey, R. T., and Cohen, S. (eds.): Mechanisms of Cell-Mediated Immunity. New York, John Wiley & Sons, Inc., 1974.

49. North, R. J.: Importance of thymus-derived lymphocytes in cell-mediated immunity to infection. Cell. Immunol. *7*:166, 1973.

50. Patnode, R. A., and Hudgins, P. C.: Sonic fragility of leukocytes from guinea pigs vaccinated with BCG. Am. Rev. Tuberc. *79*:323, 1959.

51. Patterson, R. J., and Youmans, G. P.: Demonstration in tissue culture of lymphocyte-mediated immunity to tuberculosis. Infect. Immun. *1*:600, 1970.

52. Patterson, R. J., and Youmans, G. P.: Multiplication of *Mycobacterium tuberculosis* within normal and "immune" mouse macrophages cultivated with and without streptomycin. Infect. Immun. *1*:30, 1970.

53. Raffel, S.: The mechanism involved in acquired immunity to tuberculosis. *In* Wolstenholme, G. E. W., Cameron, M. P., and O'Connor, C. M. (eds.): Experimental Tuberculosis. Boston, Little, Brown and Company, 1955.

54. Rees, R. J. W.: Enhanced susceptibility of thymectomized and irradiated mice to infection with *Mycobacterium leprae*. Nature *211*:657, 1966.

55. Rich, A. R.: The Pathogenesis of Tuberculosis. 2nd ed. Springfield, Ill., Charles C Thomas, 1951.

56. Sever, J. L.: Passive transfer of resistance to tuberculosis through use of monocytes. Proc. Soc. Exp. Biol. Med. *103*:326, 1960.

57. Shepard, C. C.: Use of HeLa cells infected with tubercle bacilli for the study of antituberculous drugs. J. Bacteriol. *73*:494, 1957.

58. Simon, H. B., and Sheagren, J. N.: Cellular immunity *in vitro*. I. Immunologically mediated enhancement of macrophage bactericidal capacity. J. Exp. Med. *133*:1377, 1971.

59. Suter, E.: Multiplication of tubercle bacilli within mononuclear phagocytes in tissue cultures derived from normal animals and animals vaccinated with BCG. J. Exp. Med. *97*:235, 1953.

60. Suter, E.: The multiplication of tubercle bacilli within normal phagocytes in tissue culture. J. Exp. Med. *96*:137, 1952.

61. Suter, E.: Multiplication of tubercle bacilli within phagocytes cultivated *in vitro*, and the effect of streptomycin and isonicotinic acid hydrazide. Am. Rev. Tuberc. *65*:775, 1952.

62. Suter, E.: Passive transfer of acquired resistance to infection with *Mycobacterium tuberculosis* by means of cells. Am. Rev. Respir. Dis. *83*:535, 1961.

63. Suter, E., and Ramseier, H.: Cellular reactions in infection. Adv. Immunol. *4*:117, 1964.

64. Turcotte, R., Des Ormeaux, Y., and Borduas, A. G.: Partial characterization of a factor extracted from sensitized lymphocytes that inhibits the growth of *Mycobacterium tuberculosis* within macrophages *in vitro*. Infect. Immun. *14*:337, 1976.

65. Wisseman, C. L., Jr., Waddell, A. D., and Walsh, W. T.: Mechanisms of immunity in typhus infections. IV. Failure of chicken embryo cells in culture to restrict growth of antibody-sensitized *Rickettsia prowazeki*. Infect. Immun. *9*:571, 1974.

66. Youmans, G. P., and Youmans, A. S.: Nonspecific factors in resistance of mice to experimental tuberculosis. J. Bacteriol. *90*: 1675, 1965.

67. Youmans, G. P., and Youmans, A. S.: Unpublished results.

13

Relationship Between Delayed Hypersensitivity and Immunity in Tuberculosis

INTRODUCTION

A discussion of the relationship between delayed-type hypersensitivity and acquired immunity in tuberculosis becomes primarily a consideration of the relationship of tuberculin hypersensitivity to acquired immunity in tuberculosis. This follows because tuberculoprotein, to the best of our knowledge, is the major constituent of

the tubercle bacillus to which human beings and lower animals become sensitive after infection with virulent tubercle bacilli or after vaccination with attenuated mycobacterial cells.

The question of the relation of tuberculin hypersensitivity to immunity in tuberculosis has been a controversial one almost since Koch's original observations nearly 100 years ago on tuberculin hypersensitivity.[47, 48] More

302

precisely, the controversy has centered around whether the inflammatory reaction of tuberculin hypersensitivity is responsible for the increased resistance noted in animals either infected with tubercle bacilli or made sensitive by the injection of viable attenuated mycobacterial cells. Somewhat different viewpoints on the relationship of delayed hypersensitivity and immunity in tuberculosis will be found in three recent review articles.[49, 71, 89] The possibility that tuberculin hypersensitivity might mediate increased resistance to tuberculosis probably stems primarily from the findings of Romer[69] and Hamburger.[37] These investigators noted that the intensity of the allergic reaction was dependent on the amount of antigen administered. For example, small numbers of tubercle bacilli administered to tuberculous animals cause only slight inflammatory reactions, whereas large numbers cause intense destructive inflammatory reactions. If the inflammatory reactions were not too intense, tuberculous animals clearly showed a considerably increased resistance to reinfection with virulent tubercle bacilli. Thus, it was recognized that intense reactions of tuberculin hypersensitivity were destructive and that tuberculin, therefore, could have a deleterious effect on the sensitive host. On the other hand, if these reactions were mild, it appeared reasonable to ascribe the increased resistance to infection to the beneficial effects of the inflammatory process. Rich[67] described the basis for this position as follows:

Everyone agrees that inflammation is a protective mechanism of essential importance in resistance to bacterial infection. It is well known that inflammation can wall off and prevent the spread of bacteria, and the action of the inflammatory exudate in destroying bacteria has also been thoroughly well demonstrated in many infections. Hypersensitivity endows the body with the ability to respond with a more rapid and abundant inflammation at any site at which tubercle bacilli lodge in the tissues. Bacilli that enter the tuberculous body from without, or metastasize from a lesion to distant tissues will, therefore, be met by a more prompt protective inflammation, and will be hemmed in mechanically and destroyed more effectively than in the non-hypersensitive body, in which they may proliferate and spread before a sufficient amount of inflammation develops about them to restrain their activities.

The apparently reasonable hypothesis that the inflammation of tuberculin hypersensitivity was responsible for immunity in tuberculosis gained wide acceptance and was not seriously questioned until in a critical review, Rich and McCordock[68] pointed out:

There had never been placed on record one single experiment or clinical observation that demonstrated that hypersensitivity is necessary for protection in any stage of tuberculosis or any other infection, under any condition whatsoever.

The dearth of evidence to support the popularly held view that tuberculin hypersensitivity was responsible for acquired immunity in tuberculosis led Rich and his colleagues to devise experiments to test this hypothesis. The most important of these experiments involved the desensitization of tuberculous guinea pigs by the daily administration of increasing doses of tuberculin to the point at which dermal sensitivity to tuberculin was lost. In such desensitized animals, however, immunity to reinfection with virulent tubercle bacilli was not lost. These observations were soon confirmed by a number of other investigators.[3–5, 27, 31, 40, 73, 74, 77, 80] Thus, it appeared that immunity to tuberculosis could exist in the absence of tuberculin hypersensitivity.

Rich[67] provided other evidence to support his conclusion that acquired immunity to tuberculosis and tuberculin hypersensitivity were dissociable phenomena. For example, he pointed out: 1) that there is no correlation between the degree of hypersensitivity and the degree of acquired resistance in man or in animals, and in fact, an inverse relationship can clearly be demonstrated — the higher the degree of tuberculin hypersensitivity, the greater the susceptibility to tuberculous infection; 2) that hypersensitive inflammation alone is incapable of preventing the spread of bacteria in the tissues or the development of the disease; and 3) that acquired immunity can remain intact after the tuberculin hypersensitivity has spontaneously disappeared.

These observations, which suggested the lack of relationship between tuberculin hypersensitivity and acquired immunity to tuberculosis, were supported by the subsequent findings of Choucroun,[14] who isolated a protein component of the tubercle bacillus and a carbohydrate-lipid complex. The protein component, when injected into guinea pigs in mineral oil, induced tuberculin hypersensitivity but did not bring about any significantly

increased resistance to tuberculous infection. Similar findings were reported by Raffel,[63] who found that the induction of a high degree of tuberculin hypersensitivity by injecting guinea pigs with wax D and tuberculoprotein isolated from tubercle bacilli was not accompanied by an increased resistance to infection with virulent tubercle bacilli.

MYCOBACTERIAL IMMUNOGENS

The evidence just outlined led to the general feeling that tuberculin hypersensitivity was not responsible, after all, for immunity to tuberculosis because the two phenomena could be dissociated. This belief, in turn, provided the basis for extensive experiments by a number of investigators to isolate a nonallergenic immunizing component from mycobacterial cells. The successful accomplishment of this

mission by Crowle,[26] by Kanai and Youmans,[43] by Kanai and associates,[44] and by Youmans and Youmans[91] further emphasized the dichotomy between tuberculin hypersensitivity and immunity in tuberculosis.

NATURE OF THE IMMUNE RESPONSE

Mackaness[52] reopened the question of the relationship between acquired immunity to tuberculosis and tuberculin hypersensitivity. In a series of publications, Mackaness[53, 54] and Collins and Mackaness[18, 19] supported the proposition that tuberculin hypersensitivity may be responsible, after all, for acquired immunity in tuberculosis. Before examining and commenting on the evidence, it is necessary to review the nature of the acquired immune response in this disease and some of the factors that are involved in its genesis (see Chapter 12 for further details).

Mycobacterium tuberculosis is classified as a facultative intracellular parasite because it has the capacity to multiply within macrophages. These phagocytic cells are capable of rapidly killing and digesting most bacteria. *Listeria, Pasteurella, Brucella,* and certain fungi also are facultative intracellular parasites, although they differ profoundly from *M. tuberculosis* in other respects.

For a microorganism to grow intracellularly, it must be able to resist lethal factors produced by phagocytic cells and must have an ability to resist digestion by the battery of hydrolytic enzymes found in lysosomes of the leukocyte. In tuberculosis, this resistance to destruction is not absolute because, depending on the number of virulent tubercle bacilli injected and the route of inoculation, as many as 50 percent of the mycobacterial cells injected may be killed or rendered nonviable within a few days.[34, 35] The remaining intracellular bacilli multiply and may eventually reach such large numbers that the phagocytic cells in which they reside are killed and the destructive lesions of tuberculosis may appear (see Chapters 7, 8, 9, 10, 11, 12, and 14).[11, 64, 65, 67]

It has long been recognized that once animals are infected with tubercle bacilli, they become much more resistant to reinfection. Furthermore, animals, including man, vaccinated with viable cells of attenuated mycobacterial strains such as bacillus Calmette-Guérin (BCG) or the H37Ra strain acquire a much greater resistance to infection.[67, 70, 88] This actively acquired immune state is characterized not only by an increased capacity of macrophages to kill tubercle bacilli but also by the development by these cells of an ability to inhibit the intracellular multiplication of the parasite. In fact, intracellular bacteriostasis is the major manifestation of acquired immunity to tuberculosis, and tubercle bacilli may remain viable but nonmultiplying with cells in vivo for years. Rich[67] pointed this out many years ago. In spite of extensive investigation, the actual mechanism, or mechanisms, whereby phagocytic cells of immunized animals are able to exert such control over intracellular tubercle bacilli remains largely unknown, although recent evidence suggests that lymphocytes may be the primary cells mediating this effect.[51, 62] More will be said about this in the paragraphs that follow (see also Chapters 7, 8, 9, 10, 11, 12, and 14).

A strictly cellular basis for immunity to tuberculosis is also supported by the fact that macrophages obtained from tuberculous or immunized animals may be more motile and metabolize at faster rates. In addition, large numbers of lysosomes accumulate in the cytoplasm, and these cells are more actively phagocytic.[28, 29, 53] Thus, acquired immunity in tuberculosis might conceivably result merely from the more efficient functioning of these "activated" macrophages and, in particular, those activated by the inflammatory process of tuberculin hypersensitivity.

Such a mechanism would not necessarily involve an immunologic process and, therefore, would not necessarily be specific. In this connection, it has been documented that animals immunized with attenuated mycobacterial cells may also show an increased resistance to infection with other facultative intracellular parasites.[52, 53, 55, 78, 79] This has led to the conclusion that so-called cellular immunity to infection with facultative intracellular parasites is nonspecific.[53, 54] In addition, a possible underlying immunologic basis for this type of nonspecific immune response was revealed by Mackaness.[53, 54] He showed that once the nonspecific immunity engendered by injection of a facultative intracellular parasite has waned, it can be recalled rapidly by administration of a booster injection in a fashion analogous to the recall of antibody production by the reinjection of an antigen. Mackaness noted that the recall of increased resistance could be brought about only by the injection of the same species of microorganism used in the original vaccine. However, the recalled immune mechanism was apparently equally effective for the prevention of infection due to either the homologous or a heterologous facultative intracellular parasite. He concluded that acquired cellular immunity was an immunologic mechanism specifically engendered and recalled, but one that was nonspecific in action (see Chapters 7, 8, 9, 10, 11, 12, and 14).

Furthermore, Mackaness felt that the immunologic basis for the nonspecific action of increased resistance to tuberculosis is provided by tuberculin hypersensitivity.[54] In other words, acquired cellular immunity to tuberculosis is merely another manifestation of delayed tuberculin hypersensitivity. The rationale for this position is based on the following: 1) The two phenomena coexist after vaccination of animals with viable attenuated mycobacterial cells. 2) Experimentally, there is usually a direct relationship between the degree of delayed hypersensitivity and the degree of immunity when animals are vaccinated with viable mycobacterial cells. 3) Both are recalled when a booster injection of the cells used for vaccination is given. 4) Both can be adoptively transferred with T-lymphocytes from vaccinated animals, but not with serum.

The theory that acquired immunity in tuberculosis is just another manifestation of delayed hypersensitivity finds some support from the fact that viable attenuated mycobacterial cells are far more effective immunizing agents than killed cells (see Chapter 8). This much greater immunizing capacity of viable attenuated mycobacterial cells has generally been ascribed to the capacity of these cells to multiply to a limited extent in vivo, thereby producing a greater mass of immunogen (see Chapter 8). Presumably, the same reasoning could be applied to the development of tuberculin hypersensitivity.

From the foregoing the generally accepted current picture of acquired immunity to tuberculosis can be summarized as follows: 1) It is merely another manifestation of tuberculin hypersensitivity. 2) It is specifically induced and recalled, but is nonspecific in action. 3) Only one stable immunogen, which is found in killed as well as viable attenuated mycobacterial cells, need be involved. 4) The greater capacity of viable cells to immunize against infection resides in their ability to multiply in vivo.

MULTIPLE RESPONSE THEORY OF IMMUNITY IN TUBERCULOSIS

We have been led to question each one of the four hypotheses just stated, not only because of our own experi-

ence but also because of evidence derived from the work of others. We feel there are alternatives that provide better explanations for the manifestations of acquired immunity in tuberculosis. These alternative hypotheses are: 1) Killed mycobacterial cells are never as immunogenic as viable attenuated cells; that is, regardless of the number of killed cells used to immunize, there will always be a smaller number of viable cells that are more effective (see Chapter 8). 2) In vivo multiplication is not a requisite for the higher immunizing capacity of living mycobacterial cells. 3) The greater efficacy of viable mycobacterial cells for immunization is due to the presence of a highly active but labile immunizing component. 4) The immunizing capacity of killed cells is due to the presence of weakly immunogenic cell wall components. 5) Tuberculin hypersensitivity is not involved in the specific immune response. 6) There is both a specific and a nonspecific immune response when viable attenuated cells are used to immunize. When killed cells are used, only the nonspecific response is activated (see Chapter 8).

If the six hypotheses are correct, it follows that not only do tubercle bacilli contain more than one immunizing substance, but animals are capable of activating more than one immune mechanism in response to immunization with viable cells.

Evidence to support the validity of the conclusion just stated has been presented in a previous report[94] and in reviews.[90, 92, 93, 95] Most of our attention here will be focused on the relationship between tuberculin hypersensitivity and immunity in tuberculosis and on the specificity of immunity to tuberculosis. The question of specificity is important because, if immunity to tuberculosis is due to the allergic inflammatory response to tuberculin, the immune response must of necessity be nonspecific. Thus, evidence for the specificity of immunity to tuberculosis would argue against a role for tuberculin hypersensitivity.

Unfortunately, most of the experiments used to provide the data purporting to show the identity of tuberculin hypersensitivity and immunity to tuberculosis have employed animals immunized with intact viable tubercle bacilli. If, as we believe,[90, 92-95] various substances in the tubercle bacillus can induce differing immune responses, one would expect all of the possible responses to occur in animals immunized with viable cells because all of the biologically active substances would be present in these cells. Thus, immunity and tuberculin hypersensitivity would appear together and tend to parallel each other to a greater or lesser degree. However, no matter how great the parallel between the appearance of the two, this cannot be used as evidence for a causal relationship.

More meaningful experiments than those using animals vaccinated with intact viable cells are those attempting to abolish one immune response and then measuring the effect of the treatment on the other response. Certainly, anti-inflammatory agents, such as the corticosteroids, and lympholytic agents, such as antilymphocyte serum, reduce both immunity and tuberculin hypersensitivity when administered to vaccinated animals. This is to be expected because all lymphocyte functions would be affected by such agents. However, as we have already noted, when Rich[67] specifically desensitized vaccinated animals with tuberculin, there was no reduction in immunity to tuberculous infection, even though skin reactivity to tuberculin was lost. Mackaness[54] has questioned Rich's conclusions because, as he correctly points out, lack of dermal hypersensitivity to tuberculin does not mean that no sensitive lymphocytes are present in the animal. We now know that dermal sensitivity can be lost because of a reduction in the number of circulating lymphocytes, even though fully reactive lymphocytes frequently can be found compartmentalized in other parts of the body (see Chapter 7).

IMMUNIZING FRACTIONS OF TUBERCLE BACILLI

Other investigators have approached the problem through fractionating tubercle bacilli by chemical or physical means, such as breakage of the cells and separation of cellular components by centrifugation. The components have then been tested for their capacity to induce both immunity to tuberculous infection and tuberculin hypersensitivity (see Chapter 7).

We already have noted that when Raffel[63] injected guinea pigs with wax D and tuberculoprotein, they became highly tuberculin-sensitive but showed no increased resistance to infection. Mackaness[54] feels that the results obtained by Raffel may be misleading because, owing to the prolonged course of the disease in these experiments and the large challenge dose of virulent cells, the control animals eventually may have become tuberculin-sensitive and equally as immune as the animals rendered tuberculin-sensitive and immune with viable BCG cells. This response would be the result of stimulation of the host by the infecting dose of virulent tubercle bacilli. In Chapter 15 and elsewhere,[95] we have pointed out the lack of validity of this criticism; however, this criticism cannot be leveled at the experiments of Reggiardo and Middlebrook,[66] who produced tuberculin hypersensitivity in guinea pigs by injection of an extract of BCG cells. This hypersensitivity was not accompanied by an increased resistance, when the guinea pigs were challenged aerogenically with small numbers of virulent tubercle bacilli.

Some investigators have studied the capacity of immunizing materials obtained from attenuated mycobacterial cells to induce tuberculin hypersensitivity in both mice and guinea pigs. Crowle[26] has reported on a polysaccharide extracted from killed mycobacterial cells that will produce a significant increased resistance to tuberculous infection in mice. This material, however, did not induce tuberculin hypersensitivity in either mice or guinea pigs (see Chapter 11).

We[81, 83-86] have extensively investigated the allergenicity of ribosomal and RNA vaccines prepared from mechanically broken viable cells of the attenuated H37Ra strain of *M. tuberculosis*. We found that guinea pigs vaccinated subcutaneously with carefully washed ribosomal fraction material were completely negative when skin-tested 6 to 12 weeks later with large amounts of purified protein derivative (PPD). Mice vaccinated subcutaneously or intraperitoneally with either ribosomal fraction or mycobacterial ribonucleic acid (RNA) were negative when footpad-tested with PPD at intervals of up to eight weeks after vaccination; however, after challenge with virulent tubercle bacilli, these animals exhibited a pronounced immune response. In fact, the immune response quantitatively was equivalent to that produced by the viable attenuated H37Ra cells from which the RNA was prepared. Furthermore, attempts to recall and make manifest a low degree of tuberculin hypersensitivity by injecting graded doses of viable attenuated mycobacterial cells intravenously into animals previously vaccinated with ribosomal fraction or mycobacterial RNA completely failed.[91] These last experiments were done to answer the criticism that failure to elicit dermal hypersensitivity in animals at time of challenge does not eliminate the possibility that a low degree of hypersensitivity may be present and can be recalled by the challenge dose of virulent tubercle bacilli rapidly enough to account for the immunity. We[91] also failed to elicit systemic shock in mice vaccinated with myco-

bacterial RNA or ribosomal material, by the intravenous injection of large amounts (2 mg) of PPD.

More recently, Neiburger and coworkers[59] have extended these studies and have shown that not only are mice vaccinated with mycobacterial RNA vaccine footpad-negative but also that when stimulated with PPD, spleen cells from these animals failed to bring about inhibition of migration of macrophages. In addition, spleen cells from these animals did not produce, under any conditions of culture, migration inhibition factor (MIF) when exposed to PPD in tissue culture (see Chapter 9).

Finally, as shown by Casavant and Youmans,[12] guinea pigs vaccinated with mycobacterial RNA vaccine display no dermal hypersensitivity to PPD; also, their lymphocytes fail to react with PPD to bring about inhibition of macrophage migration, and they do not produce MIF when exposed to PPD in tissue culture. However, spleen cells taken from both mice and guinea pigs vaccinated with viable attenuated H37Ra cells will bring about inhibition of macrophage migration when added to cultures of macrophages from nonimmunized animals and will also produce MIF when exposed to PPD in vitro.[12] It is of some importance that this same mycobacterial RNA vaccine, when mixed with PPD in vitro and injected into guinea pigs, will serve as a potent adjuvant for the induction of tuberculin hypersensitivity.[12] The hypersensitivity was evidenced by elicitation of strong dermal reactions with PPD, showing a characteristic mononuclear cellular infiltrate upon section and staining. Also, the hypersensitivity could be passively transferred with cells but not with serum. Thus, even though it was a potent immunologic adjuvant for the induction of delayed hypersensitivity to tuberculoprotein, mycobacterial RNA vaccine itself did not induce tuberculin hypersensitivity (see Chapter 9).

In view of the evidence, it is difficult to arrive at any conclusion other than that tuberculin hypersensitivity and acquired immunity to tuberculosis are separate immune responses that are directed toward different components of the mycobacterial cell. However, other evidence can be provided to support the separateness of the two phenomena. For example, rifampin, a potent immunosuppressive drug, when administered to mice during the vaccination period has no effect on the immune response produced by mycobacterial RNA vaccine.[81] This same drug will profoundly suppress the induction of tuberculin hypersensitivity in mice vaccinated with viable H37Ra cells (see Chapter 10).[82, 87]

INVERSE RELATIONSHIP BETWEEN IMMUNITY AND TUBERCULIN HYPERSENSITIVITY

At least in human beings, there is essentially an inverse relationship between dermal hypersensitivity to tuberculin and the incidence of disease. This was commented on many years ago by Rich[67] and more recently was re-emphasized by the results of the British vaccine study using BCG.[39] In this study, among nonvaccinated control subjects, there was a much higher incidence of active disease in those who exhibited the highest degrees of dermal tuberculin sensitivity than in those who had a low degree of dermal tuberculin hypersensitivity. It is now well recognized that persons infected with *M. tuberculosis* who exhibit high degrees of tuberculin hypersensitivity are at greater risk of developing active progressive disease than persons exhibiting low degrees of dermal tuberculin hypersensitivity. A lack of correlation between development of tuberculin hypersensitivity in human beings and immunity to tuberculosis has been noted in other BCG vaccination trials.[1, 20-22]

In addition, it has been fully documented that allergic inflammation per se is not sufficient to prevent dissemination of bacteria in the tissues or the development of progressive disease.[67]

It is also of interest to point out that animals of species that develop delayed hypersensitivity with ease (for example, human beings and guinea pigs) are highly susceptible to tuberculosis, whereas animals (such as the mouse and the rat) that have a much lower capacity to develop delayed hypersensitivity are far more resistant. If tuberculin hypersensitivity is responsible for acquired immunity, the opposite relationship would be expected. In this respect, it has been shown that various strains of mice vary widely in their capacity to develop delayed hypersensitivity to protein antigens.[38] One inbred strain, C57Bl/6, developed hypersensitivity to protein antigens more rapidly and to a greater degree than any of a number of other mouse strains tested.[38] We have found[96] that this strain is far more susceptible to tuberculous infection than a number of other strains that develop delayed hypersensitivity less readily. So the parallel between a high degree of delayed hypersensitivity and a high degree of susceptibility to tuberculous infection can be demonstrated experimentally within individual strains of a single species of animal.

SPECIFICITY OF THE IMMUNE RESPONSE

We have pointed out that the question of specificity is of importance when studying the relationship between tuberculin hypersensitivity and immunity to tuberculosis because, if the increased resistance is due solely to tuberculin hypersensitivity, the immunity should be nonspecific. We have already noted that Mackaness and coworkers have, in fact, postulated that immunity in tuberculosis is specifically engendered but nonspecific in action. A number of investigators, however, have clearly shown that although nonspecific resistance can be produced by vaccination with mycobacterial cells to challenge with heterologous microorganisms, this immunity is quantitatively much less than that conferred by the homologous microorganisms.[16, 23-25, 51] In addition, it has been shown that mycobacterial RNA vaccine in mice produced no increased resistance to *Klebsiella pneumoniae*,[24] *Listeria monocytogenes*,[24, 25] *Salmonella typhimurium*,[97] *Staphylococcus aureus*,[76] or *Pseudomonas aeruginosa*.[76] Also, it has been demonstrated that animals vaccinated with mycobacterial cells show no increased resistance to another facultative intracellular parasite, *Pasteurella tularensis*, whereas animals vaccinated with attenuated strains of *P. tularensis* show a high degree of resistance to infection with fully virulent *P. tularensis*;[15] in other words, immunity here is specific.

ACQUIRED IMMUNITY TO OTHER FACULTATIVE INTRACELLULAR PARASITES

If delayed hypersensitivity to tuberculoprotein is responsible for acquired immunity to tuberculosis, one would expect that delayed hypersensitivity would also be responsible for the acquired immunity observed with other facultative intracellular parasites. However, Osebold and associates[61] failed to demonstrate any parallel between the degree of hypersensitivity of mice to listeria antigens and resistance to infection. Halliburton and Blazkovec[36] failed to show any temporal relationship in guinea pigs between development of delayed hypersensitivity to listeria antigens and increased resist-

ance to infection. Frenkel and Caldwell[33] also found that there was a great deal of specificity in the immune response to a wide variety of bacteria, viruses, and protozoa.

IN VITRO STUDIES

It is well recognized that the direct inhibition of macrophage migration by lymphocytes obtained from immunized animals and exposed to antigen, or indirect inhibition of MIF produced from sensitive lymphocytes stimulated with antigen in vitro, is a correlate of delayed hypersensitivity.[30]

Immunity to tuberculosis can also be investigated in vitro.[62] Macrophages obtained from nonimmunized animals can be maintained as monolayers on coverslips in vitro. These living cells can be infected with virulent tubercle bacilli by adding the tubercle bacilli to the tissue culture medium. The tubercle bacilli are phagocytosed and multiply within the macrophages. By removing coverslips at intervals after infection and staining these by the Ziehl-Neelson method, the number of tubercle bacilli within the macrophages can be counted under the microscope and the average number per macrophage calculated. It becomes feasible, therefore, to measure the effect of a variety of factors on the rate of growth of virulent tubercle bacilli within macrophages (see Chapter 12).

Using this technique, Patterson and Youmans[62] found that virulent tubercle bacilli multiplied just as rapidly within mouse peritoneal macrophages obtained from animals immunized with viable attenuated mycobacterial cells as they did within macrophages obtained from nonimmunized mice. It was not until spleen cells (lymphocytes) obtained from mice vaccinated with viable attenuated mycobacterial cells were added to the tissue culture system that an inhibition of the rate of multiplication of the intracellular virulent tubercle bacilli was noted. These results provided direct evidence that lymphocytes, not macrophages, were responsible for the immune response to tuberculosis. Lefford and coworkers[51] provided additional direct evidence for the involvement of lymphocytes in immunity to tuberculosis by showing that specific immunity to tuberculosis in rats could be adoptively transferred to nonvaccinated recipient rats, using thoracic duct lymphocyte suspensions that were free of macrophages.

More recently, Lefford[50] has passively transferred immunity to tuberculosis, using lymphocytes from immunized mice. In Lefford's study, however, the adoptively immunized animals did not manifest immunity until 14 days after they had received the lymphocytes. This finding suggests that the recipient mice may actually have been actively immunized by the transfer of residual, viable mycobacterial cells present in the donor animals.

Patterson and Youmans[62] also found that lymphocytes obtained from immunized mice, when stimulated with specific antigen, would elaborate and secrete a substance into the tissue culture medium. This substance (lymphokine), when added to macrophages infected with virulent tubercle bacilli, brought about inhibition of the growth of the intracellular tubercle bacilli (see Chapter 12).

The availability of these in vitro techniques—MIF assay and assay of mycobacterial growth inhibitory factor (MycoIF) — along with the knowledge that a lymphokine is apparently involved in the mediation of both tuberculin hypersensitivity and acquired immunity to tuberculosis, allowed us to approach the study of the relationship of tuberculin hypersensitivity to immunity in tuberculosis in another way. It would follow that if MIF is the mediator of tuberculin hypersensitivity, as appears to be the case,[30] and if tuberculin hypersensitivity is respons-

ible for acquired immunity to tuberculosis, then MIF should be the lymphokine that brings about the inhibition of intracellular multiplication of tubercle bacilli in vitro.

RELATION BETWEEN MIGRATION INHIBITORY FACTOR AND MYCOBACTERIAL GROWTH INHIBITORY FACTOR

We have investigated the relationship between MIF and MycoIF extensively. Initially, Neiburger and associates[59] vaccinated separate groups of mice with either viable H37Ra cells or mycobacterial RNA vaccine. Only spleen cells from mice vaccinated with viable H37Ra mycobacterial cells produced MIF when stimulated either in vitro or in vivo with PPD. However, both groups of mice were equally immune to challenge intravenously with virulent tubercle bacilli. Thus, no sign of tuberculin hypersensitivity could be elicited with PPD in animals vaccinated with the RNA material; yet these animals were just as immune to infection as the animals vaccinated with the H37Ra viable cells. Klun and Youmans,[46] confirming the findings of Patterson and Youmans,[62] found that lymphocytes from mice vaccinated with both H37Ra cells and mycobacterial RNA, when stimulated in vitro with H37Ra cells or with mycobacterial RNA, would produce MycoIF. However, when lymphocytes from the same animals were stimulated in vitro with PPD, only the cells from mice immunized with H37Ra cells produced MIF. Klun and coworkers[45] extended these observations and investigated the relationship between mouse MycoIF and MIF in supernatant fluids from stimulated mouse lymphocyte cultures. This was done by examining the same lymphocyte supernatant fluid for the presence of both MIF and MycoIF. Although in certain experiments lymphocyte supernatant fluids were found to have both MIF and MycoIF activity, MIF could be found in certain of the lymphocyte supernatant fluids that did not contain MycoIF. Conversely, MycoIF was found in some lymphocyte supernatant fluids that did not contain MIF. The results indicated that MycoIF and MIF were separate substances, therefore suggesting tuberculin hypersensitivity and immunity to tuberculosis are mediated by separate lymphokines.

Cahall and Youmans[6-8] extended these observations, using highly active MycoIF partially purified by gel filtration. These preparations also were tested for MIF activity. In no case using this more purified material was there any inhibition of macrophage migration. These results provided further support for the conclusion that mouse MIF and mouse MycoIF are separate substances.

More recently, Mayo and colleagues[56] have shown that peripheral blood lymphocytes obtained from guinea pigs infected with *Salmonella typhimurium*, when stimulated with *S. typhimurium* antigens, would produce macrophage migration inhibitory factor (MIF). Macrophages exposed to this MIF, however, did not exhibit an enhanced phagocytic or bactericidal activity against virulent *S. typhimurium*. These findings provide further evidence for the lack of a role for MIF in immunity to infection.

Further data on the role of lymphocytes and lymphocyte products on immunity to infection can be found in several sources.[9, 10, 17, 32, 41, 42, 57, 58, 72, 75]

CONCLUSIONS

In view of the evidence as outlined here, it is impossible to come to any conclusion other than that reactions of tuberculin hypersensitivity play little, if any, role in acquired immunity to tuberculosis. To the extent that mild tuberculin reactions might bring about the activation of macrophages, resistance to infection can be increased. This is insignificant, however, compared to the high degree of specific immunity that can develop in animals after infection with virulent tubercle bacilli after vaccination with viable attenuated mycobacterial cells or with mycobacterial RNA (see Chapters 8, 9, and 10).

However, we cannot leave a discussion of the relationship of delayed hypersensitivity to immunity to tuberculosis without considering the possibility that delayed hypersensitivity to some component of the tubercle bacillus other than tuberculoprotein might play a significant role, especially because Ortiz-Ortiz and coworkers[60] and Baker and associates[2] have shown that guinea pigs will develop hypersensitivity to ribosomal protein after the administration of ribosomal material. To date, however, there is nothing to suggest that this delayed hypersensitivity to ribosomal protein plays any role in the immunity that develops in animals after administration of RNA preparations.

Another possibility should be mentioned. We have seen that the major immunogen of the tubercle bacillus can be found in an RNA preparation. Recently, Casavant and Youmans[13] reported that delayed hypersensitivity to the polynucleotides poly A:U and poly U can develop in guinea pigs. Although we have been unable to obtain any evidence that delayed hypersensitivity can develop to mycobacterial RNA in guinea pigs vaccinated with RNA vaccine, this possibility must be kept in mind.

Thus, our assessment of the relationship between delayed hypersensitivity and immunity to tuberculosis leads us to the conclusion that although tuberculin hypersensitivity plays little or no role in the immune response, we cannot completely rule out delayed hypersensitivity to other constituents of the tubercle bacillus, although we feel that this last possibility is unlikely. A more reasonable view would be that delayed hypersensitivity and immunity to tuberculosis are entirely separate processes, initiated by animals in response to various components of the tubercle bacillus. Both phenomena involve a cellular type of immune response, and both are mediated by thymus-derived lymphocytes. Because different lymphokines appear to be involved, it is also reasonable to hypothesize that separate T-lymphocyte populations mediate the two phenomena. Confirmation or denial of these possibilities will require future experimentation. Fortunately, from the technical standpoint, the way seems clear to a resolution of the mechanisms of acquired immunity to tuberculosis in the not too distant future.

REFERENCES

1. Aronson, J. D.: Protective vaccination against tuberculosis with special reference to BCG vaccination. Am. Rev. Tuberc. *58*:255, 1948.
2. Baker, R. E., Hill, W. E., and Larson, C. L.: Delayed hypersensitivity reactions provoked by ribosomes from acid-fast bacilli. I. Ribosomal isolation, characterization, delayed hypersensitivity, and specificity. Infect. Immun. *6*:258, 1972.
3. Birkhaug, K.: Allergy and immunity (iathergy) in experimental tuberculosis. Statistical interpretation of degree of tuberculosis in superinfected allergic and desensitized anergic (iathergic) guinea pigs. Acta Tuberc. Scandinav. *11*:199, 1937.
4. Boquet, A.: Influence des réactions hyperergiques d'épreuve et de l'anergie provoquée (désensibilisation) sur l'évolution de la tuberculose expérimentale. C. R. Soc. Biol. (Paris) *112*:1168, 1933.
5. Branch, A., and Kropp, G. V.: The desensitization of tuberculous guinea pigs with unheated tuberculin. Am. Rev. Tuberc. *35*:247, 1937.
6. Cahall, D. L., and Youmans, G. P.: Conditions for production, and some characteristics, of mycobacterial growth inhibitory factor produced by spleen cells from mice immunized with viable cells of the attenuated H37Ra strain of *Mycobacterium tuberculosis*. Infect. Immun. *12*:833, 1975.
7. Cahall, D. L., and Youmans, G. P.: Macrophage migration inhibitory activity of mycobacterial growth inhibitory factor and the effect of a number of factors on mycobacterial growth inhibitory factor activity. Infect. Immun. *12*:851, 1975.
8. Cahall, D. L., and Youmans, G. P.: Molecular weight and other characteristics of mycobacterial growth inhibitory factor produced by spleen cells obtained from mice immunized with viable attenuated mycobacterial cells. Infect. Immun. *12*:841, 1975.
9. Cameron, C. M., and van Rensburg, J. J.: Inhibition of macrophage migration in *Salmonella* immunity. Onderstepoort, J. Vet. Res. *42*:15, 1975.
10. Campbell, P. A.: Immunocompetent cells in resistance to bacterial infections. Bacteriol. Rev. *40*:284, 1976.
11. Canetti, G.: The Tubercle Bacillus in the Pulmonary Lesion of Man. New York, Springer Publishing Co., Inc., 1955.
12. Casavant, C. H., and Youmans, G. P.: The adjuvant activity of mycobacterial RNA preparations and synthetic polynucleotides for induction of delayed hypersensitivity to purified protein derivative in guinea pigs. J. Immunol. *114*:1014, 1975.
13. Casavant, C. H., and Youmans, G. P.: The induction of delayed hypersensitivity in guinea pigs to poly U and poly A:U. J. Immunol. *114*:1506, 1975.
14. Choucroun, N.: Tubercle bacillus antigens. Biological properties of two substances isolated from paraffin oil extract of dead tubercle bacilli. Am. Rev. Tuberc. *56*:203, 1947.
15. Claflin, J. L., and Larson, C. L.: Infection-immunity in tularemia: Specificity of cellular immunity. Infect. Immun. *5*:311, 1972.
16. Collins, F. M.: Recall of immunity in mice vaccinated with *Salmonella enteritidis* or *Salmonella typhimurium*. J. Bacteriol. *95*:2014, 1968.
17. Collins, F. M.: Vaccines and cell-mediated immunity. Bacteriol. Rev. *38*:371, 1974.
18. Collins, F. M., and Mackaness, G. B.: The relationship of delayed hypersensitivity to acquired antituberculous immunity. I. Tuberculin sensitivity and resistance to reinfection in BCG-vaccinated mice. Cell. Immunol. *1*:253, 1970.
19. Collins, F. M., and Mackaness, G. B.: The relationship of delayed hypersensitivity to acquired antituberculous immunity. II. Effect of adjuvant on the allergenicity and immunogenicity of heat-killed tubercle bacilli. Cell. Immunol. *1*:266, 1970.
20. Comstock, G. W.: Community research in tuberculosis, Muscogee County, Georgia. Public Health Rep. *79*:1045, 1964.
21. Comstock, G. W., and Palmer, C. E.: Long-

term results of BCG vaccination in the southern United States. Am. Rev. Respir. Dis. *93*:171, 1966.

22. Comstock, G. W., and Sartwell, P. E.: Tuberculosis studies in Muscogee County, Georgia. IV. Evaluation of a community-wide x-ray survey on the basis of six years of observations. Am. J. Hyg. *61*:261, 1955.

23. Coppel, S., and Youmans, G. P.: Specificity of acquired resistance produced by immunization with *Listeria monocytogenes* and listeria fractions. J. Bacteriol. *97*:121, 1969.

24. Coppel, S., and Youmans, G. P.: Specificity of acquired resistance produced by immunization with mycobacterial cells and mycobacterial fractions. J. Bacteriol. *97*:114, 1969.

25. Coppel, S., and Youmans, G. P.: Specificity of the anamnestic response produced by *Listeria monocytogenes* or *Mycobacterium tuberculosis* to challenge with *Listeria monocytogenes*. J. Bacteriol. *97*:127, 1969.

26. Crowle, A. J.: Trypsin-extracted immunizing antigen of the tubercle bacillus: A practical vaccine? Adv. Tuberc. Res. *18*:31, 1972.

27. Cummings, D. E., and Delahant, A. B.: Relationships between hypersensitiveness and immunity in tuberculosis. Transactions of the National Tuberculosis Association, 1934, p. 123.

28. Dannenberg, A. M., Jr.: Cellular hypersensitivity and cellular immunity in the pathogenesis of tuberculosis: Specificity, systemic and local nature, and associated macrophage enzymes. Bacteriol. Rev. *32*:85, 1968.

29. Dannenberg, A. M., Jr., Meyer, O. T., Esterly, J. R., and Kambara, T.: The local nature of immunity in tuberculosis, illustrated histochemically in dermal BCG lesions. J. Immunol. *100*:931, 1968.

30. David, J. R., and David, R. R.: Cellular hypersensitivity and immunity. Inhibition of macrophage migration and the lymphocyte mediators. Prog. Allergy *16*:300, 1972.

31. Follis, R. H., Jr.: The effect of preventing the development of hypersensitivity in experimental tuberculosis. Bull. Johns Hopkins Hosp. *63*:283, 1938.

32. Fowles, R. E., Fajardo, I. M., Leibowitch, J. L., and David, J. R.: The enhancement of macrophage bacteriostasis by products of activated lymphocytes. J. Exp. Med. *138*:952, 1973.

33. Frenkel, J. K., and Caldwell, S. A.: Specific immunity and nonspecific resistance to infection: *Listeria,* protozoa, and viruses in mice and hamsters. J. Infect. Dis. *131*:201, 1975.

34. Gray, D. F., and Cheers, C.: The steady state in cellular immunity. I. Chemotherapy and superinfection in murine tuberculosis. Aust. J. Exp. Biol. Med. Sci. *45*:407, 1967.

35. Gray, D. F., and Cheers, C.: The steady state in cellular immunity. II. Immunological complaisance in murine pertussis. Aust. J. Exp. Biol. Med. Sci. *45*:417, 1967.

36. Halliburton, B. L., and Blazkovec, A. A.: Delayed hypersensitivity and acquired cellular resistance in guinea pigs infected with *Listeria monocytogenes*. Infect. Immun. *11*:1, 1975.

37. Hamburger, F.: Ueber Tuberkuloseimmunität. Beitr. z. Klin. d. Tuberk. *11*:259, 1909.

38. Han, S., and Weiser, R. S.: Systemic tuberculin sensitivity in mice. I. Factors contributing to active tuberculin shock. J. Immunol. *98*:1152, 1967.

39. Hart, P. D., Sutherland, I., and Thomas, J.: The immunity conferred by effective BCG and vole bacillus vaccines, in relation to individual variations in induced tuberculin sensitivity and to technical variations in the vaccines. Tubercle *48*:201, 1967.

40. Higginbotham, M. W.: A study of heteroallergic reactivity of tuberculin-desensitized tuberculous guinea pigs, in comparison with tuberculous and normal guinea pigs. Am. J. Hyg. *26*:197, 1937.

41. Hsu, H. S., and Mayo, D. R.: Interactions between macrophages of guinea pigs and salmonellae. III. Bactericidal action and cytophilic antibodies of macrophages of infected guinea pigs. Infect. Immun. *8*:165, 1973.

42. Jones, T., and Youmans, G. P.: The *in vitro* inhibition of growth of intracellular *Listeria monocytogenes* by lymphocyte products. Cell. Immunol. *9*:353, 1973.

43. Kanai, K., and Youmans, G. P.: Immunogenicity of intracellular particles and cell walls from *Mycobacterium tuberculosis*. J. Bacteriol. *80*:607, 1960.

44. Kanai, K., Youmans, G. P., and Youmans, A. S.: Allergenicity of intracellular particles, cell walls, and cytoplasmic fluid from *Mycobacterium tuberculosis*. J. Bacteriol. *80*:615, 1960.

45. Klun, C. L., Neiburger, R. G., and Youmans, G. P.: Relationship between mouse mycobacterial growth-inhibitory factor and mouse migration-inhibitory factor in supernatant fluids from mouse lymphocyte cultures. J. Reticuloendothel. Soc. *13*:310, 1973.

46. Klun, C. L., and Youmans, G. P.: The effect of lymphocyte supernatant fluids on the intracellular growth of virulent tubercle bacilli. J. Reticuloendothel. Soc. *13*:263, 1973.

47. Koch, R.: Fortsetzung der Mittheilungen über ein Heilmittel gegen Tuberkulose. Deutsche Med. Wochenschr. *17*:101, 1891.

48. Koch, R.: Weitere Mittheilungen über ein Heilmittel gegen Tuberkulose. Deutsche Med. Wochenschr. *16*:1029, 1890.

49. Lefford, M. J.: Delayed hypersensitivity and immunity in tuberculosis. Am. Rev. Respir. Dis. *111*:243, 1975.

50. Lefford, M. J.: Transfer of adoptive immunity to tuberculosis in mice. Infect. Immun. *11*:1174, 1975.

51. Lefford, M. J., McGregor, D. D., and Mackaness, G. B.: Immune response to *Mycobacterium tuberculosis* in rats. Infect. Immun. *8*:182, 1973.

52. Mackaness, G. B.: Cellular resistance to infection. J. Exp. Med. *116*:381, 1962.

53. Mackaness, G. B.: The immunological basis of acquired cellular resistance. J. Exp. Med. *120*:105, 1964.

54. Mackaness, G. B.: The immunology of antituberculous immunity. Am. Rev. Respir. Dis. *97*:337, 1968.

55. Mackaness, G. B., and Blanden, R. V.: Cellular immunity. Prog. Allergy *11*:89, 1967.

56. Mayo, D. R., Hsu, H. S., and Lim, F.: Interactions between salmonellae and macrophages of guinea pigs. IV. Relationship between migration inhibition and antibacterial action of macrophages. Infect. Immun. *18*:52, 1977.

57. Mitsuhashi, S., Sato, I., and Tanaka, T.: Experimental salmonellosis. Intracellular growth of *Salmonella enteritidis* ingested in mononuclear phagocytes of mice, and cellular basis of immunity. J. Bacteriol. *81*:863, 1961.

58. Nathan, C. F., Karnovsky, M. K., and David, J. R.: Alterations of macrophage functions by mediators from lymphocytes. J. Exp. Med. *133*:1356, 1971.

59. Neiburger, R. G., Youmans, G. P., and Youmans, A. S.: Relationship between tuberculin hypersensitivity and cellular immunity to infection in mice vaccinated with viable attenuated mycobacterial cells or with mycobacterial ribonucleic acid preparations. Infect. Immun. *8*:42, 1973.

60. Ortiz-Ortiz, L., Solarolo, E. B., and Bojalil, L. F.: Delayed hypersensitivity to ribosomal protein from BCG. J. Immunol. *107*:1022, 1971.

61. Osebold, J. W., Pearson, L. D., and Medin, N. I.: Relationship of antimicrobial cellular immunity to delayed hypersensitivity in listeriosis. Infect. Immun. *9*:354, 1974.

62. Patterson, R. J., and Youmans, G. P.: Demonstration in tissue culture of lymphocyte-mediated immunity to tuberculosis. Infect. Immun. *1*:600, 1970.

63. Raffel, S.: Chemical factors involved in the induction of infectious allergy. Experientia *6*:410, 1950.

64. Raleigh, G. W., and Youmans, G. P.: The use of mice in experimental chemotherapy of tuberculosis. I. Rationale and review of the literature. J. Infect. Dis. *82*:197, 1948.

65. Raleigh, G. W., and Youmans, G. P.: The use of mice in experimental chemotherapy of tuberculosis. II. Pathology and pathogenesis. J. Infect. Dis. *82*:205, 1948.

66. Reggiardo, Z., and Middlebrook, G.: Delayed-type hypersensitivity and immunity against aerogenic tuberculosis in guinea pigs. Infect. Immun. *9*:815, 1974.

67. Rich, A. R.: The Pathogenesis of Tuberculosis. 2nd ed. Springfield, Ill., Charles C Thomas, 1951.

68. Rich, A. R., and McCordock, H. A.: An enquiry concerning the role of allergy, immunity and other factors of importance in the pathogenesis of human tuberculosis. Bull. Johns Hopkins Hosp. *44*:273, 1929.

69. Römer, P. H.: Spezifische Ueberempfindlichkeit und Tuberkuloseimmunität. Beitr. z. Klin. d. Tuberk., Würzb. *11*:79, 1908.

70. Rosenthal, S. R.: BCG Vaccination against Tuberculosis. Boston, Little, Brown and Company, 1957.

71. Salvin, S. B., and Neta, R.: A possible relationship between delayed hypersensitivity and cell-mediated immunity. Am. Rev. Respir. Dis. *111*:373, 1975.

72. Sato, I., Tanaka, T., Saito, K., and Mitsuhashi, S.: Inhibition of *Salmonella enteritidis* ingested in mononuclear phagocytes from liver and subcutaneous tissue of mice immunized with live vaccine. J. Bacteriol. *83*:1306, 1962.

73. Selter, H., and Weiland, P.: Der Einfluss einer Tuberkulin-Densensibilisierung auf die Tuberkuloseimmunität. Ztschr. f. Tuberk. *74*:161, 1935.

74. Siegl, J.: Allergie und Immunität bie der Tuberkulose. Beitr. z. Klin. d. Tuberk. *84*:311, 1934.

75. Simon, H. B., and Sheagren, J. N.: Cellular immunity *in vitro*. I. Immunologically mediated enhancement of macrophage bactericidal capacity. J. Exp. Med. *133*:1377, 1971.

76. Smith, R. L., Wysocki, J. A., Bruun, J. N., De Courcy, S. J., Jr., Blakemore, W. S., and Mudd, S.: Efficacy of ribosomal preparations from *Pseudomonas aeruginosa* to protect against intravenous pseudomonas challenge in mice. J. Reticuloendothel. Soc. *15*:22, 1974.

77. Thayer, J. D.: Desensitization in the treatment of tuberculous guinea-pigs. Tubercle *19*:365, 1938.

78. Weiss, D. W.: Enhanced resistance of mice to infection with *Pasteurella pestis* following vaccination with fractions of phenol-killed tubercle bacilli. Nature *186*:1060, 1960.

79. Weiss, D. W., Bonhag, R. S., and Parks, J. A.: Studies on the heterologous immunogenicity of a methanol-insoluble fraction

of attenuated tubercle bacilli (BCG). I. Antimicrobial protection. J. Exp. Med. *119*:53, 1964.

80. Wilson, G. S., Schwabacher, H., and Maier, I.: The effect of desensitisation of tuberculous guinea-pigs. J. Pathol. Bacteriol. *50*:89, 1940.

81. Youmans, A. S., and Youmans, G. P.: The effect of metabolic inhibitors and hydroxylamine on the immune response in mice to mycobacterial ribonucleic acid vaccines. J. Immunol. *112*:271, 1974.

82. Youmans, A. S., and Youmans, G. P.: The effect of metabolic inhibitors on the formation of antibody to sheep erythrocytes, on development of delayed hypersensitivity, and on the immune response to infection with *Mycobacterium tuberculosis* in mice. Infect. Immun. *19*:212, 1978.

83. Youmans, A. S., and Youmans, G. P.: Factors affecting immunogenic activity of mycobacterial ribosomal and ribonucleic acid preparations. J. Bacteriol. *99*:42, 1969.

84. Youmans, A. S., and Youmans, G. P.: Immunogenic activity of a ribosomal fraction obtained from *Mycobacterium tuberculosis*. J. Bacteriol. *89*:1291, 1965.

85. Youmans, A. S., and Youmans, G. P.: Immunogenic mycobacterial ribosomal and ribonucleic acid preparations: Chemical and physical characteristics. Infect. Immun. *2*:659, 1970.

86. Youmans, A. S., and Youmans, G. P.: Preparation of highly immunogenic ribosomal fractions of *Mycobacterium tuberculosis* by use of sodium dodecyl sulfate. J. Bacteriol. *91*:2139, 1966.

87. Youmans, A. S., Youmans, G. P., and Cahall, D. L.: Effect of rifampin on immunity to tuberculosis and on delayed hypersensitivity to purified protein derivative. Infect. Immun. *13*:127, 1976.

88. Youmans, G. P.: Acquired immunity in tuberculosis. J. Chronic Dis. *6*:606, 1957.

89. Youmans, G. P.: Relation between delayed hypersensitivity and immunity in tuberculosis. Am. Rev. Respir. Dis. *111*:109, 1975.

90. Youmans, G. P.: The role of lymphocytes and other factors in antimicrobial cellular immunity. J. Reticuloendothel. Soc. *10*:100, 1971.

91. Youmans, G. P., and Youmans, A. S.: Allergenicity of mycobacterial ribosomal and ribonucleic acid preparations in mice and guinea pigs. J. Bacteriol. *97*:134, 1969.

92. Youmans, G. P., and Youmans, A. S.: Immunizing antigens of mycobacteria. *In* Nowotny, A. (ed.): Cellular Antigens. New York, Springer-Verlag, 1972.

93. Youmans, G. P., and Youmans, A. S.: *Mycobacterium tuberculosis* immunogens. Ann. Sclavo *13*:706, 1971.

94. Youmans, G. P., and Youmans, A. S.: Nonspecific factors in resistance of mice to experimental tuberculosis. J. Bacteriol. *90*:1675, 1965.

95. Youmans, G. P., and Youmans, A. S.: Recent studies on acquired immunity in tuberculosis. Curr. Topics Microbiol. Immunol. *48*:129, 1969.

96. Youmans, G. P., and Youmans, A. S.: Response of vaccinated and nonvaccinated syngeneic C57Bl/6 mice to infection with *Mycobacterium tuberculosis*. Infect. Immun. *6*:748, 1972.

97. Youmans, G. P., and Youmans, A. S.: Unpublished observations.

Pathogenesis of Tuberculosis

INTRODUCTION

In previous chapters, we have considered at length the response of human and animal hosts to infection with virulent tubercle bacilli or to the injection of certain products of *Myco-bacterium tuberculosis*. We have noted that in certain species of animals, such as human beings, guinea pigs, and rabbits, rather distinctive, though nonspecific, cellular changes may occur. Thus, the development of epithelioid cells and giant cells and the formation of the tubercle are hallmarks of, but not pathognomonic of, tuberculosis in the human being. In addition, we have examined, in detail, immunologic responses of human beings and lower animals to infection with virulent or attenuated mycobac-terial cells or with certain products of those cells.

We have noted that there are two major immunologic responses: first, acquired immunity to infection; and, second, the development of tuberculin hypersensitivity. We have also concluded that these two immunologic responses are both of a cellular nature and are mediated by T-lymphocytes. They appear to be separate and distinct immunologic responses to tuberculous infection, probably mediated by different populations of T-cells.

The cellular changes referred to above, and the two major immunologic responses in particular, play an enormously important role in the development of tuberculous disease. In fact, whether overt disease occurs at all undoubtedly depends primarily upon the interplay between these two immunologic manifestations in each infected person. It is our hope, then, to examine in this chapter the development of tuberculous infection and disease and, in particular, to delineate the role of these immunologic factors in determining the progress of the disease. We believe that it is quite possible, providing we have a clear understanding of the nature of the immunologic forces involved, to construct a picture of the pathogenesis of tuberculosis in human beings that is reasonably simple and that will provide an explanation for the appearance of the many manifestations of tuberculous disease, which superficially appear not only to be complex but also to have no meaningful basis.

It is essential to realize, and for us to keep in mind, that tuberculous infection may occur in two general types of persons or animals. First, tuberculous infection may occur in those persons or animals that have had no previous experience with the tubercle bacillus; that is, they have never been infected or diseased. Second, tuberculous infection may occur in those persons who have had previous experience with the tubercle bacillus; that is, have previously been infected, have previously been diseased, or have previously been vaccinated with BCG vaccine. Conceivably, such persons even may have been infected at some prior time with a closely related mycobacterial species, such as *Mycobacterium kansasii* or *M. intracellulare*. We also can define these two types of persons or animals in other terms; that is, they are those persons or animals who have never reacted immunologically to *M. tuberculosis*, or those persons who at some previous time in their existence have reacted immunologically to mycobacterial cells. Those persons or animals who have had such a previous experience, and therefore have immunologically reacted to the presence of the tubercle bacillus, will possess a greater or lesser degree of acquired cellular immunity to infection, in addition to a greater or lesser degree of tuberculin hypersensitivity to the proteins of the tubercle bacillus. The presence of cellular immunity to infection, or of tuberculin hypersensitivity, or both will make a profound difference in how the person or animal responds to infection with the tubercle bacillus.

PRIMARY TUBERCULOSIS

When infection with *Mycobacterium tuberculosis* takes place in a person or an animal that has had no previous experience with the tubercle bacillus, it is referred to as a *primary infection* or *primary disease*. Since infection usually takes place by way of the lower respiratory tract, the lung is usually the first organ involved, and it is here that the initial major manifestations of disease will usually occur. *M. tuberculosis* can produce infection and disease in almost every tissue and organ in the body, but such disease is most commonly the result of dissemination from an initial pulmonary focus. Although multiplication of the tubercle bacillus will take place in other tissues, it proceeds most rapidly in the lung. Therefore, the sequence of events that follows infection of the lung with *M. tuberculosis* can be used as an example of what may occur following infection of any organ or tissue. In primary pulmonary tuberculous infection, one or more mycobacterial cells will lodge within an alveolus, where they will be rapidly phagocytosed by segmented neutrophils and alveolar macrophages. Because of their high resistance to destruction, these virulent mycobacteria multiply within these macrophages almost as rapidly as they do in an artificial culture medium. However, the maximum rate of multiplication is still quite slow; therefore, the increase in numbers of virulent tubercle bacilli will be slow. This accounts for the fact that the appearance of symptoms or of an observable pathologic condition due to the infection may require several weeks. When the numbers of tubercle bacilli become significantly large, an inflammatory cellular reaction will appear. It follows, then, that the primary tuberculous infection, at least early in the course of the infection, is characterized by being pneumonic.

In spite of the cellular reaction, there is little or no resistance to the multiplication of the tubercle bacilli, and very soon after infection, dissemination from this focus of infection will occur. This dissemination is primarily by way of the lymphatics, and there is early, extensive involvement of the regional (hilar) lymph nodes. At the same time, there is spillover from the lymphatics into the bloodstream, with a seeding of virulent tubercle bacilli in almost all of the organs and tissues of the body. There would, of course, be a reseeding of other portions of the lungs, which, in some cases, will lead to more extensive pulmonary disease.[4, 7] Thus, in primary pulmonary tuberculosis, the disease may become a generalized infection within a few hours and certainly within a few days. The initial pulmonary focus at this time may not be demonstrable roentgenographically. Most of the disseminated tubercle bacilli will be taken up by mononuclear phagocytes residing in organs rich in these cells. Within these cells, the tubercle bacilli multiply almost as readily as they multiply at the site of the initial focus of infection in the lung. Therefore — and this must be emphasized — primary pulmonary tuberculosis, or primary tuberculosis, regardless of the portal of entry of the tubercle bacillus, is actually a disease of the reticuloendothelial system. It is not customary to think of primary tuberculosis as a widely disseminated disease of the reticuloendothelial system, nor do the textbooks of pathology or medicine emphasize this point.

The focus of attention is usually on the more easily discernible initial focus — the pulmonary lesion. It is worth pointing out here that this picture of the development of primary infection in tuberculosis differs in no way from the picture one encounters with infection due to other facultative intracellular parasites. For example, primary histoplasmosis and primary coccidioidomycosis show similar patterns. The initial focus of infection in both of these diseases is pulmonary, and dissemination of the parasite occurs in the same way — the parasites multiply intracellularly within mononuclear phagocytes, and the infection is primarily one of the reticuloendothelial system.

In spite of the intense cellular reaction that occurs at each site of deposition of a tubercle bacillus, whether in the lung or some other tissue, there is relatively little resistance to the multiplication of the tubercle bacilli. Whenever restriction of growth of virulent tubercle bacilli occurs, it is probably a consequence of a lower oxygen tension in certain tissues or cells (see Chapters 2 and 5). For example, the progression of tuberculous disease, as indicated by the rate of multiplication of the virulent tubercle bacilli, is much slower in organs such as the liver and spleen than it is in the lung. Again, this slower rate of multiplication of the tubercle bacilli in the liver and spleen is probably due to the fact that oxygen tension is lower in these organs than in the alveoli of the lung. In a small proportion of persons suffering from primary tuberculous infection, the process described above will continue until widespread tuberculous disease is present. If no treatment is given, this may easily result in death. However, in the majority of persons who acquire primary tuberculous infection, after a period of a few days or a few weeks, the following dramatic changes will occur. The rate of multiplication of the virulent tubercle bacilli markedly decreases; the pneumonic process will resolve; and the dissemination of tubercle bacilli by way of the lymphatics and bloodstream to other organs will cease. The same changes also occur in all other tissues where tubercle bacilli may have come to reside. Resolution of the disease process will then begin and may proceed to such a point that in many persons, little or no residue of the infection will remain. In some — and this occurs primarily in infants and children — all that may remain of the disease process may be what is called a *Ghon complex;* that is, a small calcified nodule in the lung and enlarged hilar lymph nodes.

Coincident with the changes just described and with the control of the infection, two immunologic manifestations appear. First, the affected individual will become tuberculin-positive. In other words, he will now show a reaction of delayed hypersensitivity to certain low molecular weight proteins or polypeptides that are found in the tubercle bacillus (see Chapter 7). We have already pointed out in Chapters 3 and 4 that mycobacteria markedly promote induction of delayed hypersensitivity to proteins, so it is no wonder that they exert the same effect for their own protein constituents. Second, the macrophages, within which the tubercle bacilli previously were able to multiply so readily, now have acquired the ability to markedly inhibit the multiplication of virulent tubercle bacilli. Therefore, since the tubercle bacilli are unable to grow within the cells, the disease process is arrested, and with time, many of the virulent cells are destroyed. In other words, the diseased person has now become immunized as a consequence of his immunologic reaction to the infection. This type of immunity is known as acquired cellular immunity to infection (see Chapters 6, 8, 9, 10, and 11). The nature of this acquired cellular immunity to infection has been reviewed in detail in Chapter 12. The essential point to

keep in mind here is that the control and resolution of primary tuberculosis depends mainly upon the immune response to the tubercle bacillus by the infected person. Even adequate chemotherapy, as effective as it is today, cannot do the entire job. The chemotherapy will retard multiplication of virulent tubercle bacilli and, in this manner, provide more time for the infected host to mount a powerful and long-lasting immune response. It is the immune response of the host which brings about eventual control of the disease rather than the chemotherapy.

We mentioned above that another immunologic manifestation, tuberculin hypersensitivity, also develops at approximately the same time as the acquired cellular immunity to infection. We then can reasonably ask the question: Why do not the majority of patients with primary tuberculosis develop the inflammatory reaction and the localized tissue destruction that so commonly occur in tuberculin sensitive human beings or in animals exposed to tubercle bacilli or their products? As a matter of fact, in a small proportion of persons with primary tuberculosis, extension and progress of the disease, if it is not halted by the forces of cellular immunity to infection, will show the destructive lesions so commonly associated with reinfection tuberculosis. However, since the majority of persons who develop primary tuberculosis do not have many manifestations such as these, we can only conclude that in the majority, the forces of acquired cellular immunity to infection develop rapidly and control the infection before reactions of delayed hypersensitivity can bring about much tissue destruction. Quantitative factors — that is, the number of tubercle bacilli and the degree of delayed hypersensitivity — probably also play an important role.

From the previous discussion, it is clear that primary tuberculosis is a disease that occurs in persons who have never been exposed to tubercle bacilli and therefore are not tuberculin sensitive, nor do they have any acquired cellular immunity to infection. Until acquired immunity develops as a consequence of the primary tuberculous disease, primary tuberculosis is, for the most part, a nondestructive disease process, with rapid dissemination of the infecting microorganisms to other organs and tissues. It is primarily a disease of the reticuloendothelial system.

REINFECTION TUBERCULOSIS

On the other hand, reinfection (secondary, adult) tuberculosis is a disease that occurs in persons who have been previously infected; therefore, it occurs in those persons who are tuberculin-sensitive, and it occurs in spite of the presence of acquired cellular immunity. Reinfection tuberculosis may come about as a result of recrudescence of an old infection (endogenous) or by reinfection from an active case (exogenous). Regardless of the source of the infecting tubercle bacilli, the initial lesion of reinfection tuberculosis is characterized by the occurrence of necrosis and by being circumscribed (localized). The necrosis is the result of the destructive nature of the inflammatory reaction of tuberculin hypersensitivity. The lesion is circumscribed, and therefore localized, because of cellular immunity that, operating in all of the adjacent tissues and within the lymphatic system that drains the lesion, prevents multiplication of tubercle bacilli and prevents the dissemination of tubercle bacilli by way of the lymphatics to other organs and tissues. Such disease may progress, however, by extension to adjacent tissues, as these become necrotized as a consequence of allergic inflammation. In the lung, spread of the infection may also occur when a bronchus is eroded and infected material from the lesion enters (bronchogenic spread) or by way of the bloodstream if a blood vessel is eroded (hematogenous spread).

The reasons for the local breakdown of resistance that may lead to a necrotic focus and tuberculous disease are not well known. It is known that any factor, such as age, degenerative disease, immunosuppressive therapy, and obstructive pulmonary disease, that lowers resistance to infection will promote the development of tuberculous disease in previously infected people. Therefore, there must be a local breakdown in cellular immunity to infection, which then permits growth of tubercle bacilli to the point where enough tuberculoprotein is produced to elicit a local necrotizing allergic reaction. Since necrosis is an outstanding feature of reinfection tuberculosis, the resolution of the disease process becomes far more difficult than that of a primary infection, which usually is overcome by acquired cellular immunity before the allergic state develops to the point where extensive necrosis occurs. It should be evident that when necrosis occurs, acquired cellular immunity to infection will vanish in the necrotic area because neither macrophages nor lymphocytes — the two cells primarily responsible for acquired immunity to infection — can function or survive. The lack of blood supply and sufficient oxygen makes the necrotic areas unsuitable places for lymphocytes and macrophages to function.

VARIABILITY IN THE MANIFESTATIONS OF PRIMARY AND REINFECTION TUBERCULOSIS

In connection with the picture of pathogenesis of primary and reinfection tuberculosis just presented, it is important to point out that in reinfection tuberculosis, the pathologic and clinical picture may vary from one that resembles full-blown reinfection disease, all the way to one that is closely similar to primary infection. The variability of this picture undoubtedly represents different levels of delayed tuberculin hypersensitivity and of acquired cellular immunity to infection that may be present in different persons at different times and at different ages. A great deal depends upon the extent of the previous exposure and, therefore, upon the amount of cellular immunity to infection and tuberculin hypersensitivity that may have developed. There also may be marked variability in the relative amount of tuberculin hypersensitivity and the acquired cellular immunity to infection that will develop in different persons. It is also of interest that typical primary tuberculosis is most frequently seen in infants and children. In adults, on the other hand, the primary infection—primary in the sense that this is the first exposure to virulent tubercle bacilli — may frequently more closely resemble reinfection tuberculosis than typical primary infection. This alternate picture in adults can probably be ascribed to two factors. First, the greater immunologic competency of adults may result in a much more rapid development of both acquired cellular immunity to infection and of tuberculin hypersensitivity in an infected person. Therefore, the manifestations of tuberculin hypersensitivity with focal necrosis may be more evident. Second, adults, by virtue of having lived much longer, have had a much greater chance to have been exposed to and infected with mycobacteria of other species that are widely distributed in nature (see Chapter 18). A high proportion of young adults (college students and medical students) are highly sensitive to proteins from *Mycobacterium intracellulare,* for example, or to a number of other atypical mycobacteria (see

Chapter 18). We also recognize from experimental studies that cross reactions may occur between protein antigens found in these mycobacteria and those found in *M. tuberculosis.* Such persons, even though never exposed to *M. tuberculosis,* might well have become sensitized by virtue of these atypical infections, to the point that, when exposed to *M. tuberculosis,* they would develop an allergic reaction to the tuberculoprotein found in *M. tuberculosis.* Some cellular immunity to infection with *M. tuberculosis* undoubtedly would also develop; thus, conditions might well prevail in which these persons, when infected with tubercle bacilli, might show, to varying degrees, the picture of reinfection tuberculosis.

DORMANCY OF TUBERCLE BACILLI

In connection with the pathogenesis of tuberculosis and especially when considering reinfection tuberculosis, it is important to realize that tubercle bacilli may remain viable but dormant within tissues of human beings, or animals for that matter, for many months, for years, or for even a lifetime. This follows from the fact that the acquired immune response will inhibit the multiplication of the tubercle bacilli but apparently will not confer on the cells the capacity for destruction of all of the tubercle bacilli. Therefore, tubercle bacilli within macrophages located in small tubercles in a lymph node, for example, or in the lung may be held in check for long periods but are perfectly capable of again metabolizing and dividing if local immunity is lowered. Evidence for this type of infection is provided by the fact that tuberculin hypersensitivity persists in many persons for years following a primary infection, even though all signs of tuberculous disease have disappeared. Also, a majority of the cases of tuberculosis that occur in human beings in the United States today are found in older people. These undoubtedly represent recrudescences of infection acquired many years before, possibly as young adults. It is important to differentiate between tuberculous infection, which can be defined as the presence of viable and frequently nonmultiplying virulent tubercle bacilli within the cells or tissues of a host, and tuberculous disease due to viable, multiplying tubercle bacilli within cells or tissues or necrotic foci and which produce overt manifestations of disease. Tuberculous infection is far more prevalent than tuberculous disease in human beings today. (For further discussion of this subject, see Chapters 5, 16, and 18.)

There is a firm experimental foundation showing that tubercle bacilli may persist for long periods in vivo in a viable but nonmultiplying state. This state has been demonstrated in infected mice, either as a consequence of drug treatment[12-16] or because of the forces of cellular immunity to infection.[3, 22, 23, 28] Hart and Rees,[8] in some very ingenious experiments, have shown that the tubercle bacilli, which in vivo are nonmultiplying, are still fully viable.

IMMUNE SUPPRESSION IN TUBERCULOSIS

To many readers of this chapter, the preceding description of the pathogenesis of tuberculosis may appear to be too much of a simplification. In one respect, this is perfectly correct because we have made no attempt to describe the many manifestations of tuberculous disease, nor have we dwelt upon many of the factors that influence the course of the disase. In addition, there has been little or no reference to the many and varied pathologic changes that may take place as a consequence of the disease or

to the differing picture of tuberculous disease, depending upon the particular tissue or tissues involved. This simplification of the picture of the pathogenesis of tuberculosis has been deliberate because we wish to focus attention upon the two major immunologic responses that are the determining factors in whether tuberculosis progresses or whether the spread of the disease is halted. After all, these two immunologic responses and the degree to which they function are the major factors that determine whether frank tuberculous disease will develop. Progression of tuberculous disease can only take place in the presence of inadequate cellular immunity to infection. Once progression does occur, all other manifestations, both clinical and pathologic, are secondary manifestations. For those readers who are interested, the many and varied clinical manifestations of tuberculosis can be found well described in textbooks of medicine;[1, 9] the gross and microscopic pathologic changes are well described in textbooks of pathology[19] and in other books[2, 10, 18, 27] and monographs.[17] These sources should be consulted by anyone wishing further information on the manifestations of tuberculous disease or the tissue changes that may occur.

However, since we are primarily concerned here with basic immunologic responses of the host to tuberculous infection, we are interested in the state of these immunologic responses in the face of overt tuberculous disease, or in disseminated, progressive tuberculosis in the human being. It has been known for many years that patients with far-advanced and particularly disseminated tuberculosis may suffer a loss of dermal hypersensitivity to tuberculin. In other words, they become anergic.[18] More recent studies have shown that this loss of hypersensitivity may not be restricted only to those patients with far-advanced overwhelming or terminal disease. In fact, it has been shown that in the majority of patients with tuberculosis, their cellular immune responses may be depressed. This depressed immune state may be manifested by reduced dermal hypersensitivity to tuberculin or by a reduction in the capacity of peripheral blood lymphocytes to react to tuberculin.[11, 26, 29] Also, a significant number of patients may have reduced capacity to react to other antigens that elicit delayed-type hypersensitivity, such as mumps vaccine and candida antigen. In addition, significant numbers of patients may lose the capacity to develop delayed hypersensitivity to dinitrochlorobenzene.[6, 11, 25] This, of course, indicates a considerable reduction in the capacity of such patients to develop cell-mediated immunity. Skin test reactivity to the tuberculin, however, may be maintained even in the face of a lack of capacity to respond to sensitization to dinitrochlorobenzene. On the other hand, patients may lose capacity to react to tuberculin, even though the disease does not seem to be extensive enough to bring about an anergic state.[21, 24, 29, 30] Of course, negative skin tests will be seen most commonly in severe tuberculous infection. It is of interest that many patients with tuberculosis who have a negative skin test may regain the capacity to show dermal reactivity to tuberculin following adequate chemotherapy.[29, 30] This is regarded as a good prognostic sign, since the patient can then make use of his own immune defensive forces.

The lack of capacity of some patients to react to tuberculin is of great importance, however, in another respect. It means that a negative skin test cannot be relied upon to exclude tuberculosis. At one time, it was thought that no one with tuberculosis would react negatively to tuberculin unless he had far-advanced, severe disease; therefore, a negative tuberculin test in the face of a pulmonary lesion, for example, or even what might be disseminated tuberculosis, has been taken as evidence that the dis-

ease cannot be tuberculosis. This has led to some tragic errors in diagnosis in which persons with negative tuberculin tests, but with widespread tuberculosis, have not received chemotherapy because in view of the negative tuberculin test, it was thought that the disease must have another etiology.[5]

It must also be kept in mind that dermal hypersensitivity to tuberculin can be lost in various states of immune suppression. Immune suppression of cellular immunity may occur in a number of viral infections (such as measles), in certain malignant states (such as lymphoreticular malignancies), in Hodgkin's disease, or in patients undergoing immunosuppressive therapy (for example, with steroids for a nontuberculous condition). Therefore, the diagnostic significance placed upon a negative tuberculin test should not be too great. Conversely, of course, a positive tuberculin test does not necessarily mean tuberculous disease.

The common occurrence of immunosuppression in tuberculosis raises another very interesting point. In those patients from whom evidence of immunosuppression is obtained, for example, by a negative tuberculin test or by a failure of peripheral lymphocytes to respond to stimulation with PPD, is the immunosuppression the result of the active tuberculous infection, or is the disease a consequence of immunosuppression due to some factor other than tuberculosis? In other words, what is the cause and effect relationship? It is well known that certain conditions such as pregnancy (see Chapter 7), aging (see Chapter 7),[6, 20, 25] or malnutrition may lower the capacity of persons to develop cellular immunity. Persons who fall into one of these categories and develop tuberculosis are usually regarded as having done so because of a lowering of cellular immunity to infection. On the other hand, in many patients with tuberculosis, predisposing immunosuppressive factors cannot be detected.[29] In such diseased persons, the question just stated remains unanswered. However, as we have just pointed out, patients who are either partially or completely anergic, and who respond to treatment with chemotherapeutic agents usually find their capacity to show cellular immune reactions restored.[29, 30] This certainly supports the argument that regardless of the factors involved in the initiation of tuberculous disease, progressive disease does tend to maintain an anergic state, whether partial or complete. Thus, tuberculous infection itself has, or can have, a suppressive effect on cellular immunity and, therefore, upon the capacity of a person to mount an adequate defense to the invading microorganisms.

REFERENCES

1. Beeson, P. B., and McDermott, W. (eds.): Textbook of Medicine. 14th ed. Philadelphia, W. B. Saunders Co., 1975.
2. Canetti, G.: The Tubercle Bacillus in the Pulmonary Lesion of Man. New York, Springer Publishing Co., Inc., 1955.
3. Fenner, F., Martin, S. P., and Pierce, C. H.: The enumeration of viable tubercle bacilli in cultures and infected tissues. Ann. N.Y. Acad. Sci. 52:751, 1949.
4. Fok, J. S., Ho, R. S., Arora, P. K., Harding, G. E., and Smith, D. W.: Host-parasite relationships in experimental airborne tuberculosis. V. Lack of hematogenous dissemination of *Mycobacterium tuberculosis* to the lungs in animals vaccinated with bacille Calmette-Guérin. J. Infect. Dis. 133:137, 1976.
5. Grieco, M. H., and Chmel, H.: Acute disseminated tuberculosis as a diagnostic problem. A clinical study based on twenty-eight cases. Am. Rev. Respir. Dis. 109:554, 1974.
6. Gross, L.: Immunological defect in aged population and its relationship to cancer. Cancer 18:201, 1965.
7. Harding, G. E., and Smith, D. W.: Host-parasite relationships in experimental airborne tuberculosis. VI. Influence of vaccination with bacille Calmette-Guérin on the onset and/or extent of hematogenous dissemination of virulent *Mycobacterium tuberculosis* to the lungs. J. Infect. Dis. 136:439, 1977.
8. Hart, P. D., and Rees, R. J. W.: Effect of macrocyclon in acute and chronic pulmonary tuberculous infection in mice as shown by viable and total bacterial counts. Br. J. Exp. Pathol. 41:414, 1960.
9. Harvey, A. M., Johns, R. J., Owens, A. H., and Ross, R. S. (eds.): The Principles and Practice of Medicine. 19th ed. New York, Appleton-Century-Crofts, 1976.
10. Long, E. R.: The Chemistry and Chemotherapy of Tuberculosis. 3rd ed. Baltimore, The Williams & Wilkins Company, 1958.
11. Malaviya, A. N., Sehgal, K. L., Kumar, R., and Dingley, H. B.: Factors of delayed hypersensitivity in pulmonary tuberculosis. Am. Rev. Respir. Dis. 112:49, 1975.
12. McCune, R., Deuschle, K., and McDermott, W.: The delayed appearance of isoniazid antagonism by pyridoxine *in vivo*. Am. Rev. Tuberc. 76:1100, 1957.
13. McCune, R., Lee, S. H., Deuschle, K., and McDermott, W.: Ineffectiveness of isoniazid in modifying the phenomenon of microbial persistence. Am. Rev. Tuberc. 76:1106, 1957.
14. McCune, R. M., Deuschle, K., Jordahl, C., Des Prez, R., Muschenheim, C., and McDermott, W.: The influence of streptovaricin used alone and with isoniazid in an experimental tuberculous infection in animals, and some clinical observations. Am. Rev. Tuberc. 75:659, 1957.
15. McCune, R. M., Tompsett, R., and McDermott, W.: The fate of *Mycobacterium tuberculosis* in mouse tissues as determined by the microbial enumeration technique. II. The conversion of tuberculous infection to the latent state by the administration of pyrazinamide and a companion drug. J. Exp. Med. 104:763, 1956.
16. McCune, R. M., Jr., and Tompsett, R.: Fate of *Mycobacterium tuberculosis* in mouse tissues as determined by the microbial enumeration technique. I. The persistence of drug-susceptible tubercle bacilli in the tissues despite prolonged antimicrobial therapy. J. Exp. Med. 104:737, 1956.
17. Medlar, E. M.: The behavior of pulmonary tuberculous lesions. A pathological study. Am. Rev. Tuberc. 71(Suppl.): 1, (March, Part II) 1955.
18. Rich, A. R.: The Pathogenesis of Tuberculosis. 2nd ed. Springfield, Ill., Charles C Thomas, 1951.
19. Robbins, S. L.: Pathologic Basis of Disease. Philadelphia, W. B. Saunders Co., 1974.
20. Roberts-Thomson, I. C., Whittingham, S., Youngchaiyud, U., and Mackay, I. R.: Ageing, immune response, and mortality. Lancet 2:368, 1974.
21. Sayed, H., Hershfield, E., Gurwith, M., and Schollenberg, E.: Cell-mediated reactions in tuberculosis (Abstract). Clin. Res. 21:1053, 1973.

22. Sever, J. L., and Youmans, G. P.: The enumeration of nonpathogenic viable tubercle bacilli from the organs of mice. Am. Rev. Tuberc. *75*:280, 1957.
23. Sever, J. L., and Youmans, G. P.: Enumeration of viable tubercle bacilli from the organs of nonimmunized and immunized mice. Am. Rev. Tuberc. *76*:616, 1957.
24. Thomas, J. W., Naiman, S. C., and Clements, D.: Lymphocytic transformation with phytohemagglutinin: II. In the tuberculous patient. Can. Med. Assoc. J. *97*:836, 1967.
25. Waldorf, D. S., Willkens, R. F., and Decker, J. L.: Impaired delayed hypersensitivity in an aging population. J.A.M.A. *203*:831, 1968.
26. Waxman, J., and Lockshin, M.: *In vitro* and *in vivo* cellular immunity in anergic mili-

ary tuberculosis. Am. Rev. Respir. Dis. *107*:661, 1973.
27. Willis, H. S., and Cummings, M. M.: Diagnostic and Experimental Methods in Tuberculosis. 2nd ed. Springfield, Ill., Charles C Thomas, 1952.
28. Yamamura, Y., Walter, A., and Bloch, H.: Bacterial populations in experimental murine tuberculosis. I. Studies in normal mice. J. Infect. Dis. *106*:211, 1960.
29. Zeitz, S. J., Ostrow, J. H., and Van Arsdel, P. P., Jr.: Humoral and cellular immunity in the anergic tuberculosis patient. J. Allergy Clin. Immunol. *53*:20, 1974.
30. Zeitz, S. J., Ostrow, J. H., and Van Arsdel, P. P., Jr.: Immunologic features of the anergic tuberculosis patient (Abstract). J. Allergy *49*:93, 1972.

15

Experimental Models of Tuberculous Disease

INTRODUCTION

In earlier chapters of this book (Chapters 8, 9, 10, 11, 12, and 13), we have dealt extensively with the immunizing potency of viable and killed mycobacterial cells and of certain components of the tubercle bacillus. In these earlier chapters, when discussing our own results and the results of others, we have said very little about the reliability and validity of the procedures used to test the immunizing power of mycobacteria and mycobacterial components. We have, more or less, let the reader assume that the methods used were suitable, although we did point out (in Chapter 8) the lack of validity in comparing the im-

munizing power of two vaccine preparations, utilizing only a single immunizing dose of both, or of either one alone. We stressed that it is always essential to do dose-response titrations before the potency of two vaccine preparations can be validly compared.

Examination of the results and the experimental procedures published by different investigators can only lead to the conclusion that the methods used experimentally to evaluate the immune response to tuberculosis in different laboratories are not equally reliable (reproducible) or valid (actually measures the immune response). One major factor is the failure of many investigators to realize the numerous factors that can affect the outcome of

327

TABLE 15–1. **Possible Combinations of Vaccine Test System Variables***

Animal species	Mouse, guinea pig, rabbit
Route of vaccination	Intradermal, subcutaneous, intraperitoneal
Amount of vaccine	Low, medium, high
Vaccination-infection interval	4 weeks, 6 weeks, 8 weeks
Route of infection	Intravenous, intraperitoneal, respiratory
Level of infection	Low, medium, high.
Infection-sacrifice interval	4 weeks, 6 weeks, 8 weeks
Virulence of infecting strain	Low, medium, high
Response measured	Survival, spleen weight, microbial enumeration

*Possible combinations = 3^9 = 19,683

Modified from Smith, D W., Wiegeshaus, E. H., Stark, R. H., and Harding, G. E.: Models for potency assay of tuberculosis vaccines. *In* Chamberlayne, E. C. (ed.): Status of Immunization in Tuberculosis in 1971. DHEW Publication No. (NIH) 72-68, 1972.

an immunization experiment. A number of these factors have been given by Smith and coworkers[84] and will be found listed in Table 15–1. Failure to recognize the important influence that might result from the action of such uncontrolled variables on the outcome of an experiment could account for many of the disparate results obtained by different investigators when testing the same vaccine preparation.

Smith and colleagues[84] conducted an experiment under the auspices of the World Health Organization in which they distributed five different vaccines to a number of different laboratories around the world and asked them to assess the immunizing potency of these vaccines, using whatever in vivo test systems they usually employed. Table 15–2 shows the conditions of this experiment in terms of fixed and not-fixed parameters of each vaccine.

In this study, it should be noted that each investigator used one vaccine dose only, that the vaccination challenge interval was the same for all, that the challenge strain of virulent tubercle bacilli was the same for all, but that a number of other factors were not standardized. The particular vaccine preparations employed in this study apparently were shipped from Dr. Smith's laboratory and presumably were the same for all laboratories. These vaccines are listed in Table 15–3.

Following completion of the experiment, the vaccines were ranked by each laboratory in order of effectiveness. Apparently each laboratory used its own criteria for evaluating effective prevention of tuberculous disease. The results of the study are shown in Tables 15–4 and 15–5. The laboratories did not agree on the relative potency of the five vaccines.

To Smith and his coworkers,[84] the implications of these findings were very clear. In their own words, they were:

1) Disagreement between laboratories about the efficacy of tuberculosis vaccines is in part due to differences in test systems in which they are measured; 2) laboratories cannot build upon the work of another laboratory that uses a different test system, and 3) it has not been established that the response measured by one laboratory and termed immunity is related to a different response measured by another laboratory and also termed immunity.

Smith and coworkers[84] felt that these studies clearly point to the basic problem that each investigator studying immunity to tuberculosis uses a different test system for measuring the immune status of an animal. They felt that the results of this investigation have demonstrated that the potency of a vaccine varies with the test system in which it is measured; and yet, as they point out, we do not know which, if any, of these systems pre-

TABLE 15–2. **Collaborative Experiment Design***

Parameters Fixed	Parameters Not Fixed
Vaccination dose	Test animal
Vaccination-challenge interval	Vaccination route
Challenge strain	Challenge route
	Challenge-sacrifice interval
	Response to infection measured

*Participating laboratories—Czechoslovakia, Hungary, Japan, England, Rumania, West Germany, Soviet Union, France, Denmark, United States.
From Smith, D. W., Wiegeshaus, E. H., Stark, F. H., and Harding, G. E.: Models for potency assay of tuberculosis vaccines. *In* Chamberlayne, E. C. (ed.): Status of Immunization in Tuberculosis in 1971. DHEW Publication No. (NIH) 72-68, 1972.

TABLE 15–3. **Collaborative Experiment Vaccines**

VACCINES	
A	BCG—Live
B	*Mycobacterium avium*—Live
C	H37Rv—Formalin killed in saline
D	H37Rv—Formalin killed in oil
E	H37Rv—Extraction residue in oil

From Smith, D. W., Wiegeshaus, E. H., Stark, R. H., and Harding, G. E.: Models for potency assay of tuberculosis vaccines. *In* Chamberlayne, E. C. (ed.): Status of Immunization in Tuberculosis in 1971. DHEW Publication No. (NIH) 72-68, 1972.

dicts the efficacy of a tuberculosis vaccine for man.

We do not have space here for a detailed analysis of this study, nor for a subsequent one, similar in nature and under the control of this same group,[84] that gave essentially similar results. We should point out here, though, that the validity of the data generated by the first study is completely vitiated by the fact that only one vaccination dose from each vaccine preparation was used. It is impossible to compare two immunizing preparations on the basis of single doses. We have seen in Chapter 8 that unless dose-response curves are obtained as a result of using multiple immunizing doses, valid comparisons are impossible. This has also been emphasized by Jesperson and coworkers[34, 35] and stems from the fact that if single doses are arbitrarily selected, vaccines that actually differ markedly in their immunizing power may appear to be equally effective. Stated another way, a weak vaccine at a higher dose may well appear superior to a smaller dose of a very much more effective vaccine. In Chapter 8, Figures 8–1 and 8–3 clearly reveal this (pp. 228 and 230).

TABLE 15–4. **Results from 7 of 21 Test Systems in the Collaborative Experiments**

Test System	Vaccines Ranked According to Efficacy					
	MOST ACTIVE ————————————————→ LEAST ACTIVE					
II	A	D	C	NV	E	B
III	A	C	B	E	D	NV
V	C	A	B	E	D	NV
VII	B	C	A	D	NV	E
IX	D	A	E	B	C	NV
XI	A	D	E	C	NV	B
XVII	E	NV	C	A	D	B

From Smith, D. W., Wiegeshaus, E. H., Stark, R. H., and Harding, G. E.: Models for potency assay of tuberculosis vaccines. *In* Chamberlayne, E. C. (ed.): Status of Immunization in Tuberculosis in 1971. DHEW Publication No. (NIH) 72-68, 1972.

TABLE 15–5. **Ranking of Potency of Formalin-Killed H37Rv Suspended in Saline or in Oil**

19 test systems reported a significant difference in potency for the two vaccines,

BUT

12 reported the saline vaccine was superior to the oil vaccine, and

7 reported the oil vaccine was superior to the saline vaccine.

Modified from Smith, D. W., Wiegeshaus, E. H., Stark, R. H., and Harding, G. E.: Models for potency assay of tuberculosis vaccines. *In* Chamberlayne, E. C. (ed.): Status of Immunization in Tuberculosis in 1971. DHEW Publication No. (NIH) 72-68, 1972.

The results of the study by Smith and colleagues[84] could just as easily be interpreted, because of the single dose of each vaccine employed, as indicating that the vaccine doses used were of approximately equal potency and, regardless of the testing methods used, their position in the ranking of immunizing effectiveness was just a matter of chance. Since there is a large inherent error in any in vivo model used for the testing of immunizing potency, this could easily happen. In the subsequent experiment by Smith and coworkers[84] just referred to, two vaccinating doses were employed; however, no meaningful dose-response curve can be obtained with only two doses of any agent..

While it is obvious that the potency of a given vaccine may vary depending upon the assay method employed, when comparisons are made between vaccines, the *relative* potency of the vaccines can be determined almost independent of the methods employed, provided graded immunizing doses are used and adequate dose-response curves are constructed.

It must be granted that variations in one or more of the factors listed in Table 15–1 may seriously affect the reliability, validity, and sensitivity of a procedure designed to test the immune response of an animal species to vaccine preparations. However, the influence of all of these factors can be minimized, providing the investigator has a clear understanding of the mechanisms of immunity in tuberculosis and, therefore, a clear understanding of what he is actually trying to measure. We have seen in Chapters 8, 9, 10, 11, and 12 that the major manifestation of immunity to tuberculosis is inhibition of mycobacterial multiplication within cells of the reticuloendothelial system. Therefore, in any test for immunity, the procedure used should be one that will correctly reflect the increase in capacity of the cells of the reticuloendothelial system to inhibit the intracellular multiplication of tubercle bacilli. With this objective clearly in mind, it is not too difficult to devise, regardless of the animal species involved, a reliable, valid, and sensitive method for the measurement of immunity to tuberculosis.

Two general procedures have been employed by microbiologists to measure, on the one hand, the virulence of microorganisms and, on the other, the resistance of the human host to infection. The first is to record the percentage of animals that respond as a function of the challenge doses (the quantal response). In other words, experimental animals are injected with a wide range of infecting doses of a given microorganism, and the percentage of animals that respond to each dose is plotted in an appropriate manner against the infecting dose. The second procedure is to determine the time required between infection of hosts with a single dose and the appearance of a detectable reaction (the graded response), such as death or some other easily measured manifestation of infection. In experimental models of tuberculous disease, the most commonly used response has been the graded response. The reason for this stems from the fact that in most experimental animals, there is only a very narrow range of doses of tubercle bacilli that will give a uni-

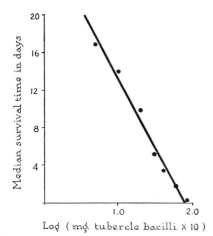

Log (mg. tubercle bacilli X 10)

FIGURE 15–1. The effect of the size of the infecting dose of *M. tuberculosis* (H37Rv) on the median survival time (Semilog plot). (From Youmans, G. P., and Youmans, A. S.: The relation between the size of the infecting dose of tubercle bacilli and the survival time of mice. Am. Rev. Tuberc. 64:534, 1951.)

form response. In tuberculosis, at least in mice, the response to tuberculous infection tends to be a somewhat "all-or-none" phenomenon. Within a rather narrow range of large doses, all of the animals will show a response; however, with doses only slightly smaller, not all of the animals will respond. This all-or-none type of response in mice is illustrated in Figure 15–1. The curve shown is constructed from actual experimental laboratory data. When less than 0.25 mg per mouse was administered intravenously (not shown in Figure 15–1), the distribution of deaths was not uniform, and a median survival time could not be calculated.[102]

On the other hand, if a single suitably selected infecting dose of a given strain of *M. tuberculosis* is injected into animals, a record can be kept of the response of the animals to this infection, usually in terms of death. Other responses, such as lung density,[10] omentum weight,[29, 73] time of appearance of tubercle bacilli in the spleen,[95] or development of an ulcer following injection of tubercle bacilli into the skin of guinea pigs,[71] can be used. The average response of a group of animals so infected will then be a

function of the virulence of the culture of *M. tuberculosis* used, on the one hand, and the resistance of the host, on the other. In this way, virulence of different strains of tubercle bacilli can be measured, or the effect of a variety of factors, including vaccination, on host resistance can be determined. The details of these methods of measuring host response to infection and their mathematic basis can be found in the excellent reviews by Meynell and Meynell,[55] by Shortley and Wilkins,[79] and by other authors.[6, 20]

In the following discussion, we will be dealing primarily with the response to tuberculous infection in the laboratory mouse. Other animals, such as guinea pigs,[13-16, 21, 22, 81, 91, 92] rabbits,[38, 43, 44, 57, 70, 85, 89] rats,[24, 25, 86] chickens,[87] hamsters,[11, 36] dogs,[19, 26-28] and rhesus monkeys,[4, 74, 75] can also be used; however, the labor and expense of handling and maintaining such larger animals makes them less suitable laboratory animals than the laboratory mouse. Some further reference to guinea pigs and rhesus monkeys will be made below, but as already stated, the major emphasis of our discussion will be on the use of the laboratory mouse.

Although we have already stated that the designing of a reliable, valid, sensitive measure of host response to virulent tubercle bacilli and, therefore, to the measurement of the degree of immunity in mice is not too difficult, there are certain factors that are very important to keep in mind and that must be standardized in an appropriate manner before the in vivo assay system is ready for use. These factors are: 1) the virulence of the strain of tubercle bacillus to be employed and, in particular, an understanding of what is required to maintain the virulence at a constant level; 2) the route of inoculation of the challenge dose of virulent tubercle bacilli; 3) depending upon the route of inoculation, the size (number of tubercle bacilli) of the challenge dose; 4) the strain of mouse to be employed; and 5) the measurement of the response of the experimental animals to tuberculous infection.

VIRULENCE OF MYCOBACTERIA USED FOR CHALLENGE

Mycobacterial strains may vary somewhat in virulence. However, most any moderately or highly virulent strain can be employed if an appropriate infecting dose is selected. How to make this selection of a suitable infecting dose is outlined here.

The most important reason for failure to obtain a uniform response in mice infected with *Mycobacterium tuberculosis* arises from the failure to realize that cultures of virulent cells regularly mutate and produce mutant cells of much reduced virulence. This has been emphasized by Baker and colleagues,[2] by McKee and coworkers,[54] and by Youmans and his coworkers.[96] It is, therefore, of the utmost importance to circumvent the replacement of virulent cells with mutant cells of reduced virulence. This can be done most effectively by growing the microorganisms on the surface of the modified Proskauer and Beck synthetic medium (see Chapter 2), or any other liquid medium. These cultures should be subcultured at least every 5 to 7 days, and care must be taken to utilize for subculture the filmy type of surface growth of the virulent cells. Frequently, islands of a piled-up, more waxy type of growth will appear in these flasks. These are mutants, which are much less virulent and should not be used for infecting animals. The mutant waxy-appearing cells will, in a matter of a few weeks, almost completely replace the virulent cells in the surface pellicle. Other methods can also be used. Once a fully virulent culture is obtained, suspensions can be prepared by slow freezing[23] and maintained at $-70°$ C, then reconstituted as

needed. This process has been claimed by Grover and coworkers[23] to result in fully viable and virulent suspensions of cells when reconstituted. Further details on the maintenance of virulence of mycobacterial cultures can be found in Kanai[37] and in Youmans and Youmans.[100] If cells of a fully virulent strain are serially subcultured in a liquid medium containing a dispersing agent, such as Tween 80, virulence will rapidly become reduced. There is no way in which the fully virulent cells in such a culture can be selected for transfer.

ROUTE OF INJECTION OF THE INFECTING DOSE

One would hardly expect that there would be much controversy over the route to use for injecting the challenge dose of virulent tubercle bacilli when testing for the development of immunity in mice, and in fact, the intravenous route has been the one most commonly employed. However, one school of thought espouses the position that the intravenous route is unsuitable because, in human beings, tuberculosis is a pulmonary disease and the natural route of infection of human beings with tubercle bacilli is by way of the lungs. Therefore, any experimental procedure that does not use the intrapulmonary route for challenge cannot provide information on the effectiveness of a vaccination procedure for the prevention of tuberculosis in human beings. This argument is, of course, a spurious one and merely reveals a lack of understanding of the pathogenesis of tuberculosis. We have concluded in Chapter 14 that although the initial infection with *Mycobacterium tuberculosis* in human beings in most cases is in the lung, the microorganisms are rapidly disseminated throughout the body, setting up what is actually a disease of the reticuloendothelial system. From the evidence presented in Chapters 9 and 10, it is also clear that the cells of the reticuloendothelial system (the macrophages), together with T-lymphocytes, are responsible for mediating immunity to tuberculosis. Therefore, the intravenous route of injection that most directly introduces the challenge infecting dose to the cells responsible for immunity to tuberculosis is to be preferred. In addition, an infecting dose can be more uniformly distributed to the various cells of the reticuloendothelial system by the intravenous route. Other routes, such as the intrapulmonary (by inhalation of an aerosol containing virulent tubercle bacilli), subcutaneous, intracerebral, or intraperitoneal, lead to far less uniform distribution of the infecting inoculum and, therefore, to an experimental setup in which there is apt to be a greater variation in the response of different animals to infection.

The argument that the intrapulmonary route of infection should be employed because it is the natural route of infection in man does have some validity, when the purpose of a vaccine protection experiment is solely to determine how well the vaccine protects against aerosol infection of an animal with virulent cells of *Mycobacterium tuberculosis*. It would be reasonable to insist that all vaccines be tested for their ability to protect against aerogenic infection with *M. tuberculosis* before they are used in man. However, for this purpose, it would be much better to conduct such experiments with subhuman primates because of their much greater resemblance to man, both in physiology and in response to tuberculous infection. Such studies have been done, for example, in rhesus monkeys,[4, 22] and it is quite clear that following subcutaneous vaccination with BCG or mycobacterial RNA, an increased resistance to intrapulmonary infection can be detected.

However, in basic studies on the nature of the immune response to tuberculosis in mice, the intravenous route of infection is to be preferred. First of all, as we have already stated, more uniform distribution of the infecting virulent tubercle bacilli can be made to the organs that harbor the most reticuloendothelial cells. Second, the primary organ affected—or the "target organ," if one prefers — is the lung, and by the intravenous route a relatively uniform seeding of the lung with virulent tubercle bacilli can be done with ease. At least it can be done with much greater ease than by use of the intrapulmonary route, where complicated and expensive apparatus are needed to assure the production of an aerosol containing the desired number of virulent tubercle bacilli. In addition, for the purpose of safety, appropriate chambers in which animals can be housed for a period to inhale the desired number of tubercle bacilli are needed. This of course can be done; however, it is merely a far more complicated and less safe procedure that, in the long run, does not provide any more information on the immune status of the infected mouse than can be obtained by the much simpler intravenous route of administration of the infecting dose.

In fact, not only is the infecting of animals such as the mouse by the aerosol route fraught with expense, trouble, and danger to personnel, but it can, under certain circumstances, provide misleading results. It has been demonstrated by a number of investigators[4, 22, 23, 82, 83, 93] that following an intracutaneous or subcutaneous inoculation with BCG vaccine in guinea pigs, rabbits, or monkeys, when a challenge infecting dose of virulent tubercle bacilli is administered by aerosol, an increased resistance to such infection in the vaccinated animals can be detected. This is not the case, however, in mice. A number of studies[42, 83, 107] have shown that following BCG vaccination of mice by the intraperitoneal or subcutaneous routes, no indication of increased immunity to infection can be detected in these animals when the challenge infecting dose is administered by the pulmonary route. Yet, as we will see in Chapter 17, when human beings are given BCG vaccine by the intracutaneous or subcutaneous route, there is a marked increase in resistance to infection with virulent tubercle bacilli that happen to lodge in the lung. The mice previously referred to that had been vaccinated by the intraperitoneal or subcutaneous route can be shown, however, to be much more resistant to infection with virulent tubercle bacilli that are administered by the intravenous route, and this includes a markedly increased resistance to infection of the pulmonary tissue seeded with these intravenously administered tubercle bacilli. No fully adequate explanation has been offered for the paradoxical response of mice. We can surmise that for some reason, in the mouse, the small number of tubercle bacilli that arrive in the alveoli of the mouse when aerosol infection is used do not provide enough of a stimulus to the lymphatic and reticuloendothelial systems of the mouse to set off the secondary, or recall, immune response, which is so important for the control of tuberculous infection in these animals. We will see later on in this chapter that the major immune response in mice actually consists of rapid recall of the immunity engendered by the vaccinating procedure. In the other animals — the guinea pig, rabbit, monkey, and man — apparently, the pulmonary infecting dose either encounters fully immune cells or rapidly stimulates the secondary immune response. No systematic study has been made of the nature of this difference in response between mice and other animals. It should be clear, however, that the aerosol method of administering challenge doses of virulent tubercle bacilli to vaccinated mice might well result in a very effective vaccine for human use being labeled inactive because it did not control the pulmonary infecting dose.

By using the intravenous route for challenge, we can be more certain of maintaining the validity of our testing procedure; that is, we are directly challenging the cells responsible for inhibiting the multiplication of tubercle bacilli in the immune response, and we are increasing to a maximum the reliability of our testing procedure (i.e., the reproducibility of our test). Data showing the very high degree of reproducibility of infection that is produced in mice by the intravenous route has been published by Youmans and Youmans.[105] Table 15–6, taken from that publication, shows the response of nonvaccinated mice to a standard infecting dose of tubercle bacilli over a five-year period. There was no significant deviation in the mean survival time from experiment to experiment over this extended period.

SIZE OF THE INFECTING DOSE OF VIRULENT TUBERCLE BACILLI

Probably equally, if not more, controversial has been the question of the size of the infecting dose of virulent tubercle bacilli used to assess immunity to tuberculosis. It is necessary when using the intravenous route, and evaluating the immune response by recording survival time, to use numerically relatively large numbers of virulent human-type tubercle bacilli, in the range of 10^6 to 10^7 viable cells.[72] This has been necessary because of the innate capacity of mice to rapidly develop immunity to a challenge dose of virulent tubercle bacilli. Because of this capacity, large infecting doses of intravenously administered tubercle bacilli must be used in order to get a uniform response, in terms of mortality, in control nonvaccinated mice. Great difficulty is encountered in assessing the magnitude of the immune

TABLE 15–6.   **Median Survival Times in Days of Groups of Strong A Strain Mice Injected Intravenously with 1.0 mg of the H37Rv Strain of *M. tuberculosis***

Year	JAN.	FEB.	MAR.	APR.	MAY	JUNE	JULY	AUG.	SEPT.	OCT.	NOV.	DEC.	Yearly Means
1950		12.5	13.5	15.0	15.0	14.0	13.0			13.0	13.0	13.5	13.57
		13.0	14.5	16.0	14.0	14.0	13.5			12.5		11.5	
			14.0		14.0	13.5				.11.5			
			15.0		12.5								
1951	12.5	12.0		14.5	15.5	11.5	14.5	15.0	12.5	14.5	12.5	14.0	13.53
	14.0	12.5		14.0	13.5	11.5		16.0	15.0	14.0	12.5		
	14.0					11.0		16.0	12.0	13.0	11.5		
						13.5				14.5	13.0		
										15.5			
1952	16.0	13.0	12.0	12.0	11.0	11.5	12.5	13.0	14.5	13.0	15.0	13.5	13.11
	14.0	14.5	12.5	14.5	12.5	14.5	14.5	10.0	14.5	14.0	12.5	10.5	
	14.0	13.5	11.0	12.5	12.0	13.5			10.5	11.5	11.5	15.5	
	13.0	14.5	15.0	13.0	14.0				12.5	13.5	14.5		
		12.0			13.5					13.5			
1953	15.5	13.0	11.5	14.5	12.5	12.5	13.0	12.5	13.0	13.5	13.0	14.5	12.70
	11.5	12.5	14.5	12.0	12.0	11.5	12.0		13.0	14.0	14.5	13.5	
	14.0	12.0		12.5	14.5	10.5	10.5		12.5	12.0		12.0	
	12.0	12.5		13.0	12.0	12.5	11.5		14.5	12.5			
					13.5		15.0			11.5			
					10.0								
1954	18.0	14.5	14.0	12.0	14.0	15.0	13.5	12.0	13.0	13.5	13.0	14.5	13.47
	14.0	13.5	13.0	12.0	13.5		12.5	10.5	13.5	12.0	14.0	12.5	
	13.5		12.5	13.5	14.0		11.5	12.5	11.0	14.5	14.5	12.0	
									15.0	19.5		14.0	
										12.0		14.0	
Monthy means	14.0	13.10	13.21	13.40	13.21	12.53	12.88	13.05	13.13	13.43	13.11	13.25	

From Youmans, G. P., and Youmans, A. S.: Response of mice to standard infecting doses of *Mycobacterium tuberculosis* var. *hominis*. Proc. Soc. Exp. Biol. Med. *90*:238, 1955.

response if an immune response to the challenge infection occurs in a significant portion of the nonvaccinated control mice. It is essential in these animals to use an infecting dose large enough to produce a uniform distribution of deaths, or other responses. This can only be done if the infecting dose is large enough to overwhelm any immune response before it can have a significant effect on the end point being used. Death is the usual end point, and we will frequently refer to the normal distribution of death in future discussions. In immunized mice, on the other hand, having once already developed an immune response, the recall of immunity will be so rapid that a significant number of the animals will not die as soon as the controls, and therefore, the proportion of animals that live beyond the time that the control animals die can be used as a measure of the immune response. This will be examined in greater detail in the last section of this chapter on the evaluation of the immune response, but it is essential to mention it here to set the stage for a discussion of the validity of using numerically large infecting doses intravenously in mice.

The doses of infecting virulent tubercle bacilli of the magnitude mentioned in the preceding paragraph have been derogatorily referred to by a number of investigators as "massive." The implication, of course, is that they are so large that no valid information can be obtained from their use on the immune status of the infected animals. The argument is also made that such numerically large infecting doses are completely out of line with the number of tubercle bacilli human beings inhale when they become naturally infected. Human beings under natural conditions probably do not inhale more than a few tubercle bacilli.

These arguments are, of course, specious. When measuring the response of animals to an infectious agent, it is only necessary that the number of microorganisms used be small enough so that each viable cell of the infecting inoculant can multiply exponentially for a long enough period that the host can respond in a typical manner. The lethal number of tubercle bacilli for most strains of mice is about 10^{10} cells (see Fig. 15–1).[102] This allows, then, virulent cells of a 10^7 inoculum to increase some three or four logs in number before death will occur; this is time for many cell divisions. Actually, if there is an allowance for the infecting microorganism to increase in number by only one log, in most circumstances, this would be enough to obtain a true measure of the host response. The book by Meynell and Meynell[55] and the review of Shortley and Wilkins[79] should be consulted for the experimental basis for such statements and for the mathematic treatment of data generated by graded response measurements. Of course, if too large an infecting dose (approximately 10^{10} cells) is used, the animals will be overwhelmed and die almost immediately (see Fig. 15–1). On the other hand, it is important not to use too small an infecting dose, or the immune response to the infection in the controls will be so great that no distinction can be made between vaccinated and control animals. Thus, an infecting dose cannot be too large, or the secondary immune response may be overwhelmed; at the same time, it cannot be too small, or it will be impossible to differentiate between a primary immune response in the control animals and the secondary immune response in the vaccinated animals. More will be said about this when we discuss evaluation of the immune response. Actual examples will be shown to illustrate the important point that when using intravenous administration, the infecting dose must not be too small or too large. However, statements to the effect that an infecting dose, at least of the H37Rv strain, of 10^6 or even 10^7 cells is massive and too large are completely incorrect. There is actually a range of doses somewhere between 10^6 and 10^7 cells that can be used for the detection of the immune response in the vaccinated mice when the H37Rv strain of *M. tuberculosis* is used.

What we have said applies primarily, however, to situations in which mortality or some other objective and measurable pathologic reaction is the end point. When small numbers of tubercle bacilli are injected intravenously into vaccinated and normal mice and the results evaluated in terms of actual numbers of tubercle bacilli in the lung or other organ at various times after infection, the use of numerically large numbers of tubercle bacilli may make the counting of the number of viable tubercle bacilli in various organs, after sacrifice of the mice, more difficult and laborious. On the other hand, small infecting doses may not trigger the secondary immune response. In such cases, measurements of the primary response can be made (see p. 345).

The generalizations that we have made regarding the suitable size of an inoculum of *M. tuberculosis* for challenge of vaccinated mice can be better understood and can be validated by examination of some actual data. Figure 15–2 shows the distribution of deaths of nonvaccinated control mice, as compared with mice that had been vaccinated intraperitoneally two to eight weeks earlier with viable cells of the attenuated H37Ra strain of *M. tuberculosis*. It can be seen that the deaths of over 90 percent of the 295

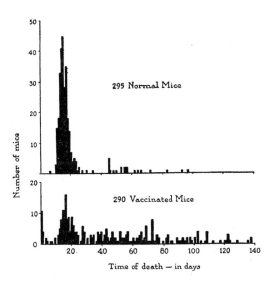

FIGURE 15–2. Distribution of deaths of normal mice and mice vaccinated with 1.0 mg of the H37Ra strain following challenge with 1.0 mg of the virulent H37Rv strain of *Mycobacterium tuberculosis*. (From Youmans, G. P., and Youmans, A. S.: The measurement of the response of immunized mice to infection with *Mycobacterium tuberculosis* var. *hominis*. J. Immunol. 78:318, 1957).

control mice followed the expected normal frequency distribution pattern. These results are similar to those shown for some 2,123 normal mice infected intravenously with a 1 mg dose of the virulent H37Rv strain over a five-year period (see Table 15–6). However, the median survival time (13.84 days) of the 2,123 mice, with an average weight of 18 to 22 grams, differed significantly from the median survival time (18.7 days) of the nonvaccinated mice shown in Figure 15–2. This difference in survival between the two groups of nonvaccinated mice can be accounted for by the fact that following vaccination there was a two- to eight-week waiting period in which both controls and vaccinated animals gained appreciably in weight. These older, heavier mice are always somewhat more resistant to infection. This illustrates the necessity of using, as controls for such vaccination, experiments, mice selected from the same population of animals as mice used for the vaccination. Only about half of the vaccinated mice showed a distribution of deaths similar to that of the controls. The remainder lived much longer; their deaths were distributed over approximately another 110 days.

From the data shown in Figure 15–2, it can be seen that the deaths of the vaccinated mice are distributed so anormally that neither the mean nor the median would be suitable measures of the average response. Actually, nearly half of the vaccinated mice died at approximately the same time and in the same manner as did over 90 percent of the controls; these vaccinated animals were judged, therefore, to have had little or no increased resistance to infection — in other words, little or no immunity. The increased resistance (immunity) of the remainder of the vaccinated mice, however, was evident from the prolonged survival.

The distribution of deaths of the vaccinated animals shown in Figure 15–2 is bimodal. This bimodal response is more clearly illustrated in Figure 15–3 in which the cumulative percent mortality has been plotted against time of death in days, using the same data that was used in Figure 15–2. Actually, in the light of our knowledge of the course of the tuberculous infection in mice, such a bimodal response would be expected.[62, 99] To recapitulate, those animals that succumb early have an acute infection and die as a consequence of rapid multiplication of the tubercle bacilli in the lungs with the formation of numerous, necrotic, exudative lesions.

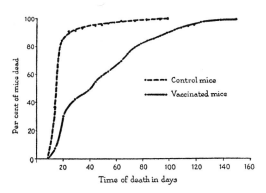

FIGURE 15–3. Distribution of cumulative percent of deaths of normal mice and mice vaccinated with 1.0 mg of the H37Ra strain following challenge with 1.0 mg of the virulent H37Rv strain of *Mycobacterium tuberculosis.* (From Youmans, G. P., and Youmans, A. S.: The measurement of the response of immunized mice to infection with *Mycobacterium tuberculosis* var. *hominis.* J. Immunol. *78:*318, 1957.)

Those animals that die later suffer from a more chronic type of infection in which there is little or no multiplication of tubercle bacilli in any of the organs and in which death appears to be less a consequence of multiplication of tubercle bacilli than the result of the massive proliferative cellular reaction occurring in the lungs. The increase in resistance to infection engendered in mice by vaccination has little or no beneficial effect on the course of the early acute infection (see Figure 15–2). The major effect of vaccination is to bring about cessation of multiplication of the virulent tubercle bacilli and, therefore, change the pulmonary infection from the acute progressive disease to a chronic tuberculous infection (see Chapter 8). When deaths of vaccinated mice are recorded, this will be noticed as a shift in the number of mice in the early acute-infection group into the longer-life, chronic-infection group because the secondary immune response has brought about the cessation of multiplication of the tubercle bacilli. Therefore, a more valid method for the estimation of the immune response is to measure the number of mice that are shifted from the acute-infection population into the chronic-infection group by vaccination. We have done this, using the data shown in Figure 15–2, by selecting 30 days as the length of time vaccinated animals should survive in order to be considered to have

some increased immunity to infection. We chose that time period because the data in Figures 15–2 and 15–3 showed that over 90 percent of the control animals had succumbed to the acute infection within 30 days and because the 30-day period appears to be the time at which a division between the two mouse populations could be clearly noted.

We now come back to the question of the influence of size of the infecting dose on the response of vaccinated mice to infection with *M. tuberculosis* and to the consideration of the proper means of selecting a suitable dose of a virulent culture of *M. tuberculosis* for such challenge.

We can see (see Fig. 15–1) that when normal mice are infected intravenously with doses of tubercle bacilli between 0.5 and 8.0 mg, a linear relationship is observed between the logarithm of the infecting dose and the median survival time. This means that with all these doses, the tubercle bacilli in the infected animals are multiplying at the same exponential rate until death of the animal. However, when the infecting dose is lower than 0.5 mg, the survival of nonvaccinated mice is prolonged and the distribution of deaths becomes anormal and resembles the distribution of deaths which occurs in vaccinated mice challenged with the 1 mg dose of tubercle bacilli (see Fig. 15–2). Consequently, when such small infecting doses are employed in normal mice, the response to the infection can be evaluated in the same manner as that employed for vaccinated mice infected with larger doses, since the division point in time between the two populations is approximately the same regardless of the state of resistance of the mice or the size of the infecting dose. In Table 15–7 we have tabulated data from experiments in which both vaccinated and nonvaccinated mice were challenged with different numbers of tubercle bacilli 28 days after vaccination with the H37Ra strain. Using the cut-off period of 30 days, which we derived from the data shown in Figure 15–2, we have recorded the number of mice that survived less than 30 days (D-30) and the number of mice that survived longer than 30 days (S-30). The median survival times of the mice that died within the 30 days have also been included. From the data in this table (15–7), it can be seen that with challenge doses of greater than 1.0 mg (10^7

cells), the response of the controls was so similar to that of the immunized mice that no evidence of immunity could be detected. These are the data, then, that provide the basis for our earlier statement in this chapter that very large doses of infecting tubercle bacilli cannot be used to challenge vaccinated mice because the secondary immune response will not appear soon enough or be of sufficient magnitude to affect the course of the infection. This table (15–7) also shows that when an infecting dose of 0.25 mg or less was used, the survival pattern of the nonvaccinated mice began to approach that of the vaccinated mice. Hence, measurement of the immune response is impossible because of the rapid immune response of the nonvaccinated mice to the infecting dose itself. These data, in turn, validate our previous statements to this effect.

These kinds of data illustrate two very important points. First, there is only a narrow range of infecting doses

TABLE 15–7. **The Effect of the Size of the Challenge Dose of *Mycobacterium tuberculosis* on the Survival of Strong A Mice Vaccinated with Strain H37Ra**

Challenge Dose (mg)	Vaccinated	No. of Mice D-30*	No. of Mice S-30†	Percent of Mice D-30 Mice	Percent of Mice S-30 Mice	Median Survival Time of D-30 Mice (95 Percent Confidence Limits)
0.065	No	22	27	44.9	55.1	24.0 (23 to 25)
0.125	No	48	43	62.7	37.3	20.0 (19 to 21)
0.25	Yes	3	16	16.0	84.0	
0.25	No	13	6	68.5	31.5	16.0 (14 to 18)
0.5	Yes	7	31	18.4	81.6	16.5 (14 to 20)
0.5	No	32	9	78.1	21.9	17.0 (16 to 18)
1.0	Yes	15	18	45.5	54.5	18.0 (16 to 20)
1.0	No	33	6	84.7	15.3	14.5 (12 to 17)
1.5	Yes	24	5	82.8	17.2	15.7 (14 to 18)
1.5	No	39	1	97.5	2.5	12.5 (12 to 13)
2.0	Yes	35	2	94.6	5.4	11.0 (10 to 12)
2.0	No	38	0	100.0	0.0	11.2 (10.6 to 12)
3.0	Yes	26	0	100.0	0.0	6.8 (6.3 to 7.3)
3.0	No	36	0	100.0	0.0	6.8 (6.3 to 7.3)
4.0	Yes	34	0	100.0	0.0	1.3 (1 to 1.6)
4.0	No	37	0	100.0	0.0	3.2 (2.5 to 3.9)

*D-30, death occurred in less than 30 days.
†S-30, survived 30 days or longer.
From Youmans, G. P., and Youmans, A. S.: The measurement of the response of immunized mice to infection with *Mycobacterium tuberculosis* var. *hominis*. J. Immunol. 78:318, 1957.

that can be used validly to measure the immune response of mice when larger infecting doses are administered intravenously and, second, that selection of an infecting dose to use in a given mouse strain or in a given laboratory can only be done after measurements of the dose-response relationships in both vaccinated and nonvaccinated mice, such as those shown in Table 15–7.

Other investigators have also noted that somewhat larger doses of virulent tubercle bacilli were better for measuring the immune response in animals than small doses. Swedberg[90] for example noted that in mice, challenge infecting doses of the Ravenel strain of *Mycobacterium bovis* of intermediate size were better for detecting immunity than either small or very large doses. Schwabacher and Wilson[76] and Smith and coworkers[80] also reported that better evidence of acquired immunity could be obtained in mice when they were challenged with large rather than very small infecting doses of virulent human-type tubercle bacilli. The basis for the findings of these other investigators is undoubtedly the same as that previously outlined where we used our own results as an example. It is also of interest to note that the principles derived here apply not only to mice but also to other animals. Swedberg[90] has shown that more accurate measurements of immunity in guinea pigs can be made by the intravenous administration of larger doses of virulent tubercle bacilli, not smaller doses. Opie and Freund[58] found that the intravenous administration of small doses of a highly virulent bovine culture (Ravenel) was a satisfactory method for the measurement of acquired resistance to tuberculous infection in rabbits. Since the Ravenel strain is far more virulent for rabbits than is the H37Rv strain for mice, the small doses used by Opie and Freund were, in terms of virulence of the culture, comparable to the larger doses of the H37Rv strain.

It follows, then, that the use of the terms "large," "small," or "massive" in reference to the number of tubercle bacilli used to challenge vaccinated animals may be very misleading. The number of tubercle bacilli may be numerically large, but depending upon the virulence of the strain of *Mycobacterium* and the nature of the mouse strain employed or the species of animal used, a distribution of deaths may occur that is characteristic of the distribution obtained with smaller infecting doses. On the other hand, what may appear to be a small infecting dose may give a distribution of death characteristic of that obtained when a numerically large inoculum is used. For example, Swedberg,[90] after determining the response in terms of time of death of mice to intravenous infection with different amounts of the Ravenel strain of *Mycobacterium bovis*, chose as a standard challenge inoculum a dose of 0.06 mg. Because of the higher virulence of the Ravenel strain for mice, the inoculum produced an essentially normal distribution of deaths. An 0.06 mg inoculum of the H37Rv strain in Strong A mice (see Table 15–7), however, gives us a distinctly anormal distribution of deaths and is considered a small challenge inoculum. Therefore, to reiterate, the proper challenge infecting dose of tubercle bacilli to be used for testing the immunity of mice to tuberculosis can be selected only after a determination of the response of a particular strain of mouse, or species of animal, being employed to different numbers of cells of the strain of virulent *Mycobacterium* to be used. In terms of total weight of culture or number of tubercle bacilli, the most suitable dose may be numerically either small or large.

THE CHOICE OF MOUSE STRAIN

There is relatively little to discuss concerning the choice of mouse strain, except to point out that a wide variety of allogeneic strains of mice have been used for assessment of the immune response to mycobacteria and mycobacterial fractions. Although differences among these strains in the capacity to develop immunity to tuberculosis have been noted,[12, 60, 106, 108] apparently all of them can be used, providing close attention is paid to selecting the proper infecting dose of virulent tubercle bacilli (as outlined in the preceding section). It has also been noted that male mice respond somewhat better to immunization than do female mice.[31, 103] This may be a consequence of the fact that male mice tend to gain weight more rapidly. Some people prefer to use female mice because of their greater docility, which makes them easier to handle.

A number of syngeneic strains of mice have been tested for their susceptibility to tuberculosis,[12, 60] and somewhat more recently, Youmans and Youmans[106] have shown that the C57Bl/6 strain is more capable of mounting an immune response to mycobacterial cells and to RNA vaccine than are a number of allogeneic strains.

EVALUATION OF THE IMMUNE RESPONSE IN EXPERIMENTAL ANIMALS

In the preceding pages there has been, of necessity, some discussion of the evaluation of the response of mice to vaccination, and particularly of the selection of a proper challenge dose of the infecting culture of virulent tubercle bacilli. However, many of the details involved in the proper evaluation of an immune response remain to be covered. In the following paragraphs, we will discuss evaluation of the immune response not only in mice but also in guinea pigs, which still remain useful animals for this purpose under certain circumstances. We will also look at the evaluation of the response of subhuman primates to vaccination and challenge.

Much of our knowledge regarding the nature of the host-parasite interaction in experimental tuberculosis in mice, guinea pigs, rabbits, and monkeys has come from the intensive efforts during the period from approximately 1940 to 1955 to find suitable chemotherapeutic agents for the treatment of tuberculosis in human beings. The success of these efforts has been documented by the development of drugs such as streptomycin, para-aminosalicylic acid, isoniazid, ethionamide, and rifampin.[100] Most of the studies conducted during this period in the experimental chemotherapy of tuberculosis made use of the mouse as an experimental model, although Rich and Follis,[69] Feldman,[13, 14] and Feldman and Hinshaw[15, 16] pioneered in this field by using guinea pigs. The objective of these chemotherapeutic studies was to determine whether a given drug would, when administered to an experimental animal infected with *Mycobacterium tuberculosis*, favorably influence the course of the disease. Since many thousands of compounds had to be tested for their antituberculous activity, it was necessary to devise reliable and valid methods for the response of mice and guinea pigs to infection with tubercle bacilli. (For a detailed review of the experimental chemotherapy of tuberculosis, see Youmans and Youmans.[100])

When the heyday of chemotherapy had passed and investigators again became interested in the response of the host to vaccination against tuberculosis, many of the same methods that were used to test for the chemotherapeutic activity of chemical compounds, or some modification of these, were found to be equally suitable for the detection of the immune response. We have seen that the immune response, when it develops, brings about a favorable influence on the course of infection by inhibiting the multiplication of virulent tubercle bacilli. This is also the primary mode of action of most of the chemotherapeutic agents in use today. They provide the body with more time to cope with the infection by retarding multiplication of the virulent tubercle bacilli. It would be reasonable to expect that experimental models of infection useful for measuring the antimycobacterial action of drugs would also be useful for the measurement of acquired immunity to tuberculosis.

Immune forces, though, do not have the magnitude of effect on virulent tubercle bacilli that can, for example, be exerted by optimal doses of isoniazid or rifampin. Therefore, the detection of this weaker antituberculous activity of the body requires very careful attention to numerous factors, many of which we have already mentioned, such as the species of animal, route of inoculation of the challenge infecting dose of *M. tuberculosis,* and the number of tubercle bacilli injected. Also, the magnitude of the immune response is significantly affected by the nutrition of the animal, the genetic constitution of the experimental animal, intercurrent infection with unrelated bacteria, and even by the conditions under which the animals are housed.[62]

Mice

Many factors involved in the evaluation of the immune response to tuberculosis in the mouse have been dealt with in earlier sections of this chapter — the importance of the mouse strain, the route of inoculation of the challenge dose, and the size of the challenge dose of virulent tubercle bacilli. We concluded that a mouse strain that readily develops immunity to tuberculosis should be employed and, since males respond better than females, that male animals should be used. We also concluded that if the results were going to be evaluated in terms of the survival time, the best route of inoculation for the challenge dose is intravenous and that the size of the infecting dose should be neither too small nor too

large. If too small, the immune response of control animals to the challenge dose of tubercle bacilli might mask differences between vaccinated and control animals. If the challenge dose is too large, the immunity developed as a result of vaccination might be completely overwhelmed.

Mice are vaccinated with whatever preparation the investigator wishes to use, and the route of vaccination is usually subcutaneous or intraperitoneal. Other routes, however, can be employed if the investigator so wishes. After sufficient time has elapsed for immunity to develop, the mice can be challenged intravenously with virulent human-type tubercle bacilli, the challenge dose having been carefully selected by preliminary experimentation (see p. 334). The animals are kept under observation, and the time of death of each animal from the tuberculous infection is recorded. It is wise to autopsy each dead animal in order to confirm death as being due to tuberculosis.

If the proper challenge dose has been selected and the immunized animals have shown an immune response, the great majority of the control animals will die within 30 days, and the times of death will be normally distributed (see Fig. 15–2). On the other hand, a significant proportion of the vaccinated animals will live longer than 30 days, and their deaths will occur over a prolonged period. The degree of immunity developed by the immunized animals can be assessed by calculating the proportion of animals that live more than 30 days. The handling of such data has been fully analyzed by Youmans and Youmans.[101, 104]

This pattern of survival follows from the nature of the immune response in mice. There seems to be among certain investigators a misconception of this immune response. Their assumption is that the pattern of response is similar to the example shown in Figure 15–4. This purely hypothetical curve shows that while the rate of multiplication in both control and vaccinated animals is expo-

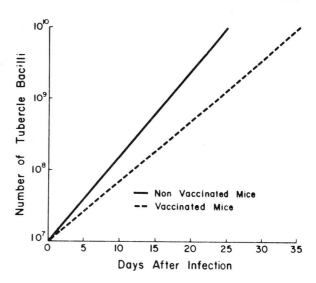

FIGURE 15–4. Diagrammatic representation of manner in which tubercle bacilli do *not* multiply in vaccinated mice. (From Youmans, G. P., and Youmans, A. S.: Relative effectiveness of living and non-living vaccines. *In* Chamberlayne, E. C. (ed.): Status of Immunization in Tuberculosis in 1971. DHEW Publication No. (NIH) 72-68, 1972.)

nential, the exponential growth is at a slower rate in vaccinated animals than in the controls. This, however, is a completely incorrect view of what actually happens to larger doses of virulent tubercle bacilli in vaccinated animals. What actually happens is illustrated in Figure 15–5. This purely graphic representation shows that the initial rate of multiplication of virulent tubercle bacilli in both control and vaccinated animals is the same. Multiplication continues at this rate in the controls until all, or nearly all, of the animals are dead; of course, the distribution of deaths will be normal. In some of the vaccinated animals, however, depending upon the degree of immunity, multiplication of the infecting virulent tubercle bacilli will be slowed or halted; then these animals will go on to survive a prolonged period. In Figure 15–5, we have shown hypothetical times when this inhibition of multiplication of tubercle bacilli might begin. With a high secondary immune response, inhibition of multiplication of tubercle bacilli would begin early, and

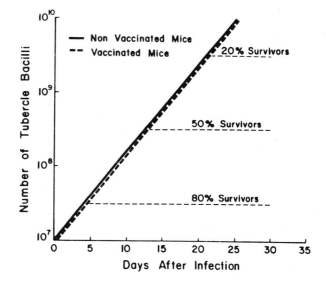

FIGURE 15–5. Diagrammatic representation of manner in which tubercle bacilli *do* multiply in vaccinated mice. (From Youmans, G. P., and Youmans, A. S.: Relative effectiveness of living and non-living vaccines. *In* Chamberlayne, E. C. (ed.): Status of Immunization in Tuberculosis in 1971. DHEW Publication No. (NIH) 72-68, 1972.)

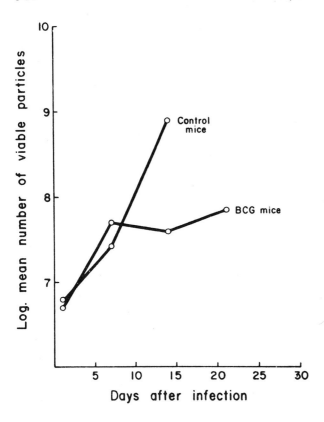

FIGURE 15–6. Multiplication of virulent tubercle bacilli in the lungs of vaccinated and nonvaccinated mice. (Modified from Niffenegger, J., and Youmans, G. P.: The effect of macrocyclon on the multiplication of tubercle bacilli in the lungs and spleen of mice. Br. J. Exp. Pathol. 4:403, 1960.)

the majority of the animals would survive greater than 30 days. With a moderate secondary immune response, the inhibition of multiplication would occur later, and perhaps only 50 percent of the animals would survive for more than 30 days. With a very low immune response, only a few of the animals would survive longer than 30 days because marked inhibition of multiplication in these few would not begin until much later. The validation of this picture of what happens to virulent tubercle bacilli in vaccinated animals is provided by Figure 15–6, which is taken from data acquired in an actual experiment with mice vaccinated with BCG. Figure 15–7, taken from Smith and colleagues,[82] also indicates a similar pattern of multiplication of *M. tuberculosis* may occur in vaccinated guinea pigs. The reason for this pattern of multiplication of virulent tubercle bacilli in vaccinated animals derives from the fact that the

major effect of vaccination is to prime the animal, so that it will respond with a rapid secondary immune response in response to the stimulus of the larger infecting dose of virulent tubercle bacilli. At the time vaccinated animals are challenged (usually three to six or more weeks after vaccination), there is apparently not enough immunity to affect the multiplication of these larger doses of virulent tubercle bacilli immediately. Therefore, the degree of the immune response will be determined by the rapidity with which a secondary immune response is mounted. Thus, with the use of the proper challenge infecting dose, this mounting of the secondary immune response can be measured by noting the number or proportion of animals that survive greater than, in this case, 30 days. Other cut-off points can be chosen, depending upon the experimental conditions.[30, 32]

In the final analysis, then, what is

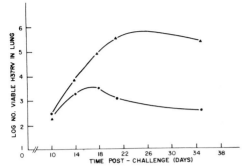

FIGURE 15–7. Plot of the mean of the logarithm of the number of H37Rv organisms recovered from the lungs of guinea pigs infected by the respiratory route. Nonvaccinated group, (▲); BCG-vaccinated group, (●). (From Smith, D. W., McMurray, D. N., Wiegeshaus, E. H., Grover, A. A., and Harding, G. E.: Host-parasite relationships in experimental airborne tuberculosis. VI. Early events in the course of infection in vaccinated and nonvaccinated guinea pigs. Am. Rev. Respir. Dis. *102*:937, 1970.)

really measured following infection of vaccinated animals is the heterogeneity in the response to infection induced by vaccination. We wind up with two populations of mice: in one, the immune response is so weak that the animals behave much like the controls, while in the other, the secondary immune response is so strong that the multiplication of virulent tubercle bacilli is inhibited and the mice survive for prolonged periods. We[101] and others[30, 32] have shown that this is a very reliable and valid method for measuring the immune response of mice to vaccination with BCG, H37Ra cells, and immunogenic components of the tubercle bacillus. (See Chapters 6, 7, 8, 9, 10, 11, 12, and 13 for details and references.) It is possible by this procedure, using approximately 10^7 tubercle bacilli for challenge, to detect the immune response produced, for example, by only nanograms of mycobacterial RNA, or by viable H37Ra cells (see Chapter 9).

It is also possible to detect the immune response to vaccination in mice by using the enumeration technique (to be described in the next section) when discussing the measurement of the immune response in guinea pigs by challenging them either by using the intrapulmonary route with aerosols of either large or small numbers of tubercle bacilli or by using intravenous injection of either large or small numbers of tubercle bacilli. Usually, at appropriate times after challenge, the lungs, and the spleens and livers if desired, are removed, homogenized, diluted appropriately, and aliquots of each dilution plated on a suitable medium. After an appropriate incubation period, the colonies of tubercle bacilli can be counted. A graph can then be constructed from data collected at different times after infection, and this will show the actual rate of multiplication of the tubercle bacilli in vivo. In this manner, comparisons can be made between nonvaccinated and vaccinated animals. This procedure has been used rather extensively by certain investigators both for assessing response of mice to vaccination and for detecting the effect of antimycobacterial drugs. References[8, 9, 17, 40-42, 45-53, 56, 64-67, 77, 78] and Figure 15–8 show the kind of data which are frequently derived when using small doses of virulent tubercle bacilli intravenously. In experiments such as these, since the numbers of tubercle bacilli used for infection are very small, apparently residual immunity from the primary immune response to the vaccination procedure can be detected, and the bacterial growth curves resemble those hypothesized in Figure 15–4 since some inhibition of multiplication is frequently seen almost from the time animals are infected. Such small infecting doses also do not appreciably stimulate the secondary immune response, at least not for a considerable period of time, so this enumeration technique, which uses very small numbers of tubercle bacilli to infect mice, is very sensitive. When the enumeration technique is used following intravenous administration of larger doses of virulent tubercle bacilli, the growth curves resemble those in Figure 15–6. We have already pointed out earlier in this chapter, though, that

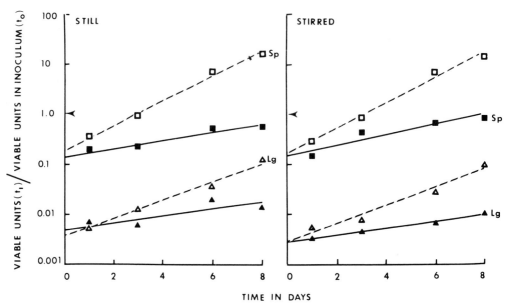

FIGURE 15–8. Change in viable numbers of *M. tuberculosis* H37Rv relative to the intravenous inoculum (10^5 viable units = 1.0 on graph) in normal mice (dashed lines) or BCG-vaccinated mice (solid lines). Spleen (squares) and lung (triangles) populations for D-8 stationary culture (left) or for D-8 stirred culture (right). (From Collins, F. M., Wayne, L. G., and Montalbine, V.: The effect of cultural conditions on the distribution of *Mycobacterium tuberculosis* in the spleens and lungs of specific pathogen-free mice. Am. Rev. Respir. Dis. *110*:147, 1974.)

in mice the use of the intrapulmonary route of infection will not allow the detection of any immunity in mice that will show a good immune response when challenged intravenously.

We should point out here, though, that regardless of whether one measures the primary immune response by using small infecting doses of virulent tubercle bacilli or measures the secondary immune response by using larger numbers of tubercle bacilli, both are valid measures of the immunity produced by a given vaccine. If an animal shows a primary immune response following vaccination, then when given a sufficient stimulus, it will show a secondary immune response. On the other hand, an animal in which a secondary immune response can be detected must, at some prior time, have shown a primary immune response. Therefore, viewed in proper perspective, the use of small numbers of challenge tubercle bacilli or the survival time technique, which uses larger infecting doses of

tubercle bacilli, should provide equally valid measurements of the immune response in mice.

Guinea Pigs

Ever since the time of Koch, the guinea pig has been the favorite animal for studying experimental infections with *Mycobacterium tuberculosis*. The high susceptibility of the guinea pig to infection, its ability to develop delayed hypersensitivity, and its capacity to develop at least some immunity to infection have made this animal a favorite. However, the large size of guinea pigs and the labor and expense of maintaining significant numbers for long-term studies have discouraged their use, especially since it has been revealed that the mouse is an equally suitable animal for studies on the pathogenesis of tuberculosis and the mechanisms of the acquired immune state.[34, 35, 61, 62, 97–99, 101]

However, guinea pigs are still useful,

especially when a different animal species is needed to confirm the immunizing power of a potential vaccine that has been found effective in mice or to study antituberculous drugs that have been shown to be effective in mice. It is, therefore, worthwhile to outline some of the standard procedures that are used for evaluating the immune response in these animals.

Interestingly enough, the pathogenesis of the experimental disease in guinea pigs has not been as systematically investigated as it has been in the mouse. However, it is clear from the available evidence that primary tuberculosis in the guinea pig is much the same as that in the mouse. That is, following subcutaneous or intraperitoneal injection of virulent tubercle bacilli into guinea pigs (the routes most commonly employed), Soltys and Jennings[88] have shown that both *M. tuberculosis* and *M. bovis* spread rapidly throughout the body of the animal. The rapidity of the spread is influenced to a considerable degree by the number of tubercle bacilli injected. When a small dose was injected, tubercle bacilli were found to reach the spleen somewhere between 48 and 96 hours after inoculation. With larger doses of tubercle bacilli, the mycobacteria could be found in the spleen as early as one hour after infection. Other organs, such as the liver, kidney, and lungs, were also invaded by tubercle bacilli in about the same time. Interestingly enough, the brain was the last organ to be invaded, tubercle bacilli being found there only after 24 hours. The blood could be shown to contain tubercle bacilli only during the first few hours after infection. Thus, early dissemination of tubercle bacilli from the focus of infection is very similar to that noted in man and in mice (see Chapter 14). Because of the absence of acquired immunity at this time, there is little or no tendency toward localization of the infecting dose.

As the disease develops, it is worth noting that in the mouse, regardless of the route of inoculation, the lung is the organ mainly involved in the tuberculous process, whereas in the guinea pig, almost regardless of the route of inoculation, the lung is less involved and the spleen and liver appear to bear the brunt of the infection. Swedberg,[90] however, has shown that following intravenous injection of small doses of virulent tubercle bacilli, the lung will be primarily involved. For further information on the pathogenesis of tuberculosis and the gross and microscopic pathology of the disease, the publications of Cobbett and colleagues,[7] Krause,[39] Willis,[94] Perla,[59] Francis,[18] Bjerkedal,[5] and Rich[68] should be consulted.

As with mice, evaluation of the results of infection with tubercle bacilli, whether in control or in vaccinated animals, can be determined by keeping records of the times of death and then comparing the average survival times of vaccinated and normal animals. However, when guinea pigs are injected subcutaneously or intraperitoneally, the distribution of deaths does not appear to be normal and, furthermore, especially with smaller inocula, deaths may occur over periods up to or in excess of six to ten months. The length of time that is required with small infecting doses for all of the animals to die imposes a severe burden upon most laboratories. Swedberg,[90] on the other hand, found that by injecting guinea pigs intravenously, the distribution of deaths was much more uniform and, depending upon the virulence of the strain of tubercle bacilli used and the number of tubercle bacilli injected, would occur over a period of only 30 to 50 days. Although the protective effect of BCG vaccination could be measured by Swedberg using the intravenous route, this has not been utilized by other investigators.

Feldman[13, 14] and Feldman and Hinshaw,[15, 16] on the other hand, preferred to evaluate the results of the therapy of tuberculous guinea pigs with chemotherapeutic agents by determining after an appropriate time the relative amounts of pathology found in the various organs and the lymph nodes. This, of course, is a purely subjective analysis of the extent of disease and carries with it considerable error. Furthermore, even as there are marked differences in survival among infected guinea pigs, the amount of disease in the various organs can vary markedly from animal to animal. For this reason, Feldman and Hinshaw developed a simple and convenient recording method for the extent of lesions in the organs and tissues of guinea pigs infected with *M. tuberculosis*.

A schematic representation of the various organs of the guinea pig can be printed upon the record card of each animal by means of a large rubber stamp measuring approximately 2 in. by 4 in. (see Fig. 15–9). At the time of autopsy an observer records the lesions noted grossly, by sketching the approximate size and form with a red pencil. If the disease is too extensive for the lesions to be recorded individually, the whole organ is colored red. Marginal notes can be made at this time to indicate approximate size and appearance of organs. These authors feel that the cards demonstrate the gross patho-

logic appearance with minimal effort and in a much clearer manner than could possibly be achieved by any verbal description, regardless of how carefully or extensively it might be written. When such cards are arranged for display, the comparative effectiveness of various drugs or of vaccination is clearly evident (see Fig. 15–10). After fixation of tissues, the amount of microscopic pathology can be recorded in the same manner.

Furthermore, the amount of tuberculous disease in different tissues can be assigned varying numeric values. By this scheme (see Tables 15–8 and 15–9) the maximal value of tuberculosis in any one animal cannot exceed 100. This would be the correct numeric index should there be extensive and severe progressive tuberculosis in the spleen, liver, and lung and signs of progressive tuberculosis in the tissues at the site of inoculation or the contiguous lymph nodes or both. Less severe disease of a progressive character can be graded either moderate or slight, and the proper numeral assigned for the involvement of the different organs. When this scoring and recording has been finished and the proper calculations completed,

Key of Symbols

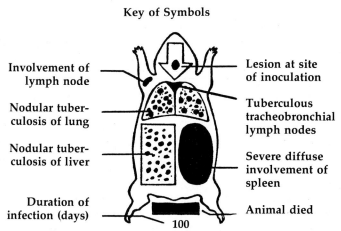

Involvement of lymph node	Lesion at site of inoculation
Nodular tuberculosis of lung	Tuberculous tracheobronchial lymph nodes
Nodular tuberculosis of liver	Severe diffuse involvement of spleen
Duration of infection (days)	Animal died

100

FIGURE 15–9. Schematic representation of a guinea pig showing the organs usually affected in inoculation tuberculosis. The amount of disease recorded for the spleen, lungs, and liver is indicated. (From Feldman, W. H., and Hinshaw, H. C.: Chemotherapeutic testing in experimental tuberculosis. Suggested outline of laboratory procedures for testing antituberculosis substances in experimentally infected animals. Am. Rev. Tuberc. *51:*582, 1945.)

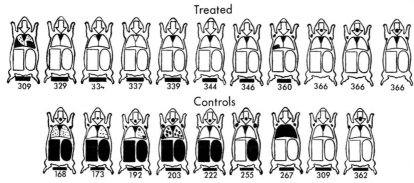

FIGURE 15–10.   Use of the outline drawing (see Fig. 15–9) to record the amount of tuberculosis in an actual experiment. (From Feldman, W. H., and Hinshaw, H. C.: Chemotherapeutic testing in experimental tuberculosis. Suggested outline of laboratory procedures for testing antituberculosis substances in experimentally infected animals. Am. Rev. Tuberc. *51*:582, 1945.)

scores of animals vaccinated with any vaccine can be compared with the scores of the nonvaccinated controls. Once again, this subjective evaluation has a large margin of error, but it has been used successfully by a number of investigators.

Attempts have also been made to measure the extent of the disease in guinea pigs by weighing, following sacrifice, the omentums of treated and control animals[29, 73] or by determining the time of appearance of tubercle bacilli in the spleen.[95] These methods, though, have generally been regarded as being appreciably less valid than the method of Feldman and Hinshaw just described.

It is more common, at this time, when studying the result of vaccination in guinea pigs to infect the animals by the pulmonary route by allowing them to inhale aerosols of tubercle bacilli. The dosage of tubercle bacilli can be adjusted and the animals allowed to inhale very small numbers of tubercle bacilli. This method has been explored and validated, particularly by Smith and his colleagues,[23, 82, 83, 93] and these publications should be referred to for the technical details and citations of the earlier literature. Following infection in this manner, animals can be sacrificed at intervals and the degree of infection assayed in two ways. One, actual counts of the gross lesions that can be

TABLE 15–8.   **Key Table for Evaluating by Gross Appearance the Extent and Character of Tuberculous Lesions in Experimentally Infected Guinea Pigs***

Extent of Involvement in Tissues Examined	Spleen	Lung	Liver	Site of Inoculation and Contiguous Lymph Nodes	If Lung Is Negative, Examine Tracheobronchial Lymph Nodes
Extensive	35	30	25	10	10
Moderate	20	20	20	10	10
Slight	10	10	10	10	10
Maximal values = 100 total	35	30	25	10 (If lung is negative)	10

*Assign the highest number corresponding to the description of the lesion in each tissue.
From Feldman, W. H.: A scheme for numerical recording of tuberculous changes in experimentally infected guinea pigs. Am. Rev. Tuberc. *48*:248, 1943.

TABLE 15–9. **Key Table for Evaluating Histologically the Extent and Character of Tuberculous Lesions in Experimentally Infected Guinea Pigs***

Extent and Character of Lesions in Section Examined	Spleen	Lung	Liver	Site of Innoculation and Contiguous Lymph Nodes	If Lung Is Negative, Examine Tracheobronchial Lymph Nodes
Progressive lesions present					
Extensive involvement	35	30	25	10	10
Moderate	20	20	20	10	10
Slight	10	10	10	10	10
Nonprogressive lesions only					
Fibrosis, hard tubercles	3	3	2	1	1
Fibrosis or calcification only	1	1	1	1	1
Maximal values = 100 total	35	30	25	10	10 (If lung is negative)
If only inactive lesions, maximal values less than 10	3	3	2	1	1 (If lung is negative)

*Assign the highest number corresponding to the description of the lesion in each tissue.
From Feldman, W. H.: A Scheme for numerical recording of tuberculous changes in experimentally infected guinea pigs. Am. Rev. Tuberc. *48*:248, 1943.

seen in the lungs can be recorded, and second, portions of the lungs can be cut out, weighed and homogenized. Dilutions are then prepared in a suitable medium and an agar base plating medium inoculated with aliquots of these dilutions. Following an incubation period of two to three weeks, the colonies can be counted, and the actual numbers of tubercle bacilli at each time can be calculated. From such data, curves can be constructed that will show the actual rate of growth of tubercle bacilli in vaccinated animals as compared with control animals. Figure 15–7, taken from Smith and co-workers,[82] shows such a comparison. Smith found that bacterial counts obtained in this manner correlated well with the survival time of animals similarly infected. The labor involved in such determinations is enormous; for this reason, some investigators may hesitate to use it, especially when sufficiently adequate comparisons can prob-

ably be made from analysis of·survival time data.[22]

Monkeys

We have already pointed out that monkeys can be used for experimental purposes in tuberculosis because they are highly susceptible and they respond well to vaccination. However, because of their large size, their high cost and problems concerned with maintenance, there are very few places that can afford to invest heavily in vaccination programs using subhuman primates. This work can best be done in primate centers where the efforts of many are devoted exclusively to the care, handling, and management of these animals. However, data obtained from the vaccination of subhuman primates against tuberculosis can be very useful, particularly for the evaluation of vaccines that appear to have some potential for use in human beings. A number of studies have been carried out in which monkeys have been vaccinated with BCG cells and with certain components of tubercle bacilli.[1, 3, 4, 33, 63, 74, 75] These papers should be consulted for technical details.

REFERENCES

1. Anacker, R. L., Brehmer, W., Barclay, W. R., Leif, W. R., Ribi, E., Simmons, J. H., and Smith, A. W.: Superiority of intravenously administered BCG and BCG cell walls in protecting rhesus monkeys (*Macaca mulatta*) against airborne tuberculosis. Z. Immunitäetsforsch. *143*:363, 1972.

2. Baker, M. J., Schlosser, M. E., and White, H. J.: A method for evaluating antitubercular activity in mice. Ann. N. Y. Acad. Sci. *52*:678, 1949.

3. Barclay, W. R., Anacker, R. L., Brehmer, W., Leif, W., and Ribi, E.: Aerosol-induced tuberculosis in subhuman primates and the course of the disease after intravenous BCG vaccination. Infect. Immun. *2*:574, 1970.

4. Barclay, W. R., Busey, W. M., Dalgard, D. W., Good, R. C., Janicki, B. W., Kasik, J. E., Ribi, E., Ulrich, C. E., and Wolinsky, E.: Protection of monkeys against airborne tuberculosis by aerosol vaccination with bacillus Calmette-Guerin. Am. Rev. Respir. Dis. *107*:351, 1973.

5. Bjerkedal, T.: Host-agent interaction in experimental tuberculosis in guinea pigs, with special reference to the effects of BCG vaccination. Am. J. Hyg. *79*:86, 1964.

6. Boyd, W. C.: Fundamentals of Immunology. 3rd ed. New York, Interscience Publishers, Inc., 1956.

7. Cobbett, L., Griffith, A. S., and Griffith, F.: Additional investigations of bovine and human viruses. *In* Second Interim Report of the Royal Commission Appointed to Inquire into the Relations of Human and Animal Tuberculosis. Vol. III, Part II. London, Wyman, 1907.

8. Collins, F. M., and Montalbine, V.: Relative immunogenicity of streptomycin-sensitive and -resistant strains of BCG. Infect. Immun. *8*:381, 1973.

9. Collins, F. M., Wayne, L. G., and Montalbine, V.: The effect of culture conditions on the distribution of *Mycobacterium tuberculosis* in the spleens and lungs of specific pathogen-free mice. Am. Rev. Respir. Dis. *110*:147, 1974.

10. Crowle, A. J.: Lung density as a measure of tuberculous involvement in mice. Am. Rev. Tuberc. *77*:681, 1958.

11. Dennis, E. W., Goble, F. C., Berberian, D. A., and Frelih, E. J.: Experimental tuberculosis of the Syrian hamster (*Cricetus auratus*). Ann. N.Y. Acad. Sci. *52*:646, 1949.

12. Donovick, R., McKee, C. M., Jambor, W. P., and Rake, G.: The use of the mouse in a standardized test for antituberculous activity of compounds of natural or synthetic origin. II. Choice of mouse strain. Am. Rev. Tuberc. *60*:109, 1949.

13. Feldman, W. H.: The chemotherapy of tuberculosis — Including the use of streptomycin. The Harben Lecture, Lecture No. 2. An evaluation of the efficacy in tuberculosis of sulfonamides, sulfones and certain other substances. J. R. Inst. Public Health Hyg. *9*:297, 1946.

14. Feldman, W. H.: A scheme for numerical recording of tuberculous changes in experimentally infected guinea pigs. Am. Rev. Tuberc. *48*:248, 1943.

15. Feldman, W. H., and Hinshaw, H. C.: Chemotherapeutic testing in experimental tuberculosis. Suggested outline of laboratory procedures for testing antituberculosis substances in experimentally infected animals. Am. Rev. Tuberc. *51*:582, 1945.

16. Feldman, W. H., and Hinshaw, H. C.: Effects of streptomycin on experimental tuberculosis in guinea pigs: A preliminary report. Proc. Staff Meeting Mayo Clin. *19*:593, 1944.

17. Fenner, F., Martin, S. P., and Pierce, C. H.: The enumeration of viable tubercle bacilli in cultures and infected tissues. Ann. N.Y. Acad. Sci. *52*:751, 1949.

18. Francis, J.: Tuberculosis in Animals and Man; a Study in Comparative Pathology. London, Cassell, 1958.

19. Francis, J.: Tuberculosis in the dog, with special reference to experimental bronchogenic tuberculosis. Am. Rev. Tuberc. *73*:748, 1956.

20. Frenkel, J. K.: Models for infectious diseases. Fed. Proc. *28*:179, 1969.

21. Glover, R. E.: The effects of (a) freeze-drying and (b) low temperature on viability of *Mycobacterium tuberculosis*. J. Pathol. Bacteriol. *58*:111, 1946.

22. Good, R. C., Youmans, G. P., Youmans, A. S., and McCarroll, N. E.: Immunogenic activity of mycobacterial RNA in guinea pigs. Abstracts of the Annual Meeting of the American Society for Microbiology, 1977. p. 86.

23. Grover, A. A., Kim, H. K., Wiegeshaus, E. H., and Smith, D. W.: Host-parasite relationships in experimental airborne tuberculosis. II. Reproducible infection by means of an inoculum preserved at −70 C. J. Bacteriol. *94*:832, 1967.

24. Grumbach, F.: Chimiothérapie antituberculeuse expérimentale chez le rat blanc. Ann. Inst. Pasteur (Paris) 98:485, 1960.

25. Grumbach, F., Grosset, J., and Canetti, G.: L'inactivation de l'isoniazid chez le rat. Son incidence sur les résultats de chimiothérapie de la tuberculose dans cette espèce. Ann. Inst. Pasteur (Paris) 98:642, 1960.

26. Gunn, F. D., Mills, M. A., Shepard, C. C., and Barth, E. E.: Experimental pulmonary tuberculosis in the dog. Reinfection. Am. Rev. Tuberc. 47:78, 1943.

27. Gunn, F. D., and Sheehy, J. J.: Experimental tuberculosis in the dog. Comparison of lesions in puppies and in mature dogs. Am. Rev. Tuberc. 61:77, 1950.

28. Gunn, F. D., Sheehy, J. J., Colwell, C. A., and Mills, M. A.: Experimental pulmonary tuberculosis in the dog. BCG immunization. Am. Rev. Tuberc. 46:612, 1942.

29. Han, E. S., Kelly, R. G., and Woodruff, C. E.: Use of the guinea pig omentum as an index of the effectiveness of antimicrobials in experimental tuberculosis. Am. Rev. Tuberc. 68:583, 1953.

30. Hoyt, A., Dennerline, R. L., Moore, F. J., and Smith, C. R.: Tubercle bacillus wax as an experimental vaccine against mouse tuberculosis. Am. Rev. Tuberc. 76:752, 1957.

31. Hoyt, A., Moore, F. J., Knowles, R. G., and Smith, C. R.: Sex differences of normal and immunized mice in resistance to experimental tuberculosis. Am. Rev. Tuberc. 75:618, 1957.

32. Hoyt, A., Moore, F. J., and Thompson, M. A.: Analysis of mixed distributions in antituberculosis vaccine assays. Am. Rev. Respir. Dis. 86:733, 1962.

33. Janicki, B. W., Good, R. C., Minden, P., Affronti, L. F., and Hymes, W. F.: Immune responses in rhesus monkeys after bacillus Calmette-Guerin vaccination and aerosol challenge with *Mycobacterium tuberculosis*. Am. Rev. Respir. Dis. 107:359, 1973.

34. Jespersen, A., and Bentzon, M. W.: The acquired resistance to tuberculosis induced by BCG vaccine assayed by a quantitative method on red mice (*Clethrionomys* g. *glareolus Schreb.*) I. Vaccination effect of BCG strains strongly or weakly virulent for hamsters. Acta Tuberc. Scandinav. 44:253, 1964.

35. Jespersen, A., and Bentzon, M. W.: The acquired resistance to tuberculosis induced by BCG vaccine assayed by a quantitative method on red mice (*Clethrionomys* g. *glareolus Schreb.*) II. Vaccination effect of BCG strains strongly or moderately virulent for hamsters. Acta Tuberc. Scandinav. 44:276, 1964.

36. Jespersen, A., and Bentzon, M. W.: The virulence of various strains of BCG determined on the golden hamster. Acta Tuberc. Scandinav. 44:222, 1964.

37. Kanai, K.: Review. Acquired resistance to tuberculous infection in experimental model. Jpn. J. Med. Sci. Biol. 20:21, 1967.

38. Karlson, A. G., and Feldman, W. H.: Sulfapyridine in avian tuberculosis. The effect of sulfapyridine on the bacillaemia of rabbits infected experimentally with avian tubercle bacilli. Am. Rev. Tuberc. 42:146, 1940.

39. Krause, A. K.: Studies on tuberculous infection. VI. Tuberculosis in the guinea pig after subcutaneous infection, with particular reference to the tracheo-bronchial lymph nodes. Am. Rev. Tuberc. 4:135, 1920.

40. Larson, C. L., Ribi, E., Wicht, W. C., List, R. H., and Goode, G.: Resistance to tuberculosis in mice immunized with BCG disrupted in oil. Nature 198:1214, 1963.

41. Larson, C. L., and Wicht, W. C.: Infection of mice with *Mycobacterium tuberculosis*, strain H37Ra. Am. Rev. Respir. Dis. 90:742, 1964.

42. Larson, C. L., and Wicht, W. C.: Studies of resistance to experimental tuberculosis in mice vaccinated with living attenuated tubercle bacilli and challenged with virulent organisms. Am. Rev. Respir. Dis. 85:833, 1962.

43. Lurie, M. B.: Resistance to Tuberculosis: Experimental Studies in Native and Acquired Defense Mechanisms. Cambridge, Harvard University Press, 1964.

44. Lurie, M. B.: The use of the rabbit in experimental chemotherapy of tuberculosis. Ann. N.Y. Acad. Sci. 52:627, 1949.

45. Mackaness, G. B.: Resistance to intracellular infection. J. Infect. Dis. 123:439, 1971.

46. Mackaness, G. B., and Blanden, R. V.: Cellular immunity. Prog. Allergy 11:89, 1967.

47. Mackaness, G. B., Blanden, R. V., and Collins, F. M.: Host-parasite relations in mouse typhoid. J. Exp. Med. 124:573, 1966.

48. Mackaness, G. B., Smith, N., and Wells, A. Q.: The growth of intracellular tubercle bacilli in relation to their virulence. Am. Rev. Tuberc. 69:479, 1954.

49. McCune, R., Deuschle, K., and McDermott, W.: The delayed appearance of isoniazid antagonism by pyridoxine *in vivo*. Am. Rev. Tuberc. 76:1100, 1957.

50. McCune, R., Lee, S. H., Deuschle, K., and McDermott, W.: Ineffectiveness of isoniazid in modifying the phenomenon of microbial persistence. Am. Rev. Tuberc. 76:1106, 1957.

51. McCune, R. M., Deuschle, K., Jordahl, C., Des Prez, R., Muschenheim, C., and McDermott, W.: The influence of streptovaricin used alone and with isoniazid in an experimental tuberculous infection in animals, and some clinical observations. Am. Rev. Tuberc. *75*:659, 1957.

52. McCune, R. M., Jr., and Tompsett, R.: Fate of *Mycobacterium tuberculosis* in mouse tissues as determined by the microbial enumeration technique. I. The persistence of drug-susceptible tubercle bacilli in the tissues despite prolonged antimicrobial therapy. J. Exp. Med. *104*:737, 1956.

53. McCune, R. M., Jr., Tompsett, R., and McDermott, W.: The fate of *Mycobacterium tuberculosis* in mouse tissues as determined by the microbial enumeration technique. II. The conversion of tuberculous infection to the latent state by the administration of pyrazinamide and a companion drug. J. Exp. Med. *104*:763, 1956.

54. McKee, C. M., Rake, G., Donovick, R., and Jambor, W. P.: The use of the mouse in a standardized test for antituberculous activity of compounds of natural or synthetic origin. I. Choice and standardization of culture. Am. Rev. Tuberc. *60*:90, 1949.

55. Meynell, G. G., and Meynell, E.: Theory and Practice in Experimental Bacteriology. 2nd. ed. Cambridge, The University Press, 1970.

56. Morrison, N. E., and Collins, F. M.: Restoration of T-cell responsiveness by thymosin: Development of antituberculous resistance in BCG-infected animals. Infect. Immun. *13*:554, 1976.

57. Muschenheim, C., Forkner, C. E., and Duerschner, D. R.: Effect of N'-dodecanoylsulfanilamide and of sulfapyridine on experimental tuberculosis in rabbits. Proc. Soc. Exp. Biol. Med. *45*:556, 1940.

58. Opie, E. L., and Freund, J.: An experimental study of protective inoculation with heat killed tubercle bacilli. J. Exp. Med. *66*:761, 1937.

59. Perla, D.: Experimental epidemiology of tuberculosis. The elimination of tubercle bacilli in the feces, bile, and urine of infected guinea pigs. J. Exp. Med. *45*:1025, 1927.

60. Pierce, C., Dubos, R. J., and Middlebrook, G.: Infection of mice with mammalian tubercle bacilli grown in Tween-albumin liquid medium. J. Exp. Med. *86*:159, 1947.

61. Raleigh, G. W., and Youmans, G. P.: The use of mice in experimental chemotherapy of tuberculosis. I. Rationale and review of the literature. J. Infect. Dis. *82*:197, 1948.

62. Raleigh, G. W., and Youmans, G. P.: The use of mice in experimental chemotherapy of tuberculosis. II. Pathology and pathogenesis. J. Infect. Dis. *82*:205, 1948.

63. Ribi, E., Anacker, R. L., Barclay, W. R., Brehmer, W., Harris, S. C., Leif, W. R., and Simmons, J.: Efficacy of mycobacterial cell walls as a vaccine against airborne tuberculosis in the rhesus monkey. J. Infect. Dis. *123*:527, 1971.

64. Ribi, E., Anacker, R. L., Brehmer, W., Goode, G., Larson, C. L., List, R. H., Milner, K. C., and Wicht, W. C.: Factors influencing protection against experimental tuberculosis in mice by heat-stable cell wall vaccines. J. Bacteriol. *92*:869, 1966.

65. Ribi, E., Brehmer, W., and Milner, K.: Specificity of resistance to tuberculosis and to salmonellosis stimulated in mice by oil-treated cell walls. Proc. Soc. Exp. Biol. Med. *124*:408, 1967.

66. Ribi, E., and Larson, C.: Immunological properties of cell wall versus protoplasm from mycobacteria. Zbl. Bakt. I Abt. Ref. *194*:673, 1964.

67. Ribi, E., Larson, C., Wicht, W., List, R., and Goode, G.: Effective nonliving vaccine against experimental tuberculosis in mice. J. Bacteriol. *91*:975, 1966.

68. Rich, A. R.: The Pathogenesis of Tuberculosis. 2nd ed. Springfield, Ill., Charles C Thomas, 1951.

69. Rich, A. R., and Follis, R. H., Jr.: The inhibitory effect of sulfanilamide on the development of experimental tuberculosis in the guinea pig. Bull. Johns Hopkins Hosp. *62*:77, 1938.

70. Rist, N., Bloch, F., and Hamon, V.: Action inhibitrice du sulfamid et d'une sulfone sur la multiplication *in vitro* et *in vivo* du bacille tuberculeux aviaire. Ann. Inst. Pasteur (Paris) *64*:203, 1940.

71. Rubbo, S. D., and Pierson, B. J.: A rapid method of screening antituberculous agents in the guinea pig. Am. Rev. Tuberc. *68*:48, 1953.

72. Sattler, T. H., and Youmans, G. P.: Unpublished results.

73. Saz, A. K., Johnston, F. R., Burger, A., and Bernheim, F.: Effect of aromatic iodine compounds on the tubercle bacillus. Am. Rev. Tuberc. *48*:40, 1943.

74. Schmidt, L. H.: Some observations on the utility of simian pulmonary tuberculosis in defining the therapeutic potentialities of isoniazid. Proceedings of a Symposium on Tuberculosis in Infancy and Childhood. Am. Rev. Tuberc. *74*(Supplement):138, 1956.

75. Schmidt, L. H., Hoffman, R., and Jolly, P. N.: Induced pulmonary tuberculosis in the rhesus monkey: Its usefulness in evaluating chemotherapeutic agents. Transactions of the 14th Conference on Chemotherapy of Tuberculosis (Atlanta,

Georgia). Veterans Administration, Army/Navy, Washington, D. C., 1955.

76. Schwabacher, H., and Wilson, G. S.: Inoculation of minimal doses of tubercle bacilli into guinea pigs, rabbits, and mice. Tubercle 18:492, 1937.
77. Sever, J. L., and Youmans, G. P.: The enumeration of nonpathogenic viable tubercle bacilli from the organs of mice. Am. Rev. Tuberc. 75:280, 1957.
78. Sever, J. L., and Youmans, G. P.: Enumeration of viable tubercle bacilli from the organs of nonimmunized and immunized mice. Am. Rev. Tuberc. 76:616, 1957.
79. Shortley, G., and Wilkins, J. R.: Independent-action and birth-death models in experimental microbiology. Bacteriol. Rev. 29:102, 1965.
80. Smith, D. W., Grover, A. A., and Nungester, W. J.: Comparison of immunizing properties of BCG, ultraviolet irradiated vaccines, and various lipid antigens in rats, mice and guinea pigs. U. Mich. Med. Bull. 19:122, 1953.
81. Smith, D. W., Grover, A. A., and Wiegeshaus, E.: Nonliving immunogenic substances of mycobacteria. Adv. Tuberc. Res. 16:191, 1968.
82. Smith, D. W., McMurray, D. N., Wiegeshaus, E. H., Grover, A. A., and Harding, G. E.: Host-parasite relationships in experimental airborne tuberculosis. IV. Early events in the course of infection in vaccinated and nonvaccinated guinea pigs. Am. Rev. Respir. Dis. 102:937, 1970.
83. Smith, D. W., Wiegeshaus, E., Navalkar, R., and Grover, A. A.: Host-parasite relationships in experimental airborne tuberculosis. I. Preliminary studies in BCG-vaccinated and nonvaccinated animals. J. Bacteriol. 91:718, 1966.
84. Smith, D. W., Wiegeshaus, E. H., Stark, R. H., and Harding, G. E.: Models for potency assay of tuberculosis vaccines. In Chamberlayne, E. C. (ed.): Status of Immunization in Tuberculosis in 1971. Washington, D.C., U.S. Government Printing Office, DHEW Publication No. (NIH) 72-68, 1972.
85. Smith, M. I., Emmart, E. W., and Westfall, B. B.: The action of certain sulfonamides, sulfones and related phosphorus compounds in experimental tuberculosis. J. Pharmacol. Exp. Therap. 74:163, 1942.
86. Smith, M. I., McClosky, W. T., and Emmart, E. W.: Influence of streptomycin and promin on proliferation of tubercle bacilli in the tissues of albino rat. Proc. Soc. Exp. Biol. Med. 62:157, 1946.
87. Solotorovsky, M., Siegel, H., and Ott, W. H.: The use of avian tuberculosis in the chick for experimental studies. Ann. N.Y. Acad. Sci. 52:696, 1949.

88. Soltys, M. A., and Jennings, A. R.: The dissemination of tubercle bacilli in experimental tuberculosis in the guinea pig. Am. Rev. Tuberc. 61:399, 1950.
89. Steenken, W., Jr., Wolinsky, E., Bristol, L. J., and Costigan, W. J.: Use of the rabbit in experimental tuberculosis. I. A visual method of evaluation of antituberculous agents by serial chest roentgenograms. Am. Rev. Tuberc. 68:65, 1953.
90. Swedberg, B.: Studies in experimental tuberculosis. Investigation of some problems of immunity and resistance. Acta Med. Scandinav. (Suppl.) 139:254, 1951.
91. Weiss, D. W., and Wells, A. Q.: Vaccination against tuberculosis with nonliving vaccines. II. Vaccination of guinea pigs with phenol-killed tubercle bacilli. Am. Rev. Respir. Dis. 81:518, 1960.
92. Weiss, D. W., and Wells, A. Q.: Vaccination against tuberculosis with nonliving vaccines. III. Vaccination of guinea pigs with fractions of phenol-killed tubercle bacilli. Am. Rev. Respir. Dis. 82:339, 1960.
93. Wiegeshaus, E. H., McMurray, D. N., Grover, A. A., Harding, G. E., and Smith, D. W.: Host-parasite relationships in experimental airborne tuberculosis. III. Relevance of microbial enumeration to acquired resistance in guinea pigs. Am. Rev. Respir. Dis. 102:422, 1970.
94. Willis, H. S.: Studies on tuberculous infection. X. The early dissemination of tubercle bacilli after intracutaneous inoculation of guinea pigs of first infection. Am. Rev. Tuberc. 11:427, 1925.
95. Woodruff, C. E., Kelly, R. G., and Leaming, M. A.: Spleen-appearance time of tubercle bacilli, as related to dosage of bacilli. Am. Rev. Tuberc. 51:574, 1945.
96. Youmans, G. P., Doub, L., and Youmans, A. S.: The Bacteriostatic Activity of 3500 Organic Compounds for *Mycobacterium tuberculosis* var. *hominis*. Washington, D.C.; Chemical-Biological Coordination Center, National Research Council, 1953.
97. Youmans, G. P., and McCarter, J. C.: A preliminary note on the effect of streptomycin on experimental tuberculosis of white mice. Q. Bull. Northwestern U. Med. Sch. 19:210, 1945.
98. Youmans, G. P., and McCarter, J. C.: Streptomycin in experimental tuberculosis. Its effect on tuberculous infections in mice produced by *M. tuberculosis* var. *hominis*. Am. Rev. Tuberc. 52:432, 1945.
99. Youmans, G. P., and Raleigh, G. W.: The use of mice in experimental chemotherapy of tuberculosis. III. The histopathologic assay of chemotherapeutic action. J. Infect. Dis. 82:221, 1948.
100. Youmans, G. P., and Youmans, A. S.: Experimental chemotherapy of tuberculosis and other mycobacterial infections. In

Schnitzer, R. J., and Hawking, F. (eds.): Experimental Chemotherapy. Vol. II. New York, Academic Press, 1964.

101. Youmans, G. P., and Youmans, A. S.: The measurement of the response of immunized mice to infection with *Mycobacterium tuberculosis* var. *hominis*. J. Immunol. *78*:318, 1957.

102. Youmans, G. P., and Youmans, A. S.: The relation between the size of the infecting dose of tubercle bacilli and the survival time of mice. Am. Rev. Tuberc. *64*:534, 1951.

103. Youmans, G. P., and Youmans, A. S.: The relationship of sex to the susceptibility of normal and immunized mice to tuberculosis. Am. Rev. Respir. Dis. *80*:750, 1959.

104. Youmans, G. P., and Youmans, A. S.: Relative effectiveness of living and non-living vaccines. *In* Chamberlayne, E. C. (ed.):

Status of Immunization in Tuberculosis in 1971. Washington, D.C., U.S. Government Printing Office, DHEW Publication No. (NIH) 72–68, 1972.

105. Youmans, G. P., and Youmans, A. S.: Response of mice to a standard infecting dose of *Mycobacterium tuberculosis* var. *hominis*. Proc. Soc. Exp. Biol. Med. *90*:238, 1955.

106. Youmans, G. P., and Youmans, A. S.: Response of vaccinated and nonvaccinated syngeneic C57Bl/6 mice to infection with *Mycobacterium tuberculosis*. Infect. Immun. *6*:748, 1972.

107. Youmans, G. P., and Youmans, A. S.: Unpublished data.

108. Youmans, G. P., Youmans, A. S., and Kanai, K.: The difference in response of four strains of mice to immunization against tuberculous infection. Am. Rev. Respir. Dis. *80*:753, 1959.

16

Epidemiology of Tuberculosis

INTRODUCTION

In this chapter we will focus on the transmission of tuberculosis and the factors responsible for the development and decline of the epidemic of tuberculosis, which has afflicted mankind for more than 400 years. We will not dwell to any great extent upon the influence of such factors as sex, age, race, and season on the incidence and mortality of tuberculosis, since these have been amply covered in texts of microbiology and medicine,[4, 12, 22, 24, 40] in other books,[10, 27, 28, 34, 39] and in Chapters 6 and 14 of this book.

In the United States, the incidence of tuberculosis has decreased to the point where today probably 95 percent or more of the children reach early adulthood without having been exposed to tuberculosis. This situation is viewed by the medical profession and public health workers with great pride and complacency, although apparently the decline has taken place pretty much independently of the efforts mankind has made to control the disease. Are we entitled to view this low incidence of tuberculosis with complacency, or should we perhaps view it with apprehension, if not with alarm?

We will show in this chapter that there is some reason for concern. Only through an understanding of the factors involved in the transmission of

356

tuberculosis and of the operation of the factors leading to the rise and decline of the epidemic can we hope to cope with the problem of tuberculosis in future generations of human beings.

TRANSMISSION

Although tuberculosis can affect almost every organ and tissue of the body (see Chapter 14), the chronic form of the disease is predominantly pulmonary. The bacilli are most frequently discharged from a pulmonary focus and reach the upper respiratory tract, where they are either swallowed or discharged to the outside by spitting, coughing, or sneezing. Therefore, the causative microorganism is most commonly transmitted from an open case of pulmonary disease to other persons by way of infected droplet nuclei. These droplet nuclei are created when the diseased person coughs or sneezes. Tiny droplets of mucous expelled in this way rapidly dry and become droplet nuclei. The larger mucous particles containing tubercle bacilli settle out rapidly, but the very small droplet nuclei may remain suspended in the air, depending upon conditions, for hours. Only particles less than 10 mμ in diameter are small enough to reach the alveoli. Particles larger than this either are retained in the upper respiratory tract or will settle on the mucous membranes of the trachea and larger bronchi. In the latter situation, the particles, including those containing tubercle bacilli, will be removed by the mucociliary stream, which then propels them upward into the oropharynx, where they are usually swallowed.

Other methods of transmission are possible but seldom occur. For example, tuberculosis due to *Mycobacterium bovis* was common at one time because of the consumption of milk from tuberculous cows. This mode of transmission is uncommon in the Western Nations at the present time but is still a factor in the maintenance of tuberculous disease in certain parts of the world.

Infection can occur from the handling of infected fomites, but this is unusual. It is difficult for tubercle bacilli from such contaminated objects to reach the alveoli of the lung. Persons, of course, may introduce tubercle bacilli from contaminated objects into the mouth by way of the hands or by direct introduction of the object into the oral cavity. However, the vast majority of tubercle bacilli will be disposed of by swallowing. For the most part, the tubercle bacilli acquired in this manner will be too few to produce progressive disease by way of the intestinal tract. At one time it was felt that dust and other objects in the room occupied over a period of time by a tuberculous patient could become contaminated and be a primary source of infection. For the reasons just mentioned, this seldom occurs. Aerosols of dust contain particles that, for the most part, are too large to reach the lower respiratory tract. It would be incorrect to say that infection and disease from such a course could never occur, but they are probably rare.

Infection of man with *Mycobacterium tuberculosis* can occur by way of the skin, provided the microorganisms are artificially introduced into or below the skin. Since *M. tuberculosis* is not found widely distributed in nature, inoculation tuberculosis will occur only in persons handling infected material. It is occasionally seen in medical students, pathologists, and laboratory workers handling cultures and infected animal tissues.

However, other mycobacteria that are found widely distributed in nature, such as *Mycobacterium ulcerans* and *M. marinum*, frequently produce skin lesions (see Chapter 18). Also, microorganisms such as *M. intracellulare* that are widely distributed in soil, water, food, and elsewhere will produce disease when ingested or inhaled (see Chapter 18).

EPIDEMIOLOGIC PATTERNS

History

Tuberculosis is undoubtedly an ancient disease.[14] Indeed, man may have been afflicted ever since he evolved. Evidence of existence of tuberculosis has been found in the bones of prehistoric man found in Germany. These remains dated back to about 8,000 B.C. Typical tuberculous changes have been found in the spines of skeletons of ancient Egyptians dating from about 2,500 to 1,000 B.C.[31] Descriptions of what could be tuberculosis also have been noted in ancient Hindu and Chinese writings.[14] These ancient clinical descriptions should be interpreted with caution because many other diseases can simulate tuberculosis; only in recent years have we been able to distinguish them readily. However, the typical changes in the spines of ancient man point to the presence of tuberculosis of the bone in early populations of human beings. Furthermore, although the point is still controversial, there is strong evidence that tuberculosis existed in American Indians before Europeans populated the New World.[18-20]

If, as appears to be the case, tuberculosis appeared very early in man's evolutionary scale, its persistence until this time should not be surprising. The chronic course of tuberculosis allows ample time for transmission, and the tubercle bacillus can persist in viable form in the tissues of healthy people for many years. Thus, ideal conditions are provided for the perpetuation of the microorganism and the maintenance of the disease in human populations. It has been pointed out[5] that with infectious diseases, those that can persist in an individual for a long period of time are highly

endemic but those that are infectious only in the acute phase die out quickly after introduction into a closed society.

Primitive societies consisted of relatively small isolated collections of human beings. Diseases such as measles, influenza, smallpox, poliomyelitis, and perhaps cholera probably could not have persisted in such societies. In fact there is a reasonable basis, according to Black,[5] for assuming that many of the diseases just mentioned may have only appeared in more modern times, perhaps after the first century A.D. when populations of human beings became large enough and communication between communities commonly occurred.

Tuberculosis, therefore, is an excellent example of a disease that can persist in small isolated communities. Furthermore, as we shall soon see, although tuberculosis is endemic in such restricted populations, the disease can become epidemic when urbanization occurs and large numbers of susceptible people become involved.

Epidemic "Waves"

An understanding of the incidence and prevalence of tuberculosis must be derived from material that dates back three or four hundred years. Accurate vital statistics on incidence and mortality are only available for about the last one hundred years. Furthermore, clinical descriptions of the disease written one or more centuries ago are subject to error because there was no way the clinicians of earlier eras could distinguish tuberculosis from the many other diseases with similar manifestations. We must remember that tuberculosis was shown to be a contagious disease with certainty, and the causative agent isolated, less than one hundred years ago.[26]

Keeping in mind the inadequacies

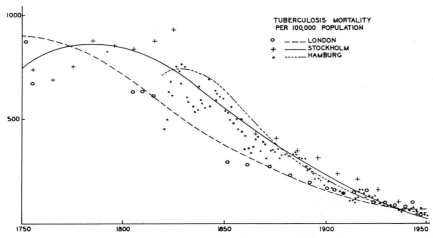

FIGURE 16–1. "Biologic phenomena exhibit cyclic patterns, and tuberculosis, as a group disease, makes no exception. The latest tuberculosis wave began its course in England in the sixteenth century, and reached a peak of mortality in London, probably before 1750. The capitals of Western Europe surmounted their peaks in the first half of the nineteenth century, those in Eastern Europe a few decades later. Statistical accuracy is wanting in early figures, but they permit identification of the general trend, which in this graph has been indicated by curves traced after considering the disparate points available." (From Grigg, E. R. N.: The arcana of tuberculosis with a brief epidemiologic history of the disease in the U. S. A., Parts I and II. Am. Rev. Tuberc. *78*:151, 1958.)

of the early data, there nevertheless appears to have been an enormous wave that has covered the last three or four hundred years (Fig. 16–1). Prior to the beginning of this wave, the disease was primarily endemic with cases appearing only sporadically. With the growth of cities that occurred as a consequence of the Industrial Revolution, the incidence and mortality of tuberculosis rapidly increased. The tuberculosis epidemic in Western Europe probably reached its peak about 1750, whereas in the United States, the peak of the epidemic was not reached until about 100 years later.[18-20] Following these peaks—in which the mortality rate reached 200 to 400 people per 100,000 population—incidence and mortality have decreased gradually until, at the present time, mortality rates in most Western Countries are below 20 per 100,000.

Idealized curves of both endemic (rural) and epidemic (urban) tuberculosis have been graphed by Grigg[18-20] and are shown in Figures 16–2 and 16–3. These graphs show that tuberculosis reached epidemic proportions in urban areas but that in rural areas the disease maintained an endemic character with a much lower incidence and much lower mortality. Grigg designed these curves to represent the major tuberculosis wave in two extreme settings, urban and rural. These two imaginary communities are assumed to remain isolated from the rest of the world and to maintain a constant level of urbanization throughout the three centuries shown. Grigg feels that the differences in mortality and morbidity, both in time and space, can be fully explained by differences in urbanization. An acute change in urbanization (e.g., as in war or in massive migration from a less tuberculous territory) will result in a minor wave superimposed upon the major wave, with successive (not synchronous) miniature peaks of mortality and morbidity. Wolff also has stressed the role of industrialization in increasing the incidence of tuberculosis.[41-43]

Grigg[18-20] pointed out that urbanization can account completely for the

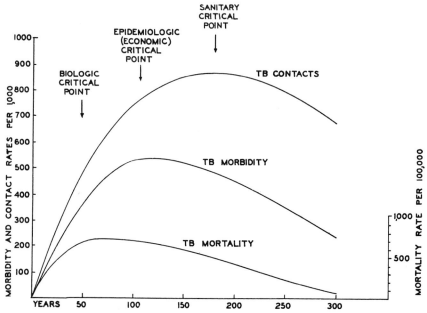

FIGURE 16–2. "This is the 'theoretical' development of a tuberculosis wave in an imaginary community (with stable degree of urbanization, and population completely isolated from the rest of the world) in which tuberculosis is assumed to appear for the first time at moment zero. Shown are the death rate (inscribed on a different scale, at right), the rate of sickness, i. e., tuberculin-positive persons, which avoids complicated definitions, and the rate of contacts, all three by reference to living population. Other intermediate curves (persons with apparent clinical disease, 'good chronics,' convalescents, *et cetera*) were not included, as they would only complicate the drawing (all follow similar, interposed pathways) without adding new information. As expected with biologic phenomena[21] all of these curves consist of two unequal segments, the ascending limb of which is comparatively steeper and shorter than the exponentially decelerated descending leg. It is also characteristic that the peaks appear in succession, not synchronously, which in real life is apt to cause confusion and/or contradictory statements. Furthermore, since theoretically the curves cannot reach the base line before infinity, the incidence of tuberculosis may decrease to the level of medical curiosities, but it is not very likely ever to become 'eradicated.' " (From Grigg, E. R. N.: The arcana of tuberculosis with a brief epidemiologic history of the disease in the U. S. A., Parts I and II. Am. Rev. Tuberc. *78:*151, 1958.

epidemic nature of tuberculosis because it acts in two major ways. First, urbanization brings about the collection of increasingly large numbers of susceptible persons in communities where there is a marked increase in mutual contact; this, in turn, permits much more ready transmission of *Mycobacterium tuberculosis* from diseased to normal persons. Second, the stress and strain of urban life may well lower natural resistance to infection. A most important point that can be derived from Figures 16–2 and 16–3 is that in spite of the gathering together of susceptible people and the greatly increased chance of transmission of *M. tuberculosis*, these factors do not continue to operate. Eventually, many years after the initiation of these events, the mortality and incidence level off and then begin a slow decline. The rate of this decline has been shown to be exponential. Also, the decline may be interrupted because of extraneous factors such as war, famine, flood, and so forth. However, the overall decline in morbidity and mortality is persistent and is still going on at the present time, although in many Western Countries it appears to be leveling off.

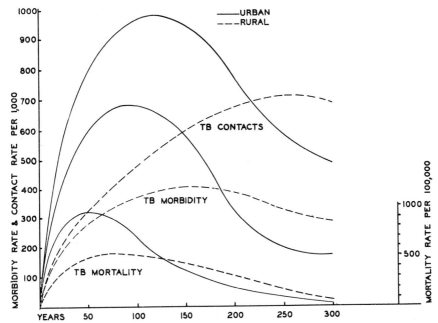

FIGURE 16–3. "Since the tuberculosis wave is the result of natural selection, its speed is proportional to the number of deaths per unit of time, and therefore, at any moment, the decrease will be commensurate with the preceding death rate. The pace of the wave is hastened by 'urbanization' because it increases the number of new contacts and raises the reactability potentials of exposed and afflicted persons (through stress and consequent alteration of corticosteroid secretions). Above curves represent the tuberculosis wave in two extreme settings (one urban, the other rural), these two imaginary communities being assumed to remain isolated from the rest of the world and to maintain a constant level of urbanization throughout the three centuries shown. These tracings, just like those in Figure 16–2, are intended only as a general outline of the phenomenon and are not for numerical comparison with observed situations. The variation in death rates between countries, or between communities, can be fully explained by the differences in urbanization, both in time and space. An acute increase in urbanization, for instance, war or massive immigration from a less tuberculized territory, will result in a reversal of the downward trend, the added deflection acting as a superimposed miniature wave, with successive (not synchronous) miniature peaks of mortality, morbidity, contacts, *et cetera*. In point of fact, observed tracings, especially in the United States, contain as a rule multiple peaks of mortality." (From Grigg, E. R. N.: The arcana of tuberculosis with a brief epidemiologic history of the disease in the U: S. A., Parts I and II. Am. Rev. Tuberc. *78*:151, 1958.)

Decline of Epidemic Tuberculosis

An explanation of the peaking of mortality and morbidity and spontaneous decline in tuberculosis has been speculated upon by a number of investigators.[6, 17, 32] Along with these researchers, Grigg[18-20] (as discussed in his excellent reviews, which should be consulted by those wishing more detailed data and more analyses) feels that the epidemic proportions that tuberculosis reached in the Western World can be accounted for by the crowding together of susceptibles under conditions conducive to dissemination of the causative organism and with native resistance to the infection reduced by the stress and strain (increased production of corticosteroids?) of modern urban and industrial life. With this part of Grigg's analysis, we have no quarrel. Grigg, though, feels that the major cause of the peaking out and the exponential decline in morbidity and mortality can be accounted for only by the building up of a more resistant population of human beings in urban communities because of the reduction in susceptibles by deaths from the disease itself. These more resistant people selected out by the disease would reproduce more-resistant offspring; therefore, the disease will naturally die out because of elimination of susceptibles and increase in number of resistant persons. This is further supported by the fact that in these epidemic periods the persons most affected and in whom there is the highest mortality are usually those in age from puberty to 35 or 40; that is to say, the most reproductive period in the life of human beings. Thus, fewer susceptible persons would be produced, hastening the selection of a more resistant population. This is an interesting theory that has also been used to explain the spontaneous decline in morbidity and mortality of other infectious deseases, such as leprosy, syphilis, and malaria.

Critical examination of the available evidence, however, can only raise serious doubts concerning the idea that natural selection of more resistant populations of human beings can account in large measure for the steady decrease in morbidity and mortality of tuberculosis. That such a selective process may play some role is readily admitted, but we feel that it is minor compared to the operation of other factors.

Statistical Considerations

Statistical considerations alone show that it would have been impossible to build up a highly resistant human population by a selective process in which the susceptibles are eliminated by death from tuberculosis. For example, if we look at the mortality rates at the height of the epidemic wave, it is estimated that these rates may have reached from 400 to 600 per 100,000 people (Figs. 16–1, 16–2, and 16–3). It is even possible that in some places, under certain circumstances, these rates may have reached 1,000 to 2,000

persons per 100,000; using these latter rates, which certainly exceed the rates that usually existed, it is easy to calculate that a mortality rate of 1,000 per 100,000 would consist of only 1 percent of the population and a rate of 2,000 per 100,000, only 2 percent. This means that the selective process would remove only 1 or 2 percent of the population per year. There is no conceivable way in which the elimination of only 1 or 2 percent of the population could significantly effect the overall resistance of the remaining 98 or 99 percent of human beings. It might be argued that the elimination of 1 or 2 percent of the human population per year, over a period of many years, would add up to a relatively large number of persons. This is entirely correct, but it is not the total number of persons eliminated that is important; rather, it is the *proportion* of persons eliminated that is meaningful. During the many years that people die in large numbers from tuberculosis, the remaining susceptibles, as well as the more resistant persons, will be reproducing. These susceptible persons presumably will have more susceptible offspring, whereas the resistant persons would have more resistant offspring. In view of the small proportion of persons who will die of tuberculosis each year, the ratio of more resistant to more susceptible in the people remaining cannot change significantly. It also has been estimated that for every death from tuberculosis, there are probably, at that point in time, ten active cases of the disease. It might be said that this group of active cases should be added to the number of persons who die of the disease because, presumably, they are highly susceptible and their reproduction rate will be much lower. Actually, persons with active disease can and do reproduce, although their rate of reproduction may perhaps be lower. Furthermore, those with active disease are not necessarily only the people who are genetically highly susceptible. Whether or not those persons who are genetically more resistant develop active disease will depend not only on their native resistance but also on many other factors. A major factor, of course, is the size of the infecting dose of tubercle bacilli (see Chapter 5). In any event, if instead of assuming a mortality rate of 1 or 2 percent, one increases the rate to 10 to 20 percent by including those persons with active disease, this higher rate would still not result in a situation that could seriously affect the ratio of more resistant to more susceptible persons in the remaining 80 or 90 percent of the population. Probably, a mortality rate of 90 percent or greater would be needed in order to bring about a marked increase in the number of remaining people who are genetically more resistant to tuberculosis.

Mini-Epidemics

Statistical considerations make it highly unlikely that selection and elimination of susceptibles could account for the marked decrease in incidence of tuberculosis in the Western Countries over the last 100 years or so; nevertheless, it would be much better to have direct evidence on whether or not persons living today who have not been exposed to tuberculosis are actually more resistant to infection with tubercle bacilli than were their forefathers. Fortunately, evidence on this point is available. Because of the marked decrease in incidence of tuberculosis in the United States over the last 100 years or so, there are many communities in which the number of people who have been exposed to tubercle bacilli is extremely low. Using the tuberculin test as the criterion of infection, the evidence obtained indicates that there are many population groups in this country in which the number of human beings infected with virulent tubercle bacilli

is 5 percent or less.[16] The remaining 95 percent (or more) have apparently never been exposed to tubercle bacilli. Also, these persons are the descendents of those who are supposed to have survived the tuberculosis epidemic of the last century and the early part of this century by virtue of their genetically greater resistance to tuberculous infection. Therefore, the descendants should comprise a genetically more resistant population of human beings that has developed because of the removal, by death from tuberculosis, of the more susceptible persons during the epidemic years. Theoretically then, if these descendants are now exposed to virulent tubercle bacilli, the incidence of active tuberculous disease in them should be much lower than it was in those more susceptible persons who accounted for most of the cases during the epidemic years. Actually, studies of mini-epidemics that have occurred recently in the United States and in other Western Countries have shown that the incidence of active disease in tuberculin-negative people today is not significantly less than it was in their forefathers of 100 years ago.[1, 2, 7-9, 11, 15, 23, 29, 30, 33, 35-38]

There have been numerous mini-epidemics, for example, in classrooms where children have been exposed to a teacher or classmate who has tuberculosis.[8, 9, 11, 23, 29, 33, 35, 36] Also, a number of such epidemics have occurred on naval vessels where naval personnel have been exposed to an unsuspected active case of tuberculosis in seamen.[15, 25]

In these mini-epidemics of tuberculosis, the contact rate, as determined by tuberculin tests, may be as high as 100 percent. The morbidity rate may range from 5 percent to as high as 20 percent of those persons exposed. This compares favorably with the percent of active cases noted during the height of the epidemic wave. Accurate morbidity data are not available for these early years, but they can be calculated from the mortality data on the basis that there are approximately 10 active cases for each death from tuberculosis. By following this procedure, we find that approximately 5 to 20 percent of the population at risk developed active tuberculosis. These figures do not differ significantly from the ones noted in many of the mini-epidemics.

Such data provide direct confirmation that there has been no significant increase in the level of genetic resistance to tuberculosis over the years by virtue of the removal from the population of the more susceptible persons by death from tuberculosis.

It is clear from the preceding discussion that selective factors have not produced a population of human beings much more resistant to tuberculosis. We cannot account for the steady decline of tuberculosis in the Western World on this basis; therefore, we will now address ourselves to an explanation that does not involve a selective process.

De-Urbanization (Suburbanization)

We already have noted that epidemic tuberculosis, with a high case-incidence and mortality rate, developed because of the urbanization that was a consequence of the Industrial Revolution. We have already noted how this urbanization provided optimal conditions for transmission of the disease among highly susceptible persons. In addition, people were required to live under deplorable conditions of sanitation and housing. These adverse conditions, together with the reduction of resistance brought about by overwork, poor nutrition, and stressful conditions, undoubtedly helped to account for the marked increase in incidence of the disease. It would be reasonable to assume that the incidence of tuberculosis engendered by these conditions would decrease with de-urbanization or with a

correction of the bad features of urbanization. It is, therefore, probably no coincidence that the topping out of the tuberculosis epidemic coincides with the beginning of the period of correction of the evils of urbanization. These corrections include better and less-crowded housing, shorter working hours, and better sanitation. All of these factors would lead to fewer chances for transmission and to less reduction of resistance. This period also was the beginning of the demands of labor for better working conditions and better pay; both of these, in turn, led to better living conditions and better nutrition. None of these events, of course, occurred all at once. Rather, they developed over a long period of time at an increasing tempo while tuberculosis incidence steadily declined.

The steadily increasing affluence of a greater proportion of the human population over these many years has been responsible for the de-urbanization, which we should probably call "suburbanization." Today, more people probably live in the suburbs than in the central parts of our cities. Living conditions as well as factors that contribute to better health, sanitation, and so forth, probably are optimal in our suburbs. In particular, the crowding so necessary for transmission of tuberculosis is at a minimum. It is our feeling that these factors alone will account in large part for the steady decrease in incidence and mortality from tuberculosis in the Western World today.

The development of effective therapy with streptomycin in 1945, followed by the utilization of a number of other drugs (see Chapter 21), has sharply accelerated the decline of tuberculosis mortality. Effective therapy, which rapidly reduces infectivity of active cases, has, of course, accelerated the downward trend in the incidence of tuberculosis. More will be said about the effect of chemotherapy on tuberculosis incidence and mortality in other portions of this book (see Chapter 21).

Active Immunization

Another factor that may have contributed to the beginning of the decline in the incidence of tuberculosis at the peak of the epidemic wave is the development of acquired active immunity by the persons infected with tubercle bacilli who did not develop significant amounts of active disease. It is not sufficiently recognized that tuberculosis is an immunizing infection in those persons who do not succumb to disease (see Chapter 8). Thus, as the epidemic developed over the years, for the reasons already given, there appeared an increasingly large pool of persons who were more resistant by virtue of active immunization. When the number of these persons reached a point where they constituted a large proportion of the human population, the incidence would naturally begin to decline. In other words, because of active immunization, there may not have been enough highly susceptible persons to maintain the previous increase in incidence of the disease; the epidemic may have run out of a sufficient number of susceptible persons to keep it going at full speed.

This development, of course, would be accelerated by a decrease in the inflow of susceptible persons from rural areas. This inflow, which persisted for many years as a consequence of urbanization, was probably mainly responsible for maintenance of the epidemic phase of the disease. To what extent active immunization may have operated to help in the decline of tuberculosis is not known. However, we might examine a somewhat analogous situation that exists today. The incidence of tuberculosis in our large cities in the United States is higher within the slum areas, where crowding and other conditions are more conducive to spread of tuberculosis and where there is a considerable retention of other negative features of urbanization that promote the development of tuberculous disease. However, the disease in these areas is not epidemic in character, although the incidence is higher than in suburban or rural areas. Also, there is a much higher proportion of persons in these areas who are infected with tubercle bacilli; that is, the number and the proportion of tuberculin positive reactions are very much higher than those found in suburbs or rural parts of the country. The occurrence of disease in these slum areas is more endemic in character than epidemic and might be compared to the pattern of disease that occurred years ago in certain primitive isolated communities (Figs. 16–1, 16–2, and 16–3). In a population where there is a high degree of tuberculous infection but a moderate degree of tuberculous disease because of the immunity that has been acquired from infection with virulent tubercle bacilli, tuberculous disease will occur most frequently in those people whose resistance has been lowered, for example, older people and chronic alcoholics. The disease does not actually become epidemic because all of the factors, especially the presence of large numbers of susceptible persons, are not operating.

Role of Infection with Atypical Mycobacteria

Fifteen years ago,[44] we speculated on the possibility that the immunity produced in human beings by widespread natural infection with atypical mycobacteria might have played a role in the steady decline in the incidence of tuberculosis in the United States:

[*M. kansasii* and *M. intracellulare* will produce in mice and guinea pigs a high degree of immunity to infection with *M.*

tuberculosis.[44] Such] . . . data do not, however, provide evidence for the immunogenicity of these microorganisms in human beings, but it does not appear unreasonable to accept, as a working hypothesis, that an appreciable degree of immunity would develop in persons naturally infected with these unclassified mycobacteria.

If, as a result of natural infection, both *M. kansasii* and *M. intracellulare* do produce a high degree of immunity in man to infection with *M. tuberculosis,* then it would follow that from 15 to 74 percent of the people of the United States may be naturally immunized against tuberculosis by the time of early adulthood, since tuberculin testing surveys indicate that these proportions of Navy recruits, depending on the state from which they came may be infected with *M. intracellulare.*[16]

Direct evidence for the presence of a large non-specifically immunized human population in the United States because of inapparent infection with unclassified mycobacteria is completely lacking. It is to be hoped that data will be accumulated in the future which will indicate whether the incidence of tuberculosis is appreciably less in people naturally infected with unclassified mycobacteria than in persons not so infected.

The very real possibility, however, that large numbers of naturally actively immunized people exist in the United States due to infection with unclassified mycobacteria raises the interesting question of what influence this situation may have had on the steady decline in incidence in tuberculosis which has been evident in this country ever since reasonably reliable morbidity rates have been available. The factors responsible for this persistent decline in incidence of this disease in the United States have never been clearly understood. In a review entitled "The Arcana of Tuberculosis,"[18-20] Grigg again has pointed out that this steady decline apparently has been independent of the efforts mankind has spent on control of the disease.

We should point out, that no matter how intriguing this hypothesis may be, it is not supported by the data obtained from the mini-epidemics mentioned earlier in this chapter. A large proportion of the persons involved in these epidemics must have been naturally infected with *M. intracellulare* and should have constituted a partially immunized population. Yet, as we have already noted, the incidence of active disease apparently did not differ from that noted a hundred or more years ago. This argues strongly against the possibility that natural infection with atypical mycobacteria may have played a large role in the steady decline in incidence of tuberculosis.

CONSIDERATIONS FOR THE FUTURE

Regardless of the reason, or reasons, for the steady decline in the incidence and prevalence of tuberculosis in the Western World, today we are faced, at least in the United States, with a situation where the great majority of our adult population have never been infected with tubercle bacilli. The proportion of persons in this category is increasing yearly, as shown by the steadily decreasing morbidity data (see Table 16–1). If the evidence provided by the mini-epidemics is valid—and we believe that it is—we are, in turn, faced with a situation in which we have a large, yearly increasing, highly susceptible population of human beings.

In view of the high proportion of susceptible persons in our population, we must be aware of the possibility that tuberculosis might again become epidemic. It would only require some massive disruption of our social and economic systems, forcing human beings again to live under crowded, unsanitary conditions. In this regard, war, of course, is the causative agent to be most feared. The effectiveness of war in this respect is fully attested to by our experiences in the First and Second World Wars. The incidence and mortality from tuberculosis increased markedly in those countries

TABLE 16–1. Morbidity and Mortality from
Tuberculosis in the United States—1965–1976

Year	Number of Reported Cases	Number of Cases of Tuberculosis Per 100,000 Population
1965	49,016	25.29
1966	47,767	24.38
1967	45,647	23.07
1968	42,623	21.33
1969	39,120	19.37
1970	37,137	18.22
1971	35,217	17.07
1972	32,882	15.79
1973	30,998	14.77
1974	30,210	14.29
1975	33,989	15.90
1976	32,105	15.00

suffering the greatest dislocations in their economy and social structures. Fortunately, these changes persisted for only a few years. When the wars were over and conditions reverted to the normal patterns of Western culture, the incidence and mortality from tuberculosis again promptly began to decline. We may not be so fortunate in the next global conflict, especially if atomic forces are unleashed.

Some authors have suggested that because of the rapid decline in tuberculosis, the disease soon would become extinct.[3, 13] In fact, Dublin[13] in 1941 predicted that tuberculosis probably would be eradicated within 20 years. A glance at Table 16–1 will illustrate the faultiness of this prediction. Part of the error that leads to such faulty predictions arises from extending the descending mortality or morbidity curves to zero without realizing that an exponential curve cannot reach zero this side of infinity. Grigg[18-20] has emphasized this point. In fact, the expected flattening out of the morbidity curve is already evident (Table 16–1). Also, the nature of the host-parasite relationship in tuberculosis (see Chapter 14) argues strongly against the possibility that tuberculosis will ever be eradicated. As long as tubercle bacilli can infect persons and

remain viable in their tissues for a lifetime, potential sources of tuberculous disease will always be with us.

The only conceivable way, at this time in which tuberculosis could be eradicated would be by the use of an antimicrobial agent so powerful that it would rapidly kill every tubercle bacillus in every person to whom it was administered. The likelihood of such a development in the foreseeable future is very small. Even if such a compound were found, tuberculosis could only be eradicated by administering it to every infected man, woman and child in the world. This in itself would pose problems almost impossible to solve.

All in all, tuberculosis will probably be with us for many centuries to come. Certain areas of the world may become almost free of the disease, but the accumulation in these areas of large numbers of susceptible persons may provide the basic requirements for future epidemics that, in turn, will restore the position of tuberculosis as "Captain of All the Men of Death."[14]

REFERENCES

1. Alpert, M. E., and Levison, M. E.: An epidemic of tuberculosis in a medical school. N. Engl. J. Med. 272:718, 1965.

2. Associated Press: TB hits 15 in Michigan nursery. Chicago Daily News, January 19, 1966.
3. Bates, J. H.: The changing scene in tuberculosis. N. Engl. J. Med. 297:610, 1977.
4. Beeson, P. B., and McDermott, W. (eds.): Textbook of Medicine. 14th ed. Philadelphia, W. B. Saunders Co., 1975.
5. Black, F. L.: Infectious diseases in primitive societies. Science 187:515, 1975.
6. Burnet, F. M.: The Background of Infectious Diseases in Man. Melbourne, Brown, Prior, Anderson Ptg. Ltd., 1946.
7. Center for Disease Control: Epidemiological notes and reports tuberculosis — California. Morbidity and Mortality 22(No. 37): 309, 1973.
8. Center for Disease Control: Epidemiological notes and reports tuberculosis —North Dakota. Morbidity and Mortality 22(No. 13):109, 1973.
9. Darney, P. D., and Clenny, N. D.: Tuberculosis outbreak in an Alabama high school. J.A.M.A. 216:2117, 1971.
10. Darzins, E.: The Bacteriology of Tuberculosis. Minneapolis, University of Minnesota Press, 1958.
11. Davies, J. W.: Epidemics of tuberculosis in Canada in the sixties. Can. Med. Assoc. J. 96:1156, 1967.
12. Davis, B. D., Dulbecco, R., Eisen, H. N., Ginsberg, H. S., Wood, W. B., and McCarty, M.: Microbiology. 2nd ed. Hagerstown, Md., Harper & Row, Publishers, 1973.
13. Dublin, L. I.: Decline of tuberculosis. Present death rates and the outlook for the future. Am. Rev. Tuberc. 43:224, 1941.
14. Dubos, R., and Dubos, J.: The White Plague. Tuberculosis, Man and Society. Boston, Little, Brown and Company, 1952.
15. (Editorial): Tuberculosis in a destroyer. J.A.M.A. 179:284, 1962.
16. Edwards, L. B., Edwards, P. Q., and Palmer, C. E.: Sources of tuberculin sensitivity in human populations. A summing up of recent epidemiologic research. Acta Tuberc. Scandivan. Suppl. 47:77, 1959.
17. Godfrey, E. S., Jr.: Epidemiology of tuberculosis. Principles of programs of tuberculosis associations. Am. Rev. Tuberc. 43:1, 1941.
18. Grigg, E. R. N.: The arcana of tuberculosis with a brief epidemiologic history of the disease in the U. S. A., Parts I and II. Am. Rev. Tuberc. 78:151, 1958.
19. Grigg, E. R. N.: The arcana of tuberculosis with a brief epidemiologic history of the disease in the U. S. A. Part III. Am. Rev. Tuberc. 78:426, 1958.
20. Grigg, E. R. N.: The arcana of tuberculosis with a brief epidemiologic history of the disease in the U. S. A. Part IV. Am. Rev. Tuberc. 78:583, 1958.
21. Grigg, E. R. N.: Essay on a fundamental law of life: The time-factor (relativity) in biological phenomena. Hum. Biol. 28:1, 1956.
22. Hoeprich, P. D. (ed.): Infectious Diseases. Hagerstown, Md., Harper & Row, Publishers, 1972.
23. Horton, R., Champlin, R. D., Rogers, E. F. H., and Korns, R. F.: Epidemic of tuberculosis in a high school. Report of eight year follow-up of students exposed. J.A.M.A. 149:331, 1952.
24. Joklik, W. K., and Willett, H. P. (eds.): Zinsser Microbiology. 16th ed. New York, Appleton-Century-Crofts, 1976.
25. Knight, V.: Tuberculosis afloat. J.A.M.A. 203:154, 1968.
26. Koch, R.: Die Aetiologie der Tuberkulose. Berl. Klin. Wochenschr. 19:221, 1882.
27. Long, E. R.: The Chemistry and Chemotherapy of Tuberculosis. 3rd. ed. Baltimore, Md., The Williams & Wilkins Company, 1958.
28. Lurie, M. B.: Resistance to Tuberculosis: Experimental Studies in Native and Acquired Defensive Mechanisms. Cambridge, Harvard University Press, 1964.
29. Mahady, S. C. F.: An outbreak of primary tuberculosis in school children. Am. Rev. Tuberc. 84:348, 1961.
30. Moore, P. E.: Puvalluttuq. An epidemic of tuberculosis at Eskimo Point, Northwest Territories. Can. Med. Assoc. J. 90:1193, 1964.
31. Morse, D., Brothwell, D. R., and Ucko, P. J.: Tuberculosis in ancient Egypt. Am. Rev. Tuberc. 90:524, 1964.
32. Pearson, K.: Tuberculosis, Heredity and Environment. London, Cambridge University Press, 1912.
33. Petter, C. K.: What price apathy — A school epidemic of tuberculosis. Diseases of the Chest 44:587, 1963.
34. Rich, A. R.: The Pathogenesis of Tuberculosis. 2nd ed. Springfield, Ill., Charles C Thomas, 1951.
35. Rideout, V. K., and Hiltz, J. E.: An epidemic of tuberculosis in a rural high school in 1967. Can. J. Public Health 60:22, 1969.
36. Rogers, E. F. H.: Epidemiology of an outbreak of tuberculosis among school children. Public Health Rep. 77:401, 1962.
37. Steiner, M., Chaves, A. D., Lyons, H. A., Steiner, P., and Portugaleza, C.: Primary drug-resistant tuberculosis. Report of an outbreak. N. Engl. J. Med. 283:1353, 1970.
38. Weber, R. E.: The Whitehall episode. National Tuberculosis Association Bulletin 47(No. 4):1961.
39. Willis, H. S., and Cummings, M. M.: Diag-

nostic and Experimental Methods in Tuberculosis. 2nd ed. Springfield, Ill., Charles C Thomas, 1952.

40. Wilson, G. S., and Miles, A.: Topley & Wilson's Principles of Bacteriology, Virology and Immunity. 6th ed. Baltimore, Md., The Williams & Wilkins Company, 1975.

41. Wolff, G.: Tuberculosis mortality and industrialization. With special reference to the United States. Part I. Am. Rev. Tuberc. *42*:1, 1940.

42. Wolff, G.: Tuberculosis mortality and industrialization: With special reference to the United States. Part II. Am. Rev. Tuberc. *42*:214, 1940.

43. Wolff, G.: Tuberculosis mortality as an index of hygienic control. Biometric contributions to the epidemiology of tuberculosis. Am. Rev. Tuberc. *34*:734, 1936.

44. Youmans, G. P., Parlett, R. C., and Youmans, A. S.: The significance of the response of mice to immunization with viable unclassified mycobacteria. Am. Rev. Respir. Dis. *83*:903, 1961.

17

Prevention of Tuberculosis

INTRODUCTION

In Chapter 16, which dealt with the epidemiology of tuberculosis, we described how the incidence of tuberculosis in the Western World has been decreasing for many years at an exponential rate. Furthermore, the beginning of this decrease antedated by many years the announcement of the discovery of the etiology of tuberculosis by Koch in 1882. Therefore, the incidence of tuberculosis had been steadily decreasing well before human beings were even aware that it was an infectious disease or that it was transmitted from person to person by way of infected droplet nuclei created from the secretions expelled by diseased persons.

We have also commented (see Chapter 16) on the many factors that contributed to this steady decline in incidence — de-urbanization, with its decreased chance for transmission of the disease; more adequate nutrition; less crowding and more sanitary conditions in factories and other places of employment; decreased work loads resulting in decreased stress; better housing and overall increase in sanitation; and of course, in more recent times, the chemotherapy of active cases of the disease.

METHODS OF PREVENTION

Sanatorium Treatment

Once the etiology of tuberculosis and mode of transmission became known, interest developed in accelerating the decline in the incidence by instituting active preventive measures. It was felt that if patients with active disease, who served as foci of infection, could be removed from the community in which they resided and isolated from susceptible persons, transmission of the disease would be prevented and reduction in the incidence of the disease achieved. Emphasis on this method of preventing the spread of tuberculosis led to, in the early part of this century, the construction in Western countries of many hospitals (sanatoria) to be used solely for the housing of patients with tuberculosis. It was hoped that in this setting, the patients would not only be prevented from transmitting disease widely through their community but also they would be in a better position to receive those benefits of medical treatment that were available.

Knowledge of the etiology of the disease rapidly led to more efficient methods for diagnosis; therefore, active cases of tuberculosis could be more readily detected and then isolated from family and friends. There is little question that the vigorous application of these practices had some impact on the occurrence of tuberculosis in the Western World. However, it is difficult to see this effect if one compares the overall rate of decline of incidence or mortality from tuberculosis prior to the institution of sanatorium treatment with the incidence and mortality in the years following (see Figure 16–1, p. 359). The reasons for this apparent contradiction are not clear. However, we can only assume that the natural forces referred to previously (and discussed in more detail in Chapter 16) exerted far more influence on the incidence of tuberculosis than did man's efforts — as well considered and logical as these efforts may have seemed to the physicians and public health workers of that time.

Chemotherapy

In any event, the era of the tuberculosis sanatorium and, for that matter, the era of large case-finding programs are now at an end. The effectiveness of chemotherapy for tuberculosis today is such that patients with active disease can be rendered noninfectious for other people within a few days or weeks after treatment is begun. There is no need to isolate patients with active disease for extended periods of time. Most patients with tuberculosis can be treated on an ambulatory basis while living at home, and bed rest is not the major feature of therapy that it once was. Chapter 21 should be consulted for the details of therapy of tuberculosis and its relationship to prevention.

There is, however, just as great a need as ever to detect the occasional person with active tuberculosis and to see that he or she is made noninfectious through treatment as rapidly as possible. The catastrophic consequences of a person with an active case of tuberculosis being introduced into a classroom or naval vessel have been detailed in Chapter 16. Therefore, physicians and public health workers should ever be on the alert for the occasional case of active tuberculosis that may still occur in any one of our communities, no matter how low the overall incidence of the disease may be.

Raising the Level of Resistance of the Population at Risk

In the past, one of the problems in regard to the prevention of tuberculosis, at least in the United States, has been the failure on the part of physicians and public health officers to allow their preventive efforts to follow logically from the nature and mode of transmission of the infectious process. The infectious case, for the most part, is the person with cavitary pulmonary disease. Bacilli are liberated from the disease process in the lung and transmitted to the upper respiratory tract where they are expelled to form droplet nuclei, which are infectious for persons who inhale them. Thus, tuberculosis is a respiratory disease that is transmitted from person to person in the same manner that all respiratory infectious diseases of human beings are transmitted. It has been generally recognized that such respiratory diseases cannot be adequately controlled by trying to prevent the transmission of the infectious agent. Prevention by controlling transmission of tuberculosis, for example, could only be accomplished if every person in this country could be completely isolated from every other person at all times. The absurdity of this kind of solution, of course, is evident. Even the isolation of active cases as practiced earlier in this century largely failed because, first, it was difficult to detect more than a small proportion of active cases and, second, it was almost impossible to keep such people isolated for the months or years required until they became noninfectious. Only a few of the most cooperative patients will submit to a program that requires their isolation from the rest of humanity for an extended period. The trauma of being shut off from family and friends for prolonged periods is more than most people can endure. Also, the cost of such programs, if applied to an entire population, is prohibitive. It is not surprising that little impact on tuberculosis morbidity can be detected from programs based on the philosophy that to prevent tuberculosis, patients should be isolated and treated until noninfectious. This also holds true for all other respiratory infectious diseases.

With most other respiratory tract infections, recognition of these facts by physicians and scientists has led to another approach — to focus preventative efforts on raising the average level of resistance of human beings to the particular parasite in question. Witness what has been accomplished in the prevention of diphtheria by the application of this principle. There is, in fact, no really effective way in which the control of a respiratory infectious disease can be accomplished except through raising the level of resistance to infection of the population at risk until significant numbers of persons will not develop disease.

In the United States in the past, a large proportion of physicians and workers have denied the usefulness of increasing the average resistance to infection to *M. tuberculosis* for a number of reasons: 1) A belief that there is no such thing as immunity in tuberculosis.[37, 42] 2) The only vaccine available (BCG) is ineffective.[37] 3) BCG vaccine, since it is a living bacterium, may be dangerous because it may cause progressive disease. 4) BCG vaccine induces the development of tuberculin hypersensitivity and, therefore, ruins the diagnostic significance of the tuberculin test. 5) Even if an effective vaccine were available, the incidence of tuberculosis is too low to justify vaccinating any but persons whose occupations involve excessive risk of contracting tuberculosis.

We will examine the validity of these reasons for refusal to use BCG vaccine in the following section of this chapter (although not exactly in this order).

VACCINATION AGAINST TUBERCULOSIS

General Principles

In Chapter 8, we discussed the development of acquired immunity in tuberculosis, and in Chapters 9, 10, and 11, considerable attention was given to a variety of immunizing substances found in mycobacterial cells. Our current knowledge concerning the nature of the specific acquired immune response in tuberculosis has been covered in detail in Chapers 10, 12, and 13. It is not our purpose here to further discuss either the immunizing agents found in mycobacterial cells or the nature of the immune response. Rather, we intend to focus upon the use of vaccination as a procedure for the prevention of tuberculosis. Our attention will be focused primarily on BCG as a vaccine, since it is currently the only available vaccine useful for administration to human beings.

At this point, though, we should deal with the first objection — i.e., is there any such thing as immunity to tuberculosis? In view of all the experimental evidence presented in previous chapters of this book, such a question would appear to be pointless. Nevertheless, even as late as 1965,[37] statements can be found in the literature that reflect a substantial body of opinion held by earlier workers in the field to the effect that there is really no such thing as immunity to tuberculosis. This feeling on the part of earlier workers stemmed from observations showing that persons with tuberculosis, even when apparently fully recovered, could reinfect themselves from tubercle bacilli harbored for months or years in a quiescent state in their own tissues. First, these earlier workers did not realize that the immune response in tuberculosis was one that primarily exerted a *bacteriostatic* effect on the virulent tubercle bacilli in the tissues, not *bacteriocidal*. Second, there was no awareness of the fact that since the potent bacteriostatic action of the specific immune response was what produced the resolution of the infection, any factor that would lower the magnitude of these immune forces would promote reactivation of the disease. Finally, there was little realization that

the prompt resolution of most cases of primary infection was a consequence of the action of specific immunity that developed in response to the infecting tubercle bacilli. In contrast to the generally held opinion, the recovery from disease is not due to so-called natural, or innate, nonspecific resistance mechanisms (see Chapter 6).

BCG Vaccine

The controlled studies on vaccination of human beings with BCG vaccine conclusively show that human beings can develop a powerful immune response to virulent tubercle bacilli.

BCG actually is a fairly recent vaccine against tuberculosis because it was not used in humans until 1921.[23] This does not mean, however, that earlier attempts to vaccinate human beings against tuberculosis were not made. Actually, almost from the time that Koch announced the discovery of the tubercle bacillus in 1882, attempts were made to use either attenuated or killed tubercle bacilli to increase resistance to tuberculosis. These attempts, of course, would have been a logical step because of the brilliant success achieved by Louis Pasteur in the immediately preceding years in the prevention of anthrax, chicken cholera, and rabies by vaccination. Also, Koch in 1891 revealed that guinea pigs infected with tubercle bacilli were appreciably more resistant to infection with virulent tubercle bacilli.[29, 30] This was manifested by what is now known as the "Koch Phenomenon." Although the Koch Phenomenon is a manifestation of an allergic hyperreactivity of guinea pig tissues to tubercle bacilli and their products, Koch clearly recognized that, at the same time, there was appreciable evidence of increased resistance to infection in the reinfected animals because the disease did not progress as rapidly and the spread to the regional lymph nodes from the site of inoculation of virulent tubercle bacilli was greatly retarded.

Early attempts to use killed bacilli for vaccination readily demonstrated, as discussed in Chapter 8, that these were not nearly as effective as vaccines composed of attenuated strains. A number of attenuated strains were developed; these included the "BOVO" vaccine (1902), which is an attenuated human tubercle bacillus, and the "Tauruman" (1904), which is an unusual combination of attenuated human and bovine tubercle bacilli.[42] However, the early demonstration that these strains were able to produce progressive tuberculous disease in guinea pigs resulted in the abandoning of their use.

The details of some of these early attempts, including the focusing of attention on killed tubercle bacilli, have been described by Rosenthal[44] and by Rich.[42]

The history of the development of BCG vaccine (bacillus Calmette-Guérin) has been vividly described by Guérin.[23] The vaccine was developed in the laboratories of Calmette between 1908 and 1921. A bovine strain of *M. tuberculosis* was grown on pieces of potato cooked at 70° C in beef bile containing 5 percent glycerine, and the medium was kept impregnated with this same liquid. The pieces of potato so treated were placed in Roux tubes, with the lower portion immersed in beef bile and glycerinated at 5 percent, and the whole was sterilized at 120° C. Two hundred and thirty-one consecutive transplants were made on this medium. After these were accomplished, it was found in 1921 that the originally virulent bovine tubercle bacillus had no pathogenicity for animals; otherwise, it appeared unchanged.

Since 1921, when BCG vaccine was first administered to a child, the use of BCG in the vaccination of human beings for the prevention of tuberculosis has been the subject of great con-

troversy. Initially, the vaccine was given orally. While great claims were made concerning its effectiveness for the prevention of tuberculosis, actual evidence was lacking. Most investigators using BCG vaccine in human beings failed to realize that it was essential to compare vaccinated subjects with a select control group of persons as nearly identical as possible in age, sex, color, social and economic values, and general environment to the vaccinated group. These should have been followed up in exactly the same way over the same period of time. Instead, the usual practice was to compare the mortality from tuberculosis in vaccinated infants with estimated mortality for nonvaccinated infants in similar surroundings or in the country as a whole. A number of investigators, such as Greenwood,[20] Greenwood and Wolff,[21] Wolff,[50, 51] Rosenfeld,[43] and Berghaus,[4, 5] pointed out that such comparisons are invalid. Statistical analyses, such as those of Greenwood, that questioned the lack of efficacy of BCG vaccine, while completely justified, had the effect as pointed out by Hart,[24] "of throwing out the baby with the bath water" because physicians and investigators in countries such as Great Britain and the United States dismissed BCG vaccine as being ineffective.[37, 42, 49] BCG vaccine, however, continued to be used in empirical fashion in a number of countries on the European continent.[47]

Furthermore, the Lubeck disaster in 1930 gave BCG a bad name. In that year, in Lubeck, Germany, some 75 infants died as the result of being given oral BCG vaccine. It was subsequently shown after extensive investigation that these tuberculosis deaths were not caused by BCG but by a virulent strain of the tubercle bacillus that had been inadvertently substituted for the BCG strain and administered to the infants.[19, 28] The overall effect of this disaster, and of the subsequent investigation, was to leave in the minds of many the thought that BCG vaccine was potentially a very dangerous vaccine to administer to human beings.

It was not until 1937 that the first prospective control trial of BCG vaccine was initiated by Aronson[2] in American Indians. In this study, the vaccinees were randomly distributed into vaccinated and control groups, and they were followed over a period of 20 years. Since that time, only some six reasonably well-controlled vaccine trials of BCG vaccine in human beings have been carried out.[9, 17, 24, 32–34, 40, 45] The effectiveness of BCG vaccine given in these six trials is listed in Table 17–1. In this table, the percent reduction in cases of tuberculosis that occurred in the vaccinated persons is compared to equivalent nonvaccinated control persons. Also in these studies, the vaccinated and nonvaccinated persons were all found to be tuberculin-negative before they were allocated to either group.

Examination of Table 17–1 shows that four of the six studies showed a relatively high degree of efficacy for BCG vaccine, whereas two showed very little efficacy. A number of reasons have been advanced for these discrepancies, particularly the discrepancy between the good result in the British BCG trial and the poor result in the United States Public Health Service trials in Georgia and Puerto Rico. These reasons have included: 1) variation in potency of the BCG strain used for vaccination, since they were different in each study;[24] 2) the inclusion in the Georgia and Puerto Rican studies of large numbers of persons who were naturally infected with atypical mycobacteria and who were therefore already at least partially immunized, since obviously, inclusion of a large number of partially immunized persons in the control groups of such trials would markedly reduce the apparent efficacy of the vaccine being tested;[24] and 3) it has been suggested that the persons involved in the Georgia and Puerto Rican trials may have been nutritionally deficient as compared with the vaccinees in Great Britain. This, however, does not seem to be a likely reason. The most reasonable explanation appears to be, as pointed out by Hart,[24] that BCG vaccination in populations of human beings that already have a broad base of infection with atypical mycobacteria would not be expected to show very

TABLE 17–1. **Six Controlled Trials of BCG Vaccination**

Intake (date)	Population Group	Reference	Vaccine	Observation Period (years)	Efficacy of BCG (percent)
1936 to 1938	N. American Indians	Aronson et al. (1958)[2]	Phipps	20	80
1937 to 1948	Chicago infants	Rosenthal et al. (1961)[45]	Tice*	12 to 23	74
1949 to 1950	Puerto Ricans	Palmer et al. (1958)[40] (U.S.P.H.S.)	N.Y. State	6 to 7	31
1949 to 1950	Georgia/Alabama	Comstock and Palmer (1966)[9] (U.S.P.H.S.)	Tice*	14	14
1950 to 1952	British urban schoolchildren	Medical Research Council (1956, 1959, 1963)[32–34]	Danish	12.5	79
1950 to 1955	S. Indian villagers	Frimodt-Møller et al. (1964)[17]	Madras	2 to 7	60

*This laboratory has issued a number of substrains, and it is not clear whether those used for the two trials were the same or different.

From Hart, P. D.: Efficacy and applicability of mass BCG vaccination in tuberculosis control. Br. J. Med. 1:587, 1967.

much of an added effect due to BCG vaccine. This is of particular importance because in the developing countries where BCG vaccine is now considered to be most useful, there may be much more natural infection with atypical mycobacteria. Comstock and Webster[10] think that this is an unlikely explanation for the failure of the Georgia and Puerto Rican studies, since all reactors to 100 TU of tuberculin were eliminated from the study. We will not discuss this in further detail here but refer the reader to detailed reviews by Hart,[24] Comstock and Webster,[10] and Topley and Wilson.[49] It is reasonable to conclude, though, from four of the studies mentioned above that when susceptible populations of human beings are vaccinated with a suitable strain of BCG vaccine, a high level of protection against subsequent infection can be expected.

The fact that BCG is a highly effective vaccine for the prevention of tuberculosis in human beings when it is administered to fully susceptible persons gives rise to the question of what person or groups of persons should be vaccinated. This matter is what Hart[24] refers to as the applicability of the vaccine. In a population of human beings where there is a heavy prevalence of infection with atypical mycobacteria and when, therefore, the population is at least partially immunized against tuberculosis, one can only expect BCG vaccination of such persons to raise the level of resistance to what it would be if they had received BCG vaccine alone. Experimentally, this has been shown to be the case by Palmer and Long.[39] One would also expect in such persons that the risk of exposure to tuberculosis would be lower because there would be fewer active cases. Therefore, the risk of exposure might possibly be so small that BCG vaccination would not be warranted. This might easily have been the case in the persons vaccinated in the Georgia/Alabama and the Puerto Rican studies of the United States Public

Health Service. On the other hand, in populations of human beings not infected with other mycobacteria and in which the prevalence of tuberculosis has decreased to a very low point because of the continued decline in incidence, the question also could be raised about the need for vaccination with BCG. The risk of exposure could be so low that vaccination might not be warranted. A paradoxical situation, therefore, is created in that in such populations of human beings, as the decrease in tuberculosis continues, the proportion of susceptible persons increases; therefore, their need for protection by vaccination should theoretically also increase. However, if this increase in the number of susceptibles is not accompanied with either a similar or an increased risk of infection, the need for vaccination also would decrease steadily over a period of time. Large areas of the United States would probably fall in this latter category because in many rural areas the incidence of tuberculosis is now small. It does not apply to certain portions of our large urban areas. Not only is the incidence of tuberculosis still high in these areas, but crowding contributes to greater ease of transmission, while other factors (see Chapter 16) contribute to greater susceptibility. In fact, in 1964 the City of New York began a program of BCG vaccination with the hope that this would reduce the incidence of tuberculosis in some of the poorer and more crowded areas of the city. This program, however, has not been continued and, in fact, was terminated a few years later without any real evaluation of the effectiveness of BCG vaccine under these conditions.

The greatest need for BCG vaccine at the present time is in the underdeveloped areas of the world where tuberculosis is still a major problem because the chances of transmission are still great and living conditions and the overall state of nutrition of the population are such as to contribute to the spread of tuberculosis. However, it is particularly in these areas that there may also be a rather heavy prevalence of infection due to atypical mycobacteria of one kind or another. One would then expect these human populations to be partially immunized, and the question arises whether vaccination would be effective. Hart[24] feels that another controlled study of the efficacy of BCG vaccine for the reduction of tuberculosis in populations of human beings in the underdeveloped countries is badly needed because we cannot really answer the question of whether BCG vaccination is useful in such situations until such a study has been conducted. In the meantime, though, from the practical standpoint, BCG vaccination is about the only preventative program that can be effectively administered to the majority of people in such countries. It is difficult to understand, though, if the underlying high prevalence of immunizing infection with atypical mycobacteria has substantially raised the resistance to tuberculosis in the people of these areas, why the incidence of tuberculosis still remains so high.

In view of this contradiction, it would appear to be reasonable that BCG vaccination is warranted in these areas solely on the basis that no matter what the prevalence of atypical acid-fast infection and, therefore, no matter how high the resistance of the population to infection with *M. tuberculosis* might be because of this atypical infection base, BCG vaccination of such persons would at least raise the average resistance of the population to infection to that degree contributed by BCG vaccination alone.[39] Depending upon the particular population group, this added degree of protection either might or might not be of significance, but in view of the fact that no other procedure is available for even partial control of tuberculosis in such countries, BCG vaccination can be justified. Hart[24] also feels that mass vaccination in the developing countries would have a beneficial, even though possibly additive, effect on the average level of resistance to tuberculosis. He makes the point that the earlier in life vaccination can be given, the better the chances for success because the proportion of susceptible individuals in a population of human beings is vastly greater early in life than later after they have been exposed to the disease or infection with mycobacteria other than *M. tuberculosis.* Youmans[53] stressed this point as early as 1957.

Tuberculin Conversion by BCG Vaccine

We must also consider briefly the objection that vaccination of human beings with BCG is undesirable because it renders tuberculin-negative people tuberculin-positive, thus destroying the diagnostic usefulness of the tuberculin test. It almost goes without saying that vaccination of human beings when the vast majority of persons are tuberculin-negative would be, first of all, undesirable and unnecessary because the risk of infection is so small. We have already commented on this. Second, since the risk of infection is so small and, therefore, the necessity for vaccination very remote, to render most of the population tuberculin-positive might hamper the detection of the occasional case of tuberculosis that might occur and certainly would render the tuberculin test of very little use in studying the epidemiology of mini-epidemics or small outbreaks.

Of course, if the efficacy of BCG vaccination in such tuberculin-negative populations is such that 80 percent of persons vaccinated will not get tuberculosis even if exposed, the question can be legitimately raised: What need would there ever be for tuberculin testing? Also, the meaningfulness of a positive tuberculin test for the detection of single isolated cases or in diagnosing pulmonary disease in a person where a lesion might be due to tuberculosis is of limited value (see Chapters 14 and 21). Therefore, the usefulness of the tuberculin test under any of the circumstances just described can be seriously questioned.

The argument that BCG vaccination should not be used because it destroys the validity of the tuberculin test is also meaningless when applied to populations of human beings where a high proportion are tuberculin-positive by virtue of previous infection with *M. tuberculosis*. In such persons it is clear that a positive tuberculin test does not necessarily mean tuberculous disease and that the detection of tuberculin hypersensitivity in a population of human beings where the majority of people have been infected and are, therefore, tuberculin-positive has little meaning. If such persons were vaccinated with BCG, their tuberculin reactivity might be somewhat augmented, but the limited usefulness of the tuberculin test as a diagnostic tool in such persons would not be affected.

On the other hand, in a population of human beings of whom a high proportion were naturally tuberculin-positive, if BCG was administered only to those who were tuberculin-negative because of their high risk of developing primary infection and disease, then, of course, BCG vaccination of such persons would greatly interfere with the usefulness of the tuberculin test for detection of recent infection with *M. tuberculosis*. In other words, if the tuberculin test converts from negative to positive in a person known to have been exposed to a tuberculous patient in the recent past, or in a person who developed pulmonary disease of unknown etiology when it was known that in the very recent past his tuberculin test had been negative, the significance of the conversion to the tuberculin-positive state is

great, since it indicates recent infection and, therefore, the possibility of the development of progressive tuberculous disease. BCG vaccination would certainly eliminate this use of the tuberculin test.

Tuberculosis Control Programs

For the reasons just given, many people feel that vaccination with BCG of persons whose risk of infection with *M. tuberculosis* is high, such as medical students, nurses, laboratory workers, and other hospital personnel, and who are tuberculin-negative is not warranted. They prefer to monitor annually the status of tuberculin sensitivity of such tuberculin-negative persons, and if conversion from negative to positive occurs, the person is treated with isoniazid. Such a procedure seems eminently reasonable because it should afford adequate protection to persons who become infected by virtue of the nature of their work, and yet it does not involve the elimination of the usefulness of the tuberculin test to determine whether infection has actually occurred. Unfortunately, most such programs fail to realize that this procedure, as logical as it appears to be, usually fails in performance because the monitoring of the tuberculin sensitivity is not done often enough. As noted previously, the most common course of action is to do tuberculin tests annually on tuberculin-negative persons and then treat the tuberculin converters by giving isoniazid. However, such programs fail to take into consideration the fact that such a person can unknowingly become infected and then develop progressive disease in as little time as six to eight weeks following the time of infection. If tuberculin tests are only done annually and if in a particular person the moment of exposure takes place within a few weeks or months after the annual tuberculin test has been administered, there will be ample time in which he or she could develop progressive disease of severe dimensions before the date of the next annual tuberculin test.

It is also not feasible to do tuberculin tests more often, say every two or three months, as would be required to fully cover the situation, because of the difficulty and expense of finding the personnel to administer the tests and because of the difficulty in getting the cooperation of the persons at risk for such frequent testing. Also, there is some evidence that frequent tuberculin tests may induce or augment tuberculin hypersensitivity.[41]

The author of this chapter has had extensive experience with the administration of such tuberculosis prevention programs to medical and dental students in one of our larger Midwest universities. While an enormous amount of effort was expended by the Student Health Service and others to administer the program and while student cooperation for the most part was good, it is the author's experience that there was no single instance in which a case of tuberculosis that developed in such students was detected because of the recent conversion of the tuberculin test. In all such cases where tuberculosis did develop — and cases of tuberculosis still do occur occasionally among medical students, dental students, nurses, and so forth — such disease was detected from examination of a routine chest x-ray taken in the course of an examination because of complaints of illness completely unrelated to those that might follow from tuberculous pulmonary disease. In the final analysis, then, these tuberculin-negative students might just as well have been vaccinated with BCG with a resulting 80 percent reduction in incidence of disease.

As a result of this large personal experience referred to in the preceding paragraph, my own recommendation would be to vaccinate those tuberculin-negative persons who are of high risk with BCG, thus achieving a significant reduction in incidence of tuberculosis and, at the same time, recommend to such persons that they get at least annual, and preferably semi-annual, chest x-rays to pick up incipient pulmonary disease in the occasional person who will develop tuberculosis in spite of vaccination with BCG.

All in all, we can only conclude that the argument against vaccination with BCG because it destroys the diagnostic usefulness of the tuberculin test is not much of an argument after all since the tuberculin test, even in people with a high risk of exposure, has relatively little value in detecting early tuberculosis.

Of course, the development of a vaccine against tuberculosis, such as the RNA vaccine described in Chapter 9, that would not induce tuberculin hypersensitivity and that is suitable for use in human beings would resolve the problem completely.

Safety of BCG Vaccine

The safety of BCG vaccine has already been discussed. However, one should be aware that local and sometimes systemic reactions do occur. These may be persistent ulcerations at the site of vaccination, and occasionally lupus erythematosus may occur. Such reactions are rare and never life threatening. Fatal BCG infections have been described but appear to occur mostly in infants and children who are immunologically deprived. Discussions of reactions to BCG will be found in some of the references.[19, 24, 32-34, 44, 49]

Recently, Lotte and associates[30a] have analyzed the adverse reactions that have occurred in approximately 1,470,-000,000 persons who were vaccinated with BCG between 1948 and 1974. The number and rate of complications per one million vaccinees are shown in

TABLE 17–2. **Adverse Reactions Following BCG Vaccination**

Serious post-BCG complications	Number of complications[a]		Rate per 1 million vaccinees
	A	B	
Abnormal BCG primary complexes	7,349	6,602	4.49
Abnormal post-BCG (non-specific) reactions (e.g., keloids, rashes, ocular manifestations, etc.)	1,894	1,838	1.25
Lesions due to BCG dissemination (some generalized and some localized)	1,128	1,072	0.72
A. *Non-fatal cases*			
Otitis and retro-pharyngeal abscesses	305	294	
Dermatological "tuberculous-like" lesions	254	242	
Lesions of bones, joints and soft tissues	295	291	
Renal lesions	2	2	
Pulmonary lesions and hilar adenitis	196	174	
Mesenteric adenitis	10	9	
Multiple adenitis (with or without hepato-splenomegaly)	30	28	
Meningitis	1	1	
B. *Fatal cases*			
Generalized lesions	35	31	
All categories of complications	10,371[b]	9,512[c]	6.46

[a]A: Total number of cases recorded and described by the authors.
  B: of which cases among subjects vaccinated from 1948 to 1974.
[b]10,371 complications concerning 9,690 patients.
[c] 9,512 complications concerning 8,874 patients.
  From Lotte, A., Wasz-Höckert, O., Poisson, N., and Dumitrescu, D.: Complications induced by BCG vaccination: A retrospective study. Bull. Int. Union Tuberc. *53*:114, 1978.

Table 17–2. The types of reactions and the fatalities also are presented in this table. One thousand seventy-two cases of disease due to dissemination of BCG were noted, and the nature of the pathologic process was confirmed bacteriologically and histologically in over half of the cases. The overwhelming majority of the disseminated lesions were found in cases from 21 European countries; the incidence in these countries (2.19 per million vaccinees) is probably due to methods of surveillance that are more precise than those used in less developed countries. This also means that, undoubtedly, a number of similar cases have occurred elsewhere in the world but have passed unrecorded.

In Western countries, BCG vaccination should be administered only to tuberculin-negative people because reactions are apt to be somewhat more frequent and severe in people who are tuberculin-positive. A great deal, though, depends upon the manner in which the vaccine is administered. The multiple puncture method of Rosenthal[44] seldom results in untoward reactions. Intradermal or subcutaneous inoculations are more apt to produce persistent draining lesions at the site of injection. In those parts of the world where it is not feasible to do tuberculin tests, BCG vaccination has been applied without consideration of the tuberculin sensitivity of the vaccinees. There seems to be no real contraindication to this, although as already noted, reactions sometimes are more severe.[24] Insofar as the development of immunity is concerned, vaccination of such tuberculin-positive persons would only serve to enhance their cellular immunity to infection.

CHEMOPROPHYLAXIS OF TUBERCULOSIS

No discussion of the prevention of tuberculosis would be complete without some consideration of chemoprophylaxis. Chemoprophylaxis literally means the administration of chemotherapeutic agents to persons at risk of infection with *Mycobacterium tuberculosis* in order to prevent infection and the subsequent development of progressive disease. Because of the lack of suitable chemotherapeutic agents, little attention was given to this approach to the prevention of tuberculosis until the advent of isoniazid in the early 1950s. Isoniazid was found to be a potent antimycobacterial agent that could be administered orally in reasonably small doses (see Chapters 20 and 21) and that appeared to have few, if any, deleterious side effects. It seemed, therefore, to be the ideal agent to administer to persons to prevent tuberculosis.

A number of controlled studies were set up by different investigators for the purpose of determining the effectiveness of isoniazid for the prevention of tuberculosis. These have been summarized by Ferebee and are shown in Table 17–3, Examination of Table 17–3,[6–8, 11, 12, 14–16, 22, 25–27, 35, 36, 38, 48] however, reveals that the term chemoprophylaxis is misleading because what was actually studied was the effect of ioniazid in the following situations: for the treatment of primary infection in children; in tuberculin converters; in contacts with known active cases who could have been presumed to be tuberculin-positive; in persons in mental institutions, that is, in older persons strongly tuberculin-positive and therefore presumed infected; and in selected populations in Alaska, Greenland, and Africa where the incidence of the disease was very high and the majority of people could be presumed to be infected.

Other terms, such as primary pro-phylaxis and secondary prophylaxis have been used in an attempt to differentiate between the prevention of infection and the prevention of disease.[13] In the same vein, some have preferred to use the terms infection prophylaxis and disease prophylaxis.[13] Actually, as Ferebee[13] points out, the term chemoprophylaxis properly should be reserved for the use of isoniazid or any other drug to prevent infection; as Ferebee also states, candidates for chemoprophylaxis under this restricted definition would be the same as those eligible for vaccination — i.e., the uninfected. Ferebee goes on to say that in her opinion only in unusual circumstances when there is a high risk of infection for a short time would the use of isoniazid to prevent infection appear to merit consideration. This would also presumably be the only condition under which Ferebee would recommend BCG vaccination.

The studies listed in Table 17–3 and general experience have shown that the use of isoniazid for the treatment of infection with *M. tuberculosis* can be highly effective for preventing the development of progressive disease or complications. However, all of these are properly considered part of the treatment of tuberculosis, whether it is treatment of an apparently inactive infection or of an active, clinical disease. The use of isoniazid for such purposes should be discussed under therapy, and a full discussion, therefore, will be found in Chapter 21.

We wish to stress that the use of isoniazid or of any other drug solely for the prevention of infection in tuberculin-negative people suffers from a number of disadvantages. First, to be effective, the drug must be taken daily over long periods of time. To obtain the cooperation either of individuals or of large numbers of people in the daily self-administration of a drug is extremely difficult. Contrast the problems here with the ease of ad-

TABLE 17–3. **Characteristics of Selected Controlled Trials of Isoniazid Prophylaxis**

Trial	Reference	Sites	Number	Randomization Unit	Admission Period
	UNITED STATES PUBLIC HEALTH SERVICE PROGRAM				
Primary tuberculosis	Ferebee et al. (1957)[15]	Pediatric clinics	2,750	Individual	Jan. 1955 to
	Mount and Ferebee (1961)[36]	29 Continental US			Dec. 1957
		1 Puerto Rico			
		1 Canada			
		1 Mexico			
Contacts of known active cases	Mount and Ferebee (1962)[35]	Health department	2,814	Household	Oct. 1956 to
		5 Continental US			April 1957
Contacts of new active cases	Ferebee and Mount (1962)[14]	Health departments	25,033	Household	Jan. 1957 to
		37 Continental US			Dec. 1959
		19 Puerto Rico			
		1 Mexico			
Mental institutions	Ferebee et al. (1963)[16]	33 hospitals	27,924	Ward or building	Oct. 1957 to May 1960
		4 schools			
Alaskan villagers	Comstock (1962)[7]	30 villages	6,275	Household	Dec. 1957 to
	Comstock et al. (1967)[8]	Bethel area			Oct. 1959
Inactive lesions	Ferebee and Mount (1962)[14]	Health departments	4,575	Individual	Sept. 1960 to
		25 Continental US			Oct. 1964
		1 Puerto Rico			
		1 Mexico			
	DANISH TUBERCULOSIS INDEX				
Greenland villagers	Groth-Peterson et al. (1960)[22]	76 Western	8,081	Village	July 1956 to
	Horwitz et al. (1966)[25]	Greenland villages			Nov. 1967
	TUBERCULOSIS CHEMOTHERAPY AND BCG CENTRE, NAIROBI, KENYA				
Contacts of new active cases	Egsmose et al. (1965)[12]	Rural area of northern Kenya	775	Household	1959 to 1961
	TUNIS MINISTRY OF HEALTH				
Community	Nyboe et al. (1963)[38]	Suburb of Tunis City	15,910	City blocks	Mar. 1958 to Aug. 1959
	YODOGAWA CHRISTIAN HOSPITAL, OSAKA, JAPAN				
Contacts of known active cases	Bush et al. (1965)[6]	Hospital clinic	2,238	Household	June 1958 —
	ROYAL NETHERLANDS NAVY				
Tuberculin converters	Veening (1968)[48]	Marine training camp	261	Individual	May 1960 —
	QUEZON INSTITUTE, MANILA, REPUBLIC OF THE PHILIPPINES				
Household contacts	Del Castillo et al. (1965)[11]	Hospital clinic	293	Household	July 1961 to Dec. 1962
	HUDSON RIVER HOSPITAL, NEW YORK STATE				
Inactive lesions	Katz et al. (1965)[26]	Mental hospital	513	Individual	April 1958 to
	Katz et al. (1962)[27]				Feb. 1964

From Ferebee, S. H.: Controlled chemoprophylaxis trials in tuberculosis. A general review. Adv. Tuberc. Res. *17*:28, 1969.

ministering BCG once and producing an increased resistance that will last for years. Also, isoniazid, for example, has been found to have serious side effects.[1, 3, 18, 31, 46, 52] A significant incidence of hepatitis, which may be severe and even fatal, has been found in persons taking isoniazid prophylactically for long periods of time. (This is also more fully discussed in Chapter 21). There is really no conceivable circumstance in which isoniazid, or any other drug available today, can be substituted with equal effectiveness for vaccination with BCG for the prevention of tuberculous infection. Once a person has become infected as indicated by positive tuberculin tests or by other criteria, then treatment with isoniazid may or may not be considered appropriate (see Chapter 21).

We wind up this brief discussion of chemoprophylaxis by pointing out that although impractical at the moment for protection against infection, the principle involved in the use of a drug such as isoniazid for prevention is exactly the same as the principle involved in the use of a vaccine such as BCG for prevention. The aim in both cases is to raise the average level of resistance of the population at risk and thereby prevent initial infection and the development of tuberculous disease. Those persons who advocate chemoprophylaxis in the pure sense, as we have described it here, for the prevention of tuberculosis and inveigh against BCG vaccination are apparently unaware that even though the means employed are different, the desired end result in both cases is the same.

We can even go further and speculate that vaccination against tuberculosis with an agent such as BCG may, in a sense, be a form of chemoprophylaxis. We have noted in Chapters 8, 9, 10, 11, 12, and 13 that acquired immunity in tuberculosis is apparently mediated by a lymphocyte product that, in some manner or another, brings about the arrest of multiplication of virulent tubercle bacilli. This substance acts as a tuberculostatic agent, although we do not know the mechanism involved, and in this respect, it is entirely similar to a number of the bacteriostatic drugs that are used for the treatment of tuberculosis. To this writer's knowledge, the concept that BCG vaccination may be a form of chemoprophylaxis has not been entertained previously. It is, however, an entirely reasonable concept in light of what we know about the nature of the acquired immune reaction in tuberculosis at the moment. With the further development of our knowledge, we may find an even closer relationship between chemoprophylaxis and vaccination against tuberculosis.

REFERENCES

1. Alarcón-Segovia, D., Fishbein, E., and Alcalá, H.: Isoniazid acetylation rate and development of antinuclear antibodies upon isoniazid treatment. Arthritis Rheum. *14*:748, 1971.
2. Aronson, J. D., Aronson, C. F., and Taylor, H. C.: A twenty-year appraisal of BCG vaccination in the control of tuberculosis. Arch. Intern. Med. *101*:881, 1958.
3. Bailey, W. C., Taylor, S. L., Dascomb, H. E., Greenberg, H. B., and Ziskind, M. M.: Disturbed hepatic function during isoniazid chemoprophylaxis. Monitoring the hepatic function of 427 hospital employees receiving isoniazid chemoprophylaxis for tuberculosis. Am. Rev. Respir. Dis. *107*:523, 1973.
4. Berghaus, W.: Die Kindertuberkulose und Calmettesche schutzimpfung im Lichte der badischen statistik. Zeitschr. Tuberk. *59*:230, 1931.
5. Berghaus, W.: Die tuberkuloseschutzimpfung von Calmette. Deutsche Med. Wochenschr. *56*:1771, 1930.
6. Bush, O. B., Jr., Sugimoto, M., Fujii, Y., and Brown, F. A., Jr.: Isoniazid prophylaxis in contacts of persons with known tuberculosis. Am. Rev. Respir. Dis. *92*:732, 1965.
7. Comstock, G. W.: Isoniazid prophylaxis in an underdeveloped area. Am. Rev. Respir. Dis. *86*:810, 1962.
8. Comstock, G. W., Ferebee, S. H., and Hammes, L. M.: A controlled trial of community-wide isoniazid prophylaxis in Alaska. Am. Rev. Respir. Dis. *95*:935, 1967.

9. Comstock, G. W., and Palmer, C. E.: Long-term results of BCG vaccination in the southern United States. Am. Rev. Respir. Dis. *93*:171, 1966.

10. Comstock, G. W., and Webster, R. G.: Tuberculosis studies in Muscogee County, Georgia. VII. A twenty-year evalution of BCG vaccination in a school population. Am. Rev. Respir. Dis. *100*:839, 1969.

11. Del Castillo, H., Bautista, L. D., Jacinto, C. P., Lorenzo, C. E., Lapuz, S., and Legaspi, B.: Chemoprophylaxis in the Philippines. A controlled pilot study among household contacts of tuberculosis cases. Bulletin Quezon Institute *7*:277, 1965.

12. Egsmose, T., Ang'awa, J. O. W., and Poti, S. J.: The use of isoniazid among household contacts of open cases of pulmonary tuberculosis. Bull. WHO *33*:419, 1965.

13. Ferebee, S. H.: Controlled chemoprophylaxis trials in tuberculosis. A general review. Adv. Tuberc. Res. *17*:28, 1969.

14. Ferebee, S. H., and Mount, F. W.: Tuberculosis morbidity in a controlled trial of the prophylactic use of isoniazid among household contacts. Am. Rev. Respir. Dis. *85*:490, 1962.

15. Ferebee, S. H., Mount, F. W., and Anastasiades, A. A.: Prophylactic effects of isoniazid on primary tuberculosis in children. A preliminary report. Am. Rev. Tuberc. *76*:942, 1957.

16. Ferebee, S. H., Mount, F. W., Murray, F. J., and Livesay, V. T.: A controlled trial of izoniazid prophylaxis in mental institutions. Am. Rev. Respir. Dis. *88*:161, 1963.

17. Frimodt-Møller, J., Thomas, J., and Parthasarathy, R.: Observations on the protective effect of BCG vaccination in a South Indian rural population. Bull. WHO *30*:545, 1964.

18. Garibaldi, R. A., Drusin, R. E., Ferebee, S. H., and Gregg, M. B.: Isoniazid-associated hepatitis. Report of an outbreak. Am. Rev. Respir. Dis. *106*:357, 1972.

19. Germany, Ministry of the Interior: Die Sauglingstuberkulose in Lübeck. Berlin, Verlag Julius Springer, 1935.

20. Greenwood, M.: Professor Calmette's statistical study of B.C.G. vaccination. Br. Med. J. *1*:793, 1928.

21. Greenwood, M., and Wolff, G.: Einige methodologisch-statistische Studien zur epidemiologie der tuberkulose. Ein beitrag zur beurteilung tuberkulose fördernder und-hemmender tuberculosis. Zeitschr. Tuberk. *52*:97, 1928.

22. Groth-Petersen, E., Gad, U., and Østergaard, F.: Mass chemoprophylaxis of tuberculosis. The acceptability and untoward side effects of isoniazid in a control study in Greenland. Am. Rev. Respir. Dis. *81*:643, 1960.

23. Guérin, C.: The history of BCG. Early history. *In* Rosenthal, S. R.: BCG Vaccination Against Tuberculosis. Boston, Little, Brown and Company, 1957.

24. Hart, P. D.: Efficacy and applicability of mass B.C.G. vaccination in tuberculosis control. Br. J. Med. *1*:587, 1967.

25. Horwitz, O., Payne, P. G., and Wilbek, E.: Epidemiological basis of tuberculosis eradication. 4. The isoniazid trial in Greenland. Bull. WHO *35*:509, 1966.

26. Katz, J., Kunofsky, S., Damijonaitis, V., Lafleur, A., and Caron, T.: Effect of isoniazid upon the reactivation of inactive tuberculosis. Final Report. Am. Rev. Respir. Dis. *91*:345, 1965.

27. Katz, J., Kunofsky, S., Damijonaitis, V., Lafleur, A., and Caron, T.: Effect of isoniazid upon the reactivation of inactive tuberculosis. Prelimary report. Am. Rev. Respir. Dis. *86*:8, 1962.

28. Kirchenstein, A.: Mit Calmettes Tuberkulose-Impfstoff BCG geimpfte Saüglinge in Riga. Zeitschr. Tuberk. *57*:311, 1930.

29. Koch, R.: Fortsetzung der Mittheilung uber ein Heilmittel gegen Tuberkulose. Deutsche Med. Wochenschr. *17*:101, 1891.

30. Koch, R.: Weitere Mittheilungen uber ein Heilmittel gegen Tuberkulose. Deutsche Med. Wochenschr. *16*:1029, 1890.

30a. Lotte, A., Wasz-Höckert, O., Poisson, N., and Dumitrescu, D.: Complications induced by BCG vaccination: A retrospective study. Bull. Int. Union Tuberc. *53*:114, 1978.

31. Maddrey, W. C., and Boitnott, J. K.: Isoniazid hepatitis. Ann. Intern. Med. *79*:1, 1973.

32. Medical Research Council: B.C.G. and vole bacillus vaccines in the prevention of tuberculosis in adolescence and early adult life. Br. Med. J. *1*:973, 1963.

33. Medical Research Council: B.C.G. and vole bacillus vaccines in the prevention of tuberculosis in adolescents. Br. Med. J. *1*:413, 1956.

34. Medical Research Council: B.C.G. and vole bacillus vaccines in the prevention of tuberculosis in adolescents. Br. Med. J. *2*:379, 1959.

35. Mount, F. W., and Ferebee, S. H.: The effect of isoniazid prophylaxis on tuberculosis morbidity among household contacts of previously known cases of tuberculosis. Am. Rev. Respir. Dis. *85*:821, 1962.

36. Mount, F. W., and Ferebee, S. H.: Preventive effects of isoniazid in the treatment of primary tuberculosis in children. N. Engl. J. Med. *265*:713, 1961.

37. Myers, J. A.: The natural history of tuberculosis in the human body. J.A.M.A. *194*: 1086, 1965.

38. Nyboe, J., Farah, A. R., and Christensen,

O. W.: Report on tuberculosis chemotherapy pilot project (Tunisia 9). WHO/TB/Techn. Information *10*:April 22, 1963.

39. Palmer, C. E., and Long, M. W.: Effects of infection with atypical mycobacteria on BCG vaccination and tuberculosis. Am. Rev. Respir. Dis. *94*:553, 1966.

40. Palmer, C. E., Shaw, L. W., and Comstock, G. W.: Community trials of BCG vaccination. Am. Rev. Tuberc. *77*:877, 1958.

41. Raj Narain, Nair S. S., Ramanatha Rao, G., Chandrasekhar, P., and Pyare Lal: Enhancing of tuberculin allergy by previous tuberculin testing. Bull. WHO *34*:623, 1966.

42. Rich, A. R.: The Pathogenesis of Tuberculosis. 2nd ed. Springfield, Ill., Charles C Thomas, 1951.

43. Rosenfeld, S.: Der statistische Beweis für die Immunisierung Neugeborener mit B.C.G. Wein. Klin. Wochenschr. *41*:800, 1928.

44. Rosenthal, S. R.: BCG Vaccination Against Tuberculosis. Boston, Little, Brown and Company, 1957.

45. Rosenthal, S. R., Loewinsohn, E., Graham, M. L., Liveright, D., Thorne, M. G., Johnson, V., and Batson, H. C.: BCG vaccination against tuberculosis in Chicago. A twenty-year study statistically analyzed. Pediatrics *28*:622, 1961.

46. Scharer, L., and Smith, J. P.: Serum transaminase elevations and other hepatic abnormalities in patients receiving isoniazid. Ann. Intern. Med. *71*:1113, 1969.

47. Sigurdsson, S., and Edwards, P. Q.: Tuberculosis morbidity and mortality in Iceland. Bull. WHO *7*:153, 1952.

48. Veening, G. J. J.: Long-term isoniazid prophylaxis. Controlled trial on INH prophylaxis after recent tuberculin conversion in young adults. Bull. Int. Union Tuberc. *41*:169, 1968.

49. Wilson, G. S., and Miles, A. (eds.): Topley and Wilson's Principles of Bacteriology, Virology and Immunity. 6th ed., Vol. 2. Baltimore, The Williams & Wilkins Company, 1975.

50. Wolff, G.: Die schutzimpfung gegen tuberkulose und die natürliche durchseuchung im lichte der statistik. Deutsche Med. Wochenschr. *56*:1644, 1930.

51. Wolff, G.: Über die Ursachen des Ruckganges der tuberkulosesterblichkeit in den Kulturstaaten. Zeitschr. Tuberk. *57*:1, 1930.

52. Wolinsky, E.: New antituberculosis drugs and concepts of prophylaxis. Med. Clin. North Am. *58*:697, 1974.

53. Youmans, G. P.: Acquired immunity in tuberculosis. J. Chronic Dis. *6*:606, 1957.

18

Disease Due to Mycobacteria Other Than *Mycobacterium tuberculosis*

HERBERT M. SOMMERS, M.D.

INTRODUCTION

It long has been recognized that acid-fast microorganisms different from *Mycobacterium tuberculosis* are sometimes associated with pulmonary disease in human beings. Until recently, little thought had been given to the possibility that some of these might be etiologically related to the pulmonary pathology, in spite of descriptions in the earlier literature of cases that supported this possibility. During about the last 25 years, we have become fully aware that a significant proportion of cases diagnosed as tuberculosis may be caused by acid-fast microorganisms so

different from *M. tuberculosis* that they represent separate mycobacterial species.

Of equal importance, and of special significance to the epidemiology and immunology of the mycobacterial diseases, is the relatively recent accumulation of evidence which strongly suggests that large numbers of persons in the United States, and probably in other countries, may become naturally infected with one or more of these mycobacteria at some period in their lives, even though the great majority of those so infected never show evidence of disease. (See Chapter 16).

For many years before the advent of

386

chemotherapy, the diagnosis of tuberculosis was made on the clinical symptoms of cough, fever, and night sweats, on a chest x-ray demonstrating a pulmonary infiltrate or cavity, and on the presence of acid-fast bacilli in the sputum. Although cultures of sputum and other clinical specimens could be obtained and in some instances *M. tuberculosis* recovered, the difficulties of preparing culture media, of decontaminating the specimen, and of following necessary safety precautions limited the number of laboratories that cultured and identified mycobacteria.

In 1944, with the discovery of streptomycin, there developed a need to recover the infecting organism from each patient, as it soon became apparent that treatment with streptomycin alone was often associated with the rapid development of resistance. For this reason, should the patient relapse during treatment, it became desirable to recover the organism to determine drug susceptibility before starting therapy.

ATYPICAL MYCOBACTERIA

As increasing numbers of cultures were made and as the incidence of disease from *Mycobacterium tuberculosis* decreased, a number of mycobacterial isolates were found that were clearly associated with disease in the patient but were obviously not typical of *M. tuberculosis* in their colonial appearance or their ability to cause disease in guinea pigs.

Timpe and Runyon in 1954[89] described atypical mycobacteria that had been isolated from 120 patients. Ninety-three of the strains were isolated by the authors from original specimens; the remainder were isolated by others and sent to the authors for examination. None of the atypical mycobacteria were pathogenic for guinea pigs following subcutaneous inoculation, although the pigmented strains produced pulmonary disease in mice following intravenous inoculation. Many of these microorganisms were etiologically related to pulmonary disease in the humans from whom they were isolated, not only because no other mycobacterium could be found in sputum but also because they were the only ones obtained from pleural fluid and diseased lung tissue. From the cultural characteristics and the development of pigmentation when exposed to light, it was possible for Timpe and Runyon to divide these atypical mycobacteria into four large groups.[89] This classification was further refined in 1965 by Runyon,[74] and it served as a framework for the classification of many of the mycobacterial species other than *M. tuberculosis*. The Runyon classification and a partial list of organisms usually considered to be in each group are given as follows:

RUNYON GROUP I. Mycobacteria in Group I are characterized by the ability to make crystals of yellow carotene pigment when actively growing cells are exposed to a strong light. Because they make pigment only when exposed to light, they are called "photochromogens" and are said to be photoreactive. Photoreactive mycobacteria include *M. kansasii*, *M. simiae*, and *M. marinum*.

RUNYON GROUP II. Organisms of Runyon Group II produce bright yellow-pigmented colonies when grown in either light or dark, although in some strains of *M. scrofulaceum*, the pigment may be intensified on exposure to light. These mycobacteria are called "scotochromogens" for their ability to make pigment in the dark. Species in the Group II scotochromogens include *M. scrofulaceum*, *M. gordonae*, *M. flavescens*, and *M. xenopi*.

RUNYON GROUP III. Runyon named the third group of organisms "nonphotochromogens." The Group III mycobacteria include a number of species, some producing small amounts of pale yellow pigment. Exposure of these lightly pigmented organisms to a bright light does not intensify the color, and hence they were designated "nonphotochromogens." Colonies of most organisms in this group appear off-white or buff in color. Species include members of the *Mycobacterium avium-intracellulare* complex, the *Mycobacterium terrae-triviale complex*, *Mycobacterium gastri*, and a group of organisms showing little or no pathogenicity for man — the *Mycobacterium nonchromogenicum* complex.

RUNYON GROUP IV. The last of Runyon's four groups of atypical mycobacteria is characterized by the ability to grow more rapidly than the other three groups, often showing mature colonies in 3 to 5 days when incubated at 37°C. This group was called "rapid growers." While a number of the species in this group show yellow pigmentation, the two species that are known to cause infection in man, *M. fortuitum* and *M. chelonei*, are nonpigmented. *M. fortuitum* and *M. chelonei* share a number of taxonomic as well as virulence characteristics and are often referred to as the *M. fortuitum-chelonei* complex. They are usually associated with infection of the skin, subcutaneous tissues, and eye.

Although Runyon's four groups of organisms were helpful in establishing a preliminary classification of the "atypical" mycobacteria, the presence of pathogenic and nonpathogenic species in the same group, e.g., scotochromogens, requires that they be speciated to distinguish between the two. The more general term might be misleading to the clinical consultant because a mycobacterium might satisfy the criteria for more than one group. The need for speciation can be illustrated by *Mycobacterium szulgai*, an organism only recently recognized to be associated with disease in humans. *M. szulgai* is scotochromogenic when incubated at 37°C, but photochromogenic when grown at 22 to 24°C. In contrast to several nonpathogenic species of scotochromogenic mycobacteria, such as *M. gordonae* and *M. flavescens*, *M. szulgai* has been found to be associated with active disease in almost all patients from whom it has been cultured.[20] For this reason, species identi-

fication can help to establish or exclude the role of an isolate in infection.

The introduction of chemotherapy for the treatment of tuberculosis resulted in a dramatic decrease in the number of new and active cases in the United States. This decrease has been accompanied by a heightened awareness of the role of mycobacteria other than *Mycobacterium tuberculosis* as the cause of disease in man. The incidence of disease from mycobacteria other than *M. tuberculosis* ranges from 1 percent to 27 percent of all mycobacterial infections, depending on the type of hospital and population served by the hospital.[65] The following section will briefly describe certain of the in vitro characteristics and clinical significance of a number of the mycobacterial species other than *M. tuberculosis*. Several of the books and review articles referred to in this chapter should also be consulted.[14, 21, 32, 105, 106]

Mycobacterium bovis

Mycobacterium bovis is the cause of tuberculosis in cattle, where it can be associated with pulmonary or extrapulmonary infection. During the early part of the twentieth century, recognition of the spread of bovine tuberculosis to humans through contaminated milk or through contact with infected cattle resulted in a highly successful compaign to control this source of infection. In 1917 it was estimated that 5 percent of the cattle in the United States were infected and that approximately 25 percent of deaths from tuberculosis in adult human beings was caused by *M. bovis*. Following the institution of a surveillance program for tuberculin testing of cattle and the disposal of positive reactors correlated with the compulsory pasteurization of milk, there was a dramatic decrease in the incidence of *M. bovis* infection in man. In the fifteen years between 1955 and 1969, fewer than two isolates a year from human sources were sent to the Center for Disease Control for confirmation of identification. Although disease from *M. bovis* in humans has been effectively controlled, occasional cases continue to occur, presumably from reactivation of previously infected humans and contact with domestic or wild animals.[35, 47, 69, 70, 99]

Recently there has been increasing interest in the use of several of the attenuated strains of bacille Calmette-Guérin (BCG) as adjuvants in the immunotherapy of cancer, particularly malignant melanoma.[6] Although BCG strains are considerably less virulent than the parent strains of *M. bovis,* when injected in large numbers into patients with advanced cancer, dissemination can occur both to local lymph nodes and the liver. Infection with granulomas in the liver can be associated with significant hepatic dysfunction, and biopsy may show a histologic appearance not unlike miliary tuberculosis.[82] (See also Chapters 4 and 16.)

Unlike most species of mycobacteria, *M. bovis* and some strains of BCG show inhibition of growth on culture media containing glycerol. Optimal recovery of clinical isolates of *M. bovis* therefore requires culture media prepared without glycerol. In culture, *M. bovis* grows more slowly than *M. tuberculosis,* but the colonial appearance of both is similar on isolation. Differentiation of *M. bovis* from *M. tuberculosis* can usually be determined by negative niacin accumulation and nitrate reduction tests, although occasional strains of BCG may be lightly positive for both these characteristics. Distinction between the two species can then be made by use of thiophene 2-carboxylic hydrazide, which inhibits the growth of *M. bovis* but not of *M. tuberculosis.*[96]

Mycobacterium kansasii

Mycobacterium kansasii is most commonly associated with pulmonary infection in man. The disease is clinically and radiologically indistinguishable from that caused by *M. tuberculosis.* Infection may also occur in the skin, in the genitourinary tract, and in joints, tendon sheaths, and lymph glands and may disseminate to many sites in patients with decreased host defense mechanisms caused by intercurrent disease or therapeutic immunosuppression.[30, 34, 36, 42, 60, 66] (See Chapters 16 and 21.)

In contrast to those with *M. tuberculosis,* patients with infections from *M. kansasii* are not highly contagious, and only rarely has more than one case been found in a family unit. In a demographic study in Chicago that involved 230 patients with disease from *M. kansasii,* Lichtenstein found them to be predominantly white, middle-aged males, living in comfortable middle-class neighborhoods. The sex, age group, race, and residential neighborhoods of these patients were in sharp contrast to a similar group of patients with disease from *M. tuberculosis.* In the latter, infection was found in younger age groups of both sexes, more frequently black and living in crowded housing units in predominantly ghetto areas (see Chapter 16).[53]

Buhler and Pollak reported the first clinical isolate of *Mycobacterium kansasii,* which was from a draining inguinal sinus.[10] *M. kansasii* is characteristically photoreactive and will grow best at 37° C, producing well-formed colonies in 10 to 14 days. The organism will also grow slowly at 24 to 26° C but not at 42° C; it produces variable amounts of nitroreductase and has the ability to rapidly hydrolyze Tween 80 within 24 to 48 hours. Organisms isolated from patients with disease produce large amounts of catalase, while those recovered from patients without evidence of infection show a much more diminished catalase activity.[93]

Reports of infections with *Mycobacterium kansasii* were first noted in Kansas City, Chicago, and Dallas, suggesting a geographic predilection for the midwestern United States. With improved laboratory procedures and more widespread knowledge of the proper identification characteristics, patients with infection from *M. kansasii* have been found in all parts of the United States and throughout the world.

The source or reservoir of the infection is not clear. Although *M. kansasii* has been isolated from tap water on several occasions,[5] it is usually not considered to be spread in this fashion. Systematic investigations have failed to show it to be widespread in water or soil samples.[102]

Pulmonary infection with *Mycobacterium kansasii* is a well-recognized cause of chronic granulomatous disease. A recent report by Francis[29] has provided insight into the natural history of the disease. In this report, Francis has described the clinical courses of four patients who had been followed without treatment for periods of 10 to 14 years after diagnosis. Three of the four patients showed slowly progressive disease in the absence of significant symptoms over a 12 to 14 year follow-up period. The subsequent use of antituberculous drugs in these three patients resulted in the rapid resolution of active disease. The fourth patient had shown evidence of progressive pulmonary disease for more than 5 years. At the end of that time there was spontaneous resolution of the disease, with clearing of the bacteriologic and roentgenologic findings. The patient remained well for an additional eight years when the report was made. These cases suggest that the usual course of the disease is to produce a destructive infection but that in some instances there can be spontaneous resolution.

Infection with *Mycobacterium kansasii* is sometimes considered "opportunistic." Although the evidence for this is not as well established as for other infectious agents, certain features suggest that opportunistic infection can occur. The geographic distribution of disease due to *M. kansasii* is not uniform, and there is little or no evidence

for transmission from open cases to contacts. In addition, the disease is seen most frequently in white males over 40 years of age. How can these puzzling features be explained — especially the lack of contagiousness, since a high degree of contagiousness is one of the outstanding features of the disease caused by *Mycobacterium tuberculosis*. A clue may lie in the low degree of pathogenicity of these microorganisms for experimental animals, even though viable cells may persist in the tissues of the animals for extended periods following injection. If pathogenicity is also very low for human beings, large numbers of human beings might become infected with atypical mycobacteria of Group I or Group III, or both, at some period in their lives, without developing clinically recognizable disease. Subsequently, an occasional infected person might, however, develop disease under conditions which would so lower local or general resistance that the atypical mycobacteria already in the body would begin to proliferate. Once a focal area of necrosis appears, the disease might become slowly progressive.

The production of disease by the mycobacteria found in Runyon's Groups I, II, III, and IV emphasizes the importance of the host susceptibility. It is probably safe to postulate that progressive disease due to these other mycobacteria probably will occur only in the abnormal host. The abnormality may be caused by other local or systemic disease or by one or more of the factors known to reduce cellular immunity to infection. In general, the mycobacteria included within the Runyon groups should be regarded as opportunists rather than as primary pathogens capable of producing progressive disease in the normal host. *Mycobacterium tuberculosis* and *Mycobacterium bovis* would fall into the latter category. In support of this theory, Ahn,[1] in a study of 232 patients with disease from *Mycobacterium kansasii*, found that they had a greater frequency of obstructive ventilatory defect than did a similar group of patients with *M. tuberculosis*. It was his interpretation that the ventilatory defect was best accounted for by previous or coexisting lung disease. The appearance of disseminated infection by *M. kansasii* is usually associated with an underlying disease (that predisposes to infection) or the administration of corticosteroids or the development of pancytopenia.[30, 36] Fraser[30] reported a patient with a renal homograft and therapeutic immunosuppression who developed cellulitis and abscesses in a foot and was thought to have a pyogenic infection. Biopsy and culture established infection from *M. kansasii*. The daily administration of prednisone and azothioprine had apparently prevented the usual cell-mediated granulomatous reaction, which resulted in an atypical pyogenic inflammatory response. A change to alternate-day prednisone therapy combined with antimycobacterial medication resulted in rapid healing of the infection without rejection of the homograph.[30]

Mycobacterium avium-intracellulare Complex

The term *Mycobacterium avium-intracellulare* refers to a group of organisms that closely resemble *Mycobacterium avium*, the organism that causes tuberculosis in fowl and swine. This group comprises a variety of mycobacteria placed together because they do not develop pigmentation when exposed to light. Many of them are closely related to *Mycobacterium avium* except that they do not cause disease in fowl. Experimentally, these microorganisms do not produce infection in guinea pigs, although some have caused infection in mice.

In this group, an organism that causes disease in humans was originally referred to as the "Battey bacillus" because of a large number of patients first recognized at the Battey State Hospital in Rome, Georgia. After reviewing taxonomic criteria, Runyon proposed the name *M. intracellulare*.[75] The similarity of *M. intracellulare* to *M. avium* and the lack of easily determined taxonomic characteristics to distinguish between the two species were two factors that led to the use of a very helpful and specific classification of the organisms. This classification is based on the use of rabbit antisera prepared against surface antigens of whole cells. Schaefer and others have described 20 separate serotypes in the *Mycobacterium avium-intracellulare* complex.[62, 79] In order to simplify the original classification, Wolinsky and Schaefer have subsequently recommended the serotypes in the *M. avium-intracellulare* complex be designated by consecutive arabic numerals (See Table 8–1).[103] Although not all of the *M. avium-intracellulare* serotypes are well-established virulent strains for humans, the similarities between the members of the group are close enough to indicate the need for a common designation recognizing both *avium* and *intracellulare* species, hence the term "*M. avium-intracellulare* complex." It is clinically important to distinguish between other species or complexes of organisms in Runyon's Group III nonphotochromogenic mycobacteria, as members of the *M. avium-intracellulare* complex are the only organisms of the nonphotochromogenic mycobacteria associated with significant progressive disease in humans.

It has been known for some time that there are close similarities in seroagglutination reactions of the higher numbered serotypes of members of the *Mycobacterium avium-intracellulare* complex and *M. scrofulaceum*. This has led to a proposal to look for intermediate strains between the two species. Many organisms that can be classified as *M. scrofulaceum* on the basis of pigment characteristics will agglutinate with specific antisera as one of the "intracellulare serotypes." While most of the members of the *M. avium-intracellulare* complex are nonpigmented,

TABLE 18–1.   **Proposed Scheme for Serotyping**
Several Mycobacterial Species

Species	Old Serotype Designations	New Serotype Designations *M. avium* Complex
M. avium	1, 2, 3	1, 2, 3
M. intracellulare	IV	4
	V	5
	VI	6
	VII	7
	Davis	8
	Watson	9
	IIIa	10
	IIIb	11
	Howell	12
	Chance	13
	Boone	14
	Dent	15
	Yandle	16
	Wilson	17
	Altman	18
	Darden	19
	Arnold	20
M. scrofulaceum	Scrofulaceum	41
	Lunning	42
	Gause	43

From Wolinsky, E., and Schaefer, W. B.: Proposed numbering scheme for mycobacterial serotypes by agglutination. Int.
J. Sys. Bacteriol. 23:183, 1973.

some can develop a pale yellow pigment on repeated subculture, and
a few can be quite pigmented from
early growth. Hawkins has proposed
the term MAIS (*M. avium-intracellulare-
scrofulaceum*) for this group of organisms and has proposed that the significance and clinical relevance of such
strains be studied in the future.[38]

Colonies of *M. avium-intracellulare*
isolated from patients with active infection are flat, thin, and spreading; this is
in contrast to the more rapidly growing,
large, butyrous, and domed colonies
that can develop in vitro with repeated
transfer. Pathogenicity is more often associated with the thin, spreading, colony type than the large domed colony.
Organisms in the *Mycobacterium avium-
intracellulare* complex do not accumulate niacin and are nitrate-reductase-
negative. They show a semiquantitative catalase of less than 40 mm but

produce catalase stable to heating at
68° C for 30 min. They cannot hydrolyze Tween 80 within 10 days.

The mode of transmission of infection by members of the *Mycobacterium
avium-intracellulare* is not clear. The organism has been isolated from the environment, which includes soil and animals as well as water. In Australia the
organisms have been isolated from
house dust, with 10 to 16 separate serotypes corresponding to those known to
cause disease in humans.[72] The organisms can also be isolated from the
secretions of normal individuals.[63]

The disease does not appear to be
highly contagious and is only rarely
transmitted from man to man, even in
close personal contacts. As judged from
the results of skin test surveys, human
infections by these bacteria are common in the Southeastern states, particularly along the Gulf of Mexico and the

middle and southern Atlantic coast, although infections have been found in all parts of the United States.

Infections from organisms in the *Mycobacterium avium-intracellulare* complex are usually pulmonary, frequently occurring in middle-aged men with pre-existing lung disease, e.g., pneumoconioses, bronchitis-emphysema, and previously diagnosed tuberculosis. A significant number of nonpulmonary infections, such as cervical lymphadenitis in children can occur and, rarely, dissemination to many organs,[83] including the lungs, liver, bones, and other sites.[77, 83] Because of certain facts — the ready availability of the organism in the environment and the evidence of hypersensitivity in a large segment of the population, but a relatively small number of patients with active disease — organisms of the *M. avium-intracellulare* complex are considered to have little inherent pathogenic potential; they are opportunists. The ability of the organism to cause disease seems to depend more upon some previous injury, disease, or defect in the host e.g., in the lung, that predisposes to invasion.

As the incidence of tuberculosis continues to decrease, infection from mycobacteria other than *Mycobacterium tuberculosis* becomes proportionately more frequent. Depending on the type of hospital, the patients served, and the interests of the medical staff, the incidence of nontuberculosis mycobacterial disease has been reported to range from 1 percent to 16 percent, with one, large, tertiary care midwestern medical center recently reporting 27 percent.[65] In this report, of the different types of non-*M. tuberculosis* infections, equal numbers were caused by *M. kansasii* and by members of the *M. avium-intracellulare* complex. This same study showed mycobacterial disease to be an opportunistic infection in patients with malignant disease; *M. tuberculosis* and other mycobacterial species were of equal virulence in this regard.

The treatment of infections from the organisms in the *M. avium-intracellulare* complex is difficult and may require a combination of 4 to 6 antimycobacterial drugs given over long periods, as well as surgery (see Chapter 21). Patients showing favorable initial response may later show relapse. In many cases there is improvement or long-term stability, even though there is not complete resolution of the disease. For further details on therapy with this group of patients, see Chapter 21.

Mycobacterium scrofulaceum

In 1956, Weed reported the isolation of pigmented mycobacteria from the enlarged cervical lymph nodes of eight children.[97] The same year, Prissick and Masson reported an additional 14 children with enlarged facial, submaxillary, and cervical lymph nodes, where the clinical picture suggested a tuberculous infection but culture of the nodes revealed a scotochromogenic mycobacterium in 10 of the total 14.[67] In 1957, Prissick and Masson proposed the name *M. scrofulaceum* for the organism.[68] Although subsequent study revealed that the name *Mycobacterium marianum* had precedence over *Mycobacterium scrofulaceum*, *M. scrofulaceum* has been retained because of the similarity of *M. marianum* to *M. marinum* and the possibility of confusing the two species.[95]

Mycobacterium scrofulaceum is most often isolated from enlarged cervical and submandibular lymph nodes of children. It is usually assumed that the portal of entry is the oropharynx. Although not common, this organism has also been isolated from inguinal lymph nodes; in one patient, a young girl, it was considered to have been the result of a vaginal infection.[2] *M. scrofulaceum* is not a common cause of lymphadenitis in adults, where *M. tuberculosis* is usually isolated. Cervical tuberculosis in adults is most commonly found in association with pulmonary infection rather than as a primary lymphadenitis.

M. scrofulaceum can colonize old tuberculous cavities in adults but there is only rarely good evidence of primary pathogenicity.[101] The inflammatory reaction caused by *M. scrofulaceum* may be granulomatous, purulent, or may show a hyperplastic response. Occasional case reports of disseminated disease from *M. scrofulaceum* in children have been associated with severe underlying disease. Several cases have shown tissue reaction characterized by the presence of large numbers of foamy macrophages.[45]

On culture media, *Mycobacterium scrofulaceum* is characterized by slowly growing, smooth colonies, usually appearing after 10 to 14 days incubation. The organism is yellow when grown in the dark, but some strains may turn a deeper yellow or an orange-yellow color when exposed to strong light. *M. scrofulaceum* does not accumulate niacin, produce nitroreductase, hydrolyze Tween 80, or produce arylsulfatase. It will give a positive urease test in three days but will not grow on medium containing 5 percent NaCl.

Although the distinct yellow pigmentation of *Mycobacterium scrofulaceum* would appear to differentiate it from the members of the *M. avium-intracellulare* complex, serologically *M. scrofulaceum* will agglutinate with antisera prepared against certain members of the *M. avium-intracellulare* complex.

The source of *Mycobacterium scrofulaceum* as the cause of human infections has not been clearly established, although scotochromogens have been found in more than half of a large series of soil samples.[102] Hypersensitivity to the purified protein derivative of the Gause strain of *M. scrofulaceum* (PPD-G) was demonstrated in 49 percent of Naval recruits, suggesting widespread exposure to the organism during youth.[25] This finding also suggests that the organism has little virulence, since most of these with a positive skin test had no history of past disease. The frequency of reactions to PPD-G of 6.0 mm or more among the recruits ranged from 22 percent for lifelong residents of the northwestern states of Oregon and Washington to 83 percent for recruits who had lived all their lives in Florida. This geographic variation provides additional evidence of the incidence of latent infection with mycobacteria in man in the United States (see Table 18–2).

TABLE 18–2. **Frequency and Mean Size of Reactions Among Navy Recruits to 0.0001 mg of PPD Antigens Prepared from Various Strains of Mycobacteria**

PPD Antigen	Prepared From	Number Tested	Reactions of 2 mm or More	
			PERCENTAGE	MEAN SIZE (MILLIMETERS)
PPD-S	*M. tuberculosis*	212,462	8.6	10.3
PPD-F	*M. fortuitum*	3,415	7.7	4.8
PPD-240	Unclassified; group 3	3,729	12.0	5.8
PPD-Y	*M. kansasii*	13,913	13.1	6.2
PPD-63	Unclassified; group 3	9,473	17.5	7.0
PPD-sm	*M. smegmatis*	14,239	18.3	5.7
PPD-ph	*M. phlei*	15,229	23.1	6.4
PPD-216	Unclassified; group 2	10,060	28.4	9.0
PPD-A	*M. avium*	10,769	30.5	6.7
PPD-B	Unclassified; (Battey type)	212,462	35.1	7.7
PPD-269	Unclassified; group 3	8,402	39.0	7.2
PPD-G	Unclassified; group 2	29,540	48.7	10.3

From Edwards, L. B.: Current status of the tuberculin test. Ann. N. Y. Acad. Sci. *106*:32, 1963.

Mycobacterium fortuitum-chelonei **Complex**

Although two separate species, *Mycobacterium fortuitum* and *Mycobacterium chelonei* ss *chelonei (borstelense)* and *Mycobacterium chelonei* ss *abscessus* (one with two subspecies), can be identified with the use of easily determined taxonomic characteristics, there is a difference of opinion as to whether the clinical disease caused by these organisms is sufficiently distinct to warrant separate speciation. The present trend is to acknowledge the similarity of the types of disease caused by the two species by combining them under the term *M. fortuitum-chelonei* complex. *M. fortuitum* appears to be composed of a fairly homogenous group of strains; *M. chelonei* contains two clusters of organisms proposed as subspecies, *M. chelonei* ss *chelonei (borstelense)* and *M. chelonei* ss *abscessus*.[51] *M. chelonei* ss *abscessus* can be differentiated from *M. chelonei* ss *chelonei* by the ability to grow on egg-base culture medium containing 5 percent NaCl.[86]

Infection with organisms of the *Mycobacterium fortuitum-chelonei* complex is usually secondary to trauma. The organisms are worldwide in distribution and are commonly found in the soil. The most frequent form of the disease is associated with cutaneous infection and abscess formation.[37, 64] Osteomyelitis following a puncture wound of the foot has also been described.[13] Several epidemics of cutaneous abscesses have been described following injection of diphtheria-pertussis-tetanus-polio vaccine, penicillin, iron, and BCG.[7, 9, 16, 19] Infections of the cornea, both from trauma and in grafts, have also been described.[100, 104, 108]

Organisms of the *Mycobacterium fortuitum-chelonei* complex are not infrequently isolated from the sputum of apparently healthy persons.[4] There have been numerous reports documenting the repeated isolation of *M. fortuitum* or *M. chelonei* from the sputum of patients with a clinical pulmonary disease that appeared similar to tuberculosis; however, proving the organisms were the cause of the infection can be difficult. Dreisin and colleagues have recently described seven patients with good evidence of progressive pulmonary infection from *M. fortuitum* or *M. chelonei*.[24] Hemoptysis, cough, and weight loss were prominent findings in 6 and rheumatoid arthritis was present in 3, an association also noted by others. One of the seven patients died of massive pulmonary hemorrhage, and caseating granulomatous inflammation was found in the lungs of two upon autopsy. Resection of a pulmonary cavity in another patient appeared to be successful but was followed by early relapse of the disease.

Disseminated infection has been described from members of the *M. fortuitum-chelonei* complex and may or may not be associated with immune suppression. Two patients under immunosuppressive therapy following renal transplantation had multiple subcutaneous abscesses and osteomyelitis, primarily in the legs.[31] Contamination of porcine heart valves with *M. chelonei* used for cardiac valve replacement resulted in two outbreaks of infection, with the infection usually involving the sternum[28] but in one patient resulting in an abscess at the base of the aorta. Aggressive antimicrobial therapy combined with resection of the infected valve appeared to have been successful in this patient.[52]

In vitro susceptibility tests to the standard antimycobacterial agents show members of the *Mycobacterium fortuitum-chelonei* complex to be uniformly resistant. Aggressive therapy with a number of these agents can show progressive sterilization of cultures and may successfully alter the course of the infection.

Only the nonpigmented species in Runyon's Group IV rapid-growing mycobacteria are known to cause disease in humans. Both *Mycobacterium fortuitum* and *Mycobacterium chelonei* will grow within 3 to 5 days at 37°C, will produce either smooth or rough, buff-colored colonies, and will give a positive test for arylsulfatase after 3 days' growth. *M. fortuitum*, but not *M. chelonei*, will reduce nitrates to nitrites. Runyon has observed that *M. fortuitum* and *M. chelonei* can be distinguished by comparing their microcolonial appearance after 24 to 36 hours incubation. On corn-meal or oleic acid agar *M. fortuitum* will show small rhizoids extending from the periphery of a microcolony, whereas *M. chelonei* will not.[76]

Mycobacterium marinum

Mycobacterium marinum was first isolated and described in 1926 by Aronson as a cause of granulomas in fish.[3] Tuberculoid skin infections associated with swimming pools were described in Sweden in 1939[40] and 1951[41], in Vancouver in 1951[17] and in San Francisco in 1953.[71] In 1954 Linell and Norden isolated an organism from the skin of patients with "swimming pool granulomas" and named it *Mycobacterium balnei*.[55] In 1959, an outbreak of cutaneous "swimming pool" granuloma occurred in an open-air, hot springs-mineral water public swimming pool in Glenwood Springs, Colorado, involving some 300 persons.[78] *Mycobacterium marinum (balnei)* was isolated in large numbers from early lesions of these patients as well as from the swimming pool water. More recently there have been a number of reports on patients with isolated skin infections following an accident that had scraped or injured a hand or arm while caring for tropical fish in a home aquarium.[39, 57] Skin infections from *M. marinum* also can be acquired from injuries to the upper and lower extremities in fresh, brackish, or sea-water environments.[44, 107]

Infection with *Mycobacterium marinum* is characterized by the appearance of single or multiple swollen red nodules appearing at the point of injury. These may enlarge and go on to ulceration and necrosis or the skin may remain intact. Some patients may develop multiple skin lesions in an ascending fashion resembling the lymphangitic spread of sporotrichosis. Infection with *M. marinum* is confined to the skin, where the temperature is 30 to 33° C, and has not been reported in the organs deep to the surface of the body. Isolation of the organism will usually occur when the culture is incubated at either room temperature or at 30 to 33° C. Incubation of cultures at 37° C will result in significant inhibition of growth or in a failure to recover the organism. All cultures obtained from the skin or biopsies of skin from suspected tuberculoid lesions should be incubated at both 30 to 33° C and 37° C. A second set of cultures at 37° C is recommended to recover *M. tuberculosis*, an organism that does not grow well at 30 to 33° C.

In culture *Mycobacterium marinum* is photochromogenic, and when incubated at 30 to 33°C, will show growth in 7 to 10 days. This is in contrast to *Mycobacterium kansasii* or *Mycobacterium simiae*, either of which requires 12 to 14 days for initial growth. Photochromogenicity, preference for growth at 30 to 33° C, and lack of nitroreductase activity are all identification characteristics helpful in separating *M. marinum* from other mycobacterial species.[85]

Infection from *Mycobacterium marinum* is usually self-limiting but may progress from 2 to 27 years. Histologically, biopsies of skin ulcers may show acute and chronic inflammation or granulomatous inflammation, including focii of caseous necrosis, giant cell formation, and epithelioid cells.

Numerous methods for treatment of *Mycobacterium marinum* have been described, including surgical excision, x-ray therapy, curettage, fulguration, liquid nitrogen cryotherapy, sulfonamides, and sulfones. Although in vitro studies have suggested that chemotherapeutic resistance is a characteristic of

M. marinum infections, isoniazid, streptomycin, and para-aminosalicylic acid have been used with apparent success.

Mycobacterium szulgai

Mycobacterium szulgai is a clinically significant mycobacterium that was first recognized as a separate species by a distinctive pattern of cell wall lipids determined by thin-layer chromatography.[43] The name of the organism recognizes Dr. T. Szulga, who developed the chromatographic method of cell wall lipid analysis for mycobacteria and thereby drew attention to the species.

Mycobacterium szulgai is unique among all species of mycobacteria in showing a scotochromogenic reaction when incubated at 37° C but a photochromogenic one when incubated at 24 to 26° C. An inadvertent rise in temperature during incubation to 30° C or higher may be sufficient to make the organism appear scotochromogenic and mask its photoreactive characteristic. The organism also shows a moderately weak nitroreductase activity and hydrolyzes Tween 80 slowly.[84]

With the exception of a single isolate cultured from a snail, all known strains of *Mycobacterium szulgai* have been associated with infections in humans. Most strains have been recovered from the sputum of patients with pulmonary disease, many with cavities. Cervical adenitis, infection in the olecranal bursa, and tenosynovitis have also occurred.[20, 59]

In contrast to other scotochromogenic mycobacteria, *Mycobacterium szulgai* is much more susceptible to first- and second-line antimycobacterial drugs. The organism is inhibited or killed by ethambutol, rifampin, ethionamide, and relatively high doses of isoniazid. Seroagglutination and agglutination absorption tests are specific for *M. szulgai* and provide an additional means of identification.[80]

Mycobacterium simiae

Mycobacterium simiae was first described in 1965 by Karasseva and colleagues during an investigation of spontaneous mycobacterial disease in monkeys.[46] Subsequently the organism was isolated from humans and described by Boisvert[8] and by Krasnow and Gross.[49] In 1971, Valdiva isolated a similar mycobacterium, which he named, *Mycobacterium habana*,[92] from the sputum of 35 patients in Havana. Comparison of the two strains by immunodiffusion and by agglutinating antibodies has shown lines of identity and identical surface antigens. Weiszfeiler and Karczag have therefore proposed the name *M. simiae* to take precedence over *M. habana*.[98]

Mycobacterium simiae has been recovered from the sputum of a number of patients, but in only a few of these has it been shown to be associated with a granulomatous tissue reaction. The organism is resistant in vitro to many of the standard antimycobacterial drugs, including isoniazid, streptomycin, para-aminosalicylic acid, ethambutol, and rifampin. Association of the organism with infection in monkeys and with the appearance of the disease in an animal caretaker raises the interesting question of transmission from animal to man.[22] Although the number of isolates and patients with infection from *M. simiae* are limited currently, as more and more laboratories learn the characteristics needed to identify this organism, it is likely there will be increasing numbers of isolates.

The laboratory identification of *Mycobacterium simiae* is based, in part, on the fact that it is usually photoreactive at the time of isolation, although this characteristic may become unstable with repeated subculture and be lost with time. Niacin accumulation can be demonstrated with adequate growth on a suitable culture medium, e.g., Lowenstein-Jensen. Differentiation between *M. simiae* and members of the *M.*

avium-intracellulare complex requires a semiquantitative catalase, usually greater than 45 mm for *M. simiae* and less than 45 mm for organisms of the *Mycobacterium avium-intracellulare* complex. In addition the urease test is positive for *M. simiae* and negative for the members of the *M. avium-intracellulare* complex.

Mycobacterium ulcerans

Mycobacterium ulcerans is the cause of chronic, slowly progressive cutaneous ulcers ("Buruli ulcer"). Disease from *M. ulcerans* was first described in 1948 in the state of Victoria, Australia, by Mac-Callum.[56] Since that time it has also been found in the northern and eastern parts of Australia as well as in Nigeria and remote areas of the Congo and Uganda.[18] It is found most commonly in rural peoples residing along the headwaters of the Congo River and along the upper reaches of the White Nile.

Infection with *Mycobacterium ulcerans* is progressive and indolent and can result in significant destruction of the skin and underlying tissues, particularly the extremities. In severe cases amputation has been necessary. The natural history of the infection is to heal by epithelialization of the surface ulcer, but without medical care this can take months or even years. In-vitro susceptibility tests have shown the organism to be resistant to isoniazid, ethambutol, para-aminosalicylic acid, and ethionamide, but susceptible to streptomycin, rifampin, cycloserine, viomycin, and kanamycin. In practice chemotherapy does not seem to be helpful. Surgical excision of the ulcer with replacement by a split-thickness skin graft appears to be the most effective treatment.[54]

Several cases have been identified in the United States, one from a physician from Nigeria who came to this country, and a second from a Peace Corp volunteer who served in Africa.[54, 90] Primary recovery of the organism by culture is difficult, requiring a tissue biopsy at the base of the ulcer near its junction with the involved subcutaneous tissue. Decontamination of the tissue biopsy should be with a mild agent, avoiding the use of 4 percent sodium hydroxide, if possible. Cultures should be incubated at 30 to 32° C for 6 to 9 months before discarding. Incubation of cultures at 37° C may inhibit or prevent growth, particularly at the time of primary isolation.

Mycobacterium xenopi

Mycobacterium xenopi was first described in 1959 by Schwabacher who found it to be the cause of granulomas in a toad, *Xenopus laevis*.[81] In 1966 it was shown to be the same organism as *M. littorale*, an organism known to cause disease in humans in England and Wales.[58]

Mycobacterium xenopi has been identified as a contaminant in hot water systems both in England and the United States.[11, 33] Gross, in reviewing the isolates of *M. xenopi* identified at one of two Veterans Administration Special Mycobacterial References Laboratories, found the organism had been recovered from 683 patients. Three or more isolates were present from 105 patients. Further study of the 105 patients revealed only 11 with clinical and bacteriologic evidence of infection from *M. xenopi*.[33] The incidence of the disease in this series of patients is in contrast to the earlier report by Marks and Schwabacher who reported that 26 of 50 isolates from patients living along the southern coast of England and Wales were considered either "clinically significant" or of "doubtful clinical significance" in the cause of pulmonary disease.[58] The organism has also been reported to cause pulmonary infection in humans in Denmark, France, Australia, and the United States; this includes the recovery of *M. xenopi* from a lung biopsy of a patient with granulomatous pneumonitis.[23, 27, 73, 87, 88] It is clinically important to distinguish patients having infection from *M. xenopi* from those having infection due to other scotochromogenic and nonphotochromogenic organisms because of the increased susceptibility of *M. xenopi* to antimycobacterial drugs, in contrast to the other scotochromogenic mycobacteria. The prognosis of a patient given a course of drug therapy, once this organism has been recovered and identified, is good.

Mycobacterium xenopi grows as a yellow-pigmented colony and, although initially classified as a Group III nonphotochromogenic mycobacterium, usually appears on primary culture as a scotochromogenic mycobacterium. The organism grows more rapidly and forms larger colonies when incubated at 42° C than 37° C. This characteristic of better growth at a temperature above 37°C is an important differential feature in separating the organism from other scotochromogenic mycobacteria. *M. xenopi* will produce detectable amounts of arylsulfatase within 5 to 7 days when incubated at 42°C, while the similar-appearing members of the *M. avium-intracellulare* complex will not.

Mycobacterium africanum

In 1968, Castets and coworkers[12] reported a series of mycobacterial isolates from patients in Dakar with pulmonary tuberculosis. These organisms appeared to occupy an intermediate position between *M. tuberculosis* and *M. bovis*. They were characterized by weak or variably positive niacin tests and showed variation in their ability to reduce nitrates to nitrites.

The following year Meissner and Schröder described an additional eight patients in Accra, Ghana, with pulmonary disease caused by organisms that had many of the characteristics described by Castets.[61] These organisms appeared similar to *M. bovis* on Lowenstein-Jensen medium in that they grew very slowly in culture and, were inhibited by 1 mcg/ml of thiophene-2-carboxylic acid hydrazide (T_2H). They also appeared similar to *M. tuberculosis* in that the niacin test was weakly positive, growth was inhibited by $25\mu g/ml$ of pyrazinamide, and the nitrate test was either positive or negative depending on the procedure used. In vitro susceptibility studies showed Meissner's strains to be susceptible to isoniazid, streptomycin, para-amino-salicylic acid, and ethambutol but relatively resistant to the thiosemicarbazones often used in Africa. The organisms were virulent for guinea pigs but not rabbits.

Until such time as these strains can be more completely identified, Meissner has proposed that they be referred to as the "african strains." No confirmed isolates of *M. africanum* have been described outside of the western coast of Africa.

NONPATHOGENIC MYCOBACTERIAL SPECIES

In addition to the foregoing mycobacteria that may cause infection, there are a number of nonpathogenic species occasionally isolated from clinical specimens that can appear on culture to be similar to strains causing disease. None of these strains are known to be photoreactive, but several are scotochromogenic and should be distinguished from disease-producing strains of *Mycobacterium scrofulaceum*, *Mycobacterium szulgai*, and *Mycobacterium xenopi*.

Mycobacterium gordonae is a slow-growing, nonpathogenic, pigmented mycobacterium that can colonize water stills, deionizers, or laboratory water taps. Not infrequently, growth of several yellow-pigmented colonies may appear on a culture after four to eight weeks, raising the question concerning the clinical significance of the organism. The differentiation of the non-pathogenic species of *M. gordonae* and *M. flavescens* from *M. scrofulaceum* and other disease-producing scotochromogenic mycobacteria is a useful and clinically important distinction.[48]

Among the non-photochromogenic mycobacteria, there are a number of nonpathogenic species that should be distinguished from the microorganisms of the *Mycobacterium avium-intracellulare* complex.[94] *Mycobacterium terrae*, an organism found in the soil and sometimes referred to as the "radish bacillus," has been reported to cause infection in humans under rare circumstances. The evidence for pathogenicity of *M. terrae* is not strong, and only a few documented cases have been reported.[15, 26] In a recent study of the numerical classification of the slowly growing mycobacteria, *M. terrae*, *M. nonchromogenicum*, and *M. novum* could not be clearly distinguished from each other and appear to belong to a single species for which the name *M. nonchromogenicum* has priority.[91] *M. gastri* has been isolated from stomach aspirates of patients unable to produce sputum specimens, but little or no evidence of pathogenicity for humans has been shown.[48] Another nonpathogenic organism that may be encountered is *Mycobacterium triviale*, an organism that has been referred to as the "atypical-atypical mycobacterium" because of the similarity of its colonial appearance to *M. tuberculosis*; it is also known as the "V" bacillus. *M. triviale* apears to be fairly distinct from similar mycobacterial species.[50, 91]

Among the rapidly growing mycobacteria, only members of the *Mycobacterium fortuitum-chelonei* complex are known to be associated with disease in man. *M. smegmatis* has been described as colonizing the genitourinary tract of humans, but it is rarely isolated from urine or other clincial specimens. Failure to isolate *M. smegmatis* may be due to a sensitivity of the organism to commonly used decontaminizing agents, e.g., 4 percent sodium hydroxide.

REFERENCES

1. Ahn, C. H., et al.: Ventilatory defects in atypical mycobacteriosis. A comparison study with tuberculosis. Am. Rev. Respir. Dis. *113*:273, 1976.
2. Andringa, C. L., and Cherry, J. A.: Bilateral inguinal adenitis due to a nonphotochromogenic atypical *Mycobacterium*. J.A.M.A. *198*:209, 1966.
3. Aronson, J. D.: Spontaneous tuberculosis in salt water fish. J. Infect. Dis. *39*:315, 1926.
4. Awe, R. J., et al.: Clinical significance of *Mycobacterium fortuitum* infections in pulmonary disease. Am. Rev. Respir. Dis. *108*:1230, 1973.
5. Bailey, R. K., et al.: The isolation of high catalase *Mycobacterium kansasii* from tap water. Am. Rev. Respir. Dis. *101*:430, 1970.
6. Bast, R. C., et al.: BCG and cancer. N. Engl. J. Med. *290*:1413, 1458, 1974.
7. Beck, A.: *Mycobacterium fortuitum* in abscesses of man. J. Clin. Pathol. *18*:307, 1965.
8. Boisvert, H.: Mycobacteries (*M. bovis* et "atypiques") identifiées a l'Institut Pasteur de Paris de 1960 1972, p. 29. The genus *Mycobacterium*. Prince Leopold Institute of Tropical Medicine, Antwerp.
9. Borghaus, J. G. A., and Stanford, J. L.: *Mycobacterium chelonei* in abscesses after injection of diphtheria-pertussis-tetanus-polio vaccine. Am. Rev. Respir. Dis. *107*:1, 1973.
10. Buhler, V. B., and Pollak, A.: Human infection with atypical acid-fast organism. Report of two cases with pathologic findings. Am. J. Clin. Pathol. *23*:363, 1953.
11. Bullin, C. H., et al.: Isolation of *Mycobacterium xenopi* from water taps. J. Hyg. (Camb.) *68*:97, 1970.
12. Castets, M. M., et al.: Les bacilles tuberculeux de type africain. Rev. Tuberc. Pneumologie *32*:179, 1968.
13. Chang, M. S., and Barton, L. L.: *Mycobacterium fortuitum* osteomyelitis of the calcaneous secondary to a puncture wound. J. Ped. *85*:517, 1974.
14. Chapman, J. S. (ed.): The Anonymous Mycobacteria in Human, Disease. Springfield, Ill., Charles C Thomas, 1960.
15. Cianciulli, E. D.: The radish bacillus (*Mycobacterium terrae.*; Saprophyte or pathogen? Am. Rev. Respir. Dis. *109*:138, 1974.
16. Clapper, W. E., and Whitcomb, J.: *Mycobacterium fortuitum* abscess at injection site. J.A.M.A. *202*:550, 1967.
17. Cleveland, D. E. H.: Possible tuberculous skin infection from a swimming pool. Acta Dermatovener (Stockholm) *31*:147, 1951.
18. Connor, D. H., and Lunn, H. E.: Buruli ulceration. A clinicopathologic study of 38 Ugandans with *Mycobacterium ulcerans* ulceration. Arch. Pathol. *81*:183, 1966.

19. da Costa Cruz, J.: *Mycobacterium fortuitum:* A new acid fast bacillus pathogenic for man. Acta Med. *1*:297, 1938.

20. Davidson, P. T.: *Mycobacterium szulgai.* A new pathogen causing infection of the lung. Chest *69*:799, 1976.

21. David, H. L.: Bacteriology of Mycobacterioses. Public Health Service DHEW (CDC) 76–8316, 1976.

22. Donovan, W. N., et al.: *Mycobacterium simiae.* Am. Rev. Respir. Dis. *113*:55, 1976.

23. Doyle, W. M., et al.: Pulmonary disease caused by *Mycobacterium xenopei.* Am. Rev. Respir. Dis. *97*:919, 1968.

24. Dreisin, R. B., et al.: The pathogenicity of *Mycobacterium fortuitum* and *Mycobacterium chelonei* in man. A report of seven cases. Tubercle *57*:49, 1976.

25. Edwards, L. B.: Current status of the tuberculin test. Ann. N. Y. Acad. Sci. *106*:32, 1963.

26. Edwards, M. S., Huber, T. W., and Baker, C. J.: *Mycobacterium terrae* synovitis and osteomyelitis. Am. Rev. Respir. Dis. *117*:161, 1978.

27. Engbaek, H. C., et al.: *M. xenopei.* Acta Pathol. Microbiol. Scand. *69*:576, 1967.

28. Epidemiologic Surveillance, Center for Disease Control: Isolation of mycobacterial species from porcine heart valve prosthesis. Morbidity and Mortality Weekly Report *26*:42, 1977.

29. Francis, P. B., et al.: The course of untreated *Mycobacterium kansasii* disease. Am. Rev. Respir. Dis. *111*:477, 1975.

30. Fraser, D. W. et al.: Disseminated *Mycobacterium kansasii* infection presenting as cellulitis in a recipient of a renal homograft. Am. Rev. Respir. Dis. *112*:125, 1975.

31. Graybill, J. R. et al.: Disseminated mycobacteriosis due to *Mycobacterium abscessus* in two recipients of renal homografts. Am. Rev. Respir. Dis. *109*:4, 1974.

32. Grigg, E. R. N.: The arcana of tuberculosis with a brief epidemiologic history of the disease in the U.S.A. Am. Rev. Tuberc. *78*:151–172 (Parts I and II), 426–454 (Part III), 584–604 (Part IV), 1958.

33. Gross, W., et al.: *Mycobacterium xenopi* in clinical specimens. Water as a source of contamination. Am. Rev. Respir. Dis. *113*(Part 2):78, 1976.

34. Gunther, S. F., and Elliott, R. C.: *Mycobacterium kansasii* infection in the deep structures of the hand. J. Bone Joint Surg. *58*:140, 1976.

35. Habib, N. I., and Warring, F. C.: A fatal case of infection due to *M. bovis.* Am. Rev. Respir. Dis. *93*:804, 1966.

36. Hagmar, B., et al.: Disseminated infection caused by *Mycobacterium kansasii.* Acta Med. Scand. *186*:93, 1969.

37. Hand, W. L., and Sanford, J. P.: *Mycobacterium fortuitum* — A human pathogen. Ann. Int. Med. *73*:971, 1970.

38. Hawkins, J. E.: Scotochromogenic mycobacteria which appear intermediate between *Mycobacterium avium-intracellulare* and *Mycobacterium scrofulaceum.* Am. Rev. Respir. Dis. *116*:963, 1966.

39. Heineman, H. S., et al.: Fish tank granuloma. Arch. Intern. Med. *130*:121, 1972.

40. Hellerstrom, S.: Contribution à la connaissance de l'infection tuberculeuse de la peau et la muqueuse. Acta Dermatovener (Stockholm) *20*:276, 1939.

41. Hellerstrom, S.: Collected cases of inoculation lupus vulgaris. Acta Dermatovener (Stockholm) *31*:194, 1951.

42. Hepper, N. G. G., et al.: Genitourinary infection due to *Mycobacterium kansasii.* Mayo Clin. Proc. *46*:387, 1971.

43. Jenkins, P.A., et al.: Thin layer chromatography of mycobacterial lipids as an aid to classification: The scotochromogenic mycobacteria. Tubercle *53*:118, 1972.

44. Jolly, H. W., and Seabury, J. H.: Infections with *Mycobacterium marinum.* Arch. Derm. *106*:32, 1972.

45. Joos, H. A., et al.: Fatal disseminated scotochromogenic mycobacteriosis in a child. Am. Rev. Respir. Dis. *96*:795, 1967.

46. Karasseva, V., et al.: Occurrence of atypical mycobacteria in *Macacus rhesus.* Acta Microbiol. Acad. Sci. Hung. *12*:275, 1965.

47. Karlson, A. G., and Carr, D. T.: Tuberculosis caused by *M. bovis.* Report of six cases: 1954–1968. Ann. Int. Med. *73*:979, 1970.

48. Kestle, D. G., et al.: Differential identification of mycobacteria. II. Subgroups of Group II and III (Runyon) with different clinical significance. Am. Rev. Respir. Dis. *95*:1041, 1967.

49. Krasnow, I., and Gross, W.: *M. simiae* infection in the United States. Am. Rev. Respir. Dis. *111*:357, 1975.

50. Kubica, G. P., et al.: Differential identification of mycobacteria. VI. *Mycobacterium triviale* Kubica sp. nov. Int. J. Syst. Bacteriol. *20*:161, 1970.

51. Kubica, G. P., et al.: A co-operative numerical analysis of rapidly growing mycobacteria. J. Gen. Microbiol. *73*:55, 1972.

52. Levy, C., et al.: *Mycobacterium chelonei* infection of porcine heart valves. N. Engl. J. Med. *297*:667, 1977.

53. Lichtenstein, M. R., et al.: Photochromogenic mycobacterial pulmonary infection in a group of hospitalized patients in Chicago II. Demographic studies. Am. Rev. Respir. Dis. *91*:592, 1965.

54. Lindo, S. D., and Daniels, E.: Buruli ulcer in New York City. J.A.M.A. *228*:1138, 1974.

55. Linell, F., and Norden, A.: *Mycobacterium balnei:* A new acid-fast bacillus occurring in swimming pools and capable of pro-

ducing skin lesions in humans. Acta Tuberc. Scand. *33*(Suppl.):1, 1954.

56. MacCallum, P.: A new mycobacterial infection in man. J. Pathol. Bacteriol. *60*:93, 1948.

57. Mansson, T., et al.: Aquarium-borne infection with *Mycobacterium marinum*. Acta Dermatovener *50*:119, 1970.

58. Marks, J., and Schwabacher, H.: Infection due to *Mycobacterium xenopei*. Br. Med. J. *i*:32, 1965.

59. Marks, J., et al.: *Mycobacterium szulgai* — A new pathogen. Tubercle *53*:210, 1972.

60. Mayberry, J. D., et al.: Cutaneous infection due to *Mycobacterium kansasii*. J.A.M.A. *194*:233, 1965.

61. Meissner, G., and Schroder, K.: Uber soz. Afrikanische Mykobakterien — Stamme aus dem tropischen West-Afrika. Zentralblatt fur Bakteriologie, Parasitenkunde, Infektionskrankheiten und Hygiene, *I* Orig. 211 S, 69–81, 1969.

62. Meissner, G., and Anz, W.: Sources of *Mycobacterium avium* complex infection resulting in human diseases. Am. Rev. Respir. Dis. *116*:1057, 1977.

63. Mills, C. C.: Occurrence of mycobacterium other than *Mycobacterium tuberculosis* in the oral cavity and in sputum. App. Microbiol. *24*:307, 1972.

64. Offer, R. C., et al.: Infection caused by *Mycobacterium fortuitum*. Mayo Clin. Proc. *46*:747, 1971.

65. Ortbals, D. W., and Marr, J. J.: A comparative study of tuberculosis and other mycobacterial infections and their associations with malignancy. Am. Rev. Respir. Dis. *117*:39, 1978.

66. Pfuetze, K. H., et al.: Photochromogenic mycobacterial disease. Am. Rev. Respir. Dis. *92*:470, 1965.

67. Prissick, F. H., and Masson, A. M.: Cervical lymphadenitis in children caused by chromogenic mycobacteria. Can. Med. Assoc. *75*:798, (Nov. 15), 1956.

68. Prissick, F. H., and Masson, A. M.: Yellow-pigmented pathogenic mycobacteria from cervical lymphadenitis. Can. J. Microbiol. *3*:91, 1957.

69. Ranney, A. F.: The status of the state-federal tuberculosis eradication program. Proc. U.S. Animal Health Assoc. *73*:410, 1969.

70. Renner, M., and Bartholomew, W. R.: Mycobacteriologic data from two outbreaks of bovine tuberculosis in nonhuman primates. Am. Rev. Respir. Dis. *109*:11, 1974.

71. Rees, R. B., and Bennett, J. H.: Granuloma following swimming pool abrasion. J.A.M.A. *152*:1606, 1953.

72. Reznikov, M., and Dawson, D. J.: Serological investigation of strains of *Mycobacterium intracellulare* ("Battey Bacillus") isolated from house-dusts. Med. J. Aust. p 682, March 27, 1971.

73. Richter, P. E., et al.: Pulmonary disease related to *Mycobacterium xenopei*. Med. J. Aust. p 1246, June 14, 1969.

74. Runyon, E. H.: Pathogenic mycobacteria. Adv. Tuberc. Res. *14*:235, 1965.

75. Runyon, E. H.: *Mycobacterium intracellulare*. Am. Rev. Respir. Dis. *95*:861, 1967.

76. Runyon, E. H.: Identification of mycobacterial pathogens utilizing colony characteristics. Am. J. Clin. Pathol. *54*:578, 1970.

77. Saito, H., et al.: Disseminated *Mycobacterim intracellulare* infection. Am. Rev. Respir. Dis. *109*:572, 1974.

78. Schaefer, W. B., and Davis, C. L.: A bacteriologic and histopathologic study of skin granuloma due to *Mycobacterium balnei*. Am. Rev. Respir. Dis. *84*:837, 1961.

79. Schaefer, W. B.: Serologic identification and classification of the atypical mycobacteria by their agglutination. Am. Rev. Respir. Dis. *96*:115, 1965.

80. Schaefer, W. B., et al.: *Mycobacterium szulgai* — A new pathogen. Serological identification and report of five new cases. Am. Rev. Respir. Dis. *108*:1320, 1973.

81. Schwabacher, H.: A strain of mycobacterium isolated from skin lesions of a cold-blooded animal, *Xenopus laevis*, and its relation to atypical acid-fast bacilli occurring in man. J. Hyg. *57*:57, 1959.

82. Scully, R. E.: Granulomatous hepatitis due to BCG. N. Engl. J. Med. *293*:443, 1975.

83. Scully, R. E. (Ed.): Case records of the Massachusetts General Hospital. Granulomatous hepatitis. N. Engl. J. Med. *296*:1218, 1977.

84. Selva-Sutter, E. A. et al.: Differential identificiation of *Mycobacterium szulgai* and other scotochromogenic mycobacteria. J. Clin. Microbiol. *3*:414, 1976.

85. Silcox, V. A., and David, H. L.: Differential identification of *Mycobacterium kansasii* and *Mycobacterium marinum*. Appl. Microbiol. *21*:327, 1971.

86. Stanford, J. L., et al.: Studies on *Mycobacterium chelonei*. J. Med. Microbiol. *5*:177, 1972.

87. Tellis, C. J., et al.: Pulmonary disease caused by *Mycobacterium xenopi*. Two case reports. Am. Rev. Respir. Dis. *116*:779, 1977.

88. Thibier, R. et al.: Sept cas de pleuropneumopathie "*Mycobacterium xenopei*" Rev. Tuberc. *34*:632, 1970.

89. Timpe, A., and Runyon, E. H.: The relationship of "atypical" acid-fast bacteria to human disease. J. Lab. Clin. Med. *44*:202, 1954.

90. Tsang, A. Y., and Farber, E. R.: The primary isolation of *Mycobacterium ulcerans*. Am. J. Clin. Pathol. *59*:688, 1973.

91. Tsukamura, M.: Numerical classification of slowly growing mycobacteria. Int. J. Sys. Bacteriol. *26*:409, 1976.

92. Valdivia, A., et al.: *Mycobacterium habana*:

probable nueva especie dentro de las micobacterias no classificadas. Bol. Hig. Epidemiol. Habana 9:65, 1971.

93. Wayne, L. G.: Two varieties of *Mycobacterium kansasii* with different clinical significance. Am. Rev. Respir. Dis. *86*:651, 1962.

94. Wayne, L. G.: Classification and identification of mycobacteria III. Species within Group III. Am. Rev. Respir. Dis. *93*:919, 1967.

95. Wayne, L. G.: On the synonomy of *Mycobacterium marianum* Penso 1952 and *Mycobacterium scrofulaceum* Prissick and Masson 1956 and the resolution of a nomenclatural problem. Int. J. Sys. Bacteriol. *91*:257, 1969.

96. Wayne, L. G., et al.: Highly reproducible techniques for use in systematic bacteriology in the genus *Mycobacterium:* Test for niacin and catalase and for resistance to isoniazid, thiophene 2-carboxylic acid hydrazide, hydroxylamine, and p-nitrobrenzoate. Int. J. Sys. Bacteriol. *26*: 311, 1976.

97. Weed, L. A.: Nontuberculous acid-fast cervical adenitis in children. Mayo Clin. Proc. *31*:259, 1956.

98. Weiszfeiler, S. G., and Karczag, E.: Synonymy of *Mycobacterium simiae* Karasseva et al 1965 and *Mycobacterium habana* Valdivia et al 1971. Int. J. Sys. Bacteriol. *26*:474, 1976.

99. Wigle, W. D., et al.: Bovine tuberculosis in humans in Ontario. Am. Rev. Respir. Dis. *106*:528, 1972.

100. Willis, W. E., and Laibson, P. R.: Intractable *Mycobacterium fortuitum* corneal ulcer in man. Am. J. Ophthal. *72*:500, 1971.

101. Wolinsky, E.: The role of scotochromogenic mycobacteria in human disease. Ann. N. Y. Acad. Sci. *106*:67, 1963.

102. Wolinsky, E., and Rynearson, T. K.: Mycobacteria in soil and their relation to disease-associated strains. Am. Rev. Respir. Dis. *97*:1032, 1968.

103. Wolinsky, E., and Schaefer, W. B.: Proposed scheme for mycobacterial serotypes by agglutination. Int. J. Sys. Bacteriol. *23*:182, 1973.

104. Wunsch, S. E., et al.: *Mycobacterium fortuitum* infection of corneal graft. Arch. Ophthal. *82*:602, 1969.

105. Youmans, G. P.: Disease due to mycobacteria other than *Mycobacterium tuberculosis*. In Youmans, G. P., Paterson, P. Y., and Sommers, H. M., (eds.): The Biologic and Clinical Basis of Infectious Diseases. Philadelphia, W. B. Saunders Co., 1975, p. 358.

106. Youmans, G. P.: The pathogenic "atypical" mycobacteria. Ann. Rev. Microbiol. *17*: 473, 1963.

107. Zeligman, I.: *Mycobacterium marinum* granuloma. Arch. Derm. *106*:26, 1972.

108. Zimmerman, L. E., et al.: *Mycobacterium fortuitum* infection of the cornea. Arch. Ophthal. *82*:596, 1969.

19

The Laboratory Diagnosis of Mycobacterial Disease*

HERBERT M. SOMMERS, M.D.

INTRODUCTION

The diagnosis of mycobacterial infection depends on the isolation and identification of an organism from the patient. Although the demonstration of acid-fast bacteria in a stained smear from sputum, pleural fluid, or other clinical specimens is presumptive evidence of infection, the isolation and species identification are important for determining the initial drug therapy, prognosis, and in many instances, the probable source of the organism. This chapter will deal with the laboratory procedures useful for the isolation, identification, and drug susceptibility testing of mycobacteria.

---

*Portions of this chapter also appear in Mycobacterial disease. *In* Henry, John (ed.): Todd-Sanford-Davidson Clinical Diagnosis by Laboratory Methods. 16th ed. Philadelphia, W. B. Saunders Co., 1979.

SPECIMEN COLLECTION AND PREPARATION

Specimens from patients with tuberculosis usually contain mixed bacterial flora. The successful recovery of mycobacteria depends on suppression of contaminating bacteria but not significant inhibition of the mycobacteria. Methods for the collection of specimens should be directed toward minimizing the number of contaminating bacteria.

Compared to a 24-hour sputum pool, sputum specimens containing *Mycobacterium tuberculosis* show faster growth with fewer contaminants when collected early in the morning, using an ultrasonic device for nebulization. Although it has been reported that 24-hour sputum collections will ultimately yield more positive cultures than early morning specimens,[13] growth is usually slower and the contamination rate is significantly higher with the sputum pools.[11] Depending on whether there is minimal or advanced disease, there will be intermittent or continual shedding or tubercle bacilli, resulting in a positive culture on one day and a negative on the next. Krasnow and Wayne have shown that a minimum of three and not more than five early morning specimens will usually be sufficient to identify the patient with active disease (Fig. 19–1).[13]

◖ Urine specimens for the diagnosis of renal tuberculosis are best collected as a single specimen early in the morning. Three to five specimens are usually sufficient. Although 24-hour urine collections can be obtained, some laboratory workers believe tubercle bacilli can suffer an irreversible injury with prolonged exposure to urine.

Cerebrospinal fluid should be inoculated to Middlebrook 7H9 broth, American Trudeau Society (ATS)* medium, or other types of noninhibitory culture medium after centrifugation. If a pellicle is present in the cerebrospinal fluid, it should be divided into pieces for inoculation to several different types of culture medium, saving a small fragment for an acid-fast stain. Portions of tissue from surgical biopsies or autopsies should be cut into small fragments and either ground in a mortar and pestle with sterile sand or alundum powder, or homogenized briefly with a ground-glass or Teflon homogenizer. Prolonged homogenization can kill the organism from heat. The homogenized tissue should be inoculated to both selective and noninhibitory culture media to provide optimal growth and control of contaminating bacteria.

◣ Recovery of mycobacteria from a suspected tuberculous draining sinus occurs best when exudate or biopsies can be obtained. Swabs obtained from draining sites should be placed directly on culture media or in broth. Growth of mycobacteria from swabs may be inhibited by the hydrophobic nature of the lipid-containing mycobacterial cell wall, so that the mycobacteria remain in the interstices of the swab, avoiding the water-containing culture medium. Under these conditions, growth of contaminating bacteria from the drainage materials often masks the presence of mycobacteria.

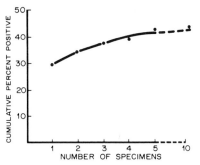

SEQUENTIAL ADMISSION SPECIMENS

FIGURE 19–1. Relationship of number of sputum specimens collected to positive cultures obtained from suspected tuberculous patients. (From Kubica, G. P., Gross, W. M., Hawkins, J. E., Sommers, H. M., Vestal, A. L., and Wayne, L. G.: Laboratory services for mycobacterial diseases. Am. Rev. Respir. Dis. *112*:773, 1975.)

*Now the *American Thoracic Society.*

DIGESTION AND CONCENTRATION

The doubling time for *Mycobacterium tuberculosis* is approximately 20 to 22 hours, while other types of bacteria in the specimen may divide every 40 to 60 minutes. The disproportionate rate of growth between the two types of microorganisms often results in the accumulation of metabolic waste products from the rapidly growing bacteria, making the culture medium unsatisfactory for mycobacteria. The successful isolation of mycobacteria is dependent upon selective suppression of nonmycobacterial-contaminating bacteria.

The high lipid content of mycobacterial cell walls makes them more resistant to killing by strong acid and alkaline solutions than most of the contaminating bacteria. Specimens submitted for recovery of mycobacteria are first treated with an alkaline or acid decontamination agent to reduce bacterial overgrowth and liquefy any mucus present to promote concentration of the organisms by centrifugation. After a carefully timed exposure of the specimen, while being mechanically shaken, the acid or alkaline solution is neutralized and then centrifuged at high speed to concentrate the mycobacteria. The centrifugal force should be as high as possible because the lipid content of the mycobacterial cell wall provides a buoyant effect and makes their specific gravity close to unity. For this reason the selective sedimentation of mycobacteria in a thick, viscous sputum specimen is difficult.

In the past, decontaminating solutions were often so strong that if exposure times were not carefully controlled, large numbers of mycobacteria were either killed or so seriously injured that they grew only very slowly or not at all. Decreasing the strength of decontamination solutions has resulted in the improved survival and recovery of mycobacteria but frequently at the price of a high incidence of culture contamination. Exposure of specimens to strong decontaminating agents such as 3 or 4 percent NaOH, or 5 percent oxalic acid, must be carefully timed to prevent excessive chemical injury. Neutralization of a strong decontaminating solution requires an equally strong acid or alkali, and often titration to a neutral end point might be incomplete with the specimen remaining either strongly alkaline or acid. Although the culture medium can act as a buffer for a moderate pH shift, an inadequately neutralized specimen can destroy the culture medium prior to the growth of any mycobacteria. The use of mild decontaminating agents, such as trisodium phosphate (TSP) or TSP with benzalkonium chloride (Zephiran Chloride*), has become an alternative in some laboratories. Specimens containing large numbers of *M. tuberculosis* can withstand the action of these agents for periods of time as long as 24 hours and still grow on culture. All specimens digested and concentrated with TSP-benzalkonium chloride should be inoculated to egg-base culture media in order to neutralize the growth inhibition characteristics of benzalkonium chloride. The concentrate should be neutralized by adding lecithin if it is to be inoculated to agar base media.[21]

In response to the increased need to recover mycobacteria for susceptibility testing, Kubica[14] developed a concentrating solution containing 2 percent NaOH and N-acetyl-L-cysteine (NALC). NALC is a mucolytic agent that liquefies mucus by splitting disulfide bonds. It does not have any antibacterial activity. Mild bacterial decontamination is effected by 2 percent NaOH, and with the mucous liquefied, the mycobacteria are sedimented by centrifugation. On occasion the concentration of NaOH has to be increased to 3 percent during periods of warm weather or for specimens from patients with large pulmonary cavities, often associated with persistent bacterial contam-

---

*Registered trademark of Winthrop Laboratories, New York, N.Y.

ination. One advantage of the NALC decontamination procedure is neutralization of the specimen by the addition of a large volume of a slightly acid (pH 6.8), phosphate buffer. The use of the buffer makes strong pH shifts less likely. It also acts as a "wash" during centrifugation, diluting any toxic substances present as well as decreasing the specific gravity of the specimen to make the sedimentation of lipid containing mycobacteria more effective. Following centrifugation, the sediment is resuspended in 0.2 percent bovine albumin, which provides a buffering and detoxifying effect on the sedimented concentrate.

Dithiothreitol (Sputolysin*) is anoth-

*Registered trademark of Calbiochem Laboratories, San Diego, Calif.

er mucolytic agent useful for concentrating mycobacteria similar in action to NALC.[24] Cetyl-pyridium chloride with NaCl has also been shown to be an effective decontaminating agent for sputum specimens transported through the mail. Mycobacteria have withstood transit times of eight days in this agent without significant loss of viability.[25]

Table 19–1 lists a number of decontamination and concentration agents in current use. The selection of one or more agents by a laboratory will depend in part on the number and types of specimens they receive and the time and numbers of technical staff available to process the specimens. Decontamination and concentrating procedures useful in laboratories receiving specimens from hospitalized patients may differ from those serving outpatient

TABLE 19–1. **Agents for Digestion and Concentration of Specimens Containing Mycobacteria**

	Comments
1. N-acetyl-L-cysteine (NALC) + 2 percent NaOH	Mild decontamination solution with mucolytic agent, NALC, to free mycobacteria entrapped in mucous. NaOH may have to be increased to 3 percent to control contamination on occasion.
2. Dithiothreitol + 2 percent NaOH*	Very effective mucolytic agent used with 2 percent NaOH. Trade name of dithiothreitol is Sputolysin. Reagent is more expensive than NALC, but it has the same advantages of NALC.
3. 13 percent trisodium phosphate + benzalkonium chloride (Zephiran)	Preferred by laboratories unable to always control time of exposure to decontamination solution. Benzalkonium chloride should be neutralized with lecithin if not inoculated to egg-base culture medium.
4. 1 percent cetyl-pyridium chloride + 2 percent NaCl**	Effective as a decontamination solution for sputum specimens mailed from outpatient clinics. *M. tuberculosis* has survived 8-day transit without significant loss of viability.
5. 4 percent NaOH	Traditional decontamination and concentration solution. Time of exposure must be carefully controlled. Four percent NaOH will effect mucolytic action to promote concentration by centrifugation.
6. 4 percent sulfuric acid	The use of 4 percent sulfuric acid when decontaminating urine specimens has improved recovery for many laboratories.
7. 5 percent oxalic acid	This is most useful in the processing of specimens that contain *Pseudomonas aeruginosa* as a contaminant.

*Shah and Dye (1966).[24]
**Smithwick, Stratigos, and David (1975).[25]

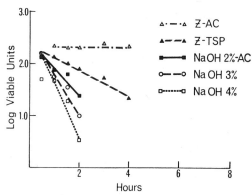

FIGURE 19–2. Death rates of tubercle bacilli in digested sputum. Z-AC = Zephiran-N-acetyl-L-cysteine; Z-TSP=Zephiran-trisodium phosphate; NaOH 2%-AC = 2% NaOH + N-acetyl-L-cysteine; 3% and 4% NaOH. (From Kubica, G. P., Gross, W. M., Hawkins, J. E., Sommers, H. M., Vestal, A. L., and Wayne, L. G.: Laboratory services for mycobacterial diseases. Am. Rev. Respir. Dis. 112:773, 1975.)

clinics. Similarly, the specimens from some patients may require the use of more than one decontaminating agent if persistent contamination occurs; e.g., specimens containing *Pseudomonas aeruginosa* may survive 2 percent NaOH-NALC and require concentration with 5 percent oxalic acid.

Krasnow and Wayne[12] have plotted the death rates with time of *M. tuberculosis* from different decontaminating agents, using split sputum specimens from patients with active tuberculosis (Fig. 19–2). The results emphasize the need for careful control of the length of time that specimens are exposed to these agents, usually recommended not to exceed 15 minutes. This is particularly true if 3 to 4 percent NaOH solutions are used. Z-AC in Figure 19–2 refers to Zephirin Chloride (benzalkonium chloride) and N-acetyl-L-cysteine. This combination exerts very little or no antimycobacterial activity but is not clinically useful due to inadequate activity against contaminating organisms.

Animal Inoculation

The inoculation of guinea pigs with neutralized concentrated sediment for the purpose of isolating *Mycobacterium tuberculosis* was an effective procedure for many years. More recently, refinements in decontamination and concentration procedures with the development of selective culture media have made the use of animals for isolation unnecessary. Although guinea pigs are quite susceptible to infection from *M. tuberculosis*, mycobacterial species other than *M. tuberculosis*, e.g., *M. kansasii* and *M. avium-intracellulare*, do not cause progressive infection in these animals and would be missed entirely. Rabbits, susceptible to infection from 0.01 mg of *M. bovis* bacilli but not from the same number of *M. tuberculosis* bacilli, are seldom used to distinguish between the two species. Although animals (including guinea pigs, rabbits, and fowl) are helpful in the research laboratory, their use in the identification of mycobacterial infections in man is no longer as important as it was in earlier years due to differences in species susceptibility and the costs involved in maintaining an appropriate colony compared to the recovery by culture.[5]

CULTURE MEDIA

Culture media for mycobacteria can be broadly grouped as those solidified from coagulated eggs ("egg-base media"), those solidified with agar ("agar-base media"), liquid media, and media containing antimicrobial agents ("selective media").

Early attempts to recover mycobacteria by culture were only partially successful until a medium solidified with coagulated eggs was used. A large number of egg-base media have been developed, each differing slightly from the next. Most egg-base media are composed of varying combinations of whole eggs, potato flour, organic and inorganic salts, and glycerol. Egg-base media are solidified by heating the liquid medium to a temperature of 85° C to 90° C for 30 to 45 minutes (inspissation). Contaminating bacteria, particularly gram-positive bacteria, are controlled in part by the addition to the medium of aniline dyes such as crystal violet and malachite green. The concentration of aniline dye in a medium is an important variable as slight increases over the specified amount can result in significant inhibition of mycobacterial growth as well as growth of contaminants. (See also Chapter 2.)

Egg-Base Culture Media

Numerous types of egg-base culture media have been described and are currently in use. The most commonly used egg-base medium for primary isolation of mycobacteria is Lowenstein-Jensen (see Table 19–2). Petragnani medium is considerably more inhibitory both for mycobacteria and nonmycobacterial organisms and should be reserved for specimens known to contain large numbers of contaminants. A less inhibitory egg-base medium than Lowenstein-Jensen is the American Trudeau Society (ATS) medium. ATS is particularly helpful in the primary isolation of mycobacteria from specimens not likely to be contaminated with other bacteria, e.g., cerebrospinal fluid, pleural fluid, and tissue biopsies.

Agar-Base Culture Media

During the 1950s Middlebrook and coworkers (as described by Russell and Middlebrook in their book[22]) developed a series of mycobacterial culture media. These media were synthesized from inorganic salts, a series of organic compounds, glycerol, and albumin. Agar-containing Middlebrook-Cohn media are transparent and have a distinct advantage as media: when scanned with a 10× low power objective, or a dissecting microscope, growth of *M. tuberculosis* after 10 to 14 instead of after 18 to 24 days incubation

can be seen. The isolation of mycobacterial colonies from mixed cultures is also facilitated when agar-containing plates are used in contrast to the tubes or prescription bottles commonly filled with egg-base culture media. Middlebrook-Cohn 7H9 broth medium is a popular liquid culture medium, and both 7H10 and 7H11 agar are widely used for primary isolation and susceptibility testing. Medium 7H11 differs from 7H10 only by the addition of 0.1 percent casein hydrolysate, a compound found to improve the rate and amount of growth of mycobacteria resistant to isoniazid.[4] Both 7H10 and 7H11 contain malachite green, but in much smaller quantities than in egg-base media (Table 19–2). Although most culture media will yield more and larger colonies of mycobacteria when incubated in 5 percent to 10 percent CO_2, the Middlebrook-Cohn media *must* be incubated in CO_2 for optimal recovery of bacilli.

Exposure of the 7H10 or 7H11 culture media to strong light or storage of the media at 4° C for more than four weeks may be associated with partial deterioration and release of formaldehyde. The presence of formaldehyde results in a very inhibitory medium with little or no growth of mycobacteria.[18] Laboratories using 7H10 or 7H11 culture media are urged to prepare their own from commercially available components or to assure the source, age, and conditions of handling of prepared media obtained from outside sources.

Both Middlebrook-Cohn 7H10 and 7H11 can be used for mycobacterial drug susceptibility testing, although 7H11 is preferred. Incorporation of antimycobacterial agents in the medium after sterilization and just before it solidifies reduces the loss of drug activity that can occur with some agents during the long heating period used in preparing inspissated egg-based media. The components of commonly used nonselective culture media are listed in Table 19–2.

TABLE 19–2. **Nonselective Mycobacterial Isolation Media**

Medium	Components	Inhibitory Agent
Lowenstein-Jensen	Coagulated whole eggs, defined salts, glycerol, potato flour	0.025 gm/100 ml malachite green
Petragnani	Coagulated whole eggs, egg yolks, whole milk, potato, potato flour, glycerol	0.052 gm/100 ml malachite green
American Trudeau Society medium	Coagulated fresh egg yolks, potato flour, glycerol	0.02 gm/100 ml malachite green
Middlebrook 7H10	Defined salts, vitamins, co-factors, oleic acid, albumin, catalase, glycerol, dextrose	0.0025 gm/100 ml malachite green
Middlebrook 7H11	Defined salts, vitamins, co-factors, oleic acid, albumin, catalase, glycerol, 0.1 percent casein hydrolysate, dextrose	0.0025 gm/100 ml malachite green

Selective Culture Media

Mycobacterial culture media containing antimicrobial agents to suppress bacterial and fungal contamination have been used for many years. Although certain antimicrobial agents will reduce bacterial contamination, they can exert significant growth inhibition on mycobacteria as well. Despite the inhibition of growth of some mycobacterial species, the use of selective culture media can result in greatly improved recovery of mycobacteria. The names and components of several selective culture media are listed in Table 19–3.

One of the more commonly used selective culture media was developed by Gruft, who added penicillin, nalidixic acid, and RNA to Lowenstein-Jensen medium.[7] Petran and Vera[20] found that a medium containing cyclohexamide, lincomycin, and nalidixic acid was also effective in the control of fungal and bacterial contaminants. By varying the amount of each of these three agents, the medium could be prepared using either Lowenstein-Jensen or 7H10 medium (see Table 19–3).

The culture medium, Selective 7H11, is a modification of an oleic acid agar medium first described by Mitchison.[19] It contains four antimicrobial agents and was originally developed to be used for sputum specimens without exposure to a decontaminating agent. McClatchy[16] suggested the carbenicillin be reduced from 100 to 50 μg/ml and that 7H11 medium be used instead of oleic acid agar, calling this modification, Selective 7H11. Several reports comparing Selective 7H11 medium with Lowenstein-Jensen and 7H11 have shown a distinct increase in recovery of mycobacteria when used in combination with the NALC–2 percent NaOH decontamination and concentration procedure.

STAINING FOR ACID-FAST BACILLI

The mycobacteria have a unique characteristic, i.e., binding the stain carbolfuchsin so tightly it resists destaining with strong de-colorizing agents such as alcohols and strong acids. (See Chapters 2 and 4.) The "acid-fast" staining reaction of mycobacteria, along with their beaded and slightly curved shape, is a valuable aid in the early detection of infection and in the monitoring of therapy (see Chapters 2, 3, 4, and 17). The finding of acid-fast bacilli in the sputum, combined with a history of cough and weight loss and a chest x-ray showing a pulmonary infil-

TABLE 19–3. Selective Mycobacterial Isolation Media

Medium	Components	Inhibitory Agents		
Gruft modification of Lowenstein-Jensen	Coagulated whole eggs, defined salts, glycerol, potato flour, RNA-17 mg/100 ml	0.025 50 35	gm/100 ml units per ml μg per ml	malachite green penicillin nalidixic acid
Mycobactosel* 1. Lowenstein-Jensen	Coagulated whole eggs, defined salts, glycerol, potato flour	0.025 400 2 35	gm/100 ml μg/ml μg/ml μg/ml	malachite green cycloheximide lincomycin nalidixic acid
2. Middlebrook 7H10	Defined salts, vitamins, co-factors, oleic acid, albumin, catalase, glycerol, and dextrose	0.0025 360 2 20	gm/100 ml μg/ml μg/ml μg/ml	malachite green cycloheximide lincomycin nalidixic acid
Selective 7H11 (Mitchison's medium)	Defined salts, vitamins, co-factors, oleic acid, albumin, catalase, glycerol, dextrose, and casein hydrolysate	50 10 200 20	μg/ml μg/ml units/ml μg/ml	carbenicillin amphotericin B polymyxin B thrimethropin lactate

*Mycobactosel is the registered trademark of Bioquest Laboratories, Cockeysville, Md.

trate, is often considered presumptive evidence of active tuberculosis and sufficient cause to initiate therapy.

It has been estimated that there must be 10,000 acid-fast bacilli per ml of sputum to be detected by microscopy.[30] Patients with extensive active disease will shed large numbers of mycobacteria and show a good correlation between a positive smear and a positive culture of sputum specimens. In patients with minimal or with less active disease, the correlation of positive smears to positive cultures may be only 60 to 70 percent, the cultures offering a more sensitive method of detecting small numbers of organisms.

Acid-fast stains are also useful in following the response to drug therapy of patients with active disease. After antituberculous drugs are started, cultures will become negative before smears. This indicates that the bacilli are injured sufficiently to prevent replication, but not binding of the stain. With continued drug treatment, more organisms are killed and fewer shed, so that following the number of stainable organisms in the sputum during treatment can provide an objective measure of response before the results of cultures are available from 3 to 6 weeks later.[8] *It should be emphasized that for the first few months after starting therapy, not all stainable organisms are viable.* Should the number of organisms seen in smears fail to decrease after therapy is started, the possibility of drug resistance must be considered. Additional cultures should be taken and drug susceptibility studies obtained. Two types of acid-fast stains are frequently used:

1. The carbolfuchsin stains, so-called because of the reagent formed by mixing the stain fuchsin with the disinfectant phenol (carbolic acid). Two procedures using carbolfuchsin stains are in common use:
    a. the Ziehl-Neelsen, or "hot stain" and
    b. the Kinyoun, or "cold stain."
2. The fluorochrome dye, auramine 0,

sometimes used in combination with a second fluorochrome stain, rhodamine.

Because of the small size of the organism and the low contrast in the color of the organism and the bright background, smears stained by carbolfuchsin must be scanned with the 100× oil-immersion objective, thereby greatly restricting the area of a slide that can be viewed in a given period of time. In comparison, smears stained with auramine 0 can be scanned using a 25× objective. Fluorochrome-stained mycobacteria appear bright yellow against a dark background, obtained by counterstaining with potassium permanganate, permitting the slide to be scanned under lower magnification without losing sensitivity. The sharp visual contrast between the brightly colored mycobacteria and the dark background offers the advantage of scanning a larger area of the specimen smear during the same time necessary for looking at the carbolfuchsin stain. For this reason, the fluorochrome stain will often result in the detection of mycobacteria in smaller numbers per slide then when using a carbolfuchsin stain.

Fluorochrome-stained smears require a strong blue light source for illumination, either a 200 watt mercury vapor burner or a strong blue light source with a fluorescein isothiocyanate filter. Modifications of the auramine 0 staining procedure include the addition of rhodamine, to give a more golden appearance to the mycobacteria, or the use of acridine orange[27] as a counterstain to stain the background red to orange.

Enthusiasm for the carbolfuchsin and fluorochrome-staining methods varies between laboratories, with different workers strongly partial to one method or the other. Specificity for mycobacteria seems to be the same for both procedures, with the exception of one reported series of 15 strains of *Mycobacterium fortuitum.* In this series, 5 of the 15 isolates did not stain with auramine 0, but all 15 stained with carbolfuchsin.[10] Reports differ as to which one of the two types of stain will bind to nonviable bacilli for the longest period of time. These differences probably reflect differences in attention to detail shown to staining and microscopy by individual laboratories. As mentioned above, when using the auramine 0 stain, a significantly larger area of the smear can be scanned in the same period of time used to scan a carbolfuchsin-stained smear. For this reason the fluorochrome stain offers the possibility of greater sensitivity. Because some workers are hesitant to give up carbolfuchsin stains, laboratories may scan smears by the fluorochrome method and then confirm positive slides by destaining and restaining with a carbolfuchsin stain.[26] Once microbiologists have become familiar with the auramine 0 stain, they usually prefer the fluorochrome method to carbolfuchsin stains.

Reports from examination of stained smears from clinical specimens should provide some quantitation of the number of organisms present on a smear as there can be a relationship to the number of acid-fast bacilli present and the degree of activity of the disease. The National Tuberculosis Association recommends the following method:[5]

Number of Bacilli	Report
0	No acid-fast bacilli found
1 to 2 in entire smear	Report number found and request additional specimens
3 to 9 in entire smear	Rare, or +
10 or more in entire smear	Few, or ++
1 or more per oil-immersion field	Numerous, or +++

The use of the sputum smear as a screening procedure for the diagnosis of pulmonary tuberculosis has recently been criticized following the finding by several large laboratories that up to 55 percent of specimens with positive smears failed to grow mycobacteria in culture. A review of the clinical symptoms and chest X-rays in many of these patients failed to show supporting clinical evidence for tuberculosis. The point has been made that as the incidence of tuberculosis decreases, the predictive value of a positive smear will also decline. Thus, carried to the extreme, if there were no tuberculosis, 100 percent of the positive smears would be false positives.[2] As techniques for detecting mycobacteria become more sensitive, the finding of commensal mycobacteria that may be more susceptible than *M. tuberculosis* to the decontamination and concentrating procedures will contribute to the higher incidence of positive smears and negative cultures. Important factors in the reliability of the predictive value of the smear include the presence or absence of abnormal findings on a chest x-ray, the clinical history, the patient's symptoms, and the number of bacilli present on the smear. As might be expected, there is a positive correlation between increasing numbers of bacilli and incidence of active infection.

The similarities and differences between the Ziehl-Neelsen, Kinyoun, and fluorochrome stains are listed in Table 19–4. It should be remembered that the auramine 0 or auramine-rhodamine fluorochrome stains are not fluorescent antigen-antibody reactions. Fluorescent-tagged antibodies useful for the identification of individual species of mycobacteria have been described but are not in widespread use, nor are they commercially available.[9]

INCUBATION OF CULTURES

Most mycobacteria show growth stimulation when incubated in an atmosphere of increased concentration of carbon dioxide. Studies have suggested that the optimal concentration of CO_2 is

TABLE 19–4.   Acid-Fast Staining Procedures

Ziehl-Neelsen Stain	Kinyoun Stain	Auramine Fluorochrome Stain
Carbol-fuchsin: Dissolve 3.0 gm of basic fuchsin in 10.0 ml of 90 to 95 percent ethanol. Add 90 ml of 5 percent aqueous solution of phenol.	**Carbol-fuchsin:** Dissolve 4.0 gm of basic fuchsin in 20 ml of 90 to 95 percent ethanol and then add 100 ml of a 9 percent aqueous solution of phenol.	**Phenolic auramine:** Dissolve 0.1 gm auramine 0 in 10 ml of 90 to 95 percent ethanol and then add to a solution of 3 gm of phenol in 87.0 ml of distilled water. Store the stain in a brown bottle.
Acid-alcohol: Add 3.0 ml of concentrated HCl *slowly* to 97.0 ml of 90 to 95 percent ethanol, in this order. Solution may get hot!	**Acid-alcohol:** Add 3.0ml of concentrated HCl *slowly* to 97.0 ml of 90 to 95 percent ethanol, in this order. Solution may get hot!	**Acid-alcohol:** Add 0.5 ml concentrated HCl to 100 ml of 70 percent alcohol.
Methylene blue counterstain: Dissolve 0.3 gm of methylene blue chloride in 100 ml of distilled water.	**Methylene blue counterstain:** Dissolve 0.3 gm of methylene blue chloride in 100 ml of distilled water.	**Potassium permanganate:** Dissolve 0.5 gm potassium permanganate in 100 ml of distilled water.
Procedure: 1. Cover heat-fixed, dried smear with a small rectangle (2x3 cm) of filter paper.* 2. Apply 5 to 7 drops of carbol-fuchsin stain to thoroughly moisten filter paper. 3. Heat the stain-covered slide to steaming but do not allow to dry. Heating may be done by gas burner or over an electric-staining rack. 4. Remove paper with forceps, rinse with water, and allow to drain. 5. Decolorize with acid-alcohol until no more stain appears in the washing (2 min). 6. Counterstain with methylene blue (1 to 2 min). 7. Rinse, drain, and air dry (1 to 2 min). 8. Examine with 100× oil immersion objective. Bacilli are stained red and the background light blue.	**Procedure:** 1. Cover heat-fixed, dried smear with a small rectangle (2x3 cm) of filter paper.* 2. Apply 5 to 7 drops of carbol-fuchsin to thoroughly moisten filter paper. Allow to stand for 5 min. Add more stain if paper dries. Do not steam! 3. Remove paper with forceps, rinse with water, and allow to drain. 4. Decolorize with acid-alcohol until no more stain appears in the washing (2 min). 5. Counterstain with methylene blue (1 to 2 min). 6. Rinse, drain, and air dry (1 to 2 min). 7. Examine with 100× oil immersion objective. Bacilli are stained red and the background light blue	**Procedure:** 1. Cover heat-fixed, dried smear with carbol auramine and allow to stain for 15 min. Do not heat or cover with filter paper. 2. Rinse with water and drain. 3. Decolorize with acid-alcohol (2 min). 4. Rinse with water, drain. 5. Flood smear with potassium permanganate for 2 min and not more than 4 min. 6. Rinse with tap water. Drain. 7. Examine with 25× objective using a mercury vapor burner and BG-12 filter or a strong blue light. Mycobacteria are stained yellowish-orange against a dark background.

*To avoid the transfer of bacilli from one slide to another, never blot smears dry. Stain smears on a rack. Do not use jars between 8 percent and 12 percent (Fig. 19–3). Increased CO_2 tension is a requirement for the proper use of 7H10, 7H11, and Selective-7H11 culture media, and it will also improve recovery of the number and size of colonies of mycobacteria on egg-base culture media.[1, 6] Candle extinction jars are not acceptable for this purpose, which is best served by a CO_2 incubator. The CO_2 concentration in the incubator should be monitored and recorded in the quality control chart on a daily basis.

M. *tuberculosis* will grow slowly when cultures are incubated at 37° C. In contrast, M. *marinum* and M. *ulcerans*, organisms causing disease of the skin, should be incubated at 30° C to 32° C for optimal recovery. Incubation of cultures at 37° C for the recovery of M. *marinum* or M. *ulcerans* will greatly delay or even prevent their growth. Simi-

larly, specimens containing M. *xenopi* will show optimal growth and recovery when incubated at 42° C. If incubators for 30° C to 32° C are not available, cultures from skin infections or other sources thought to contain M. *marinum* should be placed in a temperature-monitored box or container at 24° C and positioned away from heating or cooling air currents. Incubation of cultures at this temperature can offer a valuable identification characteristic to other species of bacteria (e.g., *Pseudomonas aeruginosa*) as well as mycobacteria (see also Chapter 18).

IDENTIFICATION

Laboratories receiving only occasional clinical specimens for mycobacteria may find the technical effort required to maintain competence for all services in

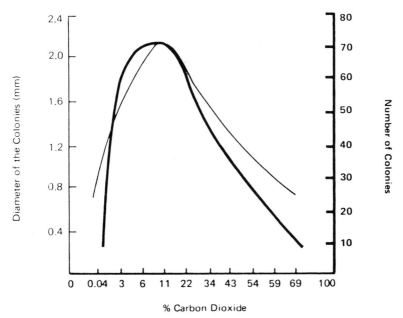

FIGURE 19–3. Effect of CO_2 on the growth (colony size and number of colonies) of M. *tuberculosis* on primary isolation from sputum. (Modified from Beam, R. E., and Kubica, G. P.: Stimulatory effects of carbon dioxide on the primary isolation of tubercle bacilli on agar-containing medium. Am. J. Clin. Pathol. 50:395, 1968. Reproduced from David, H. L.: Bacteriology of the mycobacterioses. Atlanta, Ga., USPHS Center for Disease Control, Mycobacteriology Branch, DHEW Publication No. (CDC) 76-8316.)

the mycobacterial laboratory to be expensive and not cost-effective. Other laboratories will find that the number of specimens and patients seen in their institution require that they be able to offer complete identification as well as susceptibility testing. In order to help each laboratory decide how far they should go in establishing mycobacterial services, the College of American Pathologists has suggested four "extents" of service. A similar list of "Levels of Proficiency" has subsequently been suggested by the American Thoracic Society. These two lists are compared in Table 19–5, where the similarities are readily apparent.[3, 15]

Metabolic Characteristics

The characteristics found helpful in the identification of mycobacteria are listed in Table 19–6 and in the appendix to this chapter. Additional characteristics useful in the classification of mycobacteria may be found in chapters or

laboratory manuals prepared by Runyon, Karlson, Kubica, and Wayne,[21] Vestal,[27] and David.[5] Most laboratories will be primarily interested in establishing the identification of *Mycobacterium tuberculosis*. This can be done for the majority of isolates by determining the following:

1. The optimal temperature and rate of growth
2. Photoreactivity
3. Niacin accumulation
4. Reduction of nitrates to nitrites
5. Catalase production
   a. Heat-stable
   b. Semiquantitative

Although not a common problem, certain strains of the *M. bovis* (BCG mutants) can accumulate small quantities of niacin and produce nitroreductase, thereby resembling *M. tuberculosis*. These strains can be distinguished from *M. tuberculosis* by inhibition of growth on medium containing 1 or 5 μg/ml of thiophene-2-carboxylic hydrazide. The

TABLE 19–5. **Suggested Limits of Mycobacteriological Services**

Extents of Service College of American Pathologists	Levels of Proficiency American Thoracic Society
1. No mycobacteriologic procedures performed.	1. Collection and transportation of specimens; preparation and examination of smears for acid-fast bacilli.
2. Acid-fast stain of exudates, effusions, and body fluids, with inoculation and referring of cultures to reference labs.	2. Detection, isolation, and identification of *Mycobacterium tuberculosis*. Determination of susceptibility of mycobacteria to the primary antimycobacterial drugs.
3. Isolation of mycobacteria; identification of *Mycobacterium tuberculosis* and preliminary identification of the atypical forms as photochromogens, scotochromogens, nonphotochromogens and rapid growers. Drug susceptibility testing may or may not be performed.	3. Identification of mycobacteria other than *M. tuberculosis* and performance of susceptibility testing on all antimycobacterial drugs.
4. Definitive identification of mycobacteria isolated to the extent required to establish a correct clinical diagnosis and to aid in the selection of safe and effective therapy. Drug susceptibility testing may or may not be performed.	

majority of the remaining mycobacteria listed in Table 19–6 can be classified by determining the hydrolysis of Tween 80, the presence of arylsulfatase after three days' incubation, the presence or absence of urease, the ability to grow on medium containing 5 percent NaCl, and the ability to incorporate soluble iron salts to give a rusty color to the bacterial colonies. (For details of how to determine many of these identification characteristics, see the appendix to this chapter.)

Immunologic Procedures

In addition to laboratory procedures determining metabolic characteristics useful for mycobacterial species identification, four different immunologic procedures have proved helpful in the study of mycobacteria, i.e., agglutination of bacterial cells by rabbit serum antibodies, precipitin reactions in agar diffusion, immunofluorescence procedures, and tuberculin testing of sensitized animals.

Agglutinating antibodies, which are developed by injection of killed mycobacteria into rabbits, have been very helpful in separating the members of the *Mycobacterium avium-intracellulare* complex into 17 different serotypes. Agglutination studies have shown a very close relationship between the members of the *M. avium-intracellulare* complex and the three serotypes of *M. scrofulaceum*, a species that by colonial and metabolic characteristics would seem reasonably unrelated.[23] Seroagglutination studies are also very helpful to confirm unusual or uncommonly isolated species such as *Mycobacterium szulgai*. The restricted availability of agglutinating antisera has limited the use and application of the procedure to reference laboratories and research centers.

Immunodiffusion procedures have also been applied to the study of relatedness of different species. Although useful in determining the similarities or differences of antigens between two bacterial strains, this technique has not found widespread application in the clinical laboratory identification of mycobacteria.[29]

A third immunologic procedure that has been applied to the study of mycobacteria is immunofluorescence. Species-specific fluorescent-tagged antisera have been used in direct antigen-antibody immunofluorescent staining studies. Although the procedure has been found to be promising, no commercial source of antisera is available.[9] Cross reactions can occur, limiting the usefulness of the technique.

The fourth type of immunologic procedure, which has had wide application to the study of mycobacteria, is the testing of skin hypersensitivity to protein extracts of different species of mycobacteria. The use of tuberculin tests and the significance of positive and negative tuberculin reactions have been covered in detail in Chapters 7 and 14.

SUSCEPTIBILITY TESTING OF MYCOBACTERIA

Random drug resistance in mycobacteria is independent of exposure to the agent. The frequency of drug-resistant mutants in a culture of tubercle bacilli has been estimated to be between 1 in 10^5 to 10^7 bacteria for isoniazid and 1 in 10^6 to 10^8 for streptomycin.[5] If two drugs, isoniazid and streptomycin, are both given, the incidence of resistance will be the product of the two separately, or 1 out of every 10^{15} organisms. The importance of the incidence of spontaneously resistant mutants becomes apparent when it is known that an open pulmonary cavity may have a total bacillary population of 10^7 to 10^9 mycobacteria. If such patients are treated with a single antituberculous agent, their cultures will soon be populated only with resistant organisms and treatment will

TABLE 19–6. Identification Characteristics of Mycobacteria

Organism	Optimum Isolation Temperature and Rate of Growth in Days	Pigmentation Growth in Light	Pigmentation Growth in Dark	Niacin Test	Nitrate Reduction
M. tuberculosis	37°C, 12 to 25	buff	buff	+	3 to 5+
M. africanum	37°C, 31 to 42	buff	buff	V	V
M. bovis	37°C, 24 to 40	buff	buff	V	—
M. ulcerans	32°C, 28 to 60	buff	buff	—	—
M. kansasii	37°C, 10 to 20	yellow	buff	—	1 to 5+
M. marinum	31 to 32°C, 5 to 14	yellow	buff	V	—
M. simiae	37°C, 7 to 14	yellow[4]	buff	+	∓
M. szulgai	37°C, 12 to 25	yellow to orange	yellow – 37°C buff – 25°C	—	+ (weak)
M. scrofulaceum	37°C, 10 or more	yellow	yellow	—	—
M. gordonae	37°C, 10 or more	yellow to orange	yellow	—	—
M. flavescens	37°C, 7 to 10	yellow	yellow	—	+
M. xenopi	42°C, 14 to 28	yellow	yellow	—	—
M. intracellulare avium complex	37°C, 10 to 21	buff to pale yellow	buff to pale yellow	—	—
M. gastri	37°C, 10 to 21	buff	buff	—	—
M. terrae complex	37°C, 10 to 21	buff	buff	—	1 to 5+
M. triviale	37°C, 10 to 21	buff	buff	—	1 to 5+
M. fortuitum	37°C, 3 to 5	buff	buff	—	2 to 5+
M. chelonei					
ss borstelense	37°C, 3 to 5	buff	buff	V	—
ss abscessus	37°C, 3 to 5	buff	buff	V	—
M. smegmatis	37°C, 3 to 5	buff to yellow	buff to yellow	—	1 to 5+

Key to results: + = 84 percent of strains positive; ± = 50 to 84 percent; ∓ = 16 to 49 percent; = 16 percent of strains positive; V = variable; blank spaces = little or no data.
[1] Numbers indicate millimeters of bubbles.
[2] INH-resistant strains may be negative.
[3] Positive (most) in 24 to 48 hours.
[4] Photochromogenicity unstable with repeated subcultures.
Reproduced with the permission of Sommers, H. M.: The identification of mycobacteria. Lab. Med. 9(2):34, 1978.

TABLE 19–6. **Identification Characteristics of Mycobacteria**—*Continued*

Catalase Semi-quantitative[1]	Catalase pH 7.0 68°C	Tween 80 Hydrolysis 10 Days	Arylsul-fatase 3 Days	Urease	Resistance to T_2H 1 µg/ml	Growth on 5 percent NaCl	Iron Uptake
<40[2]	−	∓	−	+	+	−	−
<20	−	−	−		+	−	−
<20	−	−	−	+	−	−	−
>50	+	−	−		+		
>50	+	+[3]	−	+	+	−	−
<40	∓	+	∓		+	−	−
>50	+	−	−	−	+		
>50	+	∓	∓	+	+	−	−
>50	+	−	−	+	+	−	−
>50	+	+	−	−	+	−	−
>50	+	+	−	+	+	+	−
<40	+	−	±	−	+	−	−
<40	+	−	−	−	+	−	−
<40	−	+	−	+	+	−	−
>50	+	+	−	−	+	−	−
>50	+	+	∓		+	+	+
>50	+	±	+	+	+	+	+
>50	+	−	+	+	+	−	−
>50	+	−	+	+	+	+	−
>50	±	+	−		+	+	+

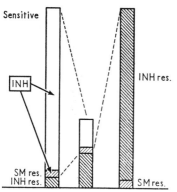

FIGURE 19–4. Emergence of isoniazid (INH) resistance with single-drug therapy. SM = streptomycin. (From Crofton, J.: Some principles in the chemotherapy of bacterial infections. Br. Med. J. 2:137, 1969.)

fail (Figs. 19–4 and 19–5). Patients with tuberculosis must be treated with two or preferably three drugs to prevent the rapid selection of drug-resistant tubercle bacilli.

Clinically, it has been found that if more than 1 percent of a patient's tubercle bacilli are resistant to a drug in vitro, therapy with that drug will not be effective in vivo. For this reason, the mycobacterial susceptibility test must determine the *number* of bacilli susceptible and resistant to each drug. The

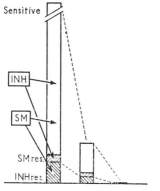

FIGURE 19–5. Preventing resistance by combined chemotherapy. (From Crofton, J.: Some principles in the chemotherapy of bacterial infections. Br. Med. J. 2:137, 1969.)

inoculum should be adjusted so that the number of naturally resistant mutants will not mislead the laboratory worker to interpret the culture as resistant. At the same time, there must be a sufficiently dilute inoculum so that the incidence of drug resistance in the range of 1 percent can be determined. For optimal results, such an inoculum will result in 100 to 300 colony-forming units on each quadrant of a four quadrant Petri plate. Because it is difficult to standardize an inoculum of mycobacteria, particularly *M. tuberculosis*, it is usually necessary to inoculate two sets of susceptibility test plates, the first with a 10^{-2} or 10^{-3} dilution of a barely turbid broth culture and the second set with a hundredfold dilution of the inoculum used for the first set. This procedure is known as the *proportional susceptibility testing method.*

Twelve drugs are used in the treatment of tuberculosis. Four are considered "primary" and include streptomycin, isoniazid, rifampin, and ethambutol; the remaining eight — ethionamide, capreomycin, kanamycin, cycloserine, *p*-aminosalicylic acid, thiacetazone, viomycin, and pyrazinamide — are considered secondary and are used only when resistance develops to the primary drugs (see Chapters 20 and 21). The suggested concentrations of the drugs used for mycobacterial susceptibility testing are listed in Table 19–7.

The mycobacterial susceptibility test is performed using plastic Petri plates divided into four quadrants. Five ml of agar is placed in each quadrant. The medium in the first quadrant does not contain any antimycobacterial agent and acts as a growth control. The other three quadrants contain dilutions of the drugs to be tested. Although drugs have been incorporated in inspissated egg-base media in the past, most laboratories now prefer using either 7H11 or 7H10 as a base medium, adding the drugs after cooling the agar to 45° C. Adding the drugs after cooling to the medium decreases the loss of activity of

TABLE 19–7. Drug Concentration for Susceptibility Testing Using 7H10 Agar or 7H11 Agar

Drug	Drug Concentration (µg/ml) 7H10	7H11
Isoniazid	0.2, 1.0	0.2, 1.0
PAS	2.0	8.0
Streptomycin	2.0	2.0
Rifampin	1.0	1.0
Ethambutol	6.0	7.5
Ethionamide	5.0	10.0
Kanamycin	5.0	6.0
Capreomycin	10.0	10.0
Cycloserine	20.0	30.0
Viomycin	5.0	10.0
Pyrazinamide	50*	–

*At pH 5.5
Reproduced with permission from McClatchy, J. K.: Susceptibility testing of mycobacteria. Lab. Med. 9(3):47, 1978.

an agent that can occur in an egg-base medium during inspissation. An additional loss of drug activity may occur in egg-base media with binding of some agents to egg albumin and other proteins.

A simplified method for preparing drug susceptibility plates that does not require the weighing and dilution of each drug has been described using

filter paper discs containing the primary antituberculous drugs.[28] Discs are available from microbiologic supply sources. With this method, preparation of drug-containing media is facilitated by placing a drug-containing disc in one quadrant of the plate and adding 5 ml of 7H11 or 7H10 agar. The drug from the disc diffuses into the medium and results in the recommended concentration to be tested. Since each disc is marked with the name and concentration of the drug it contains, labeling errors are eliminated as well as errors that can occur in weighing, dilution, and measuring of drug solutions.[29] A suggested schedule for the use of drug-containing paper discs in the preparation of testing plates is given in Table 19–8.

The *direct mycobacterial susceptibility* test is inoculated from digested and concentrated sputum found to be positive for acid-fast bacilli. The *indirect susceptibility* test is inoculated from colonies isolated from a primary culture. The direct test will usually give good results only if large numbers of mycobacteria are present in the specimen. The advantage of the direct susceptibility test is an earlier report, 3 to 4 weeks,

TABLE 19–8. Distribution of Drug-Containing Discs for Susceptibility Tests

Plate Number	Quadrant Number		Amount of Drug per Disc (µg)	Final Drug Concentration (µg/ml)
1	I	Control #1	–	0
	II	Isoniazid	1	0.2
	III	Isoniazid	5	1.0
	IV	Rifampin	5	1.0
2	I	Streptomycin	10	2.0
	II	Streptomycin	50	10.0
	III	Ethambutol	25	5.0*
	IV	Ethambutol	50	10.0*
3	I	Para-aminosalicylic acid	10	2.0
	II	Para-aminosalicylic acid	50	10.0
	III	Control #2	–	0
	IV	–	–	–

*Improved correlation with clinical response has been noted with ethambutol concentrations of 7.5 and 15 µg/ml. These can be achieved by using 1.5 of 25 µg discs in each quadrant for the 7.5 µg/ml concentration and a 25 and 50 µg disc for the 15 µg/ml concentration.
Reproduced with permission of Kubica, G. P., et al.: Laboratory services for mycobacterial diseases. Am. Rev. Respir. Dis. 112:773, 1975.

TABLE 19–9. **Reading and Reporting of Susceptibility Test Results**

Amount of Growth	Report
Confluent (> 500 colonies)	++++
Almost confluent (200 to 500 colonies)	+++
100 to 200 colonies	++
50 to 100 colonies	+
< 50 colonies	Actual number

Reproduced with permission from McClatchy, J. K.: Susceptibility testing of mycobacteria. Lab. Med. 9(3):47, 1978.

in contrast to the indirect test, which may take up to 8 weeks. The disadvantage of the direct susceptibility test is that it usually requires a large number of mycobacteria for successful growth and is often overgrown by large numbers of contaminating bacteria. The *indirect mycobacterial susceptibility* test is performed on a broth subculture from a colony isolated from the primary culture. This makes the possibility of contamination much less likely but may add an additional three to four weeks to the time necessary to obtain susceptibility results.

To perform the test, susceptibility plates are inoculated with three drops in each quadrant, of a 10^{-2} and 10^{-4} dilution of a barely turbid broth culture for the indirect test, or three drops of undiluted and a tenfold dilution of the smear positive concentrate for a direct test. If large numbers of mycobacteria are seen on the stained smear (greater than 10 per oil-immersion field with carbolfuchsin stain, or more than 250 per 250× field with fluorochrome staining) a 1:10 and 1:100 dilution of the sputum concentrate is made for incubation. Plates are incubated in individual cellophane bags in CO_2 at 37° C and interpreted at weekly intervals for three weeks. Incubation of ethambutol-containing media for more than three weeks may result in the appearance of microcolonies following the inactivation of the drug. Interpretation of the inoculated plates should include either

an estimate or a direct count of the total number of colonies on the control and drug-containing media (Table 19–9). All colonies, even those showing inhibition of growth on drug-containing media, should be counted and related to the number of colonies on the control quadrant. The control quadrant should contain the same number of colonies as inoculated to the test quadrants. Therefore, the percentage of resistant colonies can be readily calculated from the two sets of plates inoculated with dilutions of organisms either ten- or one hundredfold apart.

Susceptibility studies are not indicated for all mycobacterial isolates, as the incidence of primary drug resistance (defined as a drug-resistant organism isolated from a previously untreated patient) is less than 3 to 5 percent. Even if primary resistance to one drug is present, treatment with the recommended triple drug therapy will pro-

TABLE 19–10. **Indications for Susceptibility Studies for Mycobacteria Isolates**

A. May not be indicated for previously untreated patients.
B. Should be obtained under the following conditions:
  1. Sputum-positive patients who have had previous chemotherapy (relapsed or retreatment cases).
  2. Patients on therapy whose sputum reverts to positive.
  3. Patients whose sputum smears do not convert to negative within two to three months of treatment.
  4. Patients whose cultures do not convert to negative within four to six months of treatment.
  5. Patients with increasing numbers of tubercle bacilli seen in smears after an initial decrease.
  6. Patients with mycobacterial infections other than *Mycobacterium tuberculosis.*
  7. Patients suspected of having primary resistance:
    a. Tuberculosis patients who have lived abroad.
    b. Persons possibly infected by patients with drug-resistant tuberculosis.

Reproduced with permission from McClatchy, J. K.: Susceptibility testing of mycobacteria. Lab. Med. 9(3):47, 1978.

vide coverage. Susceptibility tests should be routinely performed on bacterial isolates from patients who have shown relapse while on drug therapy. The probability of induced resistance in this group of patients is high. Other indications for performing antimycobacterial drug susceptibility tests are given in Table 19–10. If susceptibility tests are not performed on isolates obtained from patients previously seen by a laboratory, at least one culture should be saved for six months or a year should the patient not respond to therapy. Controls for mycobacterial susceptibility studies should be run with each set of test cultures and should include both susceptible, resistant, as well as intermediately susceptible strains, e.g., *M. kansasii* resistant to 0.2 μ/ml of isoniazid but susceptible to 1.0 μ/ml. Further details for determining antimycobacterial drug susceptibility tests can be found in Runyon et al.,[21] Vestal,[27] Kubica et al.,[15] and McClatchy.[17]

REFERENCES

1. Beam, R. E., and Kubica, G. P.: Stimulating effects of carbon dioxide on the primary isolation of tubercle bacilli on agar containing medium. Am. J. Clin. Pathol. 50:395, 1968.
2. Boyd, J. C., and Marr, J. J.: Decreasing reliability of acid-fast smear techniques for detection of tuberculosis. Ann. Intern. Med. 82:489, 1975.
3. College of American Pathologists: Extents of Service, Special Mycobacteriology Survey. Survey Manual, Skokie, Ill., 1978.
4. Cohn, M. L., Waggoner, R. F., and McClatchy, J. K.: The 7H11 medium for the culture of mycobacteria. Am. Rev. Respir. Dis. 98:295, 1968.
5. David, H. L.: Bacteriology of the mycobacterioses. Public Health Services, DHEW (CDC) 76-8316, 1976.
6. Gruft, H., and Loder, A.: Enhancing effects of carbon dioxide on the primary isolation of acid-fast bacilli in a modified Lowenstein-Jensen medium. App. Microbiol. 22:944, 1971.
7. Gruft, H.: Isolation of acid-fast bacilli from contaminated specimens. Health Lab. Sci. 8:79, 1971.
8. Hobby, G. L., Holman, A. P., Iseman, M. D., and Jones, J. M.: Enumeration of tubercle bacilli in sputum of patients with pulmonary tuberculosis. Antimicrob. Agents Chemother. 4:94, 1973.
9. Jones, W. D., Jr., Beam, R. E., and Kubica, G. P.: Fluorescent antibody techniques with mycobacteria. II. Detection of *Mycobacterium tuberculosis* in sputum. Am. Rev. Respir. Dis. 95:516, 1967.
10. Joseph, S. W.: Lack of auramine-rhodamine fluorescence of Runyon Group IV mycobacteria. Am. Rev. Respir. Dis. 95:114, 1967.
11. Kestle, D. G., and Kubica, G. P.: Sputum collection for cultivation of mycobacteria. An early morning specimen or the 24- to 72-hour pool? Am. J. Clin. Pathol. 48:347, 1967.
12. Krasnow, I., and Wayne, L. G.: Sputum digestion. I. The mortality rate of tubercle bacilli in various digestion systems. Am. J. Clin. Pathol. 45:352, 1966.
13. Krasnow, I., and Wayne, L. G.: Comparison of methods for tuberculosis bacteriology. Appl. Microbiol. 18:915, 1969.
14. Kubica, G. P., Dye, W. E., Cohn, M. L., and Middlebrook, G.: Sputum digestion and decontamination with N-acetyl-L-cysteine-sodium hydroxide for culture of mycobacteria. Am. Rev. Respir. Dis. 87:775, 1963.
15. Kubica, G. P., Gross, W. M., Hawkins, J. E., Sommers, H. M., Vestal, A. L., and Wayne, L. G.: Laboratory services for mycobacterial diseases. Am. Rev. Respir. Dis. 112:773, 1975.
16. McClatchy, J. K., Waggoner, R. F., Kanes, W., Cernick, M. S., and Bolton, T. L.: Isolation of mycobacteria from clinical specimens by use of Selective 7H11 medium. Am. J. Clin. Pathol. 65:412, 1976.
17. McClatchy, J. K.: Susceptibility testing of mycobacteria. Lab. Med. 9(3):39, 1978.
18. Miliner, R. A., Stottmeier, K. D., and Kubica, G. P.: Formaldehyde: A photothermal activated toxic substance produced in Middlebrook 7H10 medium. Am. Rev. Respir. Dis. 99:603, 1969.
19. Michison, D. A., Allen, B. W., Carroll, L., Dickinson, J. M., and Aber, V. P.: A selective oleic acid albumin agar medium for tubercle bacilli. J. Med. Microbiol. 5:165, 1972.
20. Petran, E. I., and Vera, H. D.: Media for selective isolation of mycobacteria. Health Lab. Sci. 8:225, 1971.
21. Runyon, E. H., Karlson, A. G., Kubica, G. P., and Wayne, L. G.: *Mycobacterium. In* Lennette, E. H., Spaulding, E. H., and Truant, J. P. (eds.): Manual of Clinical Microbiology. 2nd ed., Washington, D.C., American Society for Microbiology, 1974, p. 148.
22. Russell, W. F., and Middlebrook, G.: Chemotherapy of Tuberculosis. Springfield, Ill., Charles C Thomas, 1961.
23. Schaefer, W. B.: Serologic identification of the atypical mycobacteria and its value in

epidemiologic studies. Am. Rev. Respir. Dis. 96:115, 1967.

24. Shah, R. R., and Dye, W. E.: The use of dithiothreitol to replace N-acetyl-L-cysteine for routine sputum digestion. Am. Rev. Respir. Dis. 94:454, 1966.

25. Smithwick, R. W., Stratigos, C. B., and David, H. L.: Use of cetylpyridium chloride and sodium chloride for the decontamination of sputum specimens that are transported to the laboratory for the isolation of *Mycobacterium tuberculosis.* J. Clin. Microbiol. 1:411, 1975.

26. Smithwick, R. W.: Laboratory Manual for Acid-fast Microscopy. Atlanta, Ga., U.S. Dept. Health, Education and Welfare, Public Health Service, Center for Disease Control, Mycobacterial Reference Section, 1975.

27. Vestal, A. L.: Procedures for the Isolation and Identification of Mycobacteria. U.S. Dept. Health, Education and Welfare, Public Health Service Publication No. (CDC) 75-8230.

28. Wayne, L. G., and Krasnow, I.: Preparation of tuberculosis drug susceptibility testing media using drug impregnated discs. Tech. Bull. Reg. Med. Tech. 36:767, 1966.

29. Wayne, L. G.: Phenol-soluble antigens from *Mycobacterium kansasii, Mycobacterium gastri,* and *Mycobacterium marinum.* Infect. Immun. 3:36, 1971.

30. Yeager, H., Lacy, J., Smith, L. R., and LeMaistre, C. A.: Quantitative studies of mycobacterial populations in sputum and saliva. Am. Rev. Respir. Dis. 95:998, 1967.

Appendix: Identification Procedures

1. **Determination of temperature preference, growth rate, and photoreactivity**
2. **Niacin accumulation**
3. **Reduction of nitrates to nitrites**
4. **Catalase activity**
5. **Hydrolysis of Tween 80**
6. **Arylsulfatase production**
7. **Growth inhibition by thiophene-2-carboxylic acid hydrazide (T$_2$H)**

Determination of Temperature Preference, Growth Rate, and Photoreactivity

Different species of clinically significant mycobacteria can show variation both in their rate and ability to grow at various temperatures. *Mycobacterium marinum* and *M. ulcerans*, both species that are associated with infection of the skin, grow best at 30° C to 32° C and very poorly, or not at all, at 37° C. In contrast, *M. tuberculosis* shows optimal growth at 37° C and grows slowly at 30° C to 32° C. *M. avium* shows the best growth at 42° C to 45° C, the body temperature of birds, in which the organism is the major cause of pulmonary tuberculosis.

Pigment production by mycobacteria is an important identification characteristic depending on whether the culture is grown in light or dark or on whether the pigment is stimulated only after exposure to light. Yellow pigment production in photochromogenic mycobacteria is the result of yellowish-orange carotene crystals produced by actively metabolizing mycobacteria following exposure to a bright light. The type of pigment produced by mycobacteria when grown in the dark is not known.

Media and Reagents

1. Temperature preference and rate of growth

Any nonselective culture medium can be used, either in tubed slants or Petri plates. Petri plates are preferable, as developing colonies can be examined by dissecting microscope or low-power microscopy more easily than when using culture tubes. Lowenstein-Jensen, American Trudeau Society, 7H10, or 7H11 media are all acceptable.

2. Pigment production

Noninhibitory culture media known to be friendly to the growth of the test organism are all acceptable. Selective or antimicrobial-containing media should not be used, as inhibitory agents may interfere with pigment formation. Lowenstein-Jensen and ATS media are both good for determining photochromogenicity.

Procedure

1. Temperature preference and rate of growth

A well-isolated colony of the test organism is subcultured to a 7H9 broth and incubated several days, or until the medium is faintly turbid. The broth is then diluted to 1:100, and isolation streaks are made to the test medium to obtain isolated colonies. The inoculation should be sufficiently dilute to produce individual colonies in order to accurately determine the rate of growth. An inoculum of large numbers of slowly growing myco-

425

bacteria may form a visible colony within a few days after only several divisions and may give an erroneous impression of the true growth rate. When testing strains of mycobacteria thought to be a species other than *M. tuberculosis*, a lightly inoculated culture tube or plate should be left at room temperature to screen for Group IV rapidly growing organisms. To determine the growth rate of mycobacteria, three cultures should be inoculated and incubated at 30° C, 37° C, and 42° C. If a 30° C incubator is not available, 24° C to 25° C (room temperature) may be used if the cultures are placed in a closed box and protected from heating or cooling drafts. The temperature in the box should be monitored daily.

2. **Pigment production**

A broth culture of test organisms diluted sufficiently to result in isolated colonies is inoculated to three Lowenstein-Jensen culture tubes. Two are carefully wrapped with aluminum foil to exclude all light and the third is left exposed to the ambient light in the incubator. Cultures thought to be photochromogenic should be incubated at 37° C; those considered to be scotochromogenic should be inoculated in duplicate and incubated at both 24° C to 26° C and 37° C.

Several days after growth is first noted on the light exposed control tube, the foil-wrapped tubes are examined for growth. If there is evidence of colony formation or early growth, one of the two foil-wrapped tubes is exposed to a strong light source. A 100-watt tungsten bulb or fluorescent equivalent is adequate, with exposure for 3 to 5 hours after loosening the cap of the culture tube. Following exposure of the culture to the light, it is returned to the incubator and inspected after 24 and 48 hours.[1]

Color changes, especially subtle ones, are compared to the culture tube exposed to ambient light and to the foil-wrapped culture tube that had not been exposed to light.

Interpretation

1. **Temperature preference and rate of growth**

M. tuberculosis will show a preference for optimal growth at 37° C with very poor or minimal growth at 30° C or 42° C. *M. marinum* and *M. ulcerans* will show growth best at 30° C and very poor or minimal growth at 37° C, particularly on primary isolation. *M. xenopi* will usually show significantly better growth at 42° C than when incubated at 37° C. *M. fortuitum* and *M. chelonei* will show growth in 3 to 5 days at 37° C and in 4 to 7 days at 22° C to 24° C. Large, mucoid colonial variants of the *M. intracellulare-avium* complex may show what appears to be rapid growth at 37° C, but when streaked for isolated colonies, a more characteristic growth rate of 10 to 14 days is found.

2. **Pigment formation**

Many species of mycobacteria are normally lightly pigmented, e.g., members of the *M. intracelullare-avium* complex. Runyon has termed these organisms "nonphotochromogenic," meaning only that exposure to light does not make the pigment more intense. Mycobacterial species that are photochromogenic include *M. kansasii*, *M. marinum*, *M. simiae*, and *M. szulgai*, the latter only when grown at 22° C to 24° C.

Scotochromogenic mycobacterial species — those that make pigment when incubated in the dark — include *M. scrofulaceum*, *M. gordonae*, *M. fluorescens*, *M. xenopi*, and *M. szulgai*, the latter only when incubated at 37° C. Non- or only lightly pigmented mycobacterial species include *M. tuberculosis, M. bovis, M. ulcerans, M. fortuitum, M. chelonei,* and certain of the species of the Group III nonphotochromogenic mycobacteria.

Controls

1. *M. kansasii* for photochromogenic organisms
2. *M. scrofulaceum* for scotochromogenic organisms
3. *M. szulgai* at 24° C and 37° C for photochromogenic and scotochromogenic control
4. *M. tuberculosis* for a buff-colored, nonpigmented organism

REFERENCES

1. Wayne, L. G., and Doubek, S. R.: The role of air in the photochromogenic behavior of *M. kansasii.* Am. J. Clin. Pathol. 42:431, 1964.

Niacin Accumulation

Niacin is formed as a metabolic byproduct by all mycobacteria, but most species possess an enzyme that converts free niacin to niacin ribonucleotide. *M. tuberculosis, M. simiae,* occasional strains of *M. marinum* and *M. chelonei,* as well as a number of strains of *M. bovis,* lack this enzyme and will accumulate niacin as a water-soluble byproduct in the culture medium. The amount of niacin present in culture medium will be a reflection of the number of colonies on the medium and the age of the culture.[3, 4]

In the chemical test for niacin described by Runyon, nicotinic acid reacts with cyanogen bromide in the presence of a primary amine (aniline) to form a yellow compound.[5] Other forms of the test have been described but are generally not considered to be as sensitive as the Runyon test.[1]

Media and Reagents

1. Lowenstein-Jensen culture medium or 7H10 or 7H11 media supplemented with 0.1 percent potassium aspartate.
2. Sterile water or 0.85 percent saline
3. 4 percent aniline
   a. colorless aniline — 4 ml
   b. 95 percent ethyl alcohol — 96 ml
   Store in brown bottle in refrigerator. If solution turns yellow, discard and prepare fresh solution.
4. 10 percent cyanogen bromide
   a. Cyanogen bromide — 5 gm

Dissolve in 50 ml of distilled or deionized water. Store in refrigerator in brown bottle with tightly fitting cap. If precipitate forms, warm to room temperature and redissolve before use. Solution is volatile and may lose strength on storage. (NOTE: Cyanogen bromide is a tear gas and should be used in a safety cabinet vented to the outside. In acid solutions, cyanogen bromide may hydrolyze to hydrogen cyanide, a very toxic gas. Always discard solutions containing cyanogen bromide into germicides mixed with 2 to 4 percent NaOH.)

Procedure

The test is performed by adding 1.0 ml of either sterile water or saline to the slant of a mature culture on Lowenstein-Jensen, 7H10, or 7H11 medium containing a number of well-formed colonies. Since niacin must be extracted from the medium, the mycobacterial culture should not occlude the entire surface of the medium. If this has happened, scrape part of the bacterial growth to one side, allowing the extracting fluid to be in direct contact with the culture medium. Allow the extracting fluid to cover the surface of the culture medium for 15 to 30 minutes, then remove 0.5 ml of the fluid and place in a clean, screwcap test tube.

Add 0.5 ml of aniline and then 0.5 ml of cyanogen bromide. If niacin has been extracted from the culture, a yellow color will appear in the extract within a few minutes.

Reagent-impregnated filter paper strips have been developed that simplify the test after the extraction has been made. These strips are sensitive and work well when instructions are followed carefully. When using the paper strips, be sure to place both the extract from the culture and the reagent-containing paper strip in a screw-capped tube and tighten the top firmly. The reaction consists of the evolution of cyanogen chloride gas given off from the top of the paper strip, which reacts with the niacin in the extracting fluid at the bottom of the tube. The tube containing the extracting fluid and test strip must be tightly closed to prevent any loss of the cyanogen chloride gas. Do not use strips that have become discolored, as the reagents may have undergone some degree of deterioration and will not be reliable.[2, 6]

Interpretation

The appearance of a yellow color in the extracting fluid indicates the presence of niacin. Negative tests on niacin-positive organisms can occur if there is insufficient growth and therefore inadequate accumulation of niacin in the medium to be detected. Cultures where there appears to be an inadequate amount of growth should be reincubated for an additional 2 to 4 weeks or make a subculture that will have a minimum of 50 or more colonies. A negative test can also occur if there is bacterial growth covering the entire surface of the culture medium thereby preventing extraction of niacin from the culture medium. When this occurs, scrape the confluent bacterial growth to one side with an inoculating needle or spatula allowing the eluting fluid to come in contact with the culture medium.

Controls

Reagent controls should be added to a tube of uninoculated culture medium. *Mycobacterium tuberculosis* should be used as a positive control. *Mycobacterium intracellulare* should be used as a negative control.

REFERENCES

1. Gangadharam, P. R., and Droubi, D. S.: A comparison of four different methods for testing the production of niacin in mycobacteria. Am. Rev. Respir. Dis. *104*:437, 1971.
2. Kilburn, S. O., and Kubica, G. P.: Reagent impregnated paper for detection of niacin. Am. J. Clin. Pathol. *50*(4):530, 1968.
3. Konno, K.: New chemical method to differentiate human type tubercle bacilli from other mycobacteria. Science *124*:985, 1956.
4. Konno, K., Kotaro, O., Yoko, S., Shigenori, T., and Sutemi, O.: Niacin metabolism in mycobacteria. Am. Rev. Respir. Dis. *93*:41, 1966.
5. Runyon, E. H., Selin, M. J., and Hawes, H. W.: Distinguishing mycobacteria by the niacin test. Am. Rev. Tuberc. *79*:663, 1959.
6. Young, W. D., Maslansky, A., Lefar, M. S., and Kronish, D. P.: Development of paper strip test for the detection of niacin produced by mycobacteria. Appl. Microbiol. *20*:939, 1970.

Reduction of Nitrates to Nitrites

The presence of the enzyme nitroreductase is an important identification characteristic for mycobacteria. *M. tuberculosis*, *M. kansasii*, *M. szulgai*, and *M. fortuitum* all reduce nitrates to nitrites. Other species that produce nitroreductase include *M. flavescens*, *M. terrae*, *M. triviali* and *M. chelonei*.

Mycobacteria containing nitroreductase can derive oxygen from nitrates and other reduction products. The chemical reaction is

$$NO_3^- + 2\bar{e} \longrightarrow NO_2 + H_2O$$
$$\text{Nitrate} \qquad\qquad \text{Nitrite}$$

The presence of nitrite in the test medium is detected by the addition of sulfanilamide and N-naphthylethylenediamine in an acid pH. If nitrites are present, they form a red diazonium dye.[4]

Reagents

1. M/100 $NaNO_3$ in pH 7.0, M/45 phosphate buffer

$NaNO_3$	0.085 gm
KH_2PO_4	0.117 gm
Na_2HPO_4 $12H_2O$	0.485 gm
Distilled water	100.0 ml

2. 1:1 dilution of concentrated HCl (add 10 ml HCl to 10 ml H_2O — always add concentrated acid to water).

3. Dissolve 0.2 gram sulfanilamide in 100 ml water

4. Dissolve 0.1 gram N-naphthylethylenediamine dihydrochloride in 100 ml distilled water

Store reagents at 4° C and discard if any change in color occurs. A reagent-containing filter paper strip has been developed for determining the presence of nitroreductase.[1] The test is not very sensitive and, although valid when positive, should be repeated by the standard Virtanen procedure when negative.[3] (See below.)

Procedure

1. Place several drops of sterile distilled water in a sterile, screw-capped test tube.

2. Emulsify a loop or spadeful of actively growing mycobacteria from the test culture in the water.

3. Add 2 ml of the buffered sodium nitrate solution to the emulsified organisms, mix by shaking, and incubate at 37° C for two hours.

4. Acidify the test culture by adding 1 drop of the 1:1 dilution of HCl.

5. Add 2 drops of the sulfanilamide solution.

6. Add 2 drops of the N-naphthylethylenediamine solution.

Interpretation

A positive test is indicated by the development of a red color within 30 to 60 seconds. The color may vary from pink to deep red. Quantitation can be made on comparison with color standards. If no color develops, confirm as a negative test by adding a small amount of powdered zinc from the tip of an applicator stick. If a red color develops after adding the zinc, the test was a true negative. If no color develops after adding the zinc, the test was positive with the nitrate in the solution reduced beyond nitrites into colorless compounds. Since complete use of all nitrate is not common in mycobacteria, the test should be repeated.

For reasons that are not too well understood, the test for nitroreductase is not highly reproducible between laboratories. This lack of reproducibility is disappointing as the nitrate test is a key characteristic in the identification of *M. szulgai* (in one comparison almost half of over two hundred laboratories reported the organism to be nitroreductase-negative). The International Working Group of Mycobacterial Taxonomy also found the interlaboratory comparison for detecting the enzyme to lack greater than 90 percent consensus.[5] Until such time as the problems associated with the test are better understood, the test for nitroreductase should be controlled with both strong and weak positive organisms as well as one known to be negative.

Controls

Each new group of reagents should be compared with established and validated reagents before using with clinical isolates. The three following organisms should be used each time the test is determined on recent isolates:

M. tuberculosis H37Rv — strongly positive

M. kansasii — selected to be weakly positive

M. intracellulare — negative

Occasionally, colors may be pale and hard to interpret. When this happens, color standards can be prepared to help with the interpretation of the test.[2, 4]

REFERENCES

1. Quigly, H. S., and Elston, H. R.: Nitrite test strips for detection of nitrate reduction by mycobacteria. Am. J. Clin. Pathol. 53:663, 1970.
2. Vestal, A. L.: Procedures for the isolation and identification of mycobacteria. USDHEW Publication No. (CDC) 75–8230.
3. Virtanen, S.: A study of nitrate reduction of mycobacteria. Acta Tuberc. Scand. Suppl. 48:119, 1960.
4. Wayne, L. D., and Doubek, S. R.: Classification and identification of mycobacteria. II. Tests employing nitrate and nitrite as substrates. Am. Rev. Respir. Dis. 91:738, 1965.
5. Wayne, L. G., Engel, H. W. B., Grassi, C., Gross, W., Hawkins, J., Jenkins, P. A., Kappler, W., Kleeberg, H. H., Krasnow, I., Nel, E. E., Pattyn, S. R., Richards, P. A., Showalter, S., Slosarek, M., Szabo, I., Tarnok, I., Tsukamura, M., Vergmann, B., and Wolinsky, E.: Highly reproducible techniques for use in systematic bacteriology in the genus *Mycobacterium*: Tests for niacin and catalase and for resistance to isoniazid, thiophene-2-carboxylic acid hydrazide, hydroxylamine and p-nitrobenzoate. Int. J. Syst. Bacteriol. 26:311, 1976.

Catalase Activity

Most mycobacteria produce the enzyme catalase, some making larger amounts than others. Some forms of catalase are inactivated if heated to 68° C for 20 minutes while others are stable after heating to this temperature. The semiquantitation of catalase and the susceptibility to inactivation after heating to 68° C at pH 7.0 are both useful characteristics in the identification of mycobacteria. A third procedure, the "spot test," is sometimes used for a quick qualitative survey for catalase.

Organisms producing the enzyme catalase have the ability to decompose hydrogen peroxide into water and free oxygen.

$$2H_2O_2 \xrightarrow[\text{catalase}]{} 2H_2O + O_2$$

The test for mycobacterial catalase differs from the test used in the detection of catalase in other types of bacteria by employment of 30 percent hydrogen peroxide ("Superoxol") in a strong detergent solution (10 percent Tween 80). The detergent helps to disperse the hydrophobic, tightly clumped mycobacteria from large clumps to individual bacilli, maximizing the detection of the enzyme catalase.

Media and Reagents

Media

1. For the spot test, bacterial growth on egg- or agar-base media.
2. For semiquantitative and heat-stable catalase tests, growth on egg-base media only is recommended.

Reagents

1. 30 percent hydrogen peroxide (Superoxol, Merck)
2. 10 percent Tween 80, sterilized at 121° C for ten minutes and stored at 4° C. Swirl before using, should settling have occurred.
3. Just before use, mix equal amounts of 30 percent hydrogen peroxide and Tween 80 in the amounts needed. Discard any Tween-peroxide mixture left, as it is unstable and cannot be reused.
4. M/15 phosphate buffer

   a. Stock solutions
      A. Anhydrous Na$_2$HPO$_4$ 9.47 gm
         Distilled water   1000.00 m
      B. Potassium phosphate
         buffer (KH$_2$PO$_4$)   9.07 gm
         Distilled water   1000.00 m

   b. pH 7.0 phosphate buffer
      Mix 61.1 ml of solution A with 38.9 ml of solution B.
      Confirm pH 7.0 with meter.

Procedure

1. **"Spot test"**

   Add 1 to 2 drops of a freshly mixed Tween-peroxide solution to a colony of mycobacterial growth on a plate or tube of culture medium. Observe for 4 to 5 minutes for evolution of bubbles. Appearance of bubbles may be rapid (strongly positive) or slow (weakly positive). The absence of any bubbles is a negative test for catalase.

2. **Semiquantitative test**

   a. Inoculate the surface of a tube of Lowenstein-Jensen medium prepared as a "deep" with 0.1 ml of a 7-day liquid culture of the test organism.

   b. Incubate at 37°C for two weeks. Caps on the culture tube must be loose to permit easy exchange of air.

   c. Add 1.0 ml of freshly prepared Tween-peroxide solution and leave upright for 5 minutes.

   d. Measure the height of the column of bubbles above the surface of the culture medium and record on a work sheet. A column of bubbles 5 to 45 mm high is considered weakly positive. If the column of bubbles is greater than 45 mm, the test is said to be strongly positive. The absence of bubbles is considered a negative catalase test.

3. **Test for heat-stable catalase — pH 7/68° C for 20 minutes**

   a. Emulsify several colonies of the test organism in a culture tube containing 0.5 ml of M/15 phosphate buffer at pH 7.0.

   b. Place the tube in a water bath or constant temperature block at 68° C for 20 minutes.

   c. Remove the tube and allow to cool to room temperature.

   d. Add 0.5 ml of freshly prepared Tween-peroxide mixture.

   e. Watch for bubbles on the surface of the fluid. Do not discard as negative until after 20 minutes.

   f. A positive test will be associated with bubbles while a negative test will be devoid of any bubbles. Do not shake the tube, as a false impression of bubbles can develop from the presence of the detergent in the mixture.

Interpretation

In each of the tests, the presence of catalase is indicated by bubbles. The spot test is a quick and easy method for detecting the presence or absence of catalase, but it gives only a broad guide as to the amount present. The determination of heat-stable catalase is a very helpful characteristic in the identification of the nonpigmented mycobacteria. Heat-labile catalase is a characteristic of *M. tuberculosis, M. bovis, M. gastri,* and occasional strains of the *M. intracellulare-avium* complex.

The semiquantitative test for catalase is useful in distinguishing strains that are strongly positive for catalase from those with small amounts and is particularly helpful for the identification of INH-resistant *M. tuberculosis* (negative).

Controls

1. *Mycobacterium kansasii* for strongly positive semiquantitative and heat-stable catalase.

2. *Mycobacterium tuberculosis* H37Rv — for weakly positive semiquantitative and heat-labile catalase.

3. *Mycobacterium tuberculosis* — INH-resistant — for negative "spot test" and semiquantitative catalase.

REFERENCES

Kubica, C. P., Jones, W. D. Abbott, V. D., Beam, R. E., Kilburn, J. O., and Cater, J. C., Jr.: Differential identification of mycobacteria. I. Tests on catalase activity. Am. Rev. Respir. Dis. *94*:400, 1966.

Hydrolysis of Tween 80

The enzymatic hydrolysis of Tween 80 is an important characteristic in the differentiation of mycobacteria.[2] With rare exceptions, species of those groups that hydrolyze Tween 80 within 10 days are not clinically significant (for example, the "tap water" bacilli, *M. gastri*, *M. terrae* complex, and *M. triviale*), while species more likely to be of clinical importance (*M. scrofulaceum* and members of *M. intracellulare-avium* complex) are negative.

Tween 80 is the trade name for the detergent polyoxyethylene sorbitan monooleate. Certain mycobacteria possess a lipase that splits Tween 80 into oleic acid and polyoxyethylated sorbitol, which modifies the optical characteristics of the test solution from a straw yellow (produced by light passing through the intact Tween 80 solution) to a pink color. Although pink is the color of the neutral red indicator, the color change is not the result of a pH shift, as the oleic acid formed by hydrolysis is neutralized by the buffer in the solution. A color change indicates the hydrolysis or destruction of the Tween 80 molecule rather than a significant change in hydrogen ion concentration.

Materials and Reagents

1. Phosphate buffer, 0.067 M, pH 7.0   100 ml
2. Tween 80   0.5 ml
3. Neutral red, 0.1 percent aqueous (NOTE: It is important to add sufficient neutral red dye, as the dye activity as supplied is often less than 100 percent. For example, if the actual dye content is 85 percent, dissolve 0.1 gm in 85 ml rather than in 100 ml water in order to achieve a 0.1 percent solution.)

Mix the three reagents and dispense 3 to 5 ml amounts in screw-capped test tubes. Autoclave and store in the refrigerator in a light-proof container to protect from spontaneous hydrolysis. This substrate is stable for only 2 to 4 weeks.

A Tween 80 hydrolysis test concentrate is commercially available and is reported to be equivalent to the standard substrate.[1]

Procedure

1. Place a 3 mm loopful of actively growing mycobacterial bacilli in the Tween 80 substrate. (Inasmuch as there is no nitrogen source in the substrate, organisms used for testing must be mature and actively metabolizing).
2. Incubate at 35° C to 37° C for 10 days.
3. Observe for color change initially in 3 days and daily thereafter. If *M. kansasii* is suspected, there may be a positive reaction within 3 to 6 hours.

Interpretation

A positive test is shown by a change in color of the substrate from straw-yellow to pink.

Control

Rapid positive — *M. kansasii*
Delayed positive — *M. gordonae*
Negative — *M. scrofulaceum*

REFERENCES

1. Kilburn J. O., O'Donnell, K. F., Silcox V. A., and David, H. L.: Preparation of a stable mycobacterial Tween-hydrolysis test substrate. Appl. Microbiol. 26:826, 1973.
2. Wayne, L. G., Doubek, J. R., and Russell, R. L.: Classification and identification of my-

The Laboratory Diagnosis of Mycobacterial Disease   433

cobacteria. I. Tests employing Tween 80 as substrate. Am. Rev. Respir. Dis. *90*:588, 1964.

Arylsulfatase Test

Arylsulfatases can aid in the identification of mycobacteria as this group of enzymes is secreted by certain mycobacteria.[4] Members of the *M. fortuitum-chelonei* complex are unique in that they produce sufficient arylsulfatase to produce a positive test within 3 days. Small quantities may also be produced by *M. xenopi, M. szulgai, M. marinum, M. kansasii, M. gordonae,* and members of the *M. avium-intracellulare* complex among others. The 3-day test is less helpful in identifying slowly growing species in that they grow too slowly to produce consistently reliable results, as there appears to be a direct relationship to bacterial mass. The test is most useful for the identification of the *M. fortuitum-chelonei* complex of organisms.

Arylsulfatase is an enzyme that splits free phenolphthalein from the tripotassium salt of phenolphthalein disulfate.

In the test described by Wayne,[3] the phenolphthalein salt is incorporated in oleic acid agar and the test is performed by adding a small amount of an alkaline solution of sodium carbonate to the surface of a three-day-old culture. A positive test is indicated by the development of a purple color.

The test can also be performed by using a 0.001 M solution of the phenolphthalein salt in 7H9 broth. A 0.003 M tripotassium phenolphthalein disulfate solution has been advocated to detect smaller quantities of the enzyme with incubation periods increased to as much as 14 days.[1, 2]

Materials and Reagents

1. Substrate

    A. Tripotassium phenolphthalein disulfate   65 mg

    B. Glycerol   1 ml

    C. Dubos oleic agar base (Bio-Quest Laboratory)   100 ml

Incorporate the phenolphthalein and glycerol into 100 ml of melted Dubos agar and dispense 5 ml into 16 × 125 mm screw-capped culture tubes. Let harden in upright position and store in the refrigerator. A dehydrated medium is commercially available as "Wayne Arylsulfatase Agar."

2. Sodium carbonate, 1 M

Add 5.3 gm to 100 ml water.

Procedure

1. Prepare a bacillary suspension of the organism to be tested and inoculate one or two drops into a tube of substrate.

2. Incubate at 35° C to 37° C for 3 days.

3. Add 1 ml of sodium carbonate solution and observe for a color change.

Interpretation

The development of a pink color at the top of the medium is a positive test, indicating the release of free phenolphthalein.

Controls

    Positive control — *M. fortuitum*
    Negative control — *M. tuberculosis*

REFERENCES

1. Kubica, G. P., and Vestal, A. L.: The arylsulfatase activity of acid-fast bacilli. I. Investigation of stock cultures of mycobacteria. Am. Rev. Respir. Dis. *83*:728, 1961.
2. Kubica, G. P., and Ridgon, A. L.: The arylsulfatase activity on mycobacteria. III. Preliminary investigation of rapidly growing mycobacteria. Am. Rev. Respir. Dis. *85*:737, 1961.
3. Wayne, L. G.: Recognition of *Mycobacterium fortuitum* by means of a three-day phenolphthalein sulfatase test. Am. J. Clin. Pathol. *36*:185, 1961.

4. Whitehead, J. E. M., Wildy, P., and Engback, H. C.: Arylsulfatase activity of mycobacteria. J. Pathol. Bacteriol. 65:451, 1953.

Growth Inhibition by Thiophene-2-Carboxylic Hydrazide (T₂H)

The distinction between *Mycobacterium tuberculosis* and *M. bovis* can sometimes be difficult since up to 30 percent of the *M. bovis* BCG strains may accumulate small amounts of niacin. Other *M. bovis* strains may induce weakly positive tests for nitrate reduction. One identification characteristic that has been found to be helpful in differentiating between *M. tuberculosis* and *M. bovis* is the ability of thiophene-2-carboxylic acid hydrazide to inhibit the growth of the latter but not the other species of mycobacteria.[1] This characteristic provides an important distinction between *M. bovis* and other mycobacterial species, especially *M. tuberculosis*.

Media and Reagents

Thiophene-2-carboxylic acid hydrazide is incorporated in 7H10 or 7H11 agar in concentrations of 1 and 5 μg/ml (available from Aldrich Chemical Co., Milwaukee, Wisconsin). Previous recommendations to use a concentration of 10 μg/ml were found to inhibit some strains of *M. tuberculosis*. The medium can be dispensed in plastic Petri plates divided into biplates or quadrants.

Procedure

Inoculate a barely turbid broth culture of the test organism to media containing 1 and 5 μg/ml of T₂H and to the same medium not containing the drug. Streak the inoculum to achieve isolated colonies. Incubate in 5 to 8 percent CO_2 for 14 to 21 days and examine for growth.

Interpretation

A positive test for growth inhibition will show good growth of the test organism on the drug-free medium and lack of growth on the T₂H-containing medium. Although an international collaborative study has suggested that the test is highly reproducible with the concentration of 1.0 μg/ml, many laboratories find it advisable to use a second concentration of 5 μg/ml to confirm results with the lower concentration.[2]

Controls

Positive control — *Mycobacterium bovis*

Negative control — *Mycobacterium tuberculosis* (H37Rv)

REFERENCES

1. Harrington, R., and Karlson, A. G.: Differentiation between *M. tuberculosis* and *M. bovis* by in-vitro procedures. Am. J. Vet. Res. 27:1193, 1967.
2. Wayne, L. G., Engel, H. W. B., Grassi, C., Gross, W., Hawkins, J., Jenkins, P. A., Kappler, W., Kleeberg, H. H., Krasnow, I., Nel, E. E., Pattyn, S. R., Richards, P. A., Showalter, S., Slosarek, M., Szabo, I., Tarnok, I., Tsukamura, M., Vergmann, B., and Wolinsky, E.: Highly reproducible techniques for use in systematic bacteriology in the genus *Mycobacterium*: Tests for niacin and catalase and for resistance to isoniazid, thiophene-2-carboxylic acid hydrazide, hydroxylamine, and p-nitrobenzoate. Int. J. Syst. Bacteriol. 26:311, 1976.

20

The Chemical Structures, Properties, and Mechanisms of Action of the Antituberculous Drugs

LEONARD DOUB, B.S.

INTRODUCTION

Any accounting of the major achievements of the twentieth century must surely include the near conquest by drugs of bacterial disease. These drugs have two main sources: synthetic substances from the chemical laboratory and antibiotics produced by microorganisms. In application, both sources have roots in the late nineteenth century, with the synthetics being the first to achieve success. Sulfanilamide and the related sulfa drugs were discovered in the third decade of the twentieth century and were the first substances found which really controlled bacterial disease. Their success pointed the way and made reasonable the huge investments of time and capital required to develop the antibiotics early in the next decade, penicillin being the first great success.[38, 71]

Emboldened by their achievements

435

with the sulfa drugs, chemists, pharmacologists, and microbiologists turned early in the 1940s to developing drugs for tuberculosis. This work began with the sulfones (for a summary, see Feldman's Harben Lectures[22] and Chapter 21) and was eventually to culminate in isoniazid, currently accepted as perhaps the single most important antituberculous drug. An important early consequence of this intensive effort was the development of reliable test methods (see Chapter 15) and of criteria for the treatment of human disease (see Chapter 21). Thus, when streptomycin was discovered in 1944,[84] it was quickly and decisively shown to be active first in experimental tuberculosis, then in man.[23, 37, 107, 108]

The success of streptomycin as the first antituberculous drug gave further impetus to the massive search already underway for new antibiotics. This search had been triggered by the triumph of penicillin. An unplanned consequence of the great effort was that often more than one group of investigators, in their screening of microorganisms to produce antibiotics, turned up the same type of organism and the same antibiotics. A similar redundancy occurred in the synthetics. The rationales that governed the search for new compounds were widely known and acted upon. Consequently, it happened repeatedly that more than one group came up with the same or similar new antituberculous drugs.

Space and continuity forbid recounting the fascinating history of the antituberculous drugs. Many drugs failed the ultimate clinical test. Of those that succeeded, it is a story of serendipity and of chemical intermediates for planned drugs, which were themselves a breakthrough — of the sulfones, which failed in tuberculosis but became the treatment of choice in the related disease, leprosy,[12] of PAS, discovered by following a rationale later found to be of doubtful validity (see under PAS); and other fascinating events. Finally

and recently, the historic synthetic and antibiotic approaches to new antituberculous drugs were joined to cause conversion of an inactive rifamycin antibiotic into an important new semisynthetic tuberculosis drug, rifampin.

The drugs that have found a place in the treatment of tuberculosis are discussed here, starting with the synthetics. Within each group, the drugs are introduced in the order of their discovery.

SYNTHETIC COMPOUNDS

P-Aminosalicylic Acid (PAS)

The substance PAS has been known for many years.[30] It was discovered to be active in experimental tuberculosis by Lehmann, having been prepared for testing purposes by Rosdahl.[50, 51] Lehmann was following up on the discovery by Bernheim[7] that salicylates and benzoates stimulated the respiration of virulent tubercle bacilli. He concluded that these acids were important metabolites, and he tested some fifty related substances for their inhibitory effect on the growth of virulent tubercle bacilli in vitro. By far, the most effective of these was PAS. The drug was found to be well tolerated in animals, and it was then tried directly in humans. As described elsewhere in this volume (see Chapter 21), PAS, while probably active in human therapy, has such a weak effect when used alone that its only use today is as a companion drug to a major drug to prevent emergence of mycobacterial resistance.

When pure, PAS and its salts are white crystalline powders. It has the structure shown in Figure 20–1. In the acid form, it is only slightly soluble in water. As the sodium salt, it is freely soluble, and the drug is usually dispensed in this form. For special uses, however, other salts have been employed.[104]

PAS has a deceptively simple struc-

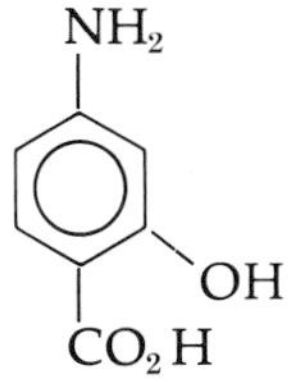

FIGURE 20–1. *P*-aminosalicylic acid (PAS).

ture, and the chemical manipulation of it holds surprises for the unwary. Solutions of the salts darken quickly in the air and, independent of air exposure, slowly decompose to *m*-aminophenol. Even the dry powdered sodium salt blackens slowly, especially if it is exposed to moisture, light, or heat. The free acid is even more unstable. It loses it carboxyl as carbon dioxide, slowly at just above room temperature and loses it quickly as a visible effervescence at 110° C to 130° C. This principal decomposition reaction is formulated in Figure 20–2 (going to the right). The reverse of this reaction (to the left) proceeds in the presence of sodium carbonate and carbon dioxide and is an important method of synthesis.[21]*

Mechanism of Action

Lehmann's original rationale leading to the discovery of PAS[50, 51] furnished, of course, necessarily the first mechan-

_____

*This procedure is the one used originally to prepare PAS.[30] However, the structure was not identified in the original patent, and it was incorrectly identified in the summarizing literature of the day. PAS for test in tuberculosis originally was prepared by a difficult route. It was only after PAS became prominent in tuberculosis treatment that it was discovered to be the product of this simple reaction.

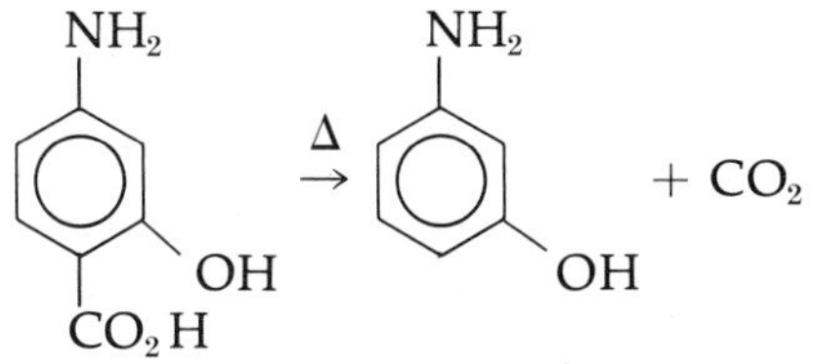

ism of action to be proposed for the drug. This rationale rests on Bernheim's work and shows that salicylate and benzoate are utilized in respiration uniquely by virulent mycobacteria and not by avirulent ones; it assumes that these substances are important metabolites and that PAS exerts its effect by interfering with their utilization. Furthermore, according to Ratledge and Brown,[11, 78] salicylic acid actually occurs as an integral part of mycobactin, an iron-transporting substance unique to mycobacteria. This mechanism has the virtue that it accounts for the great specificity of PAS for the inhibition of growth of virulent mycobacteria but not of avirulent variants. However, the existence of this role for PAS largely has not been borne out experimentally. Youmans and colleagues[109] could detect no reversal of bacteriostasis by PAS, even when fiftyfold greater concentrations of salicylate were added. Lehmann himself could find no constant action of PAS in antagonizing the stimulating action of salicylate on respiration. An exception is the report that salicylate at high levels, ordinarily toxic to tubercle bacilli, did antagonize PAS.[40]

It was first observed by Youmans and associates,[109] and confirmed by others,[20] that the addition of PABA (*p*-aminobenzoic acid) to the culture medium reduces the bacteriostatic activity of PAS. That this is not an artifact of in vitro systems is shown by the fact that PABA reverses the suppressant activity of PAS on experimental tuberculosis in mice.[39] PAS thus meets the classical test for affecting the synthesis of folic acid-related vitamin forms as met by sulfon-

FIGURE 20–2. The principal decomposition reaction of PAS.

amides; namely, its activity is reversed competitively by PABA. (For a recent, detailed formulation of this general mechanism with associated references, see the paper by Seydel and Butte[87] and the book by Pratt.[75]) An important consequence of inhibiting the synthesis of folic acid is that the biochemical methylation reactions which depend upon it are impaired. This leads to reduced production of important methylated products such as serine, methionine, and others. It is, thus, deeply significant that the inhibition of growth of *Mycobacterium tuberculosis* by PAS is not only reversed competitively by PABA but is reversed noncompetitively by methionine.[33]

While there is thus impressive evidence that PAS is active by affecting the folic acid-related systems, much remains unexplained. In particular, the exquisite specificity of PAS for inhibition only of virulent mycobacteria and not of the saprophytic variants has no obvious explanation in a straightforward formulation of this mechanism. Nor does it explain why sulfonamides, which are good inhibitors of folate production in other bacteria, are generally either inactive or poorly active against virulent mycobacteria. In certain enterococci, PAS may actually be incorporated into a folate analog, which truly functions in the place of the normal folate.[96] Whether such a process occurs in mycobacteria is not known. If spurious folate is actually formed, and if formed, is utilized normally or is inhibitory in some systems, is also unknown. Conceivably, this putative false analog could be inhibitory to systems unique to virulent mycobacteria. More likely, to continue this speculative line, PAS itself may simply be somehow concentrated within the bacillus by some sort of active transport system unique to virulent forms. Indeed, much remains to be explained.

In an interesting elaboration of the original salicylate mechanism used by Lehmann in the discovery of PAS, Ratledge and coworkers tied salicylate into the iron transport of mycobacteria.[11, 56, 78] Salicylic acid occurs as an integral building block of mycobactin, the iron ionophore. Briefly, they postulated that PAS "probably acts as an antimetabolite of salicylic acid, not, however, by inhibiting the conversion of salicylic acid to mycobactin, but probably somewhere along the metabolic pathway of iron uptake."[11]

The theory of Ratledge and coworkers, since it is based on salicylate, again gives a basis for the great specificity in the growth-inhibiting action of PAS and stands on the absolute essentiality of iron for the functioning of all organisms. They explain away the reversal by PABA by postulating that PAS is absorbed into the mycobacterium by an active transport system which functions normally for PABA. With an excess of PABA in the medium, PAS is no longer absorbed well and is thus unable to affect the salicylate system.

On the negative side, this theory is based on data primarily from *Mycobacterium smegmatis,* normally considered insensitive to PAS, and is based on levels of PAS (500 μg per ml) some 500 to 1000 times higher than those considered bacteriostatic for most virulent mycobacteria. (For these usual levels, see the review by Youmans and Youmans.[110]) At these high levels it might be expected that systems would be inhibited which have no necessary relation to those responsible for the chemotherapeutic action of PAS (see also Chapter 4).

On balance, the evidence available at this time favors the view that PAS acts chemotherapeutically by affecting folic acid systems. The deficiency of this view — that it does not account for the specificity of PAS for mycobacteria — could be explained, perhaps, by an inversion of the rationale of Ratledge and coworkers. Possibly PAS of all PABA inhibitors is uniquely effective against virulent mycobacteria because it, *as a salicylate,* is absorbed specifically better than all other PABA inhibitors.

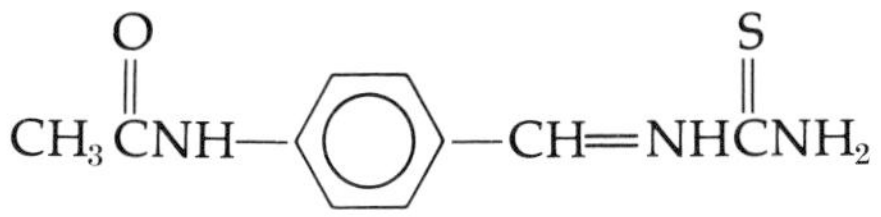

$$CH_3CNH-\langle O \rangle-CH=NHCNH_2$$

with O double-bonded above the first C and S double-bonded above the second C.

FIGURE 20–3. Thiacetazone (Contebin, Tb 1, *p*-acetaminobenzaldehyde thiosemicarbazone).

Thiacetazone

The team of Domagk (pharmacologist), and Behnisch, Mietzsch, and Schmidt, (chemists, two of whom were part of the earlier team who ushered in the sulfonamide epoch)[71] carried the legacy of that great period on to further achievements in tuberculosis therapy. Intrigued by the heightening effect on the modest antituberculous activity of certain sulfonamides and sulfones when sulfur heterocycles were combined in the molecule, this team undertook work with the sulfur heterocycle, sulfathiadiazole. Chemical intermediates in the synthesis of these thiadiazole-containing sulfonamide derivatives were certain compounds related to thiosemicarbazones. The thiosemicarbazones turned out to have greater activity than the sulfonamides, and their mechanism of action was different. These thiosemicarbazones are reaction products of araldehydes and semicarbazide. When the aryl group is phenyl, substitution of the phenyl group profoundly affects the activity of the thiosemicarbazone. After comparison of many derivatives, *p*-acetylamino benzaldehyde thiosemicarbazone was selected as the best among them. The structure is given in Figure 20–3. This work, revealed first in 1946,[19] is summarized in English.[5, 18]

Thiacetazone is a pale yellow, finely crystalline powder, melting with decomposition at about 230° C. The compound is almost insoluble in water and is only sparingly soluble in the usual organic solvents.[5]

Mechanism of Action

Thiacetazone suppresses the growth of *Mycobacterium tuberculosis* both in vitro and in vivo at low concentrations,[18] but how it acts is not known.

Liebermeister established that thiacetazone easily forms a copper complex. He proposes that this complex is the active form of thiacetazone. This copper complex forms from the traces of copper present in in vitro and in vivo systems.[53] In support of this theory is the observation that the growth-inhibiting effect of the thiosemicarbazones on mycobacteria is noticeably increased by the addition of even the slightest amounts of copper sulfate. Presumably, this theory, to be useful, would require that the copper complex of thiacetazone resemble the actual biochemical carriers of copper and interfere with their function; otherwise, no net increase in understanding is gained, and we are faced with the equally involved problem of determining what the mechanism of action is of the copper complex of thiacetazone.

Thiacetazone has been thought to have a number of subtle effects on the host that contribute to its antituberculous chemotherapeutic action. For more on this involved subject, see the review by Protivinsky.[76]

Thiacetazone is cross-resistant to other classes of antituberculous compounds that contain the thioamide grouping but are otherwise widely different chemically; namely, ethionamide and its congeners and thiocarbanilides. This usually is taken to indicate that the compounds share some common features of mode of action. However, this cross-resistance has some unusual features and limitations.[31, 80] For this reason, if the mechanisms of action are indeed similar for these separate classes, there are nevertheless some important differences.

Pyrazinamide

Pyrazinamide was first used in experimental tuberculosis in 1952 as a result of independent research in different laboratories.[49, 58, 91] It had been synthesized 15 years previously as a chemical intermediate.[16] The antituberculous activity of nicotinamide had been discovered in 1945 and later independently in 1948.[15, 65] The preparing and testing of compounds bearing a structural resemblance to nicotinamide led to pyrazinamide.[49, 58, 91]

Pyrazinamide is a white crystaline solid, mp 189 to 190° C (see Fig. 20–4). It dissolves up to approximately 1.5 percent in water to form a neutral solution. It is generally less soluble in most organic solvents.[104]

Mechanism of Action

Not a great deal is known about the way pyrazinamide acts. Its resemblance to nicotinamide has led to the suggestion that pyrazinamide affects nicotinamide or nicotinic acid metabolism.[47] The effectiveness of pyrazinamide could be due to interference in some way with the role of nicotinamide (or nicotinic acid) as a cofactor in the dehydrogenases. This would also suggest that the point of action of pyrazinamide is somewhere in the final steps of the electron transport system going to oxygen.

Besta[9] has observed that at very low concentrations, pyrazinamide greatly reduces the oxygen uptake of mycobacteria. He hypothesizes that the mycobacterium deprived of oxygen becomes more vulnerable to cellular defenses in vivo. This suggestion also must place the locus of action in the final steps of the electron transport system.

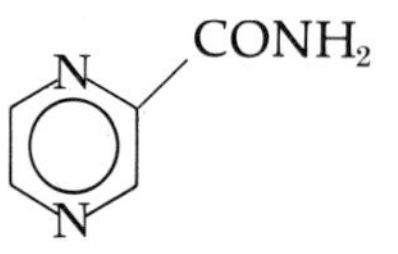

FIGURE 20–4. Pyrazinamide.

If it interferes with dehydrogenases, this action of pyrazinamide would relate to one imputed to isoniazid (see under Isoniazid in this chapter). However, such an effect of pyrazinamide on dehydrogenases must differ in some essential details from that of isoniazid because bacteria resistant to one of the drugs are not resistant to the other.[76]

Not only is the biochemical mode of action of pyrazinamide uncertain, but there has been debate about the way it exerts it effect biologically to give a chemotherapeutic response. In the usual testing media at pH 7, a level of about 250 μg per ml is needed to completely inhibit the growth of tubercle bacilli. This level is some five to eight times larger than the serum levels afforded by the maximum permissible dose in humans of 3 gm daily. McDermott and Tompsett have found that if the pH of the testing medium is lowered, the minimal inhibitory concentrations of pyrazinamide for tubercle bacilli is reduced. At pH 5 to 6, this inhibitory concentration is within the usual serum ranges for a 3 gm dose of pyrazinamide. They suggest that pyrazinamide exerts its effect in vivo in acidic loci in the body where tubercle bacilli are found, for instance, within phagocytic cells and in caseous lesions.[64]

An alternative explanation of the high effectiveness of pyrazinamide in experimental tuberculosis,[62, 63] in the face of an almost negligible bacteriostatic effect of the drug against tubercle bacilli in vitro, is explicitly contained in Besta's suggestion.[9]

Isoniazid

Isoniazid (isonicotinic acid hydrazide, INH) was first described as a chemical substance in 1912.[67] Its activity in tuberculosis was not known until 40 years later, when it was rediscovered simultaneously and independently by the research teams of three major pharmaceutical laboratories.[8, 28, 72] Each of

FIGURE 20–5. Isoniazid (INH).

these groups was working on the modification of thiosemicarbazones in an attempt to increase the antituberculous activity. Because of the tuberculostatic activity of nicotinamide, the pyridine nucleus was a prominent candidate to be incorporated in new agents. Thus (probably), each group set out to specifically make, among other pyridine aldehyde thiosemicarbazones, isonicotinic aldehyde thiosemicarbazone. Chemically, the best way to prepare this substance is to start with isonicotinic acid hydrazide. Since antituberculous testing of interesting chemical intermediates was routine in these laboratories, the remarkable activity of INH was quickly recognized.

The structure of isoniazid is given in Figure 20–5. Isoniazid is a white crystalline solid, mp 171.4° C and is about 14 percent soluble in water at room temperature. It is only slightly soluble in the usual organic solvents. Its aqueous solutions are faintly acid and are relatively stable.[104]

Mechanism of Action

The voluminous literature on this subject defies review in the space available here. Those particularly interested in the subject should refer to the review by Krishna-Murti.[44]

There is a cluster of theories that involve, in some way, the affinity of isoniazid for metals or metalloporphyrins (hemin, catalase, and so forth). The molecule is a powerful chelator of metals and, because of the nature of the hydrazine portion, is capable of reducing certain metal ions, free or complexed (as in porphyrins).

The simplest of these theories asserts that isoniazid is bacteriostatic because it complexes essential metals such as copper or iron. In this way it would interfere with the function of important oxidation-reduction enzymes that employ these metals. If indeed this is the mode of action of INH, the theory as now formulated leaves unexplained why closely related hydrazides, which complex metals equally well or better, do not show comparable antituberculous activity. (See the review of Krishna-Murti[44] for details and references). Presumably, active transport systems highly specific for isoniazid could account for the differences, but there is no evidence at hand for this specificity.

Isoniazid-resistant mycobacteria often have lost their catalase or peroxidase activity concomitant with some of their virulence in certain animals.[68, 70] This led to the hypothesis that isoniazid exerts its effect by interacting with these metalloporphyrin enzymes to give toxic breakdown products or free radicals.[101] Mutation to resistance then relieves this lethality, making the cell no longer dependent on these metalloporphyrin enzymes.

The metalloporphyrin, hemin (coenzyme for catalase and the peroxidases), antagonizes in a competitive fashion the antibacterial action of isoniazid.[25] This effect may be an artifact of extracellular destruction of isoniazid by hemin.[45] However, hemin and inorganic iron function as growth factors for some isoniazid-resistant strains.[42] Whether isoniazid affects some aspect of hemin synthesis, and thereby catalase and peroxidase activity, is unknown. (See the review by Krishna-Murti[44] and the review by Protivinsky[76] for more on metalloporphyrins as possible target substances for isoniazid action.)

Another set of mechanisms of action was probably suggested to its originators because of the great chemical similarity of isoniazid to the nicotinamide in dehydrogenase cofactors, nicotinamide adenine dinucleotide and nicotinamide adenine dinucleotide phosphate (NAD and NADP respectively; coenzyme I and coenzyme II).

One of these theories assumes that isoniazid in mycobacteria is converted to isonicotinic acid, which can replace the nicotinamide of NAD to form nicotinic acid analogs of NAD. This NAD analog then disturbs the NAD and NADP dehydrogenases.[46] This viewpoint has been elaborated as a comprehensive theory (see the review by Protivinsky[76]). Reports that isoniazid affects the oxidative and dehydrogenase systems is compatible with this theory.[66, 82]

Contrary to the above theory, another approach, while still implicating isoniazid as an inhibitor of NAD synthesis, notes that in mycobacteria, nicotinamide or nicotinic acid is not directly incorporated into NAD. A more fundamental synthetic route is used, not involving nicotinamide or nicotinic acid directly. This route goes from aspartate to quinolinic acid and directly to the half molecule nicotinamide mononucleotide (NMN); this latter would then be converted into NAD. This point of view pinpoints the action of INH as being somewhere in this sequence. It is known that INH in relatively high concentrations inhibits NAD synthesis in cell-free extracts. Whether early or late steps are affected is unknown (see the review of Krishna-Murti[44]).

Once formed, the NAD is subject to cleavage by a specific enzyme, NAD glycohydrolase. This degradative enzyme is, in turn, ordinarily held in check by an inhibitor. It is here that INH has been postulated to play a role. Isoniazid combines with the inhibitor from sensitive strains to make it inoperative and causes NAD to be degraded but does not combine with inhibitor from strains highly resistant to INH.[6] In less resistant strains the glycohydrolase inhibitor still combines with INH, but there is evidence that these cells are resistant by being less permeable to INH.[92]

It has been suggested that inter-ference with the initiation of DNA synthesis is the principal mode of action of isoniazid.[61] Interestingly, NAD repression by INH has been tied into this interference. DNA ligase, necessary for extension of polydeoxynucleotide chains, depends on NAD as a cofactor.[73] The prompt lowering of NAD levels caused by isoniazid would shortly be reflected in diminished DNA synthesis.

Three additional proposed action mechanisms for INH remain to be mentioned. First, pigment production by sensitive mycobacteria invariably accompanies isoniazid treatment.[106] Accumulation of toxic pigments might account for inhibition. Second, INH reacts readily with pyridoxal. It has been proposed that depletion of this essential material is the basis of the effect of INH on mycobacteria. Third, inhibition by isoniazid of mycolic acid synthesis has been proposed as the primary action of isoniazid.[102] Experimentally, this inhibition is a prominent feature of the action of isoniazid on the cell wall of mycobacteria. The mycolic acids are unique to mycobacteria and are major constituents of the cell walls of these bacteria. Inhibition of the synthesis of mycolic acids by isoniazid would therefore explain the high specificity of isoniazid for mycobacteria (see also Chapter 4). (For other studies supporting this hypothesis, see the book by Pratt.[75])

In summary, numerous chemical theories purporting to explain isoniazid action have been advanced. The validity of any one of these is at the moment uncertain. The majority of these theories place the primary action somewhere in the terminal steps of the oxidative sequence leading from oxygen through the dehydrogenases. It is uncertain whether this action is adequate unto itself to doom this obligatory aerobic mycobacterium or whether, as the DNA theory asserts, this action is reflected in a blocking of the ultimate regulatory machinery of the cell.

Implicit in most of these theories of isoniazid action is the idea that the biological mechanism, ultimately, is killing by the drug alone. While most experiments show INH to be only growth inhibitory to tubercle bacilli, it is, nevertheless, in some circumstances bactericidal.[17, 69, 83] Thus, there is some reason for thinking that this simplest biologic mechanism *can* apply.

The changes that lead to lethal action of isoniazid in vitro on mycobacteria seem to occur mainly in the outer envelope, including loss of mycolic acids. *M. tuberculosis* loses early its acid-fast staining reaction under the influence of isoniazid — a change usually associated with the cell envelope (see also Chapter 4). This action is accompanied by loss into the medium of carbohydrates, amino acids, and phosphate.[44] These changes in the outer wall are, of course, compatible with a bactericidal action. However, they are also compatible with loss by the pathogenic mycobacterium of the first line of defense against the immune forces of the host. This latter, more subtle effect would be shown at lower concentrations of INH because even small changes could disrupt the pathogen-host balance.

Ethionamide

This compound was prepared for tuberculosis testing by Libermann and colleagues.[52] Its antituberculous activity is described by Rist and coworkers.[80] Ethionamide was synthesized to further improve antituberculous activity of compounds arising from chemical manipulation of the structural elements of thioureas and thiosemicarbazones (see Fig. 20–6).

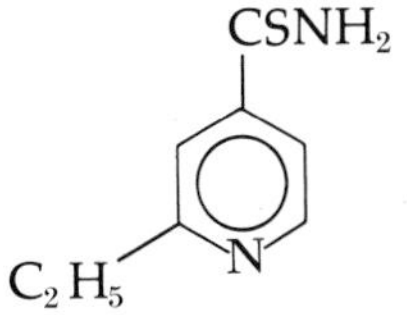

FIGURE 20–6. Ethionamide (2-ethylthioisonicotinamide).

It is a yellow crystalline solid decomposing at 164° C to 166° C. It is only sparingly soluble in water and in the majority of the usual organic solvents.[104]

Mechanism of Action

Ethionamide is cross-resistant to thioureas and thiosemicarbazones. Cross-resistance probably means that these substances share a common mode of action. It is bacteriocidal and also causes loss of acid-fastness in tubercle bacilli.[80] Ethionamide has been implicated in the inhibition of mycolic acid synthesis in mycobacteria; in this respect, it resembles isoniazid (see under Isoniazid).[103] Again reminiscent of isoniazid, ethionamide affects dehydrogenase activity in tubercle bacilli.[82]

Ethionamide is easily converted to a substituted isonicotinic acid in the cell. The isonicotinic acid hypothesis for the action of isoniazid (see under Isoniazid) has been extended to ethionamide.[88] It has been postulated that this substituted isonicotinic acid is incorporated into NAD. The same criticism must be applied to this extension as to the original theory for isoniazid — mycobacteria probably do not incorporate nicotinamide or nicotinic acid directly into NAD (see under Isoniazid).

Ethambutol

The high antituberculous activity of this synthetic compound was announced in 1961 by Wilkinson and associates.[99, 100] It was developed in a rational synthetic program. This program began with the knowledge that related diamines had slight antituberculous activity. These diamines were modified in a systematic manner by Shepherd and Wilkinson,[89] in an exploration of their postulation that these diamines were active because of their ability to chelate metal ions. The synthetic program was guided by a knowledge of

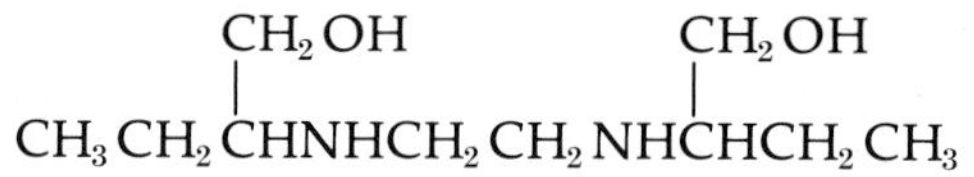

$$CH_2OH \qquad\qquad CH_2OH$$
$$| \qquad\qquad\qquad\qquad |$$
$$CH_3CH_2CHNHCH_2CH_2NHCHCH_2CH_3$$

FIGURE 20–7.   Ethambutol; (+)-2,2'-(ethylenediimino-di-1-butanol).

the types of structural changes that would increase metal chelation in this type of compound (Fig. 20–7).

Ethambutol in medical use is the dihydrochloride, a white, crystalline water-soluble solid, mp 198.5° C to 200.3° C. It is optically active; the optical isomers are either inert or only slightly effective in vitro and in vivo.

Mechanism of Action

As noted previously, the metal chelation rationale was followed by the inventors of ethambutol in developing it from diamines.[99] They noted, however, that ability to form a chelate is not enough by itself to insure antituberculous activity. Several closely related compounds capable of chelating metals equally well are inactive. They postulate that ability to form a metal chelate must occur simultaneously with the ability of the compound (or its chelate) to fit a specific enzyme template. Only in this way could the authors account for the structural and stereoisomeric selectivity exhibited by these diamines.

Subsequent experimental studies have implicated ethambutol as an inhibitor of nucleic acid metabolism, but the details of its action remain to be uncovered. Compatible with a nucleic acid connection, ethambutol is taken up by mycobacteria, whether proliferating or not, but does not injure the nonproliferating cells — i.e., it has no effect on endogenous respiration or on oxygen uptake. On the proliferating cells, growth inhibition occurs after a long delay, up to one to two days with the virulent H37Rv tubercle bacillus.[27, 48]

In cytological studies the most obvious effect of ethambutol is to cause a virtual absence of probable nuclear substance in mycobacteria exposed to it.[29] Spermidine and magnesium ion, both of which play a role in nucleic acid turnover and in maintaining the integrity of ribosomes, specifically counteract the effect of ethambutol on mycobacteria.[26] One must conclude, therefore, that ethambutol, itself a diamine, interferes with the function of polyamines and metal cations in the synthesis and stabilization of RNA. (For further details and references, see the review of Protivinsky[76] and the book by Pratt.[75])

A further study with *M. smegmatis,* while confirming the action of ethambutol upon nucleic acid and upon protein synthesis, points out an involvement with lipid metabolism. Ethambutol inhibits incorporation of methionine in lipids.[94]

Ethambutol is primarily bacteriostatic, or at most only weakly bactericidal in vitro.[17] What its biologic mechanism of action is in chemotherapy is unknown.

ANTIBIOTICS

Streptomycin and Dihydrostreptomycin

Streptomycin in a crude form was isolated from two cultures of the actinomycete, *Streptomyces griseus,* described in 1944 by Schatz and colleagues.[84] The antibiotic, while active on a wide variety of bacteria, has come to be used primarily in tuberculosis.

The early production of streptomycin from streptomyces strains was beset with difficulties. Some strains gave low yields; high-yielding mutant strains reverted, or attack of the strain by phage occurred. Finally, *Streptomyces bikiniensis,* a high-yielding strain, was selected for streptomycin production. Streptomycin can be isolated by adsorption from the crude fermentation beer by activated carbon, by alumina, or by ion-exchange resin. The antibiotic can be purified by chromatography on columns of the same materials.[79]

Dihydrostreptomycin can be obtained from streptomycin by catalytic reduction.[3]

The determination of the structure of streptomycin was the result of a massive effort in the mid-1940s. Chemists from six pharmaceutical laboratories and from groups in two universities participated in its elucidation.[79]

As is apparent from the accompanying structural formula shown in Figure 20–8,[104] streptomycin and dihydrostreptomycin differ only in the conversion of the aldehyde group of the streptose function to an alcohol.

Streptomycin and dihydrostreptomycin each have the highly basic streptidine moiety and, thus, are strong bases known only in the form of their salts, which usually are water-soluble, white, hygroscopic solids. Streptomycin is available as the sulfate and as the hydrochloride double salt with calcium chloride. Dihydrostreptomycin is available principally as the sulfate.

Both substances are relatively stable in neutral solutions. Streptomycin is rapidly inactivated by strong acid or strong base through attack on the aldehyde group. Dihydrostreptomycin is far more stable, as would be expected, because the aldehyde is no longer present.

Mechanism of Action

The literature on this subject has be-

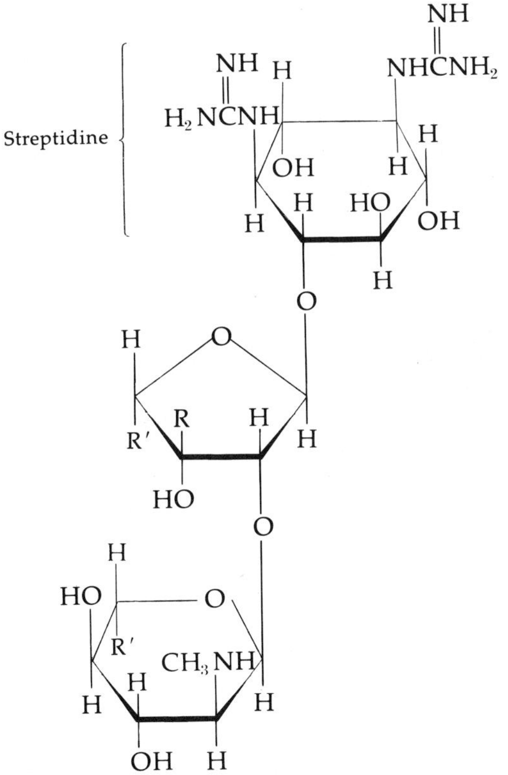

FIGURE 20–8. Streptomycin and dihydrostreptomycin (adapted from Merck Index). Streptomycin, R = CHO; dihydrostreptomycin, R = CH_2OH, for both R' = CH_2OH.

come extensive. Over the years, numerous reviews have devoted space to it. The most recent are by Schlessinger and Medoff[85] and Pratt.[75] Earlier reviews should be consulted, however, since in the excitement of covering the newer protein inhibition studies, short shrift may have been given to some of the earlier fundamental ideas.[41, 43, 110]

By far the most significant work on mechanisms of the last decade or so revolves around the effect of streptomycin on protein synthesis. Streptomycin combines with ribosomes of bacteria. The action is specific and strong and is greatly lessened in genetically mutant strains. The binding of only one molecule of streptomycin per ribosome inhibits polypeptide synthesis by the ribosome. The binding of streptomycin by the ribosome has been traced farther into the fine structure of the ribosome to a particular constituent protein. Ribosomes reconstituted using RNA and this constituent protein bind the drug; ribosomes reconstituted using RNA and the equivalent of this constituent protein taken from a resistant ribosome bind the drug clearly less. In a 70S ribosome, the binding occurs entirely to a 30S subunit; the 50S subunit displays almost no binding.

These relations have been worked out mainly in cell-free systems. The principal effect of streptomycin bound to ribosomes is to modify every measurable phase of protein synthesis and to cause miscoding. The drug, thus, is a useful tool in molecular biology research. Consequently, its mode of action has become an important area of investigation. Space forbids further coverage here of this general subject. (See the review by Schlessinger and Medoff[85] and the book by Pratt.[75])

In the intact cell, inhibition of protein synthesis is still the most prominent effect. The probable focus of this action is to inhibit the act of initiation of polypeptide synthesis on the ribosome. It is important for an understanding of lethality via this mechanism that the ribosomes must be free of m-RNA and thus available for initiation when exposed to streptomycin. Chloramphenicol, which protects the m-RNA of polyribosomes from dissociation, protects the cell from killing by streptomycin; puromycin, which promotes this dissociation, promotes killing.

It should be mentioned that some investigators credit misreading of the genetic code as an important aspect of streptomycin action (see Pratt[75]).

Two theories that precede the discovery of protein synthesis inhibition remain to be mentioned. Anand and Davis in 1960 proposed that damage to the cell membrane was the primary cause of the lethality of streptomycin.[2] According to Kogut and Lightbrown in their review,[43] none of the extensive data accumulated on this mechanism would rule it out. Nonetheless, none of these constitutes evidence in support of the theory. Conceivably, one of the proteins inhibited in the protein inhibition theory would be needed to form a complete membrane and lead to a faulty one. In this case, the two theories would coalesce.

Another important theory maintains that streptomycin exerts its effect by interacting with some component of the aerobic energy yielding reactions. This view has its basis in the frequently observed dependence of streptomycin action on aerobic metabolism (see the review by Kogut and Lightbrown[43]).

Mechanism studies tend to use streptomycin and dihydrostreptomycin data interchangeably. The strong presumption is that they behave identically in antibacterial action, as their close chemical similarity would seem to dictate.

The theory of broadest impact and greatest validity is almost certainly that of protein inhibition. It serves remarkably well at relating diverse phenomena and can explain many intricacies of action. However, it suffers a drawback of many other theories of modes of action, whether with streptomycin or other drugs. Although it is sophisticated in dealing with the proposed biochemical mechanism, it is deficient in explaining the *biologic* mechanism. For the researcher in molecular biology, it is sufficient that a mechanism apply in the particular system he employs, whether it is a cell-free system or a cell system employing non-pathogenic bacteria. To the chemotherapist the system *must* be appropriate to bacterial disease and operate in the complex milieu that is the animal body.

Inherent in most discussions of the mode of action of streptomycin is the assumption that the antibiotic is directly lethal to the bacterium. This is, of course, true of most of the bacteria studied in the test tube to establish the theory. Indeed, direct lethality may be the mode of action of streptomycin with most pathogens. However, it is not certain to apply to mycobacterial disease. Streptomycin is primarily bacteriostatic against tubercle bacilli in the test tube, and bactericidal action is not a prominent feature of its action even in experimental disease. (See the review by Youmans and Youmans, p. 441.[110]) Streptomycin is bactericidal, however, in Tween-containing media.[17]

If inhibition of protein synthesis is the fundamental mechanism of action, then it seems likely that it is not protein synthesis in general which is inhibited to give a chemotherapeutic effect in tuberculosis but rather that it is the production of specific proteins which plays a role in the pathogenicity of the tubercle bacillus. This would allow a synergism between the drug and body defense mechanism.

If protein synthesis inhibited by streptomycin were of proteins involved in cell wall synthesis, it could give lead to a change in the cell surface of the tubercle bacillus, which in turn could lead to its destruction or suppression by the macrophage in which the bacillus is located.[2] This effect would occur long before the level of streptomycin rose to that which is bactericidal without assistance. Unfortunately for this view, according to Kogurt and Lightbrown,[43] there is no reason to believe that the primary action of streptomycin is to affect the mycobacterial cell wall.

A theory has been proposed to the effect that streptomycin interferes with an aerobic electron transport mechanism.[54] This theory has its support in the dependence of streptomycin action upon aerobic metabolism.[43] Whether or not this theory has validity in the biochemical sense, it does present a plausible biologic mechanism whereby phagocytic cells could more easily suppress the growth of this obligatory aerobe. Much has been written on the great importance of oxygen to the growth of tubercle bacilli (see Chapter 2). The theory gains credibility as a chemical mechanism in that perhaps other antituberculous agents exert their effect on the terminal or near-terminal rungs of the electron transport ladder from oxygen. One prominent theory for the mode of action of isoniazid (see under Isoniazid) has this drug affecting certain dehydrogenases; furthermore, the ready oxidation-reduction capabilities of the antituberculous thiocarbamyl drugs (thiosemicarbazones, thioureas, and ethionamide) suggest the possibility that they, too, affect aerobic electron transport. This conjecture, if borne out, would be a simplifying one. The electron transport system of the tubercle bacillus would be singled out as particularly vulnerable and could be the locus of action of streptomycin, isoniazid, and the thiocarbamyl drugs — three independent classes of tuberculochemotherapeutics.

There can be little doubt that any final theory on the mechanism of action of streptomycin will be built around the striking specificity of this drug for ribosomes and its consequent effect on proteins. Not all ribosomes and proteins are affected alike. It is not known at present which of the ribosomes and proteins are tied directly into the chemotherapeutic effect of streptomycin and in what way. Even in the simplest case where direct lethality of streptomycin is taken as the measure, not much is known.[85] If the effect depends upon a harmonious concert action with the body defenses, even less is known. A quote from the review of Kogut and Lightbrown is as valid now as it was then: "Any definite conclusions on the mode of action of streptomycin are still premature."[43]

Viomycin

In 1950, unknown to each other, three different research groups discovered and isolated the substance to be known as viomycin.[4, 24, 60] It is produced by fermentation by the organism *Streptomyces pumiceus* var. *Floridae.*[104] It can be isolated from the culture medium by adsorption on, and elution from, carbon and purified by repeated precipitation from methanol. Its principal activity is against the tubercle bacillus.

The structure has proved difficult to determine. Several structures have been proposed. The most recent one, given in Figure 20–9, relates it to the closely similar members of the capromycin complex in a family of unique macrocylcic peptides.[14]

Viomycin is a strong base known only as its salts (ordinarily the sulfate), which are purple and usually soluble in water while relatively insoluble in most solvents. Aqueous solutions adjusted to pH 5 to 6 are quite stable.[104]

Mechanism of Action

Viomycin is a cyclic peptide antibiotic and is completely unrelated to the aminoglycoside antibiotics. However, its mode of action may resemble that of the aminoglycosides (see under Streptomycin).* It inhibits protein synthesis

---

*Viomycin also produces mammalian toxicity similar to that produced by the aminoglycosides (see Chapter 21). The similarity of mechanism of action and type of toxicity has led to a widespread misconception that viomycin is an aminoglycoside.

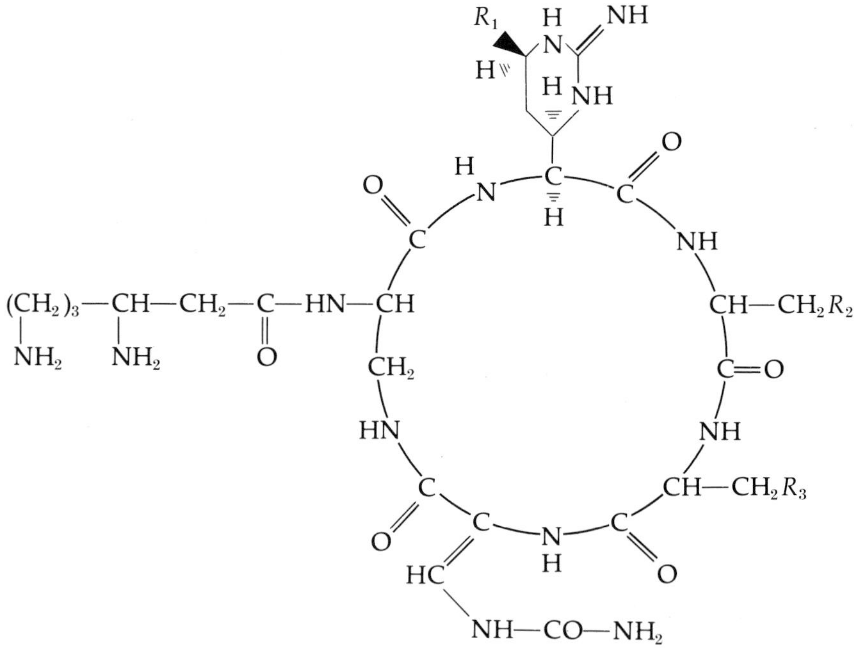

FIGURE 20–9. Viomycin and capreomycin. Viomycin, $R_1 = R_2 = R_3 = OH$; capreomycin IB, $R_1 = R_2 = H$; $R_3 = NH_2$.

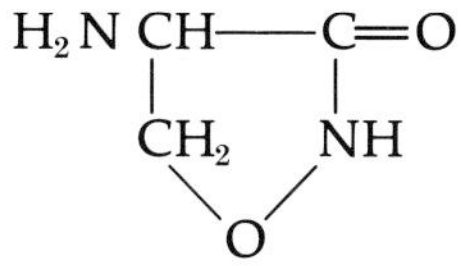

H₂ N CH——C=O

CH₂   NH

O

FIGURE 20–10. Cycloserine; D-4-amino-3-isoxazolidinone.

by binding to ribosomes as do the aminoglycosides.[105] Indeed, viomycin reduced the amount of dihydrostreptomycin bound to ribosomes.[59] There are significant differences, however. Streptomycin causes misreading of the genetic message; whereas viomycin does not. Viomycin affects both 30S and 50S ribosome subunits, while streptomycin affects only the 30S subunits.[55]

Nothing has been published regarding the biologic mechanism of action of viomycin in a chemotherapeutic setting.

Cycloserine

Cycloserine is another of the antibiotics that was discovered in several laboratories independently and simultaneously. Its discovery was announced in 1955. [13, 36, 90] It is elaborated by the organism *Streptomycin orchidaceus* and can be isolated from the fermentation beer by adsorption on ion exchange resin.

Cycloserine is a low molecular weight substance with the simple, albeit unusual, structure given in the accompanying figure (Fig. 20–10).

This structure was revealed in the original announcements.[13, 36] The projected structure has been confirmed by synthesis.[93]

Cycloserine is obtained as colorless crystals, mp 154° C to 155° C. It is amphoteric and, thus, forms salts with both acids and bases. It is soluble in water to form solutions around pH 6. Neutral and acid solutions are unstable. Solutions on the alkaline side are rather more stable.[13, 36, 104]

Mechanism of Action

Cycloserine is one of a limited number of antibiotics whose mechanism of action, both biochemical and biologic is known. Structurally, cycloserine resembles the amino acid, D-alanine. Because its cyclic structure holds the molecule in a cramped conformation suited closely to the enzyme active site, cycloserine has an even higher affinity for this D-alanine site than does D-alanine itself.[81] Consequently, cycloserine is a good inhibitor of enzyme reactions involving D-alanine.

Rando carried the description of cycloserine action a step further. He postulates that cycloserine is activated by contact with its target enzyme and forms a covalent bond with the enzyme; i.e., cycloserine is an irreversible inhibitor of D-alanine enzymes. This action increases its effectiveness greatly.[77]

D-alanine occurs in cell wall structures of many bacteria. It is not synthesized directly for this purpose but is made in the cell by racemization of the usual L-alanine by means of the enzyme, alanine racemase. Two molecules of D-alanine are subsequently coupled to give D-alanyl-D-alanine by another D-alanine-specific enzyme, D-alanyl-D-alanyl synthetase.

Cycloserine inhibits the action of both the racemase and the synthetase to effectively deprive the cell of D-alanyl-D-alanine. This latter material is ordinarily incorporated as the last two-peptide unit of an essential cell wall building block, UDP-acetylmuramyl pentapeptide.* This pentapeptide is a soluble precursor of cell wall structure, which ordinarily is polymerized and attached to the cell membrane (a reaction inhibited by vancomycin and bacitracin) and finally cross-linked to form a rigid insoluble wall (inhibited by penicillin). For an excellent recent survey of cell wall inhibition mechanisms of this class of drugs, see the book by Pratt.[75]

---

*UDP is uridine diphosphate.

Thus, the inhibition of D-alanine enzymes leads to defective cell wall structure. The biologic consequences of this chemical action varies. The cell without its protective cell wall may lyse. Cycloserine in such a case is directly bactericidal. The cell with an incomplete or defective wall would in chemotherapy fall easy prey to host defenses — a more subtle effect of cycloserine.

The mechanism just described has been worked out on gram-positive bacteria. How (and even whether) it applies to mycobacteria is not known. If it applies, it must do so with at least some differences. The cell walls of mycobacteria have gross differences from those of gram-positive bacteria, and mycobacteria are not sensitive to the cell wall inhibitors that affect later stages of cell wall synthesis, such as penicillin, vancomycin, and so forth (see Chapter 4).

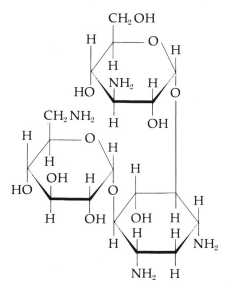

FIGURE 20–11. Kanamycin A.

Kanamycin

Kanamycin was discovered in 1957 by Japanese scientists. This work was reviewed by Umezawa, one of the principal investigators.[95] Kanamycin is produced by *Streptomyces kanamyceticus*; it can be isolated from the fermentation beer by adsorption on cation resin and purified by repeated elution and readsorption on resin (Fig. 20–11). Finally, it can be crystallized. As produced, the beers contain a mixture of closely related antibiotics, the principal component of which is kanamycin A. The structure of the kanamycin fractions was determined by the work of numerous investigators (see *Merck Index*[104]).

Kanamycin A sulfate is a white crystalline solid, soluble in water, and practically insoluble in common alcohols and nonpolar solvents.

Mechanism of Action

The mode of action of kanamycin is probably similar to that of streptomycin and other aminoglycoside antibiotics, since it interacts with the 30S ribosomal subunits, inhibits protein synthesis, and causes misreading of the genetic code. There are significant differences, however, because cross-resistance between kanamycin and streptomycin is the exception rather than the rule. The accounting for these differences is largely speculative (see p. 99 in Pratt[75]).

Capreomycin

As used in medicine, capreomycin is a mixture of four closely related substances, designated capreomycins 1A, 1B, IIA and IIB; their relative proportions are 25, 62, 3, and 6 percent respectively.[34, 35]

The mixture (as the disulfate) is a white solid that is soluble in water and practically insoluble in most organic solvents. Solutions are stable in the range of pH 4 to 8 and are unstable when strongly acidic or basic.[104] The proposed structure for the mixtures is given in Figure 20–9, which accompanies the section on viomycin.[14]

Mechanism of Action

Tubercle bacilli resistant to capreomycin are also resistant to viomycin, i.e., cross-resistant (see, for instance, Algeorge and Petre[1]). Thus, the strong chemical resemblance to viomycin and the cross-resistance both point to its sharing the same mode of action (see section on viomycin).

Rifampin

Rifampin and numerous, less important, related derivatives have been prepared by the synthetic modification of rifamycin B. The parent rifamycin B is one of at least five different antibiotics produced by *Streptomyces mediterrani*.[10] It was selected for synthetic modification, even though inactive, because it is produced by the organism in far greater quantity than the other accompanying antibiotics. Extensive synthetic modifications of rifamycin B have been made and have yielded several series of highly active derivatives. A discussion of this synthetic work is beyond the scope of this review.[10, 57, 86] The structure of rifamycin B for comparison with rifampin is given in Figure 20–12.

The particular modification that is rifampin was selected for use because of its exceptionally high activity and because it is well absorbed when given orally; most rifamycins and their derivatives are poorly absorbed when given by this route. Rifampin is very active against mycobacteria but has other impressive actions as well. In animal infections rifampin shows high activity against gram-positive infections and has achieved some application in the treatment of human meningococcal carriers (see Maggi et al.[57] and Pratt[75]). The drug has actions against certain DNA viruses and larger infectious agents of the class Chlamydozoaceae.[97] Rifampin has an immunosuppressive effect in various animal test systems and affects certain immune related systems in man, but the significance of these latter effects is not known.[75]

Rifampin is a red-orange crystalline solid, mp 183° C to 188° C with decomposition. It is a zwitterion and is only slightly soluble in water at pH above 6; at lower pH, it is much more soluble. It is soluble in most organic solvents. It is rather stable in aqueous solutions, especially when neutral or alkaline. It is, however, attacked slowly by oxygen, a reaction that can be prevented by added sodium ascorbate.[57]

Mechanism of Action

Attention here will be focused upon the effect of rifampin on bacteria. Concentrations running from 10^2 to 10^4 greater than those necessary to inhibit bacteria are needed to affect eukaryotic cells and viruses. (See Wehrli and Staehelin[97] for references and details on rifampin's wider scope of action.)

The most prominent way in which rifampin acts against bacteria, and one shown at extremely low concentrations, is an effect on the process of transcription. The drug inhibits the synthesis of RNA by inactivating the DNA-dependent RNA polymerase. This enzyme polymerizes ribonucleoside triphosphates on a DNA template. Rifampin was first shown to have this specific inhibitory effect by Hartmann and colleagues.[32] This action of rifampin in cell-free systems is brought about by the same low range of concentrations needed to affect intact bacteria, showing that there is little barrier to penetration of the bacterial cell. Quantitative measurements have shown that one mole of rifampin is bound per mole of enzyme.[97]

Rifampin is highly specific for the bacterial RNA polymerase enzyme; concentrations 10,000 times higher are needed to affect the corresponding mammalian enzyme. This accounts for the low mammalian toxicity of rifampin. Certain toxic antibiotics (actinomycin and mitomycin) also inhibit RNA polymerase, but they do it by interacting with the DNA template on which the enzyme acts, not by affecting the enzyme itself. As no specificity of template action exists, the bacterial enzyme and mammalian enzyme are equally vulner-

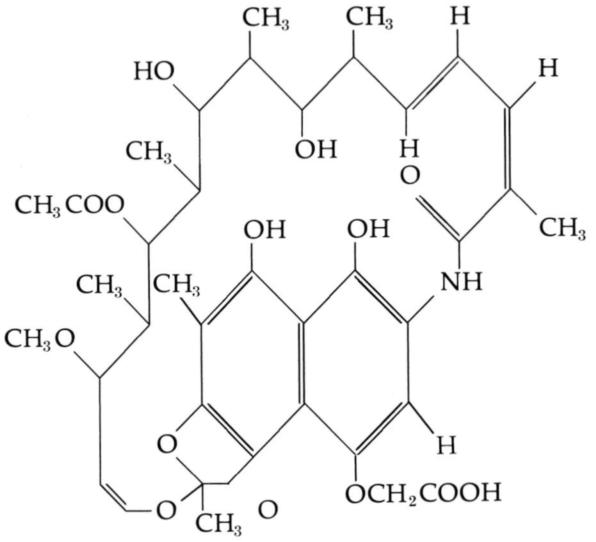

Rifamycin B

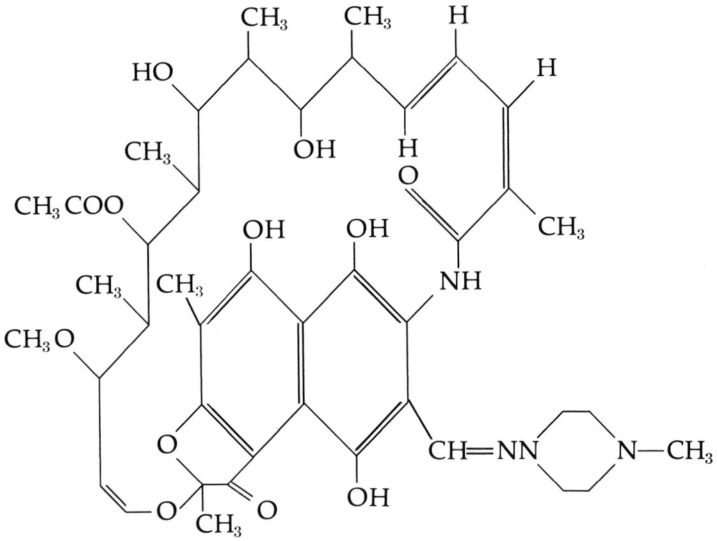

Rifampin (rifampicin)

FIGURE 20–12. Rifamycin B and rifampin (rifampicin).

able, and these antibiotics are toxic. The action of rifampin has been pinpointed to stopping the initiation of new RNA chains; RNA chains already under construction are continued to completion. When bacteria mutate to high rifampin-resistance, the RNA polymerase enzyme is no longer affected by rifampin and can no longer bind the drug.

While there is unanimity in the extensive published work on the biochemical mechanism of action of rifampin, there is no explicit reference in this literature to a biologic mechanism for rifampin action in the treatment of bacterial disease. One must suppose that in chemotherapy lethality by direct drug action is the end point of rifampin's attack on the RNA polymerase enzyme. Certainly, no reference is made to more subtle end effects, as for example, bacteriostasis or immune assistance. Rifampin, according to Pallanza and coworkers, exhibits marked bactericidal action on mycobacteria.[74] Perhaps lethality to mycobacteria is adequate to explain its chemotherapeutic effect; this reviewer is not aware of any other experimental work directed to this question.

REFERENCES

1. Algeorge, G., and Petre, A.: Some experimental aspects of cross-resistance between capreomycin and viomycin. Antibiot. Chemother. *16*:32, 1970.
2. Anand, N., and Davis, B. D.: Effect of streptomycin on *Escherichia coli*. Damage by streptomycin to the cell membrane of *Escherichia coli*. Nature *185*:22, 1959.
3. Bartz, Q. R., Controulis, J., Crooks, H. M., Jr., and Rebstock, M. C.: Dihydrostreptomycin. J. Am. Chem. Soc. *68*:2163, 1946.
4. Bartz, Q. R., Ehrlich, J., Mold, J. D., Penner, M. A., and Smith, R. M.: Viomycin, a new tuberculostatic antibiotic. Am. Rev. Tuberc. *63*:4, 1951.
5. Behnisch, R., Mietzsch, F., and Schmidt, H.: Chemical studies on thiosemicarbazones with particular reference to antituberculous activity. Am. Rev. Tuberc. *61*:1, 1950.
6. Bekierkunst, A., and Bricker, A.: Studies on the mode of action of isoniazid on mycobacteria. Arch. Biochem. Biosphys. *122*:385, 1967.
7. Bernheim, F.: Effect of salicylate on oxygen uptake of tubercle bacillus. Science *92*:204, 1940.
8. Bernstein, J., Lott, W. A., Steinberg, B. A., and Yale, H. L.: Chemotherapy of experimental tuberculosis. V. Isonicotinic acid hydrazide (Nydrazid) and related compounds. Am. Rev. Tuberc. *65*:357, 1952.
9. Besta, B.: La morfazinamide: Resultati terapeutici ed indagini sperimentali. G. Ital. Chemioter. *10*:196, 1963. (As cited in Protivinsky.[76])
10. Binda, G., Domenichini, E., Gottardi, A., Orlandi, B., Ortelli, E., Pacini, B., and Fowst, G.: Rifampin, a general review. Arzneim. Forsch. *21*:1907, 1971.
11. Brown, K. A., and Ratledge, C.: The effect of *p*-aminosalicylic acid on iron transport and assimilation in mycobacteria. Biochim. Biophys. Acta *385*:207, 1975.
12. Browne, S. G.: Leprosy. Br. Med. J *iii*:725, 1968.
13. Buhs, R. F., Putter, I., Ormond, R., Lyons, J. E., Chaiet, L., Kuehl, F. A., Wolf, F. J., Trenner, N. R., Peak, R. L., Howe, E., Hunnewell, B. D., Downing, G., Newstead, E., and Folkers, K.: D-4-amino-3-isoxazolidone, a new antibiotic. J. Am. Chem. Soc. *77*:2344, 1955.
14. Bycroft, B. W., Cameron, D., Croft, L. R., Hassanali-Walji, A., Johnson, A. W., and Webb, T.: Total structure of capreomycin IB, a tuberculostatic peptide antibiotic. Nature *231*:301, 1971.
15. Chorine, S. V.: Action of nicotinamide on bacilli of the species *Mycobacterium*. Comp. Rend. Acad. Sci. *220*:150, 1945.
16. Dalmer, O., and Walter, E.: Derivatives of pyrazine carboxylic acid and process for their production. German Patent 632257 (1936); U.S. Patent 2149279 (1939).
17. Dickinson, J. M., Aber, V. R., and Mitchison, D. A.: Bactericidal activity of streptomycin, isoniazid, rifampin, ethambutol, and pyrazinamide alone and in combination against *Mycobacterium tuberculosis*. Am. Rev. Respir. Dis. *116*:627, 1977.
18. Domagk, G.: Investigations on the antituberculous activity of the thiosemicarbazones *in vitro* and *in vivo*. Am. Rev. Tuberc. *61*:8, 1950.
19. Domagk, G., Behnisch, R., Mietzsch, F., and Schmidt, H.: Über eine neue, gegen Tuberkelbacillen *in Vitro* wirksame Verbindungsklasse. Naturwissenschaften *33*:315, 1946.
20. Donovick, R., Bayan, A., and Hamre, D.: The reversal of the activity of antituberculous compounds *in vitro*. Am. Rev. Tuberc. *66*:219, 1952.
21. Doub, L., Schaefer, J. J., Bambas, L. L., and

Walker, C. T.: Some derivatives of 4-amino-2-hydroxybenzoic acid (*p*-aminosalicylic acid). J. Am. Chem. Soc. *73*:905, 1951.

22. Feldman, W. H.: The chemotherapy of tuberculosis—including the use of streptomycin (Harben Lectures, No. 2, 1946). An evaluation of the efficacy in tuberculosis of sulfonamides, sulfones and certain other substances. J. Royal Inst. Publ. Health Hyg. *9*:297, 1946.

23. Feldman, W. H., and Hinshaw, H. C.: Effects of streptomycin on experimental tuberculosis in guinea pigs: A preliminary report Proc. Staff Meet. Mayo Clin. *19*:593, 1944.

24. Finlay, A. C., Hobby, G. L., Hochstein, F., Lees, T. M., Lenert, T. F., Means, J. A., P'an, S. Y., Regna, P. P., Routien, J. B., Sobin, B. A., Tate, K. B., and Kane, J. H.: Viomycin, a new antibiotic active against mycobacteria. Am. Rev. Tuberc. *63*:1, 1951.

25. Fisher, M. W.: The antagonism of the tuberculostatic action of isoniazid by hemin. Am. Rev. Tuberc. *69*:469, 1954.

26. Forbes, M., Kuck, N. A., and Peets, E. A.: Effect of ethambutol on nucleic-acid metabolism in *Mycobacterium smegmatis* and its reversal by polyamines and divalent cations. J. Bacteriol. *89*:1299, 1965.

27. Forbes, M., Kuck, N. A., and Peets, E. A.: Mode of action of ethambutol. J. Bacteriol. *84*:1099, 1962.

28. Fox, H. H.: The chemical approach to the control of tuberculosis. Science *116*:129, 1952.

29. Gale, G. R., and McLain, H. H.: Effect of ethambutol on cytology of *Mycobacterium smegmatis*. J. Bacteriol. *86*:749, 1963.

30. Gnehm, R., and Schmid, J.: Carbonic-acid compound of meta-amidophenol. German Patent 50835 (1889); U.S. Patent 427564 (1890).

31. Gubler, H. U., and Angehrn, P.: Sensitivity to thiocarlide and thiacetazone of far-eastern strains of *Mycobacterium tuberculosis*. Tubercle *47*:400, 1966.

32. Hartmann, G., Honikel, K. O., Knüsel, F., and Nüesch, J.: The specific inhibition of DNA-induced RNA synthesis by rifamycin. Biochim. Biophys. Acta *145*:843, 1967.

33. Hedgecock, L. W.: Antagonism of the inhibitory action of *p*-aminosalicylic acid on *Mycobacterium tuberculosis* by methionine, biotin, and certain fatty acids, amino acids, and purines. J. Bacteriol. *72*:839, 1956.

34. Herr, E. B., Haney, M. E., Pittenger, G. E., and Higgins, C. E.: Proceedings of the Indiana Academy of Science *69*:134, 1960. (As cited in Buhs et al.[13])

35. Herr, E. B., Jr., and Redstone, M. O.: Chemical and physical characterization of capreomycin. Ann. N. Y. Acad. Sci. *135*:940, 1966.

36. Hidy, P. H., Hodge, E. B., Young, V. V., Harned, R. L., Brewer, G. A., Phillips, W. F., Runge, W. F., Stavely, H. E., Pohland, A., Boaz, H., and Sullivan, H. R.: Structure and reactions of cycloserine. J. Am. Chem. Soc. *77*:2345, 1955.

37. Hinshaw, H. C., and Feldman, W. H.: Streptomycin in treatment of clinical tuberculosis: A preliminary report. Proc. Staff Meet. Mayo Clin. *20*:313, 1945.

38. Hoover, J. R. E., and Stedman, R. J.: The β-lactam antibiotics. *In* Burger, A. (ed.): Medicinal Chemistry. 3rd ed. New York, Wiley-Interscience, 1970.

39. Hubble, R. H., and Hedgecock, L. W.: Antagonism of chemotherapeutic activity of *p*-aminosalicylic acid in experimental tuberculosis by *p*-aminobenzoic acid. Proc. Soc. Exp. Biol. Med. *84*:526, 1953.

40. Ivanovics, G.: Antagonism between effects of *p*-aminosalicylic acid and salicylic acid on growth of *M. tuberculosis*. Proc. Soc. Exp. Biol. Med. *70*:462, 1949.

41. Jacoby, G. A., and Gorini, L.: The effect of streptomycin and other aminoglycoside antibiotics on protein synthesis. *In* Gollich, D., and Shaw, P. D. (eds.): Antibiotics. Vol. I. Mechanism of Action. New York, Springer-Verlag, 1967.

42. Knox, R.: Haemin and isoniazid resistance of *M. tuberculosis*. J. Gen. Microbiol. *12*:191, 1955.

43. Kogut, M., and Lightbrown, J. W.: The mode of action of streptomycin. *In* Schnitzer, R. J., and Hawking, F. (eds.): Experimental Chemotherapy. Vol. III. New York, Academic Press, 1964.

44. Krishna-Murti, C. R.: Isonicotinic acid hydrazide. *In* Corcoran, J. W., and Hahn, F. E. (eds.): Antibiotics. Vol. III. Mechanism of Action of Antimicrobial and Antitumor Agents. New York, Springer-Verlag, 1975.

45. Krüger-Theimer, E.: Chemismus der Isoniazidspaltung durch Hämin. Naturwissenschaften *42*:47, 1955.

46. Krüger-Theimer, E.: Isonicotinic acid hypothesis of the antituberculous action of isoniazid. Am. Rev. Tuberc. *77*:364, 1958.

47. Krüger-Theimer, E.: Jahres berichte. Borstel *3*:192, 1956. (As cited in Protivinsky.[76])

48. Kuck, N. A., Peets, E. A., and Forbes, M.: Mode of action of ethambutol on *Mycobacterium tuberculosis*, strain H37Rv. Am. Rev. Respir. Dis. *87*:905, 1963.

49. Kushner, S., Dalalian, H., Sanjurjo, J. L., Bach, F. L., Jr., Safir, S. R., Smith, V. K., Jr., and Williams, J. H.: Experimental chemotherapy of tuberculosis. II. The synthesis of pyrazinamides and related compounds. J. Am. Chem. Soc. *74*:3617, 1952.

50. Lehmann, J.: Chemotherapy of tuberculosis.

The bacteriostatic action of *p*-aminosalicylic acid and closely related substances upon the tubercle bacillus, together with animal experiments and clinical trials. Svenska Läkartidn *43*:2029, 1946.

51. Lehmann, J.: *Para*-aminosalicylic acid in the treatment of tuberculosis. Lancet *250*:15, 1946.

52. Libermann, D., Moyeux, M., Rist, N., and Grumbach, F.: Sur la préparation de nouveaux thioamides pyridiniques actifs dans la tuberculose experimentale. C. R. Acad. Sci. (Paris) *242*:2409, 1956.

53. Liebermeister, K.: Zur Wirkungsweise der tuberculostalischen Chemotherapeutika. Dtsch. Med. Wochenschr. *75*:621, 1950. (As cited in Protivinsky.[76])

54. Lightbrown, J. W.: Metabolic processes underlying streptomycin resistance. G. Ital. Chemioter. *4*:22, 1957.

55. Liou, Y., and Tanaka, N.: Dual actions of viomycin on the ribosomal functions. Biochem. Biophys. Res. Commun. *71*:477, 1976.

56. Macham, L. P., Ratledge, C., and Nocton, J. C.: Extracellular iron acquisition by mycobacteria: Role of the exochelins and evidence against the participation of mycobactin. Infect. Immun. *12*:1242, 1975.

57. Maggi, N., Pasqualucci, C. R., Ballotta, R., and Sensi, P.: Rifampicin: A new orally active rifamycin. Chemotherapia *11*:285, 1966.

58. Malone, L., Schurr, A., Lindh, H., McKenzie, D., Kiser, J. S., and Williams, J. H.: The effect of pyrazinamide (aldinamide) on experimental tuberculosis of white mice. Am. Rev. Tuberc. *65*:511, 1952.

59. Masuda, K., and Yamada, T.: Effect of viomycin on dihydrostreptomycin binding to bacterial ribosomes. Biochim. Biophys. Acta *435*:333, 1976.

60. Mayer, R. L., Crane, C., DeBoer, C. J., Konopka, E. A., Marsh, J. S., and Eisman, P. C.: Antibiotics from *Act. vinaceus.* Twelfth International Congress on Pure and Applied Chemistry, New York, 1951. (As cited in Welch, H.,[98] p. 161.)

61. McClatchy, J. K.: Mechanism of action of INH on *M. bovis,* strain BCG. Infect. Immun. *3*:530, 1971.

62. McCune, R. M., and Tompsett, R.: Fate of *Mycobacterium tuberculosis* in mouse tissues as determined by the microbial enumeration technique. J. Exp. Med. *104*:737, 1956.

63. McCune, R. M., Tompsett, R., and McDermott, W.: The conversion of tuberculous infection to the latent state by the administration of pyrazinamide and a companion drug. J. Exp. Med. *104*:763, 1956.

64. McDermott, W., and Tompsett, R.: Activation of pyrazinamide and nicotinamide in acid environments *in vitro.* Am. Rev. Tuberc. *70*:748, 1954.

65. McKenzie, D., Malone, L., Kushner, S., Oleson, J. J., and Subba Row, Y.: The effect of nicotinic amide on experimental tuberculosis in white mice. J. Lab. Clin. Med. *33*:1249, 1948.

66. Meadow, P., and Knox, P.: The effect of isonicotonic acid hydrazide on the oxidative metabolism of *M. tuberculosis* var. *bovis* BCG. J. Gen. Microbiol. *14*:414, 1956.

67. Meyer, H., and Malley, J.: Hydrazine derivatives of pyridine carboxylic acids. Monatsh. *33*:393, 1912.

68. Middlebrook, G.: Isoniazid-resistance and catalase activity of tubercle bacilli. Am. Rev. Tuberc. *69*:471, 1954.

69. Middlebrook, G.: Sterilization of tubercle bacilli by isonicotinic acid hydrazide and the incidence of variants resistant to the drug *in vitro.* Am. Rev. Tuberc. *65*:765, 1952.

70. Middlebrook, G., and Cohn, M. L.: Some observations on the pathogenicity of isoniazid-resistant variants of tubercle bacilli. Science *118*:297, 1953.

71. Northey, E. H.: The Sulfonamides and Allied Compounds. New York, Reinhold Publishing Corp., 1948.

72. Offe, H. A., Siefkin, W., and Domagk, G.: The tuberculostatic activity of hydrazine derivatives from pyridine carboxylic acids and carbonyl compounds. Z. Naturforsch. *7b*:462, 1952.

73. Olivera, B. M.: The DNA joining enzyme from *Escherichia coli.* Methods Enzymol. *21*:311, 1971.

74. Pallanza, R., Arioli, V., Furesz, S., and Bolzoni, G.: Rifampicin: A new rifamycin. Arzneim. Forsch. *17*:529, 1967.

75. Pratt, W. B.: The Chemotherapy of Infection. New York, Oxford University Press, 1977.

76. Protivinsky, R.: Chemotherapeutics with tuberculostatic action. Antibiot. Chemother. *17*:101, 1971.

77. Rando, R. R.: On the mechanism of action of antibiotics which act as irreversible enzyme inhibitors. Biochem. Pharmacol. *24*:1153, 1975.

78. Ratledge, C., and Brown, K. A.: Inhibition of mycobactin formation in *Mycobacterium smegmatis* by *p*-aminosalicylate. Am. Rev. Respir. Dis. *106*:774, 1972.

79. Rebstock, M. C.: Antibiotics. *In* Burger, A. (ed.): Medicinal Chemistry. 2nd ed. New York, Interscience Publishers, Inc., 1960.

80. Rist, N., Grumbach, F., and Libermann, D.: Experiments on the antituberculous activity of *alpha* ethylthioisonicotinamide. Am. Rev. Tuberc. *79*:1, 1959.

81. Roze, U., and Strominger, J. L.: Alanine ra-

cemase from *Staphylococcus aureus:* Conformation of its substrates and its inhibitor, D-cycloserine. Mol. Pharmacol. *2*:92, 1964.

82. Schaefer, W. B.: Effect of isoniazid on the dehydrogenase activity of *Mycobacterium tuberculosis.* J. Bacteriol. *79*:236, 1960.

83. Schaefer, W. B.: The effect of isoniazid on growing and resting tubercle bacilli. Am. Rev. Tuberc. *69*:125, 1954.

84. Schatz, A., Bugie, E., and Waksman, A.: Streptomycin, a substance exhibiting antibiotic activity against gram-positive and gram-negative bacteria. Proc. Soc. Exp. Biol. Med. *55*:66, 1944.

85. Schlessinger, D., and Medoff, G.: Streptomycin, dihydrostreptomycin and the gentamycins. *In* Corcoran, J. W., and Hahn, F. E. (eds.): Antibiotics. Vol. III. Mechanism of Action of Antimicrobial and Antitumor Agents. New York, Springer-Verlag, 1975.

86. Sensi, P., Maggi, N., Ballotta, R., Füresz, S., Pallanza, R., and Arioli, V.: Rifamycins. xxxv. Amides and hydrazides of rifamycin B. J. Med. Chem. *7*:596, 1964.

87. Seydel, J. K., and Butte, W.: P-aminobenzoic acid derivatives. Mode of action and structure-activity relationships in a cell-free system (*Escherichia coli*). J. Med. Chem. *20*:439, 1977.

88. Seydel, J. K., Wempe, E., and Nestler, H. J.: Experimentelle Untersuchungen zur Isonikotinsäurehypothese des Isoniazid wirkungsmodus. Arzneim. Forsch. *18*:362, 1968.

89. Shepherd, R. G., and Wilkinson, R. G.: Antituberculous agents. II. N,N-diisopropylethylene diamine and analogs. J. Med. Pharm. Chem. *5*:823, 1962.

90. Shull, G. M., and Sardinas, J. L.: PA-94, an antibiotic identical with D-4-amino-3-isoxazolidinone (cycloserine, oxamycin). Antibiot. Chemother. *5*:398, 1955.

91. Solotorovsky, M., Gregory, F. J., Ironson, E. J., Bugie, E. J., O'Neill, R. C., and Pfister, K., 3rd: Pyrazinoic acid amide — an agent active against experimental murine tuberculosis. Proc. Soc. Exp. Biol. Med. *79*:563, 1952.

92. Sriprakash, K. S., and Ramakrishnan, T.: Isoniazid-resistant mutants of *Mycobacterium tuberculosis* H37Rv: Uptake of isoniazid and properties of NADase inhibitor. J. Gen. Microbiol. *60*:125, 1970.

93. Stammer, C. H., Wilson, A. H., Holly, F. W., and Folkers, K.: Synthesis of D-4-amino-3-isoxazolidone. J. Am. Chem. Soc. *77*:2346, 1955.

94. Tsukamura, M., and Mizuno, S.: Further studies on the mode of action of ethambutol. Kekkaku *47*:37, 1972.

95. Umezawa, H.: Kanamycin: Its discovery. Ann. N. Y. Acad. Sci. *76*:20, 1958.

96. Wacker, A., Kolm, H., and Ebert, M.: Metabolism of p-aminosalicylic and salicylic acids by *Enterococcus.* Z. Naturforsch. *13b*:147, 1958.

97. Wehrli, W., and Staehelin, M.: Rifamycins and other ansamycins. *In* Corcoran, J. W., and Hahn, F. E. (eds.): Antibiotics. Vol. III. Mechanism of Action of Antimicrobial and Antitumor Agents. New York, Springer-Verlag, 1975.

98. Welch, H.: The Principles and Practice of Antibiotic Therapy. New York, Medical Encyclopedia, Inc., 1954.

99. Wilkinson, R. G., Cantrall, M. B., and Shepherd, R. G.: Antituberculous agents. III. (+)-2,2-(ethylenediimino)-di-l-butanol and some analogs. J. Med. Pharm. Chem. *5*:835, 1962.

100. Wilkinson, R. G., Shepherd, R. G., Thomas, J. P., and Baughn, C.: Stereospecificity in a new type of synthetic antituberculous agent. J. Am. Chem. Soc. *83*:2212, 1961.

101. Winder, F.: Catalase and peroxidase in mycobacteria. Possible relationship to the mode of action of isoniazid. Am. Rev. Respir. Dis. *81*:68, 1960.

102. Winder, F. G., and Collins, P. B.: Inhibition by isoniazid of synthesis of mycolic acids in *Mycobacterium tuberculosis.* J. Gen. Microbiol. *63*:41, 1970.

103. Winder, F. G., Collins, P. B., and Whelan, D.: Effects on ethionamide and isoxyl on mycolic acid synthesis in *Mycobacterium tuberculosis* BCG. J. Gen. Microbiol. *66*:379, 1971.

104. Windholz, M. (ed.): The Merck Index. 9th ed. New Jersey, Merck and Co., Inc., 1976.

105. Yamada, T., Masuda, K., Shoji, K., and Hori, M.: Analysis of ribosomes from viomycin-sensitive and -resistant strains of *Mycobacterium smegmatis.* J. Bacteriol. *112*:1, 1972.

106. Youatt, J.: A review of the action of isoniazid. Am. Rev. Respir. Dis. *99*:729, 1969.

107. Youmans, G. P.: The effect of streptomycin *in vitro* on *M. tuberculosis* var. *hominis.* Quarterly Bull. Northwestern U. Med. School *19*:207, 1945.

108. Youmans, G. P., and McCarter, J. C.: A preliminary note on the effect of streptomycin on experimental tuberculosis of white mice. Quarterly Bull. Northwestern U. Med. School *19*:210, 1945.

109. Youmans, G. P., Raleigh, G. W., and Youmans, A. S.: The tuberculostatic action of *para*-aminosalicylic acid. J. Bacteriol. *54*:409, 1947.

110. Youmans, G. P., and Youmans, A. S.: Experimental chemotherapy of tuberculosis and other mycobacterial infections. *In* Schnitzer, R. J., and Hawking, F. (eds.): Experimental Chemotherapy. Vol. II. New York, Academic Press, 1964.

21

Treatment of Tuberculosis

H. CORWIN HINSHAW, M.D., Ph.D., D.Sc.

INTRODUCTION

The preceding chapters of this volume provide an abundance of scientific data, much of which bear indirectly or directly upon therapy of tuberculosis. This should benefit the present-day, clinically oriented physicians who re-quire a considerable depth of knowledge concerning the tubercle bacillus — its attributes and actions in vivo and in vitro — and the response of the host to tuberculous infection, in order to best serve their patients and the community.

The main objective of this chapter

shall be to provide some practical guidelines and advice to the physician who faces the problem of managing a patient who may be a candidate for anti-tuberculosis therapy. The clinician is heavily dependent upon the microbiologist, the clinical pathologist, and the roentgenologist in choosing candidates suitable for therapy, in choosing appropriate therapeutic regimens, in monitoring the course of disease and in detecting the toxic consequences of therapy.

SELECTION OF PATIENTS FOR TREATMENT

Treatment for tuberculosis is no trivial matter. It involves months of faithful adherence to a program of daily medication, periodic physician surveillance, and a small calculated risk of serious toxic drug reaction. The emotional impact — apprehension and anxiety — is sometimes great and not easily allayed. The physician will not subject the patient to these risks, discomforts, and expenses unless he is convinced that his diagnosis is correct and that no other and less-complicated program can be recommended with safety.

Active Tuberculosis

Chemotherapy is indicated for every case of active tuberculosis. Inactive tuberculosis may or may not require chemotherapy. Determination of activity becomes a problem of prime importance, and the problem does not always have an easy solution. Frequently the clinician must rely upon his laboratory colleagues to provide the proof of activity, isolation of the organism in culture being essential under ordinary circumstances. Maturation of cultures involves considerable time, a matter of weeks, and in urgent situations it may be necessary to treat the patient on a provi-

sional basis while awaiting definitive laboratory confirmation. The viewing of acid-fast bacilli in sputum or other clinical material justifies treatment, but cultural confirmation must always be sought (see Chapter 19).[6, 110]

The roentgenologist frequently detects evidence of pulmonary tuberculosis, perhaps unsuspected on symptomatic or physical findings. Many lung disorders may mimic tuberculosis, making any roentgenographic finding only a provisional diagnosis — one that requires laboratory proof. A positive tuberculin skin test, followed by thorough search for acid-fast bacilli microscopically and culturally, must follow. Roentgenographic evidence of destructive (cavitary) disease or that of pneumonic type should promptly yield acid-fast bacilli, if disease is truly tuberculous.

Diagnosis by "therapeutic trial" with specific remedies is likely to lead the clinician astray and is a procedure to be avoided. The fact that a lesion resembling tuberculosis on the roentgenogram recedes following specific treatment does not establish a reliable diagnosis and does not justify continuing antituberculosis chemotherapy unless tubercle bacilli are demonstrated.

Comparison of serial films frequently is essential to evaluate tuberculosis activity and the need for treatment. Whenever possible, previous chest films should be obtained, even if great effort is required. In the event that any previous chemotherapy has been administered to the patient, the physicians previously consulted by the patient should be interrogated to learn what drugs were taken and for how long, bearing in mind the possibility that resistant bacilli have developed.

Every patient with active tuberculosis should receive treatment with at least two of the first-line drugs. The conventional period of treatment has been from 18 to 24 months. Duration and choice of drugs are discussed later on in the chapter.

Previously Treated, Reactivated Tuberculosis

Tuberculosis has often been defined as a relapsing chronic disease. Prior to the chemotherapy era, relapse was anticipated in at least one-third of all "arrested" cases.[75, 97] Patients who have completed a conventional long-term course of chemotherapy and who are apparently cured rarely relapse during the first two years following completion of treatment. There are a few well-documented reports of relapse rates five years or more after treatment. In New Delhi, Pamra and coworkers[78] reported a cumulative relapse rate of 11.6 percent within 5 years following apparently successful therapy of 543 cases. Most of the recurrent cases were revealed by symptoms and occurred during the third and fourth years. Stead and Jurgens[96] and Grzybowski and coworkers[46] provided more favorable reports, indicating that nearly all cases of relapse were due to inadequate chemotherapy; i.e., failure of compliance with prescribed medication. From this and other studies, it appears safe to predict that only 1 to 3 percent of adequately treated (long-term) apparently cured patients will suffer relapse and that symptoms will prompt the patient to seek medical advice if and when relapse occurs. Therefore, the practical clinical problem is mostly limited to those patients with far-advanced disease who have failed to comply with a recommended course of treatment or who have some predisposing disorder or resistant organisms. It remains to be seen if newer short-term and intensive treatment programs will provide equal or better results five years or more following completion of therapy.

Inactive and Obsolete Tuberculosis

Preventive therapy with isoniazid for one year has frequently been advocated for all patients whose chest roentgenogram reveals shadows indicative of possible previous tuberculous infection associated with a positive tuberculin skin test. Carried to its extreme, this recommendation would include any person with a healed (calcified) primary complex or one with minimal apical scars.[4]

Lesions of ancient tuberculosis are most frequently encountered among persons in the older age groups, over 35 years of age. These individuals are at greatest risk of suffering serious liver damage (over 2 percent), resulting from isoniazid therapy. Thus the physician is called upon to assess the risks of hepatitis and tuberculosis on the basis of the several variables involved: age, roentgenographic findings, factors predisposing to hepatitis (alcoholism, infectious hepatitis, age), and factors predisposing to tuberculosis (diabetes, gastric resection, steroid therapy, economic and social status, alcoholism, age).

Often overlooked in discussions of preventive therapy is the fact that if tuberculosis should develop and is recognized promptly, it is curable, with scarcely more effort than would have been expended in preventive chemotherapy. Treatment should be postponed until needed in persons with apparently healed tuberculosis if hepatitis is feared because of age or other predisposing factors. Serial roentgenograms are required to detect reactivation of tuberculosis and serve a double purpose in the older age groups, screening for cancer at the same time.

Tuberculous Infection Without Apparent Disease

Intensive interest has developed in "preventive therapy" of healthy persons with no demonstrated evidence of tuberculous disease but with positive tuberculin skin tests. Authorative advice that such persons should undergo prolonged chemotherapy with isoni-azid[3-5] has been tempered by information that risks of therapy are sometimes substantial.[8, 9, 19, 23, 29, 44, 53]

Discussion of this problem is important because it concerns some 14,000,000 tuberculin reactors in the United States and countless millions elsewhere. The problem may be clarified somewhat by distinguishing between 1) those persons with positive tuberculin skin tests who are believed to have had negative tests within recent years, and 2) those with reactions of unknown origin and duration. Some added factors that deserve consideration include: 1) recent exposure to infection, 2) age, 3) conditions predisposing to tuberculosis, 4) conditions predisposing to liver injury from isoniazid, 5) availability for protracted observation, and 6) the intensity of tuberculin sensitivity as measured by the size of the reaction to a standardized intracutaneous Mantoux test.[6, 62, 63, 64]

Recently Acquired Tuberculin Sensitivity

The practice of periodic tuberculin skin testing of adults, long popular among children, is gaining in the United States. The practice is advocated and sometimes required for health professionals and others believed to be exposed to communicable tuberculosis.

When a positive tuberculin skin test appears, preceded by a recorded recent (2 to 4 years) negative reaction, it should be realized that active tuberculosis may well be present, even though the chest roentgenogram does not reveal it. Primary tuberculosis often requires a few years to heal and may remain dormant long thereafter (see Chapter 14). Treatment of the patient with recently acquired tuberculin sensitivity should not be called "preventive therapy" but therapy of "inapparent tuberculosis."

It is well known, and frequently observed by thoracic surgeons, that many pulmonary lesions, including those of tuberculosis, may not be registered on chest roentgenograms. A primary lesion of pulmonary tuberculosis of considerable size and density may escape detection and only be suspected because of a recently acquired positive tuberculin skin test.

Many patients with inapparent lesions of tuberculosis should be presumed to have active disease and be encouraged to undergo therapy, usually one year of isoniazid, administered in a 300 mg dose once daily (customary adult dose). Those at special risk may be considered for two-drug therapy, at least for a few weeks. If circumstances indicate special risk of liver injury, treatment may be postponed.

Tuberculin Sensitivity of Unknown Duration

This problem is frequently encountered. It is important to adhere to the standard Mantoux test and measure the reaction dimensions. Large reactions are often associated with recent infection (see Chapters 7 and 13).

Johnson and Wildrick[65] stated that 70 percent of the 15 million tuberculin reactors in the United States were over 35 years of age, and only 5 percent were younger than 25 years. At the rate of change predicted by them, there should be 14 million reactors in 1978, and 75 percent of them would be over the age of 35 years. If we agree that the risk of isoniazid hepatitis is prohibitive for older persons with no special predisposition to tuberculosis, it must be concluded that a large majority of tuberculin reactors should not be so treated. (Toxicity of isoniazid is described in a later section of this chapter.)

In the same review, Johnson and Wildrick indicate how many patients in several categories would have to be treated to prevent one case of tuberculosis: 1) in adults, tuberculin-positive with normal chest roentgenograms, 163 cases treated should prevent one case of tuberculosis; 2) in adolescents, tuberculin-positive with normal chest roentgenograms, 110 cases treated should prevent one case of tuberculosis; 3) in previously known inadequately treated patients, 14.2 cases treated should prevent one case of relapse; and in tuberculin-negative household contacts to a recent case, 210 treated cases should prevent one case of tuberculosis, but if the household contacts were tuberculin-positive, only 48.3 cases need be treated to prevent one case of tuberculosis. The risk of developing active tuberculosis among those with positive tuberculin skin tests varies widely in different reports. Among tuberculin-positive Eskimos, 5 per 1,000 will develop active disease,[24] while in Denmark the risk is reported to be only 0.11 per 1,000.[61]

Young children, especially those of preschool age who have positive tuberculin skin tests should be considered as having inapparent, active lesions, even though x-rays are clear. Advancing disease of serious, even lethal, nature may rapidly develop, especially in those less than 2 or 3 years of age (Table 21–1).

Special consideration for therapy should also be given to persons treated with immunosuppressive drugs or large doses of corticosteroids and to those with such disorders as silicosis, Hodgkin's disease, malnutrition, or previous gastric resection. A preponderance of these patients will be in the age groups over 35 years, hence more likely to suffer liver injury from isoniazid. It has been shown[91] that there is no significant risk of tuberculosis among an asthmatic population receiving prolonged treatment with steroid drugs. Presumably the same observations can be applied to arthritics or others receiving modest doses of steroids over long periods, despite warnings that isoniazid therapy should be administered.[4]

In every instance the clinical decision must be based upon the hazards of hepatitis (sometimes serious) compared with the hazards of possible tuberculosis (curable), a statement that bears frequent repetition. To extend the argument, it may be predicted that the person who will neglect periodic chest x-ray examination—so necessary if treatment is not given — is also the person who will neglect to take isoniazid, if treatment is prescribed.

An adult with a positive tuberculin skin test but with no history of previ-

TABLE 21–1. **Mortality and Morbidity in Two Studies of Tuberculosis in Children**

	Lincoln, 1950 and 1951* (No Chemotherapy)	Hsu, 1974** (Chemotherapy)
Mortality; inapparent tuberculosis; children under 2 years of age (positive Mantoux, negative chest roentgenogram).	10.0 percent	None
Mortality; children with roentgenograms demonstrating primary pulmonary tuberculosis.	23.9 percent (90 percent of these deaths occurred within one year of diagnosis)	0.3 percent (Meningitis)
Morbidity; adult type of tuberculosis, 1 to 14 years after primary tuberculosis.	8.0 percent (age 7 years to 21 years)	None
Mortality from subsequent adult type of pulmonary tuberculosis.	31.6 percent among females 21.6 percent among males	None

*Lincoln, E. M.: Course and prognosis of tuberculosis in children. Am. J. Med. *9*:623, 1950.
**Hsu, K. H. K.: Isoniazid in the prevention and treatment of tuberculosis. A 20-year study of the effectiveness in children. J. A. M. A. *229*:528, 1974.

ous tests, no lesion seen on the roentgenogram, no history of exposure, and otherwise in perfect health is not in great danger. If the patient is younger than 35 years, the risk of isoniazid therapy is negligible. If the patient is older and especially if he or she is a moderately heavy drinker of alcohol, the risk of therapy may well exceed the risk of declining treatment. In any event, close roentgenographic observation should assure early detection to enable prompt curative therapy of any visible lesion that may develop. Observation is relatively simple in the case of a private patient who is responsible and well informed; it may be difficult in a public health clinic serving large numbers of persons of varying motivation because of social, economic, and psychologic factors beyond control.

A recently acquired tuberculin skin test is likely to be a large reaction. Lesions measuring 15 to 20 mm of induration should be considered more seriously than those that are barely positive. Some attention should be paid to the "booster effect" of repeated tests; the second test may qualify as positive (over 10 mm), when a test given a few weeks previously was in the questionable category (6 to 9 mm). Intense reactions with vesiculation in a person known to have had recent contact with a case of communicable tuberculosis provide strong indication for treatment.

Tuberculosis Exposure Without Infection

Persons who have been exposed to tuberculosis, especially household contacts, are likely to have developed a positive tuberculin skin test. If infection has not occurred prior to discovery of the active case, it is not likely to appear later. The possibility must be considered that infection has occurred, but sufficient time (3 to 8 weeks) has not elapsed for the skin reaction to have appeared. Therefore, all tuberculin-

negative contacts should be retested from 8 to 12 weeks after the last contact with a communicable case. In the difficult domestic circumstances that are found in families living under conditions of poverty, crowding, and deprivation, it may be desirable to treat all contacts, including negative tuberculin reactors. If the latter do not convert to positive reactions within three months, treatment may well be discontinued. In the meantime, it is likely that the case of active disease has undergone treatment and is no longer capable of transmitting the disease (Table 21–2).

ANTITUBERCULOSIS DRUGS: SOME FEATURES OF CLINICAL INTEREST

First-Line Drugs

Antituberculosis drugs of proven excellence with minimal and controllable side effects and with impressive antibacterial action (preferably bactericidal) are often referred to as "first-line drugs." These include streptomycin, isoniazid, ethambutol, and rifampin — listed here in order of discovery dates. If listed according to desirability and popularity, the sequence would be: isoniazid, ethambutol, rifampin, and streptomycin (Table 21–3). Aminosalicylic acid ("PAS") has now been relegated to "second-line" status.

Isoniazid ("INH")

Isoniazid (isonicotinic acid hydrazide) is the most widely used and most valuable, nearly ideal, chemotherapeutic drug for treatment of tuberculosis. It is indicated in nearly all types and all stages of tuberculosis and for all cases of tuberculous infection with but few exceptions.

Isoniazid is readily absorbed from the gastrointestinal tract, diffuses into all tissues and body cavities, is chemi-

TABLE 21–2. Risk of Developing Tuberculosis in Various Groups of Infected Individuals

Groups	Risk of Tuberculosis	Cases Per 100,000	Number of Persons Treated to Prevent 1 Case of Tb.	References
Recent tuberculin converters	1 in 30 (3.3 percent) in first year after infection	3,333.0	30.0	Am. Rev. Respir. Dis. *104*:460, 1971.
Household contacts of newly developed case				
Tuberculin-positive	1 in 37 (2.7 percent) during 10 years of observation	270.3	48.3	Bibl. Tuberc. *17*:28, 1970.
Tuberculin-negative	1 in 197 (0.5 percent) during 10 years observation	50.8	210.0	Bibl. Tuberc. *17*:28, 1970.
Previously known tuberculosis, sputum negative, inadequately treated	1 in 79 (1.3 percent) per year	1,266.0	14.2	Bibl. Tuberc. *17*:28, 1970.
Positive tuberculin reactors with abnormal pulmonary findings on chest x-rays	1 in 125 (0.8 percent) per year	800.0		Am. Rev. Respir. Dis. *104*:460, 1971.
Tuberculin-positive adolescents with normal chest roentgenograms or with calcifications	1 in 400 (0.2 percent) for initial 2.5 years of observation	204.0	110.3	Br. Med. J. *1*:973, 1963.
Tuberculin-positive adults with normal chest roentgenograms	1 in 1,215 (0.08 percent) per year	82.3	163.4	Am. Rev. Respir. Dis. *93*:171, 1966. Ann. Int. Med. *74*:761, 1971.

Adapted from Johnson, R. F., and Wildrick, K. H.: The impact of chemotherapy on the care of patients with tuberculosis (State of the Art Review). Am. Rev. Respir. Dis. *109*:636, 1974.

TABLE 21–3.   First-Line Chemotherapeutic Drugs in Treatment of Tuberculosis

Drugs	Dosage and Administration	More Frequent Adverse Reactions	Special Precautions and Observations	Remarks
Isoniazid (INH) (isonicotinic acid hydrazide)	Oral, 300 mg once daily for usual adult. Intramuscular, 5 to 10 mg/kg.	Hepatitis, age-related Peripheral neuritis, dose-related. Hypersensitivity reactions.	Serious liver damage rare under 20 to 35 years of age (See Table 21–4) Neuritis only with large doses or with renal disorders.	Most useful of all anti-tb drugs. Bactericidal. (See text for incompatible drugs.)
Ethambutol	Oral, 15 mg/kg once daily. Rarely, 50 mg/kg twice weekly. Narrow range of tolerance.	Optic neuritis, rare with 15 mg/kg. Visual impairment usually temporary. Hypersensitivity rash.	Subjective visual complaints call for tests and comparison with previous Snellen chart and color discrimination.	Beware of use in renal disease. Best companion drug to INH in long-term treatment.
Rifampin	Oral, 600 mg once daily for usual adult, taken on empty stomach (10 to 20 mg/kg.)	Hepatitis, usually temporary. Adverse immunologic reactions with intermittent doses. Gastrointestinal distress.	Interrogate and observe for liver symptoms. Check liver function.	Bactericidal, useful in retreatment and initial short-term intensive treatment.
Streptomycin	Intramuscular, usual adult dose 1.0 gm daily or twice weekly.	Neurotoxic (dose-related and cumulative), vestibular and auditory eighth cranial nerve. Hypersensitive reactions may be severe.	Avoid very prolonged treatment. Pre-treatment audiograms desirable.	Beware of use in renal function impairment. Bactericidal, useful in retreatment and initial short-term supervised intensive programs.

cally stable in vivo, and attains blood and tissue levels well above the sensitivity of most strains of tubercle bacilli. It is universally available and is not expensive (see Chapter 20).

Sensitive strains of tubercle bacilli are inhibited in vitro by concentrations of less than 0.05 μg of isoniazid per ml of culture medium. Peak blood levels 6 hours after a dose of 4.0 mg per kg body weight are from 4 to 20 times the inhibiting level (0.2 to 1.0 μg per ml). Approximately 70 percent of ingested isoniazid is excreted in the urine within 24 hours.

Peak levels of isoniazid are more significant than are minimal blood levels. Hence the conventional adult dose of isoniazid has become 300 mg once daily, instead of 100 mg 3 times daily as recommended for many years. This is equivalent to about 5 mg per kg body weight, but since the therapeutic range is so wide, most physicians prescribe the same dose for all adults. Much larger doses are well tolerated if accompanied by pyridoxine but probably offer no therapeutic advantage.

Isoniazid appears in therapeutic concentrations in cerebrospinal fluid, pleural fluid, peritoneal fluid, and bile. It appears to pass all tissue barriers, including the placenta, and is found in human milk at levels of concentration similar to those in serum.[92] Its diffusibility is related to its low molecular weght.

The mechanism of action of isoniazid against the bacillus of tuberculosis has not been determined with certainty (see Chapter 20). *M. tuberculosis* multiplies at a slow rate; hence, constantly high blood and tissue levels of an antibacterial substance are not essential.

Isoniazid is partially conjugated by acetylation in the liver to an inactive form. There is a wide variation among individuals in their ability to inactivate isoniazid. Many persons of Oriental races are rapid inactivators, a genetic trait unusual among Caucasians and Negroes.

Fortunately, the rate of inactivation is not sufficient to interfere with treatment in most cases, but occasionally it is a cause for failure of treatment. In such cases, isoniazid-sensitive bacilli continue to be found in cultures even after many months of treatment. When this occurs, it is virtually certain that either the patient has failed to take the medication or is a rapid inactivator. Cultivation of tubercle bacilli in media containing serum from the patient will determine if inactivation has occurred to a serious degree.

The neurotoxicity of isoniazid is rarely manifested as peripheral neuritis and is dose related. The 300 mg dose taken once daily for the usual adult is not likely to produce neuritis, and if larger doses are administered, neuritis is prevented by administration of pyridoxine, 10 to 25 mg once daily. High blood levels resulting from renal insufficiency have led to neurotoxicity. Neurotoxicity is said to be due to interference with metabolism of pyridoxine through competition with pyridoxal phosphate of the enzyme, apotryptophase. Peripheral neuritis may be extremely painful, intractable, and to be avoided whenever possible. Alcoholic neuritis may be intensified by isoniazid administration, and whenever a reasonable risk of neuritis exists, it is wise to administer pyridoxine with isoniazid.

Liver toxicity of serious, even lethal, degree may result from therapeutic doses of isoniazid, a potential that was overlooked or understated in medical literature from 1952 until 1972. Hepatitis caused by isoniazid is readily confused with infectious hepatitis or injury due to other drugs. Of the millions of persons treated, no less than 1 percent probably suffered liver injury and perhaps 1 in 1000 cases perished. Fortunately it is now known that serious injury is extremely rare in younger persons and is highest in older persons, especially those who consume alcohol in greater than therapeutic amounts (see Table 21–4).

TABLE 21–4.   **Estimated Hepatitis Rates Per 1,000 Persons
Receiving Isoniazid, by Age**

| | Age (Years) | | | | |
	25	35	45	55	65
Total cases of hepatitis, possible and probable	6.3	12.7	20.4	31.4	25.5
Definite, probable cases	1.3	6.9	10.9	17.5	10.5

Adapted from Comstock, G. W., and Edwards, P. Q.: The competing risks of tuberculosis and hepatitis for adult tuberculin reactors (Editorial). Am. Rev. Respir. Dis. *111*:573, 1975.

Minor hepatic dysfunction demonstrated by temporary enzyme disturbances may occur in at least 20 percent of all persons treated. Because these findings may be confusing, it is often recommended that periodic enzyme determinations be avoided unless there are symptoms of liver disorder (fatigue, anorexia, fever, gastrointestinal distress, jaundice). These symptoms should be sought in periodic patient interviews.

Liver disease due to isoniazid has been confused with surgical abdominal disorders, and exploratory laparatomy may have contributed to some of the deaths.

Histopathologic changes in the liver vary from acute hepatocellular inflammation to that of massive hepatic necrosis. If detected at an early stage and treatment is discontinued, complete recovery can be anticipated. The pathogenesis of this and other drug-induced hepatitis is obscure.

Isoniazid attained unprecedented popularity following the recommendation of a committee of the American Thoracic Society in 1967 that all persons with positive tuberculin skin reactions should receive preventive chemotherapy.[3] This recommendation would apply to about 15 million persons in the United States and countless millions elsewhere. It was estimated that during the following 5 years, about 500,000 persons were treated in the United States as recommended.[44] Subsequent events suggest that many of these received inadequate supervision, perhaps because the 1967 committee report stated that

"There are virtually no side effects [to isoniazid]."

The potential toxicity of isoniazid as recommended for preventive therapy was brought to public attention by the results of a project of the United States Public Health Service involving government employees in Washington, D.C. This project was well designed to monitor undesirable side effects. The outcome was reported in an article by Garibaldi, Drusin, Ferebee, and Gregg in 1972,[44] an excerpt of which is quoted here:

In February 1970, 2,321 Capitol Hill employees who were reactors to tuberculin began isoniazid chemoprophylaxis. During the following 9 months, 19 of these employees manifested clinical signs of liver disease. In 9 of the 19, illness began within the first 60 days of isoniazid therapy; the other 10 became ill during the ensuing 6 months. Symptoms included fatigue, anorexia, fever, and gastrointestinal distress; 13 of the 19 were jaundiced, and 2 died. Ten of the patients were women and 9 were men; their mean age was 49.4 years. They could not be linked by person to person contacts or by common associations except that each one had taken isoniazid before the onset of hepatitis. In a matched comparison group of 2,154 Capitol Hill employees who were unreactive to tuberculin and had not taken isoniazid, hepatitis developed in only one during the same 9-month period. Hepatitis did not occur during this same period in any of the 260 tuberculin reactive employees who had declined isoniazid therapy.

As a result of this tragic experiment, the subsequent medical literature contains ample confirmatory evidence that isoniazid is not devoid of serious toxic potentials. However, it has been determined that the risk can be reduced to an acceptable level by proper selection of patients — those with the least risk of toxicity and the greatest risk of serious tuberculosis. Monitoring of symptoms, and sometimes monitoring of liver function, together with the recognition that there are acceptable alternatives to preventive therapy, should reduce the prevalence of serious liver disease to a minimum without increasing risks of dangerous tuberculosis.[53]

The current recommendations for treatment of tuberculin-positive persons without evidence of disease are enumerated in previous paragraphs. As now modified by the American Thoracic Society and the United States Public Health Service,[5] the recommendations are virtually identical with those published 12 and 13 years previously.[56]

Rarely encountered adverse reactions ascribed to isoniazid include: hypersensitivity reactions, emotional disorders, optic neuritis, arthralgia, hematologic disorders, autoimmune-like disorders, and incompatibility with diphenylhydantoin ("Dilantin").[2, 6, 19, 65, 68, 80]

It must be emphasized that despite potential toxicity, millions of persons have taken isoniazid in full doses for years without harm. There is no substitute for this drug, and few remedies are so reliable and so safe.

Ethambutol

Ethambutol hydrochloride has found wide acceptance as a companion drug to isoniazid in the conventional long-term initial therapy of patients with pulmonary tuberculosis. It has largely replaced PAS in this role. Its antituberculosis activity is of modest degree, but it serves well to inhibit the appearance of isoniazid resistant bacilli.

Ethambutol is readily absorbed from the gastrointestinal tract and blood levels are not affected by food. The usual dose is 15 mg per kg of body weight. In retreatment cases higher doses, 25 mg per kg, may be chosen for a limited time. Since the range of safe dosage is rather narrow, it is necessary to adhere to the dose-weight ratio rather closely. Intermittent, closely supervised therapy has been reported to be effective and safe (50 mg per kg twice weekly).[1]

The peak serum level 2 to 4 hours after the 15 mg/kg dose is only about 3 μg per ml, scarcely higher than the minimal inhibitory concentration in vitro (1.0 to 5.0 μg/ml).

Hyperuricemia, even to the extent of producing an attack of acute gouty arthritis, has been reported repeatedly.[81, 82, 93]

Ethambutol is always administered with one or more companion drugs, isoniazid, rifampin, or streptomycin. In retreatment cases, only drugs not previously administered should be chosen, if possible. Otherwise the choice will be determined by the results of in vitro sensitivity tests.

Ethambutol, like some other antituberculosis drugs, is neurotoxic in large doses. The optic nerve is the site of injury, and fear of permanently impaired vision has retarded the acceptance of ethambutol as a routine remedy. Fortunately, adverse reactions are extremely rare and are reversible when detected promptly in patients receiving the 15 mg/kg dose, even for up to 24 months. A controlled study by the United States Public Health Service[27] reported no evidence of optic toxicity in a large series of patients. It must be remembered that visual acuity may deteriorate as a result of aging and other causes during the prolonged period of tuberculosis treatment, even if no neurotoxic drug is being administered. High blood levels due to impaired renal function or to large doses may result in retrobulbar neuritis. This complication is reversible when discovered at an early stage of development. Diminished visual acuity and loss of red-green color discrimination with narrowed visual fields require cessation of ethambutol administration. The return to normal vision may be slow, but permanent impairment is extremely rare.

Rifampin*

Rifampin appears to be one of the most potent and generally useful antituberculosis remedies since isoniazid became available in 1952. It is a semisynthetic derivative of one of the rifamycins first isolated in 1957. The several rifamycins derived from cultures of *Streptomyces mediterranei* were active against a variety of microorganisms. One of these, rifamycin SV, was modified chemically so as to be absorbed from the gastrointestinal tract; this substance was named rifampin.[72a] It is described chemically as a 3-(-4-methyl-1-piperazinyl-iminomethyl) derivative of rifamycin SV (see Chapter 20).

Rifampin has aroused great interest not only because of its impressive antibacterial action, but also because of some unusual adverse reactions. Its probable clinically bactericidal reaction against *M. tuberculosis* has raised hope that this drug, in combination with others, may serve to shorten the traditional prolonged administration of chemotherapeutic drugs in treatment of tuberculosis.[84]

Cultures of tubercle bacilli are inhibited by less than 1.0 μg of rifampin per ml of culture medium. Peak blood levels following the standard dose of 600 mg are usually about 7 μg per ml of serum with a range of 4 to 32 μg per ml, 2 to 4 hours after ingestion by a fasting patient of usual adult weight. The presence of food in the stomach delays absorption and reduces peak levels.[99]

---

*A special supplement to the journal, Chest (volume 61, #6, June, 1972), is devoted entirely to rifampin in the treatment of tuberculosis and includes early experiences in Europe, where this drug was developed and studied prior to being introduced into the United States. This issue includes 18 contributions to the literature on rifampin.

Rifampin appears in therapeutic concentrations in lung tissue and in lesions of tuberculosis, and it appears in diminished concentration in body fluids. The concentration in bile and in urine is very high, the liver and the kidneys being the principal organs for excretion of the drug. Presumably some of the amount excreted in bile may be resorbed. The drug is partially conjugated by acetylation and there is some serum binding, but the conjugated form remains active and these phenomena do not reduce its antibacterial activity.

Hepatitis, similar to that produced by isoniazid, is the most frequently encountered toxic manifestation of rifampin. This had aroused some apprehension, lest the combination of isoniazid with rifampin might result in prohibitive risk of liver dysfunction. However, extensive clinical experience has not confirmed that fear, and there are many clinical circumstances requiring maximal antibacterial activity such as that provided by the combination of rifampin with isoniazid.[77, 85] The opinion is widely held that this combination, perhaps with a third drug (usually streptomycin), may accomplish eradication of some or many tuberculous infections within a few months. (See discussion of short-term intensive therapy later in this chapter.)

The daily administration of rifampin is recommended because intermittent therapy, or any substantial interruption of therapy, has appeared to lead to a peculiar sensitization phenomenon.[112] Light-chain proteinuria, resembling that of "Bence-Jones" proteinuria, has been reported. If treatment is continued, there is danger of serious renal dysfunction. Permanent injury is avoided if urinalysis is monitored, and treatment discontinued if proteinuria appears.[48, 83]

An "influenza-like" syndrome — myalgia, malaise, headache, anorexia, low fever — is associated with circulating antibodies against rifampin.[95] Such antibodies also appear at times in the absence of symptoms.[10]

An immunosuppressive effect of rifampin has been detected, both humoral and cell-mediated, but this appears to have no adverse effect in treatment of tuberculosis.[10, 47] It seems possible that such an effect might have some symptomatically beneficial result if it reduces the systemic effects of sensitivity to tuberculin, although this would be difficult to demonstrate.

Rifampin reduces the anticoagulant effect of warfarin. Oral contraceptives are less reliable, and the effects of hypoglycemic drugs, digitalis, corticosteroids, and methadone may be altered. A teratogenic effect in experimental animals contraindicates its use in pregnancy. Alcoholic beverages may increase the risk of liver damage, such as in isoniazid therapy. Blood uric acid levels may be increased.

An orange-red discoloration of sweat, tears, urine, saliva, and feces is harmless but may be of concern to the uninformed patient.

As with many drugs, hematologic crises (including thrombocytopenia, leukopenia, and hemolytic anemia) and rare hypersensitivity crises (including urticarial and other types of skin rashes) are reported.

Despite this impressive list of possible deleterious side-effects, rifampin has become established as one of the most safe, effective, and reliable of antituberculosis remedies and may well revolutionize the management of this cumbersome disease by reducing the duration of treatment (see also discussion of short-term intensive therapeutic programs later in this chapter).

Rifampin, like other antituberculosis drugs, should not be prescribed as the sole remedy. A companion drug — ethambutol, streptomycin, or isoniazid, for example — should accompany rifampin to delay the appearance of resistant strains of bacilli. In retreatment cases, the companion drug should not be one that has been used previously, even if in vitro sensitivity tests indicate continued sensitivity (see also section on retreatment in this chapter).

The usually recommended dose is 600 mg, once daily, at least an hour before a meal or two hours after eating. Rifampin may be taken at the same time as the companion drug; one hour before breakfast every morning is usually a convenient time. In this, as in all tuberculosis chemotherapy, it is important to urge the patient to avoid any interruption of treatment. The physician should insist upon regular visits (usually once each month) to be alert for toxic reactions and to monitor clinical progress. The routine determination of serum transaminase levels is more likely to confuse than to inform the attending physician because, as in isoniazid therapy, moderate elevations frequently occur, returning to normal without alteration of treatment. However, the presence of suspected symptoms of liver dysfunction indicates the need for serum transaminase studies, and normal findings are reassuring. Renal function, at least urinalysis, should be checked periodically.[48]

Streptomycin

Although streptomycin was the first practical chemotherapeutic agent to be discovered for treatment of tuberculosis, it remains one of the most important first-line drugs.[53, 102] It is peculiarly adapted to present-day trends toward more intensive and shorter, preferably supervised, regimens. Streptomycin must be administered by intramuscular injection, which requires close professional supervision; this may be an advantage under some circumstances and a handicap under others. Streptomycin in combination with such powerful drugs as rifampin and isoniazid exerts a bactericidal, hence curative, action.

Streptomycin is a member of the aminoglycoside family of antibiotics. It is derived from cultures of the actinomycete *Streptomyces griseus*. Its action is by interference with protein synthesis of the bacterium. It is a large molecule (MW 580) and does not diffuse well into tissues and body cavities (for example, not appearing in cerebrospinal fluid in therapeutic concentration). However, it does diffuse into the pleural space and appears in bile, saliva, and milk. It is excreted in urine, and normal renal function is necessary to avoid high and toxic blood levels (see Chapter 20).

The usual dose, 15 mg per kg body weight (1.0 gm for the average adult) leads to a peak serum level of 25 to 50 μg per ml in about one hour. The minimal inhibitory concentration in vitro is about 0.2 μg per ml, 50 to 100 times less than the attainable blood level.

Very soon after the chemotherapeutic activity of streptomycin was discovered, the phenomenon of acquired resistance was reported.[109, 111] Since then, it has been a limiting factor in treatment of tuberculosis. Resistance appears within a few months and is the single step variety, but it can be delayed or prevented if a second drug, one to which the bacilli are sensitive, is added. Multiple drug therapy in active tuberculosis has become recognized as essential.

Toxicity of streptomycin has been an additional limiting factor in long-term use of the drug. Toxic potentiality is cumulative and related to both duration of therapy and to high sustained blood levels. Although daily administration yields superior results, intermittent therapy — injections two or three times weekly — are preferable in order to avoid sustained blood levels. The risk of serious neurotoxicity is greatly increased if renal clearance is diminished in cases of renal insufficiency with elevated blood urea level.[53, 87]

Neurotoxicity of streptomycin is similar to that of other aminoglycoside antibiotics. The eighth cranial nerve, both vestibular and auditory branches, is peculiarly susceptible. Onset of symptoms may be insidious, and symptoms may progress even after therapy has been discontinued. Usually vestibular symptoms will disappear eventually, even when permanent damage to the nerve can be demonstrated. The other mechanisms of balance — joint sense and visual orientation — will substitute for the functions of the semicircular canals.

Impairment of hearing is vastly more disabling and to be avoided whenever possible. Unfortunately, it cannot be prevented in those rare individuals, perhaps one in several thousand, who develop significant hearing loss after brief and conventional streptomycin treatment. Hearing loss is usually permanent in these cases. Fortunately vestibular symptoms usually, but not invariably, precede auditory symptoms; the latter is avoided if treatment is promptly discontinued when vertigo, unsteady gait, tinnitus, or dizziness is a complaint.

Rare adverse reactions, including dermatitis, drug fever, leukopenia, thrombocytopenia, hepatitis, peripheral neuritis, optic neuritis, and other disorders, have been reported. Such phenomena are probably no more commonly encountered with streptomycin than with other potent remedies of many varieties.

Streptomycin should not be combined with other ototoxic drugs or with nephrotoxic drugs, such as neomycin, kanamycin, gentamycin, viomycin, vancomycin, tobramycin, polymyxin, and colistin. In general, no two aminoglycoside drugs should be used simultaneously for prolonged periods.

Many persons have unrecognized impairment of audition and vestibular function prior to treatment. The physician can best protect the patient and himself by testing for hearing acuity and possibly for vestibular function (caloric test) prior to undertaking streptomycin treatment.

Sensitization to streptomycin is an unusual but dramatic and potentially serious complication of therapy. Impressive generalized drug rash (often of morbilliform type), and rarely even exfoliative dermatitis, is associated with fever, malaise, and sometimes striking eosinophilia. In very rare cases, a leukemoid reaction has been observed. Cessation of treatment is adequate to effect prompt return to normal. Subsequent use is not advocated, unless it is administered with extreme care and only when no alternate regimen appears to be feasible.

Nurses, pharmacists, and factory workers who handle streptomycin may develop troublesome contact dermatitis, usually affecting only the hands. The wearing of rubber gloves is adequate to prevent this uncomfortable complication.

The indications for use of streptomycin are wide, both in initial therapy and in retreatment. Its administration in combination with two other drugs for rapid, bactericidal effects in regimens of short-term (6 months) intensive therapy has yielded brilliant results.[15] Streptomycin should be considered in many situations when the disease is extensive, progressing, and the bacterial population is believed to be very high. Frequently, it can be discontinued within a short time (2 to 4 months), before toxic symptoms appear.

Retreatment of relapsing tuberculosis is always a difficult problem. In recent years, the combination of isoniazid and ethambutol has been extremely popular. In the event of relapse after this regimen, or the formerly popular isoniazid-PAS regimen, streptomycin should play a prominent role.

Second-Line Drugs

Chemotherapeutic drugs included in this category have inferior potency, are less acceptable to patients, or are prone to produce dangerous or undesirable side reactions, when compared with the first-line drugs (Table 21–5). None of those described here would ordinarily be chosen for initial therapy, unless some contraindication — such as initial drug resistance — prevented the use of at least two first-line remedies. An exception to this rule has sometimes been made during short-term intensive supervised treatment or for treatment of some of the nontuberculous mycobacterioses.

The advent of rifampin has diminished the need for use of second-line drugs, but if rifampin-resistant strains begin to appear more frequently in future years, this advantage may diminish. With four well-established first-line drugs available, it is unlikely that infections with *M. tuberculosis* will appear with organisms resistant to all four drugs.

Second-line drugs are indicated for retreatment of relapsing tuberculosis, or for initial failures when the infecting strain is not sensitive to at least two first-line drugs, or for the patient who has developed an allergy or other intolerance to preferred remedies. Whenever possible, at least one first-line drug should be combined with one or more second-line drugs in treating recurrent disease.

Aminosalicylic Acid (PAS)

The pioneer work of Lehmann,[70, 71] summarized by Birath,[13] established the efficacy of PAS as early as 1946. Soon after it was learned that tubercle bacilli acquired resistance to streptomycin, PAS became the companion drug designed to avoid streptomycin resistance. When isoniazid appeared in 1952, it was frequently combined with PAS for routine chemotherapy. Finally, when ethambutol became available, it rapidly supplanted PAS as the companion drug to isoniazid. Formerly, PAS was considered as a first-line drug because of its safety and its value in preventing appearance of resistant strains of bacilli to its companion drug. Demotion to second-line status is justified, **especially**

TABLE 21–5.   **Second-Line Chemotherapeutic Drugs Used in Treatment of Tuberculosis**

Drug	Usual Adult Dose and Method of Administration	Most Frequent Adverse Reactions	Special Precautions and Observations	Remarks
P-aminosalicylic acid (PAS)	Oral, 8 to 12 gm/day (200 mg/kg) in divided doses	Gastrointestinal irritation (dyspepsia and diarrhea); drug rash	Administer with meals; several formulations equally effective	Failure of patient to comply is cause for failure.
Pyrazinamide	Oral, 15 to 30 mg/kg/day in divided doses	Hepatitis—sometimes severe, rapid even fatal; hyperuricemia	Narrow therapeutic range—a dangerous drug, rarely used	Bactericidal in combination with aminoglycosides
Cycloserine	Oral, 0.5 to 1.0 gm/day in divided doses	Central nervous system irritant; seizures, psychosis	Contraindicated in epileptics and psychopathic personalities	Weakly effective, pyridoxine may reduce risk.
Ethionamide	Oral, 250 mg 3 to 4 times daily (after meals)	Nausea, vomiting, hepatitis, hypersensitivity, depression	Tolerance may be acquired with ascending doses	Weakly effective, few patients can tolerate.
Capreomycin	Intramuscular, 1.0 gm daily (15 mg/kg)	Audiovestibular injury, renal damage, painful injections	Resembles other aminoglycosides	Weakly effective
Viomycin	Intramuscular (see text)	Electrolyte disturbances; renal injury	Monitor electrolytes and kidney function	Avoid use with aminoglycosides
Thiacetazone	Oral, 150 mg/day, larger doses if intermittent	Nausea, vomiting, dizziness, hypersensitivity	Used only in combinations with 1 or 2 other drugs	Not available in United States; used widely in Asia and Africa
Kanamycin	Intramuscular, 1.0 gm 3 to 5 times weekly	Cumulative eighth nerve damage; curare effect	Avoid prolonged use	Rarely indicated for tuberculosis

since rifampin has become available, because of the poor acceptance of patients of PAS.

The one overpowering fault of PAS is the repugnance patients have for it. They must consume 12 to 16 gm daily of a distasteful drug that frequently causes dyspepsia and diarrhea but rarely any more serious disorder. Many investigators have found that the principal cause for chemotherapy failure in years past has been failure of patients to comply with prescription of PAS. Often 25 percent to 50 percent of all patients have abandoned therapy prematurely, and contrary to medical advice, often in a clandestine manner.

Hypersensitivity reactions to PAS are unusual, but occasionally drug fever and rash develop, usually about 4 to 6 weeks after starting treatment. In such cases there is often evidence of hepatic dysfunction, which appears to be fully reversible when treatment ceases.

Most strains of tubercle bacilli are inhibited in vitro by one μg of PAS per ml of culture medium. The usual doses of PAS (4.0 gm, 3 or 4 times daily, for the usual adult) yields a peak serum concentration of 5 to 10 times the minimum inhibitory concentration. This drug does not diffuse readily into body cavities and is barely detectable in cerebrospinal fluid. It does not penetrate well into macrophages, and perhaps this is a reason the drug has little therapeutic potential when administered alone. As previously stated, its principal use is to prevent appearance of resistant organisms to the companion drug, but there is undoubtedly some enhancement of the efficacy of the companion drug.

PAS is not compatible with aspirin; it may interfere with activity of anticoagulant drugs, and it retards the metabolism of phenytoin (Dilantin). It is not likely to be tolerated well by patients with functional or organic gastrointestinal disorders. It is best administered at mealtime, the dilution with food reducing the gastric irritation. Several formulations are available, all equally effective.

In the future, PAS will likely be used only when first-line drugs are not indicated or as a companion to any one or two first- or second-line drugs when, for any reason, more acceptable drugs are not available. It is one of the more reliable and safe remedies, tested in many thousands of patients for nearly 20 years, and it should not be forgotten.

Pyrazinamide (PZA)

Pyrazinamide (pyrazinoic acid amide) is regarded as a dangerous drug because of its frequent, severe, and even fatal damage to the liver. However, it is highly effective as a bactericidal drug against tubercle bacilli and should receive consideration in dealing with serious forms of tuberculosis that are not responsive to less toxic drugs. Toxicity is related to dosage, and cautious use in triple or quadruple regimens for limited time periods and under close supervision (preferably with other bactericidal drugs, such as streptomycin or rifampin) has been reported with favorable results. [16, 21]

Elevation of blood uric acid level should be anticipated with pyrazinamide therapy. If there is even moderate hyperuricemia prior to treatment, allopurinol should be given to prevent development of frank gouty arthritis. Many patients complain of arthralgias, even when there is no actual gout. Periodic uric acid blood level determination is advisable. [25, 94]

The principal use of pyrazinamide is in retreatment of relapsing tuberculosis and other treatment failures when, for any reason, less toxic drugs cannot be used. It has also been used for limited periods in combination with other bactericidal drugs, sometimes as a substitute for streptomycin when facilities for parenteral injections were limited.

The usual adult dose is 3.0 gm daily (40 to 50 mg/kg) in divided doses. To be alert for symptoms of liver dysfunction, patients should remain under physician surveillance. Periodic liver enzyme determinations, blood uric acid levels, blood counts, and urinalysis are desirable. Tenderness or enlargement of the liver and development of fever are to be regarded as danger signals.

Cycloserine (Seromycin)

Cycloserine, like several antituberculosis drugs, is neurotoxic — but in a peculiar manner. Its effects are upon higher brain centers, including the motor cortex and frontal lobe centers. Grand mal seizures are a complication to be feared, and any possible history of previous seizures is a contraindication. Psychopathic behavior, not always among persons with previous emotional instability, has been frequently reported.[53, 72] Lester[72] reported that 24 percent of 111 patients treated with cycloserine developed neurotoxicity of sufficient severity to require withdrawal of the drug. The most frequent symptoms were those of agitated depression (14 percent) and psychosis or tremulousness and mental confusion (8 percent).

Although a rather weak antituberculosis agent, its mode of action is unlike that of any of the other available drugs — acting on the cell wall, as does penicillin. This attribute would seem to be an asset in combination therapy in multiple drug regimens for unusually difficult cases.

The therapeutic dose range is a narrow one — 500 to 1,000 mg daily (250 mg, 2 to 4 times daily) (15 mg/kg). If more than 500 mg/day is administered, it is desirable to monitor blood levels, avoiding levels in excess of 30 μg/ml. Neurotoxicity is dose related.

The drug is contraindicated in persons with unstable emotional constitution, renal disorders, history of convulsions, and history of psychosis or suicidal tendency.

Ethionamide (Trecator-SC)

Ethionamide is related to isoniazid in chemical structure, but it is less effective, more toxic, and there is usually no cross-resistance with isoniazid-resistant tubercle bacilli. Cross-resistance with thiosemicarbazone drugs (Thiacetazone) is reported.[2]

Ethionamide is a drug of minor importance and is used only as a supplement to two or more other preparations in treatment of relapsing disease, of drug-resistant infections, and occasionally of nontuberculous mycobacterioses (*M. intracellulare*, for example, and in multiple drug regimens).

The limiting factors in administration of ethionamide are distressing anorexia, unpleasant metallic taste, nausea, vomiting, and liver injury. It has produced symptoms of central and peripheral nervous system disorders similar to those of cyloserine, with depression, psychotic behavior, seizures, and neuritis.

Oral administration in ascending doses to test the tolerance of the patient is recommended. The 250 mg dose is first prescribed once or twice daily after meals, increasing gradually to three or four times daily, as tolerated. Ordinarily, one additional dose is added each week.

Probably no more than 50 percent of the patients will be able to tolerate the unpleasant side-effects of ethionamide, but it is occasionally worth a trial for solution of difficult therapeutic problems.

Ethionamide is contraindicated in pregnancy.

Capreomycin Sulfate (Capastat)

Capreomycin is not absorbed from the gastrointestinal tract and is administered by intramuscular injection. Peak blood levels (20 to 40 μg/ml) attained one to two hours after injection of 1.0 gm are 5 to 8 times the minimal inhibitory levels in vitro.

Toxicity is the limiting factor in use of this drug. It has ototoxic properties similar to streptomycin; hence, it cannot be used in combination with any other ototoxic drug. In addition, renal irritation is commonly observed. Serious renal damage will result only if treatment is not stopped when blood urea levels become elevated. Casts, red cells, and leukocytes in the urine are common and are not considered serious if urea and creatinine levels are not affected. Hypokalemia, neuromuscular block (with ether anesthesia), eosinophilia, and hepatitis are reported.

Injection sites become painful, and sterile abscesses may result if too many injections are made at the same site.

Capreomycin will find occasional use, in combination with other antituberculosis drugs, in treatment of drug-resistant cases. It is not recommended for initial treatment or for retreatment when more acceptable remedies are available, based upon in vitro sensitivity studies.

Viomycin Sulfate (Viocin)

Viomycin is a weakly bacteriostatic drug with troublesome and sometimes dangerous side reactions. It is not an aminoglycoside but shares the toxic potentialities of such drugs as streptomycin, kanamycin, capreomycin, and others.

Neurotoxicity affecting the eighth cranial nerve, resulting in loss of vestibular sense and hearing, is to be feared if there is any significant impairment of renal function. Unfortunately renal function is sometimes injured or, if deficient, is greatly damaged by viomycin therapy. Loss of electrolytes (Na, K, P, Cl, Ca) is a unique attribute of viomycin and may lead to serious consequences, including changes in the electrocardiogram. Obviously the monitoring of these multiple metabolic and physical changes is no small task, requiring close observation, usually in a hospital.

Administration is by intramuscular injection — a painful procedure, requiring frequent change of injection site and avoidance of smaller muscle groups such as the deltoid region. Sterile ab-

scesses may result from frequent injections. Intermittent therapy twice weekly of 2.0 gm (divided into 2 injections of 1.0 gm each, 12 hours apart) is suggested.

Kanamycin Sulfate (Kantrex)

Kanamycin is mentioned frequently as an antituberculosis drug, but it is not recommended. While useful for infections with other bacteria that do not require prolonged therapy, its ototoxic qualities exclude it for prolonged administration as is required for tuberculosis. It has the other undesirable properties of the aminoglycosides: neurotoxicity, curare-like action, hypersensitivity reactions of major proportions, hematologic crises, and gastrointestinal complaints.

Thiacetazone (Tibione)

Thiacetazone, a thiosemicarbazone preparation, has been neglected in the American literature. One report, which was based upon impressions gained from a personal journey to several German tuberculosis institutions in the early post-war period, was pessimistic concerning the therapeutic potentialities of the thiosemicarbazone drug, Tibione, that had been developed by Professor Domagk.[57]

Since that time, the studies of the Medical Research Council of Great Britain (Tuberculosis and Chest Diseases Unit, London) have reported favorable results, moderate toxicity, and peculiar adaptation to conditions in the underdeveloped countries. International cooperative investigations of great magnitude have been reported; Miller and coworkers[74] have reported observations on over 4,000 patients in 10 different countries. The prevalence of reported toxic manifestations varied widely from country to country due to differences in closeness of supervision. In comparing 1,396 patients receiving thiacetazone, isoniazid, and streptomycin with 1,407 patients receiving isoniazid and streptomycin, it was obvious that thiace-tazone was of considerable toxicity. Among those taking thiacetazone, 50.3 percent were reported to have side-effects, while the other group had such effects in 30.1 percent. Those requiring departure from prescribed treatment were 19.8 percent and 6.1 percent, re-spectively. This communication quotes previous studies in Hong Kong that led to the conclusion, "The toxicity of thi-acetazone plus isoniazid with or with-out streptomycin was found to be too high to recommend their use in routine practice." However, it was also stated, "Confirmation has been received that thiacetazone-containing preparations are used in routine practice in Ethiopia, India, and Pakistan."[41]

SELECTION OF CHEMOTHERAPEUTIC REGIMEN

The clinician now has a wide choice of effective and reasonably safe antituber-culosis drugs that may be combined in several configurations. Some of these have proved their efficacy and safety in many thousands of cases throughout the world, over a period of 25 to 30 years. Others of great promise have yet to prove long-term benefit.

Single-Drug Regimens

Isoniazid, 300 mg, administered once daily for a period of one year for the adult patient, has become the standard regimen for "preventive therapy" of pa-tients with positive tuberculin skin tests and no evidence of active disease. As stated in previous discussion in this chapter, this program is recommended for many persons who are less than 35 years of age and for some of the older age groups.

Isoniazid in similar doses has been recommended in certain circumstances for tuberculin-negative persons ex-posed to tuberculosis, and it is contin-ued for a period of 3 months if the tuber-culin test remains negative at the end of that period. Should the previously nega-tive skin test become positive, treatment would continue for one year.

These two situations are virtually the only circumstances in which single-drug therapy should be chosen.

Initial Treatment of Active Tuberculosis with Two Drugs

The currently preferred treatment in many institutions in the United States and elsewhere is a program of 18 to 24 months administration of isoniazid (300 mg once daily) combined with etham-butol (15 mg/kg once daily). A high de-gree of efficacy, as measured by rate and promptness of sputum conversion, con-trol of symptoms, and clearing of roent-genographic shadows on the chest film, can be anticipated in all stages and types of active pulmonary tuberculosis and in most types of extrapulmonary tubercu-losis. Generalized hematogenous ("mil-iary") tuberculosis and meningeal tu-berculosis call for more aggressive therapy.[12]

Prior to the availability of ethambutol, the "standard" regimen was an 18 to 24 months' course of treatment using isoni-azid (300 mg daily, in one dose or divid-ed into three doses) combined with PAS (12 to 16 gm daily, divided into 3 doses). This program has been administered to many thousands of patients over a period of more than 20 years. A moder-ate number of failures have occurred, and in nearly every instance, failure was attributed to the inability or unwilling-ness of the patient to ingest such large quantities of ill-tasting, digestive-disturbing PAS.

Until recently, there were but three first-line drugs — isoniazid, PAS, and streptomycin. Any two of these should produce excellent results if continued for the 18 to 24 months. Of these three, streptomycin was least desirable because of cumulative toxic effects when administered for many months and because of the discomfort and expense involved in parenteral injections, even when given only 2 or 3 times weekly (1.0 gm). A similar dose of streptomycin given daily was shown to be more beneficial but also more toxic if continued at this dose level for more than a few weeks.[17]

With the appearance of rifampin and ethambutol, the use of PAS has diminished and the drug has been demoted to the second-line category. Now, with four excellent first-line preparations, the possible combinations of two drugs are greatly increased.[26]

Two-Phase, Intensive, and Shorter Term Treatment

The logic of exploiting the bactericidal actions of rifampin, isoniazid, and streptomycin by intensive triple-drug therapy during the initial weeks or months of treatment when the bacterial population is high, and in its vulnerable growth phase, is obvious. Ethambutol may be substituted for one of the three named drugs, with similar benefits.

After several weeks (a few months at most), when bacilli disappear from the sputum, a more conservative and better tolerated two-drug program may follow.

It is not yet entirely clear whether a total of one year or perhaps only six months of treatment will yield long-range (5 to 10 years) results comparable to the traditional two-year, two-drug regimen.

The extensive review by Johnson and Wildrick[65] and the one by Fox and Mitchison[40] provide strong support for shortening and intensifying the treatment of active pulmonary tuberculosis. A series of cooperative studies under the direction of the United States Public Health Service are in progress, but it is difficult to imagine that they will add materially to the extensive and controlled data presented in the monographic review of Fox and Mitchison.

It must be conceded that three drugs will produce more undesirable side-effects than two, but this may be ameliorated by the shorter duration of treatment.

It cannot be said that the optimum frequency, intensity, and duration of antituberculosis chemotherapy has been determined. More likely, there are multiple choices of similar value, and the choice may be determined by patient acceptance, cost, availability of necessary monitoring facilities, and, of course, by type of disease and susceptibility of the population of bacilli under attack.

Multiple drug therapy reduces the need for the protracted and expensive laboratory work of determining the sensitivity and resistance of each strain of tubercle bacilli isolated. In the underdeveloped countries it is often impractical to expend limited resources when the need for treating thousands outweighs the need for precision in treatment of a smaller number.[14, 18, 40]

Retreatment Regimens

Relapsing tuberculosis following previous chemotherapy is likely to be difficult to treat.[50] Previously administered drugs should be avoided while awaiting results of drug sensitivity investigations. It is assumed that resistance has developed, and even though in vitro sensitivity is reported, it is desirable to adminsiter at least two first-line drugs if possible. Sometimes three, even four, drugs may be administered in difficult cases, preferably those drugs with differing toxic potentialities.

Failure of initial therapy, shown by continuation of positive sputum, may require management similar to that of relapsing disease. When possible, it may be desirable to add two new drugs — ones not previously used. The cause of failure is not always clear. Failure to comply with the recommended program and to detect resistant strains and sometimes abnormally rapid inactivation of isoniazid may be at fault.

Pulmonary resection has lost favor in treatment of pulmonary tuberculosis, but it may deserve consideration in some cases of relapsing or nonresponsive disease.[52] If medical treatment appears likely to fail and if the disease is well localized to a single lobe and is of a chronic destructive nature, lobectomy may be rapidly curative. Prior to surgery, and for an extended period thereafter, chemotherapy must be administered with two or more drugs.

It is in treatment of therapeutic failures that the second-line drugs are best utilized. The choice is a difficult one because all of them are either only weakly effective or dangerously toxic.

Extrapulmonary Tuberculosis

Chemotherapy is directed toward the bacillus rather than the host and should be effective wherever the former is located. This rule holds true, with but few exceptions.[12, 42]

Tuberculous lymphadenitis is frequently diagnosed without the isolation of the organism. This should be avoided because a large proportion of these cases will be found associated with nontuberculous mycobacteria of varying drug sensitivity. At the time of biopsy, a portion of the material removed must be retained in its fresh state and sent to the microbiology laboratory. Too frequently, the entire specimen is fixed for histologic examination.

Renal tuberculosis may be associated with renal insufficiency, and most chemotherapeutic drugs must be used cautiously — preferably with intermittent doses, twice or thrice weekly, to avoid excessive blood levels. Careful monitoring of renal function is required in such cases.

Tuberculous pleuritis with effusion is considered to be extrapulmonary at times; yet it is invariably associated with pulmonary disease, probably hidden by the fluid. Intensive treatment is advised because of the frequency with which pleural effusion is followed by renal or skeletal tuberculosis, which may appear several years later.

Tuberculosis associated with a large "cold abscess," as in some types of skeletal disease, will heal more rapidly and more completely if the abscess can be drained freely.

Generalized hematogenous (miliary) tuberculous disease and tuberculous meningitis are life-threatening conditions demanding prompt and intensive therapy with bactericidal drugs. Streptomycin does not penetrate the blood-brain barrier well but should be used with two or more additional drugs — always isoniazid in large doses, probably with rifampin or ethambutol. The increased risk of intensive, high-dose therapy must be assumed when life is at stake. These infections are most frequently encountered in infants and young children, who tolerate chemotherapy well. Terminal hematogenous tuberculosis is being recognized sometimes in the elderly patient and in a more chronic form with anemia and debility. Diagnosis may be established by bone marrow biopsy. Such persons are likely to have a negative Mantoux test, and chemotherapy is not well tolerated because of limited renal excretion. The therapeutic consequences of such circumstances are obvious.[45, 89]

CHEMOTHERAPY OF OTHER MYCOBACTERIOSES

Disease caused by mycobacteria other than *M. tuberculosis* often is clinically and pathologically indistinguishable from tuberculosis. These infections are unlike tuberculosis in epidemiology, and therapy is often difficult. The importance of identifying the confusing array of pathogenic and nonpathogenic mycobacteria is stressed in Chapters 18 and 19.

Therapeutic success is dependent upon a reliable microbiologic laboratory to guide the clinician. Cultural identification and determination of sensitivity to antimicrobial agents are essential in every case.[107]

Management of the occasional progressive, destructive infection may call into play procedures that formerly were popular in treatment of tuberculosis; this applies especially to pulmonary resection. Bed rest and collapse therapy, formerly in great favor, have not previously been advocated for treatment of drug-resistant strains of mycobacteria.

The term "mycobacterioses" is gaining in usage to distinguish these infections from those caused by *M. tuberculosis*. None of the mycobacterioses is known to be communicable. All are believed to be acquired from environmental sources, although the nature of that source is usually obscure. Some of these diseases are benign and self-limited, in need of little or no specific therapy. Others are life-threatening, long-lasting, destructive, and difficult or impossible to treat effectively with specific drugs.[42] (See Chapters 16 and 18.)

Pre-existing pulmonary disease and compromised immunologic defenses are sometimes associated with pulmonary mycobacteriosis.[49, 69] Feldman and colleagues[32] in 1943 may have been the first to describe *M. intracellulare* in a man with silicosis. Others have reported mycobacterioses in miners and in sandblasters.[7, 66] Other debilitating pulmonary conditions, including tuberculosis, emphysema, and chronic bronchitis, are associated with infections of this type (see Chapter 18).

With the increasing use of cytopathogenic drugs for treatment of malignant disease and the administration of immunosuppressive drugs, we may expect to encounter more frequent infections with organisms of low virulence, including mycobacteria (see Chapter 18).

Infections with *Mycobacterium kansa-*

sii are encountered throughout the central United States more frequently than elsewhere and are reasonably responsive to chemotherapy.[51, 88] Conversion of sputum from positive to negative is more slowly achieved, and relapse is more likely to occur than in the case of infections with *M. tuberculosis*. The response to therapy is not closely related to in vitro sensitivity findings, and initial therapy with isoniazid, ethambutol, and streptomycin is advocated.[51] Superior results may be achieved with rifampin, and this will likely become the drug of choice for initial therapy, when combined with two of the other first-line drugs.

Pulmonary resection is more frequently advocated for destructive cavitary disease than for *M. tuberculosis* infections. However, with the advent of rifampin, the need for surgery is not likely to arise as frequently in the future. The principal indication for surgery would be in well-localized disease, limited to a single lobe, that has not provided consistently negative cultures within 6 to 9 months.

It has not been determined if short-course regimens, less than 18 months, may yield satisfactory long-term results in these infections.

Among the most difficult problems encountered in chemotherapy are those presented by infections with *Mycobacterium intracellulare* (the "Battey bacillus"). All strains are resistant to isoniazid, and most are relatively resistant to other antimicrobial agents.[6, 43] The usual recommendations are to administer multiple drugs (from four to six) for infections that appear to be advancing. Fortunately, many of these infections are stagnant, nonprogressive, smoldering infections with minimal symptoms, requiring no drastic therapeutic measures. When localized to a single lobe, as often occurs in these infections, pulmonary resection is the favored treatment.

Yeager and Raleigh[106] describe rather gloomy prospects for persons with *M.*

intracellulare infections; their data showed a 5-year survival rate of less than half of their series of 45. Associated diseases that may have predisposed to the infection contributed to some deaths, but about one-third of the fatal cases had progressing mycobacteriosis.

Other mycobacterial infections (described in Chapter 18) are rarely encountered, and each case presents peculiar problems. Only the microbiology laboratory can direct the clinician in selection of appropriate chemotherapeutic drugs. Unfortunately, most of these organisms are resistant to the usual antimicrobial drugs. Fortunately, these infections, although persistent, are usually benign and localized. Rarely are they of lifethreatening proportions, except in the compromised host with defective defenses (for example, immunoincompetence, immunosuppressive drug therapy, and steroid administration).

Although rarely advocated in recent times, it might be appropriate to revert to some of the "old-fashioned" therapeutic methods formerly used for treatment of tuberculosis, when one is dealing with rare cases of advancing mycobacterioses due to organisms not responding to antimicrobial drugs.

Bed rest in the reclining posture surely improves the perfusion-ventilation ratio in the upper lobes of lungs.[76] Clinical experience with thousands of cases in the pre-streptomycin era attest to the value of prolonged bed rest in management of upper lobe tuberculosis of the lungs.[52]

ADJUNCTIVE THERAPY AND SUBSEQUENT CARE

There has never been a double blind study of the effects of fatigue, overwork, loss of sleep, anxiety, malnutrition, alcoholism, and other environmental or intrinsic factors upon the progress of infectious disease in man, nor are such studies needed.

Tuberculosis, above all other common diseases, has long been recognized as being aggravated by adverse environments and bad habits. Although chemotherapy has supplanted former efforts at specific therapy — bed rest for many months, collapse therapy, and pulmonary resection — it has not supplanted common sense in living habits. Too frequently, it is implied that any tuberculosis patient may continue his habitual way of life while undergoing chemotherapy for tuberculosis. Not infrequently it has been just this habitual way of life that has been responsible for the exacerbation of an indolent tuberculous lesion. The attending physician is obligated to exert his influence to persuade the patient to secure adequate rest, to avoid all possible stress, to follow a sensible balanced diet, to discontinue smoking, to be moderate in alcohol consumption, and in every possible way, to improve the quality of his life. In the recovery phase, there is an important place for regulated physical exercise. Although "physical fitness" is difficult to define, it is not difficult to recognize, and the belief is widely held that the "fit" individual is more competent to deal with infectious diseases than is the physically inept person.

Change of climate has been a traditional recommendation during times past for treatment of tuberculosis. Such change of environment, whether to mountains, desert or seashore, involved rest and usually the regimentation of an institution (sanatorium). Furthermore, it segregated the patient with communicable tuberculosis. Physicians are now convinced that recovery is not affected by altitude, humidity, or other meteorologic elements; yet a change to a more placid environment may be beneficial when feasible.

The patient with active pulmonary tuberculosis rapidly regains his sense of well being, usually within a few weeks, after starting appropriate chemotherapy. He may then be encouraged to return to normal living and working habits. Rarely is a change of occupation or of environment necessary.

A fearsome aspect of tuberculosis has always been its communicability, and this should not be underestimated because there is no other way to contract the disease. Fortunately, chemotherapy rapidly renders the patient a safe member of society. The best index of communicability is cough because it is the droplet nuclei that transmit the disease from one person to another. Within a few weeks after institution of chemotherapy, the usual patient with active tuberculosis ceases to cough and may then be safely returned to normal social, business, and family contacts.[11]

Prior to the chemotherapy era, tuberculosis was considered to be a lifelong problem, with frequent relapses from the state of "arrested tuberculosis." This required periodic medical observation and continued supervision, occupying the time and talents of numerous public health workers in tuberculosis "followup" clinics. Now that a state of "cure" can be attained in a large majority of patients who have been treated by methods outlined in this chapter, such clinics are being abandoned. This is a logical development from the public health standpoint, but from the standpoint of personal preventive medicine, an annual general examination is recommended, at least after the age of 40 years. Such a "birthday examination" should include an x-ray examination of the chest, not only to detect tuberculosis relapse but also to search for other thoracic disorders, neoplastic and otherwise, that may be present.

HISTORICAL NOTES: TUBERCULOSIS TREATMENT (1882–1978)

Mycobacterium tuberculosis has been a most vicious and ever-present enemy of mankind since prehistoric times. Its recognition as a living entity by Koch in 1882[67] brought the culprit into view and opened the way to culture and animal inoculation. Yet more than half a century passed before the bacillus and the disease it caused in experimental animals and in man could be controlled by direct attack.[100, 101]

Meanwhile, armed with increasing knowledge about the nature and transmission of tuberculosis, great advances were made in the reduction of morbidity and mortality of tuberculosis in Europe and the United States (see Chapter 16). Epidemiologic data are fragmentary and scant prior to 1900 and even after 1900. However, it appears likely that the death rate in American cities must have been in excess of 250 per 100,000 population per year at the time of Koch's discovery in 1882. By 1900, this had been reduced to about 100 per 100,000, and when streptomycin was introduced, the death rate in the United States in 1946 was about 33 per 100,000. Before isoniazid was introduced in 1952, the death rate had again been reduced by one-third (12.4 per 100,000); this was due in large part to streptomycin and PAS. By 1975, the rate was reduced to nearly one-tenth of what it was only 13 years previously (1.5 per 100,000). Formerly the greatest microbial enemy of mankind, tuberculosis is now reduced to a state of "control" in the developed nations (see Chapter 16).

Sanatoriums, Bed Rest, and Collapse Therapy

Improved living standards, reduced crowding, improved nutrition, and knowledge of contagion surely deserve major credit for earlier declines in tuberculosis deaths. It is equally certain that improved treatment is responsible for the later and final accomplishing of tuberculosis control. In the underdeveloped nations, where tuberculosis remains a major health problem, the means of attaining control are clearly indicated — seeking the sources of contagion (diagnosis) and treatment (chemotherapy)

The sanatorium movement attained great proportions in the United States and in Europe; by 1950, facilities for diagnosis, segregation, and treatment of virtually all cases of tuberculosis were constructed. Recognizing the importance of segregating contagious disease, it became public policy in the United States to care for all needy tuberculosis cases at the taxpayer's expense, a successful form of "socialized medicine" (see Chapter 16).

In addition to serving as isolation centers, the sanatoriums became highly specialized medical and surgical hospitals. Collapse therapy was the treatment of choice, accompanied by prolonged bed rest. Pneumothorax, pneumoperitoneum, thoracoplasty, and other extrapleural collapse procedures were resorted to in all appropriate cases. Perhaps the most beneficial result of collapse therapy was the closure of tuberculous cavities in the lung, greatly accelerating the healing process when cavity closure could be attained.[52]

Pulmonary Resection

A thoroughly local method of curing tuberculosis is the surgical removal of the diseased tissue. Pulmonary resection was not practical in tuberculosis because of the frequency and serious nature of tuberculous complications, an obstacle that was overcome when chemotherapy was discovered. Beginning in the latter 1940s and continuing for nearly 20 years, pulmonary resection became the treatment of choice for localized lesions but was recommended only after several months of chemotherapy at the least. Eventually it became recognized that removal of residual foci of tuberculosis was not necessary, the resected lesions being sterilized of tubercle bacilli if treatment had continued for 12 to 18 months. Even residual cavities, formerly greatly feared as potential

sources for reactivation, were found to be sterilized in many cases. Cure of tuberculosis was attained by thorough medical treatment and pulmonary resection was only rarely required.[52, 53]

Chemotherapy of Experimental and Clinical Tuberculosis

The full story of the stages of development of chemotherapy of tuberculosis has rarely been summarized. However, the medical literature provides a complete account of the sequence of events.[13, 13a, 22a, 22b, 28a, 31]

A fascinating account of the search for antibiotics during the 50 years prior to the work of Fleming[38] was provided by Florey[39] in 1945. Pasteur and Joubert[79] in 1877 first applied the principle of antibiosis to experimental treatment of anthrax. In the same year, Cantani[22] attempted to implant a harmless microorganism that he called *"Bacterium termo"* into the lung of a patient with pulmonary tuberculosis, claiming beneficial results. The first serious attempt to make a therapeutic extract of microbial origin generally available was the manufacture of extracts from cultures of *Pseudomonas pyocyanea,* called "Pyocyanin," a product that attained some popularity for topical use from about 1900 to 1910.

In 1913 Vaudremer[98] found that extracts from cultures of *Aspergillus fumigatus* would digest the tubercle bacillus in vitro. This was followed by clinical applications to patients in "several hospitals and sanatoriums in Paris." Temporary benefit was reported, "Mais malheureusement les faits sont encore nombreux où la tuberculose poursuit son évolution."[98]

The attempted exploitation of tuberculin therapy by Robert Koch is a sad story of hasty misjudgment, possibly tainted with greed, and certainly lacking sober scientific reasoning.

Robert Koch found that gold cyanide would inhibit the growth of tubercle bacilli in dilutions as high as 1:2,000,000.[31] For the several decades thereafter, gold therapy for tuberculosis in patients was attempted, but no solid evidence of beneficial effect was reported and all of the gold salts tried were toxic.[104] It was soon found that numerous substances were bactericidal to cultures of tubercle bacilli. The most comprehensive survey is that of Youmans, Doub, and Youmans,[108] reporting the results after testing 3,500 compounds.

Writing in 1923, Calmette[20] stated the situation then as follows, "It must be recognized that up to the present, despite the great number of attempts made to discover among chemical agents a substance capable of arresting the development of experimental tuberculosis in the guinea pig and rabbit, these efforts have been in vain." Nearly a decade later, Wells and Long[105] came to a similar conclusion but made a prophetic statement.

A specific chemotherapy of tuberculosis has not been found, and it may be a long time in coming because of the inherent difficulties of the problem, but it is not a closed chapter. . . . Probably some new success with some other bacterial infection will be needed to stimulate a new attack on the more difficult problem offered by tuberculosis.

That new success was experience with the sulfonamides and compounds of the diaminodiphenyl sulfone series.[31, 35]

When sulfonamides first appeared, it was believed that their spectrum of antibacterial activity was extremely narrow. However, a slight degree of inhibition of the rate of progression of experimental tuberculosis was demonstrated for sulfonilamide[86] and for sulfapyradine.[34] The first antimicrobial substances capable of arresting well-developed experimental tuberculosis in guinea pigs was a diaminodiphenyl sulfone product known as "Promin" (P,P'-diaminodiphenylsulfone-N,N'-didextrose sulfonate).[36, 37] Following this, a large series of compounds were subjected to controlled and comparative studies over a period of about four years (1940 to 1944). A comprehensive review of these experiments (including a full bibliography) is supplied by Feldman in the Harben Lectures of 1946.[31] Not only did these experiments first prove that the disease of tuberculosis could be treated successfully by chemotherapy, but an experimental model was devised that later was used in promptly recognizing the virtues of streptomycin (see Chapter 15).[33, 55, 60]

Leprosy is sufficiently similar to tuberculosis to have prompted Faget to treat it with sulfone compounds,[28] a success that has revolutionized the treatment of leprosy and has abolished leprosariums — just as the antituberculosis drugs abolished the tuberculosis sanatoriums.

Although the sulfone drugs have been supplanted by other, less toxic substances, they were subjected to human experimentation, with promising results[59] despite their difficult toxic side-effects.

Streptomycin appeared on the scene about four years after the experimental successes with the sulfone drugs. The original report on streptomycin by Schatz and coworkers[90] was concerned with its action on gram-negative and gram-positive bacilli. *M. tuberculosis* was not mentioned in the text but was listed in a table as being sensitive to streptomycin. Within a few weeks of the announcement of the discovery of streptomycin by Schatz and colleagues, a small amount of rather crude streptomycin was made available to the Mayo Clinic group by Professor Waksman for guinea pig experiment — an amount sufficient for only four animals. The results were so spectacular that it was possible to persuade the Merck Company to make a lot that was sufficient for 20 animals (July, 1944). The publication of these results was delayed until December, 1944,[33] at the request of Professor Waksman, who wished to establish priority and to confirm the in vitro sensitivity of a virulent strain of *M. tuberculosis* supplied by Dr. Feldman.[103] The organism mentioned in the table contained in the January 1944 report was of doubtful identity, in Waksman's opinion.

Thus, within the confines of a single calendar year (1944), the antituberculosis properties of streptomycin were established for experimental animals, and human studies were already underway.[58] The clinical superiority of this substance was best demonstrated by its ability to control such diseases as tuberculous meningitis and generalized hematogenous (miliary) tuberculosis — diseases formerly considered to be almost uniformly fatal. Thus, no controlled study was needed, and applications to the problems of pulmonary tuberculosis were promptly made and cautiously reported.[55, 60, 73] The Scandinavian Journal of Respiratory Diseases published a series of three papers in 1969, summarizing these events.[13, 30, 54]

Comroe in 1978[22a, 22b] has just provided an extensive, thoroughly documented account of developments that led to chemotherapy of tuberculosis. This monograph reveals details that have escaped other historians. The social and economic significance of early investigations in tuberculosis chemotherapy are stressed by Bordley and Harvey[13a] and by Dowling.[28a]

Deaths from tuberculosis in the United States have been reduced from 100 per 100,000 population, in 1900, to 1.5 per 100,000, in 1976.

REFERENCES

1. Albert, R. K., Sbarbaro, J. A., Hudson, L. D., and Iseman, M.: High-dose ethambutol: Its role in intermittent chemotherapy: A six-year study. Am. Rev. Respir. Dis. *114*:699, 1976.
2. American Medical Association: *Drug Evaluation*. Chicago, American Medical Association, 1971.
3. American Thoracic Society: Chemoprophylaxis for the prevention of tuberculosis: A statement of an *ad-hoc* committee. Am. Rev. Respir. Dis. *96*:558, 1967.
4. American Thoracic Society: Preventive therapy of tuberculous infection. Am. Rev. Respir. Dis. *110*:371, 1974.
5. American Thoracic Society: Treatment of mycobacterial disease. Am. Rev. Respir. Dis. *115*:185, 1977.
6. American Thoracic Society: Diagnostic Standards and Classification of Tuberculosis and Other Mycobacterial Diseases. New York, American Lung Association, 1974.
7. Bailey, W. C., Brown, M., Buechner, H. A., Weill, H., Ichinose, H., and Ziskind, M.: Silico-mycobacterial disease in sandblasters. Am. Rev. Respir. Dis. *110*:115, 1974.
8. Bailey, W. C., Taylor, S. L., Dascomb, H. E., Greenberg, H. B., and Ziskind, M. M.: Disturbed hepatic function during isoniazid chemoprophylaxis. Am. Rev. Respir. Dis. *107*:523, 1973.
9. Bailey, W. C., Weill, H., and DeRowen, T. A.: The effect of isoniazid on the transaminase levels. Ann. Int. Med. *81*:200, 1974.
10. Bassi, L., DiBerardino, L., Perma, G., and Silvestri, L. G.: Antibodies against rifampin in patients with tuberculosis after discontinuation of daily treatment. Am. Rev. Respir. Dis. *114*:1189, 1976.
11. Bates, J. H., and Stead, W. H.: Effect of chemotherapy on infectiousness of tuberculosis (Editorial). N. Engl. J. Med. *290*:459, 1974.
12. Baydur, A.: The spectrum of extrapulmonary tuberculosis. West. J. Med. *126*:253, 1977.
13. Birath, G.: Introduction of para-aminosalicylic acid and streptomycin in the treatment of tuberculosis. Recollections of the last 25 years. Scand. J. Respir. Dis. *50*:204, 1969.
13a. Bordley, J., and Harvey, A. M.: Two Centuries of American Medicine. Philadelphia, W. B. Saunders Co., 1976, pp. 456–460, 795.
14. British Medical Research Council: Cooperative controlled trial of a standard regimen of streptomycin, PAS, and isoniazid and three alternative regimens of chemotherapy in Britain. Tubercle *54*:99, 1973.
15. British Medical Research Council/East Africa: Controlled clinical trial of four short-course (6 month) regimens of chemotherapy for treatment of pulmonary tuberculosis. Lancet *1*:1331, 1973.
16. British Medical Research Council/Hong Kong Chest Service: Controlled trial of 6-month and 9-month regimens of daily and

intermittent streptomycin plus isoniazid plus pyrazinamide for pulmonary tuberculosis in Hong Kong (Results up to 30 months). Am. Rev. Respir. Dis. *115*:727, 1977.

17. British Medical Research Council: Long-term chemotherapy in the treatment of chronic pulmonary tuberculosis with cavitation. Tubercle *43*:201, 1962.

18. British Thoracic and Tuberculosis Association: Short-course chemotherapy for pulmonary tuberculosis. Lancet *2*:1102, 1976.

19. Byrd, R. B., Nelson, R., and Elliott, T. C.: Isoniazid toxicity. J. A. M. A. *220*:1471, 1972.

20. Calmette, A.: Tubercle Bacillus Infection and Tuberculosis in Man and Animals: Process of Infection and Resistance; a Biological and Experimental Study. (Translated by W. B. Soper and G. H. Smith). Baltimore, The Williams & Wilkins Company, 1923.

21. Canetti, G., Grosset, J., and LeLirzin, M.: La sterilisation des lesions tuberculeuse sous chimiotherapie chez l'homme. Bull. Union Int. Tuberc. *43*:347, 1969.

22. Cantani, A.: G. Int. Sci. Med. N.S. *7*:493, 1885. (As quoted by Florey.[39])

22a. Comroe, J. H., Jr.: Pay dirt: The story of streptomycin. Part I. From Waksman to Waksman. Am. Rev. Respir. Dis. *117*:773, 1978.

22b. Comroe, J. H., Jr.: Pay dirt: The story of streptomycin. Part II. Feldman and Hinshaw: Lehmann. Am. Rev. Respir. Dis. *117*:957, 1978.

23. Comstock, G. W., and Edwards, P. Q.: The competing risks of tuberculosis and hepatitis for adult tuberculin reactors (Editorial). Am. Rev. Respir. Dis. *111*:573, 1975.

24. Comstock, G. W., Woolpert, S. F., and Baum, C.: Isoniazid prophylaxis among Alaskan Eskimos: A progress report. Am. Rev. Respir. Dis. *110*:195, 1974.

25. Cullen, J. H., Early, L. J. A., and Fiore, J. M.: The occurrence of hyperuricemia during pyrazinamide-isoniazid therapy. Am. Rev. Tuberc. *74*:289, 1956.

26. Dickinson, M. J., Ellard, G. A., and Mitchison, D. A.: Suitability of isoniazid and ethambutol for intermittent chemotherapy. Tubercle *49*:351, 1968.

27. Doster, B., Murray, F. J., Newman, R., and Woolpert, S. F.: Ethambutol in the initial treatment of pulmonary tuberculosis (U. S. Public Health Service Tuberculosis Therapy trials). Am. Rev. Respir. Dis. *107*:177, 1973.

28. Doull, J. A.: Current status of the therapy of leprosy. J. A. M. A. *173*:363, 1960.

28a. Dowling, H. F.: Fighting Infection; Conquests of the Twentieth Century. Cam-

bridge, Mass., Harvard University Press, 1977.

29. Farer, L. S.: Preventive treatment of tuberculosis. Basics of R. D. (Am. Thoracic Soc.) *2*:1, 1975.

30. Feldman, W. H.: Tuberculosis chemotherapy. Reminiscences of *in vivo* research. Scand. J. Respir. Dis. *50*:186, 1969.

31. Feldman, W. H.: The chemotherapy of tuberculosis, including the use of streptomycin (The Harben Lectures, 1946). J. R. Inst. of Public Health Hyg. *9*:267–288, 297–324, 343–363, 1946.

32. Feldman, W. H., Davils, R., Moses, H. E., and Andberg, W.: An unusual *Mycobacterium* isolated from sputum of a man suffering from pulmonary disease of long duration. Am. Rev. Tuberc. *48*:82, 1943.

33. Feldman, W. H., and Hinshaw, H. C.: Effects of steptomycin on experimental tuberculosis in guinea pigs: A preliminary report. Proc. Staff Meet. Mayo Clin. *19*:593, 1944.

34. Feldman, W. H., and Hinshaw, H. C.: Effect of sulfapyridine on experimental tuberculosis in the guinea pig. Proc. Staff Meet. Mayo Clin. *14*:174, 1939.

35. Feldman, W. H., and Hinshaw, H. C.: Sulfapyridine in experimental tuberculosis: The pathology of experimental tuberculosis and apparent toxic changes in guinea pigs treated with sulfapyridine. Am. Rev. Tuberc. *41*:732, 1940.

36. Feldman, W. H., Hinshaw, H. C., Moses, H. E.: Promin in experimental tuberculosis: Sodium p,p'-diaminodiphenylsulfone-N-N'-didextrose sulfonate. Am. Rev. Tuberc. *45*:303, 1942.

37. Feldman, W. H., Hinshaw, H. C., and Moses, H. E.: The effect of promin (sodium salt of p,p'-diaminodiphenylsulfone-N-N'-didextrose sulfonate) on experimental tuberculosis: A preliminary report. Proc. Staff Meet. Mayo Clin. *15*:695, 1940.

38. Fleming, A.: On the antibacterial action of cultures of a *Penicillium* with special reference to their use in the isolation of *B. influenzae*. Br. J. Exp. Pathol. *10*:226, 1929.

39. Florey, H. W.: The use of micro-organisms for therapeutic purposes. Br. Med. J. *2*:635, 1945.

40. Fox, W., and Mitchison, D. A.: Short-course chemotherapy for pulmonary tuberculosis. (State of the Art Review.) Am. Rev. Respir. Dis. *111*:325, 1975.

41. Fox, W., Stark, A. J., Tall, R., Bhatia, J. L., Clarke, J. H. C., Donia, T. O., Krishnaswami, K. V., and Oussedik, N.: A study of adverse reactions to high dosage intermittent thiacetazone. Tubercle *55*:29, 1974.

42. Gacad, G., and Massaro, D.: Pulmonary fi-

brosis and group IV mycobacteria infection of the lungs in ankylosing spondylitis. Am. Rev. Respir. Dis. 109:274, 1974.

43. Gangadharam, P. R. J., and Candler, E. R.: Activity of some antileprosy compounds against *Mycobacterium intracellulare in vitro*. Am. Rev. Respir. Dis. 115:705, 1977.

44. Garibaldi, R. A., Drusin, R. E., Ferebee, S. H., and Gregg, M. R.: Isoniazid-associated hepatitis: Report of an outbreak. Am. Rev. Respir. Dis. 106:357, 1972.

45. Gelb, A. F., Leffler, C., Brewin, A., Mascatello, V., and Lyons, H. A.: Miliary tuberculosis. Am. Rev. Respir. Dis. 108:1327, 1973.

46. Grzybowski, S., McKinnon, N. E., Tuters, L., Pinkus, G., and Philipps, R.: Reactivations in inactive pulmonary tuberculosis. Am. Rev. Respir. Dis. 93:352, 1966.

47. Goldstein, R. A., Un Hun Ang, Foellmer, J. W., and Janicki, B. W.: Rifampin and cell-mediated immune response in tuberculosis. Am. Rev. Respir. Dis. 113:197, 1976.

48. Graber, C. D., Patrick, C. C., and Galphin, R. L.: Light chain proteinuria and cellular mediated immunity in rifampin treated patients with tuberculosis. Chest 67:408, 1975.

49. Graybill, J. R., Silva, J., Jr., Fraser, D. W., Lordon, R., and Rogers, E.: Disseminated mycobacteriosis due to *Mycobacterium abscessus* in two recipients of renal homografts. Am. Rev. Respir. Dis. 109:4, 1974.

50. Gyselen, A., Verbist, L., Cosemans, J., Lacquet, L. M., and Vandenbergh, E.: Rifampin and ethambutol in the retreatment of advanced pulmonary tuberculosis. Am. Rev. Respir. Dis. 98:933, 1968.

51. Harris, G. D., Johanson, W. G., Jr., and Nicholson, D. P.: Response to chemotherapy of pulmonary infection due to *Mycobacterium kansasii*. Am. Rev. Respir. Dis. 112:31, 1975.

52. Hinshaw, H. C.: Diseases of the Chest. 3rd ed. Philadelphia, W. B. Saunders Co., 1969.

53. Hinshaw, H. C.: Management of tuberculosis: Altered role of the primary care physician. Post. Grad. Med. 61:52, 1977.

54. Hinshaw, H. C.: Tuberculosis chemotherapy: Reminiscenses of early clinical trials. Scand. J. Respir. Dis. 50:197, 1969.

55. Hinshaw, H. C., and Feldman, W. H.: Streptomycin in treatment of clinical tuberculosis: A preliminary report. Proc. Staff Meet. Mayo Clin. 20:313, 1945.

56. Hinshaw, H. C., and Hinshaw, H. C., Jr.: Recently acquired tuberculin sensitivity and the treatment of inapparent tuberculosis. Curr. Concepts Chest Dis. 2:1, 1962.

57. Hinshaw, H. C., and McDermott, W.: Thiosemicarbazone therapy of tuberculosis in humans. Am. Rev. Tuberc. 61:157, 1950.

58. Hinshaw, H. C., Feldman, W. H., and Pfuetze, K. H.: Present status of chemotherapy of tuberculosis. Ann. Int. Med. 22:696, 1945.

59. Hinshaw, H. C., Pfuetze, K. H., and Feldman, W. H.: Chemotherapy of clinical tuberculosis with Promin: p.p'-diaminodiphenylsulfone N-N'-didextrose sulfonate: A second report of progress. Am. Rev. Tuberc. 50:52, 1944.

60. Hinshaw, H. C., Pfuetze, K. H., and Feldman, W. H.: Treatment of tuberculosis with streptomycin: A summary of observations on one hundred cases. J. A. M. A. 132:778, 1946.

61. Horowitz, O., Wilbek, E., and Erickson, P. A.: Epidemiological basis of tuberculosis eradication. 10. Longitudinal studies on the risk of tuberculosis in the general population of a low prevalence area. Bull. WHO 41:95, 1969.

62. Houk, V. N., Kent, D. C., Sorensen, K., and Baker, J. H.: The eradication of tuberculous infection by isoniazid prophylaxis. Arch. Envir. Health. 16:46, 1968.

63. Hsu, K. H. K.: Isoniazid in the prevention and treatment of tuberculosis: A 20-year study of the effectiveness in children. J. A. M. A. 229:528, 1974.

64. Johnson, R. F., and Hopewell, P. C.: Chemotherapy of pulmonary tuberculosis. Ann. Int. Med. 70:359, 1969.

65. Johnson, R. F., and Wildrick, K. H.: The impact of chemotherapy on the care of patients with tuberculosis (State of the Art Review). Am. Rev. Respir. Dis. 109:636, 1974.

66. Kamat, S. R., Rossiter, C. E., and Gilson, J. C.: A retrospective clinical study of pulmonary disease due to "anonymous mycobacteria" in Wales. Thorax 16:297, 1961.

67. Koch, R.: As quoted by Wells, H. G.: Yale J. Biol. Med. 4:611, 1932.

68. Kutt, H., Brennan, R., Dehejia, H., and Verebely, K.: Diphenylhydantoin intoxication. A complication of isoniazid therapy. Am. Rev. Respir. Dis. 101:377, 1970.

69. Lakshminarayan, S., and Sahn, S.: Disseminated infection caused by *Mycobacterium avium*. Am. Rev. Respir. Dis. 108:123, 1973.

70. Lehmann, J.: Para-aminosalicylic acid in the treatment of tuberculosis: A preliminary communication. Lancet 1:15, 1946.

71. Lehmann, J.: The role of the metabolism of p-aminosalicylic acid (PAS) in the treatment of tuberculosis. Scand. J. Respir. Dis. 50:169, 1969.

72. Lester, W.: Treatment of drug resistant tuberculosis. Disease-a-Month; April. Chicago, Yearbook Medical Publishers. 1971.

72a. Maggi, N., Pasqualucci, C. R., and Ballotta, R.: Rifampicin, a new orally active rifamycin. Chemotherapia 11:285, 1966.

73. McDermott, W., Muschenheim, C., Hadley, S. J., Bunn, P. A., and Gorman, R. V.: Streptomycin in treatment of tuberculosis in humans. 1. Meningitis and generalized hematogenous tuberculosis. Ann. Int. Med. 27:769, 1947.

74. Miller, A. B., Nunn, A. J., Robinson, D. K., Fox, W., Somasundaram, P. R., and Tall, R.: A second international cooperative investigation into thioacetazone side effects. Frequency and geographical distribution of side effects. Bull. WHO 47:211, 1972.

75. Mitchell, R. S.: Mortality and relapse of uncomplicated advanced pulmonary tuberculosis before chemotherapy: 1,504 consecutive admissions followed fifteen to twenty five years. Am. Rev. Respir. Dis. 93:502, 1966.

76. Murray, J. F.: The Normal Lung. Philadelphia, W. B. Saunders Co., 1976.

77. Newman, R., Doster, B. E., Murray, F. J., and Woolpert, S. F.: Rifampin in initial treatment of pulmonary tuberculosis. A U.S. Public Health Service. T. T. Am. Rev. Respir. Dis. 109:216, 1974.

78. Pamra, S. P., Prasad, G., and Mathur, G. P.: Relapse in pulmonary tuberculosis. Am. Rev. Respir. Dis. 113:67, 1976.

79. Pasteur, L., and Joubert, J. F.: C. R. Acad. Sci. (Paris) 85:101, 1877. (As cited by Florey.[39])

80. Periman, P., and Venkataramani, T. K.: Acute arthritis induced by isoniazid. Ann. Int. Med. 83:667, 1975.

81. Postlethwaite, A. E., Bartel, A. G., and Kelly, W. N.: Hyperuricemia due to ethambutol. N. Eng. J. Med. 286:761, 1972.

82. Postlethwaite, A. E., Bartel, A. G., and Kelly, W. N.: Hyperuricemia induced by ethambutol. Adv. Exp. Med. Biol. 41:763, 1974.

83. Pujet, J., Hamberg, J., and Decroix, G.: Sensitivity to rifampin: Incidence, mechanism and prevention. Br. Med. J. 2:415, 1974.

84. Raleigh, J. W.: Clinical notes on rifampin. Clin. Notes Respir. Dis. 11:3, 1972.

85. Ravikrishnan, K. P., Muller, B. F., and Neuhaus, A.: Toxicity to isoniazid and rifampin in active tuberculosis patients (abstract). Am. Rev. Respir. Dis. 115:405, 1977.

86. Rich, A. R., and Follis, R. H., Jr.: The inhibitory effect of sulfanilamide on the development of experimental tuberculosis in the guinea pig. Bull. Johns Hopkins Hosp. 62:77, 1938.

87. Riggins, H., (Mc), and Hinshaw, H. C.: Streptomycin and Dihydrostreptomycin in Tuberculosis. New York, National Tuberculosis Association, 1949.

88. Rouscher, C. R., Kerby, G., and Ruth, W. E.: A ten year clinical experience with *Mycobacterium kansasii.* Chest 66:17, 1974.

89. Sahn, S. A., and Neff, T. A.: Miliary tuberculosis. Am. J. Med. 56:495, 1974.

90. Schatz, A., Bugie, E., and Waksman, S. A.: Streptomycin, a substance exhibiting antibiotic activity against gram-positive and gram-negative bacteria. Proc. Soc. Exp. Biol. Med. 55:66, 1944.

91. Schatz, M., Patterson, R., Kloner, R., and Falk, J.: The prevalence of tuberculosis and positive tuberculin skin tests in a steroid-treated asthmatic population. Ann. Int. Med. 84:261, 1976.

92. Scheinhorn, D. J., and Angelillo, V. A.: Antituberculosis therapy in pregnancy — risks to the fetus. West. J. Med. 127:195, 1977.

93. Self, T. H., Fountain, F. F., Taylor, W. J., Jr., and Sutliff, W. D.: Acute gouty arthritis associated with use of ethambutol. Chest 71:561, 1977.

94. Shapiro, M., and Hyde, L.: Hyperuricemia due to pyrazinamide. Am. J. Med. 23:596, 1957.

95. Singapore Tuberculosis Service (British Medical Research Council): Controlled trial of intermittent regimens of rifampin plus isoniazid for pulmonary tuberculosis in Singapore: The results up to 30 months. Am. Rev. Respir. Dis. 116:807, 1977.

96. Stead, W. W., and Jurgens, G. H.: Productivity of prolonged followup after chemotherapy for tuberculosis. Am. Rev. Respir. Dis. 108:314, 1973.

97. Stephens, M. G.: Followup of 1,041 tuberculous patients. Am. Rev. Tuberc. 44:451, 1941.

98. Vaudremer, A.: Action de l'extrait filtré d'*Aspergillus fumigatus* sur le bacille tuberculeux. Comp. Rendu Soc. Biol. 74:752, 1913.

99. Verbist, L., and Gyselen, A.: Antituberculosis activity of rifampin *in vitro* and *in vivo* and the concentrations attained in human blood. Am. Rev. Respir. Dis. 98:923, 1968.

100. Waksman, S. A.: The Conquest of Tuberculosis. Berkely, University of California Press, 1964.

101. Waksman, S. A.: The Antibiotic Era. Tokyo, University of Tokyo Press, 1975.

102. Waksman, S. A.: The Literature on Streptomycin, 1944–1952. New Brunswick, N. J., Rutgers University Press, 1952.

103. Waksman, S. A., Bugie, E., and Schatz, A.: Isolation of antibiotic substances from soil microorganisms, with special reference to streptothricin and streptomycin. Proc. Staff Meet. Mayo Clin. 19:537, 1944.

104. Wells, H. G.: The chemistry of tuberculosis. Yale J. Biol. Med. 4:611, 1932.

105. Wells, H. G., and Long, E. R.: The Chemistry of Tuberculosis: A Compilation and Critical Review of Existing Knowledge on

the Chemistry of the Tubercle Bacillus and its Products, the Chemical Changes and Processes in the Host, the Chemical Aspects of the Treatment of Tuberculosis (2nd ed.). Baltimore, The Williams & Wilkins Company, 1932.

106. Yeager, H., and Raleigh, J. W.: Pulmonary disease due to *Mycobacterium intracellulare.* Am. Rev. Respir. Dis. *108*:547, 1973.

107. Youmans, G. P.: The pathogenic "atypical" mycobacteria. Ann. Rev. Microbiol. *17*:473, 1963.

108. Youmans, G. P., Doub, L., and Youmans, A. S.: The Bacteriostatic Activity of 3,500 Organic Compounds for *Mycobacterium tuberculosis,* var. *Hominis.* Washington, D.C., National Research Council, 1953.

109. Youmans, G. P., and Karlson, A. G.: Streptomycin sensitivity of tubercle bacilli. Studies of recently isolated tubercle bacilli and the development of resistance to streptomycin *in vivo.* Am. Rev. Tuberc. *55*:529, 1947.

110. Youmans, G. P., Paterson, P. Y., and Sommers, H. M.: The Biologic and Clinical Basis of Infectious Diseases. Philadelphia, W. B. Saunders Co., 1975.

111. Youmans, G. P., Williston, E. H., Feldman, W. H., and Hinshaw, H. C.: Increase in resistance of tubercle bacilli to streptomycin: A preliminary report. Proc. Staff Meet. Mayo Clin. *21*:126, 1946.

112. Zierski, M.: Side effects under intermittent rifampin: A general review. Bull. Int. Union Tuberc. *48*:119, 1973.

INDEX

Page numbers in *italics* refer to figures; (t) indicates table.